CAMBRIDGE LIBRARY COLLECTION

Books of enduring scholarly value

History of Medicine

It is sobering to realise that as recently as the year in which *On the Origin of Species* was published, learned opinion was that diseases such as typhus and cholera were spread by a 'miasma', and suggestions that doctors should wash their hands before examining patients were greeted with mockery by the profession. The Cambridge Library Collection reissues milestone publications in the history of Western medicine as well as studies of other medical traditions. Its coverage ranges from Galen on anatomical procedures to Florence Nightingale's common-sense advice to nurses, and includes early research into genetics and mental health, colonial reports on tropical diseases, documents on public health and military medicine, and publications on spa culture and medicinal plants.

The Works of John Hunter, F.R.S.

The surgeon and anatomist John Hunter (1728–93) left a famous legacy in the Hunterian Museum of medical specimens now in the Royal College of Surgeons, and in this collection of his writings, edited by James Palmer, with a biography by Drewry Ottley, published between 1835 and 1837. The first four volumes are of text, and the larger Volume 5 contains plates. Hunter had begun his career as a demonstrator in the anatomy classes of his brother William, before qualifying as a surgeon. He regarded surgery as evidence of failure – the mutilation of a patient who could not be cured by other means – and his studies of anatomy and natural history were driven by his belief that it was necessary to understand the normal physiological processes before attempting to cure the abnormal ones. Volume 4 contains Hunter's works on animal physiology, with notes by the distinguished palaeontologist Richard Owen.

The Works of John Hunter, F.R.S.

VOLUME 4

EDITED BY JAMES F. PALMER

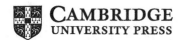

CAMBRIDGE
UNIVERSITY PRESS

CAMBRIDGE
UNIVERSITY PRESS

University Printing House, Cambridge, CB2 8BS, United Kingdom

Cambridge University Press is part of the University of Cambridge.
It furthers the University's mission by disseminating knowledge in the pursuit of
education, learning and research at the highest international levels of excellence.

www.cambridge.org
Information on this title: www.cambridge.org/9781108079600

This edition first published 1837
This digitally printed version 2015

ISBN 978-1-108-07960-0 Paperback

THE

WORKS

OF

JOHN HUNTER, F.R.S.

WITH

NOTES.

EDITED BY

JAMES F. PALMER,

SENIOR SURGEON TO THE ST. GEORGE'S AND ST. JAMES'S DISPENSARY; FELLOW
OF THE ROYAL MEDICAL AND CHIRURGICAL SOCIETY OF LONDON, ETC.

IN FOUR VOLUMES.
ILLUSTRATED BY A VOLUME OF PLATES, IN QUARTO.

VOL. IV.

LONDON:

PUBLISHED BY
LONGMAN, REES, ORME, BROWN, GREEN, AND LONGMAN,
PATERNOSTER-ROW.

1837.

PRINTED BY RICHARD AND JOHN E. TAYLOR,
RED LION COURT, FLEET STREET.

OBSERVATIONS

ON

CERTAIN PARTS

OF

THE ANIMAL ŒCONOMY,

INCLUSIVE OF SEVERAL PAPERS FROM

THE PHILOSOPHICAL TRANSACTIONS, ETC.,

BY

JOHN HUNTER, F.R.S.

WITH NOTES,

BY

RICHARD OWEN, F.R.S.,

FELLOW OF THE LINNEAN, GEOLOGICAL, AND ZOOLOGICAL SOCIETIES OF LONDON.
CORRESPONDING MEMBER OF THE ROYAL ACADEMY OF SCIENCES OF BERLIN ; OF
THE ROYAL ACADEMY OF MEDICINE AND PHILOMATHIC SOCIETY
OF PARIS ; AND OF THE ACADEMY OF SCIENCES OF
PHILADELPHIA, MOSCOW, ERLANGEN, ETC.

PROFESSOR OF ANATOMY AND PHYSIOLOGY, AND
CONSERVATOR OF THE MUSEUM OF THE ROYAL COLLEGE OF SURGEONS IN LONDON.

TO SIR JOSEPH BANKS, Bart.,

PRESIDENT OF THE ROYAL SOCIETY, &c. &c. &c.

Dear Sir,

As the following Observations were made in the course of those pursuits in which you have so warmly interested yourself, and promoted with the most friendly assistance, I should be wanting in gratitude were I not to address them to you, as a public testimony of the friendship and esteem with which I am,

Dear Sir,

Your obliged and

Very humble Servant,

JOHN HUNTER.

Leicester Square,
Nov. 9, 1786.

ADVERTISEMENT

To the First Edition of the Animal Œconomy, 1786.

———

THE nine following papers have been read at the Royal Society, and published in the Philosophical Transactions; but in a work of so general a nature, and of which physiological inquiries make so small a part, the few facts and observations which I have given upon such subjects may probably be overlooked by those who are not members of that Society. That they may be more easily procured by students in medicine, and other readers, I have, by an application to the President and Council of the Royal Society, obtained leave to reprint such of them as I consider to be connected with the principles and actions of the Animal Œconomy; and I have added such observations and remarks as have occurred to me since the time they were read before the Royal Society.

To the Second Edition of the Animal Œconomy, 1792.

———

ELEVEN of the following papers have been read at the Royal Society, and published in the Philosophical Transactions; but in a work of so general a nature, and of which physiological inquiries make so small a part, the few facts and observations which I have given upon such subjects may, probably, be overlooked by those who are not members of that Society. That they may be more easily procured by students in medicine, and other readers, I have, by an application to the President and Council of the Royal Society, obtained leave to reprint them, in this work, as being connected with the principles and actions of the Animal Œconomy; and I have added such observations and remarks as have occurred to me since the time they were read before the Royal Society.

CONTENTS.

	Page.
Preface of the Editor	i
Description of the Situation of the Testis in the Fœtus, with its descent into the Scrotum	1
Observations on the Glands situated between the Rectum and Bladder, called Vesiculæ Seminales	20
Account of the Free-martin	34
Account of an extraordinary Pheasant	44
Experiments to determine the effect of extirpating one Ovarium upon the number of Young produced	50
Case of a young Woman who poisoned herself in the first month of Pregnancy, with a description of the Uterus	55
On the Structure of the Placenta	60
Observations on the Placenta of the Monkey	71
Account of a Woman who had the Small-pox during Pregnancy, and who seemed to have communicated the same Disease to the Fœtus	74
Some Observations on Digestion	81
On the Digestion of the Stomach after Death	116
On a Secretion in the Crop of breeding Pigeons, for the nourishment of their Young	122
Observations on the Gillaroo Trout, commonly called in Ireland the Gizzard Trout	126
Experiments and Observations on Animals with respect to the power of producing Heat	131
Experiments and Observations on Vegetables with respect to the power of producing Heat	156
Proposals for the Recovery of Persons apparently drowned	165
Account of certain Receptacles of Air in Birds, which communicate with the Lungs and Eustachian Tube	176
Description of the Nerves which supply the Organ of Smelling	187
Description of some Branches of the Fifth Pair of Nerves	193
Croonian Lecture on Muscular Motion, No. I.	195
————————————————————, No. II.	224

Page.

Croonian Lecture on Muscular Motion, No. III. 242
——————————————————————, No. IV. 251
——————————————————————, No. V. 255
——————————————————————, No. VI. 267
On the Use of the Oblique Muscles 274
On the Colour of the Pigmentum of the Eye in different Animals . 277
On the Crystalline Lens, or some Facts relative to the late Mr.
    John Hunter's Preparation for the Croonian Lecture 286
Account of the Organ of Hearing in Fishes 292
Experiments on Absorption by Veins 299
Experiments and Observations on the Growth of Bones 315
Observations tending to show that the Wolf, Jackal and Dog are
    all of the same species 319
Observations on the Structure and Œconomy of Whales 331
Notes on the Anatomy of the Jerboa 393
Anatomical Description of the Amphibious Bipes of Ellis (*Siren la-
    certina*, Linn.) 394
On the Electric Property of the Torpedo 398
Anatomical Observations on the Torpedo 409
Account of the *Gymnotus electricus* 414
Observations on Bees.................................. 422
Anatomical Remarks on a New Marine Animal (*Serpula gigantea*,
    Pallas) 467
Observations on the Fossil Bones presented to the Royal Society
    by His Most Serene Highness the Margrave of Anspach 470
Descriptions of some Animals from New South Wales 481
Of the Kangaroo (*Macropus major*, Shaw) 485
Of the Potoroo (*Hypsiprymnus murinus*, Illiger) 487
Of the Hepoona Roo (*Petaurus Taguanoides*, Desmarest) 488
Of the Wha Tapoua Roo (*Phalangista Vulpina*, Geoffroy) 489
Of the Tapao Tafa (*Phascogale penicillata*, Temminck) 490
Of the Dingo (*Canis Australasiæ*) 493

PREFACE.

—————

ALWAYS an admirer of the genius of Hunter, and of late years obliged by official duties to make frequent reference to his numerous and varied productions, especially to those which are scattered through different volumes of the Philosophical Transactions and other works, I have often felt the inconvenience that resulted from the absence of a uniform edition of the whole of the extant works of that great and original thinker. When, therefore, Mr. Palmer first communicated to me his design of publishing a new edition of Hunter's works, I heard with peculiar satisfaction his intention to include in the proposed collection every memoir of the author that could be found in print, and I gladly lent my assistance, which, however, the previous assiduous researches of Mr. Palmer rendered of little moment, towards completing a list of all the published essays or observations on various parts of the 'Animal Œconomy' which had not before been included in the work so entitled. The proposal which Mr. Palmer at the same time made to me to edit this portion of the works of Hunter I declined, from a sense of the inadequacy of my powers to grapple with so vast a range of important physiological subjects as the contemplated volume must necessarily embrace, and I sincerely hoped that Mr. Palmer would have found a coadjutor better qualified than myself to do justice to this portion of his most useful and praiseworthy undertaking.

After a lapse of nearly two years Mr. Palmer again applied to me to revise the papers on the Animal Œconomy, and I then acceded reluctantly to his request, led, by the sole motive of accelerating the appearance of a much wished for edition, to a task, to which I have since dedicated a great proportion of my leisure hours, without the slightest expectation of profit or honour, the experiment having only served to convince me of the difficulty of adding the observations demanded by the progress of science to the text of Hunter in the spirit of its author, and a retrospect of my annotations leading me to suspect that often, with every wish to avoid it, I may have tacitly implied an ignorance on the part of Hunter of facts with which he was probably well acquainted, and to perceive that, in general, the addition of such details tends to overload and destroy the force of the original observations in the text.

It is with much more satisfaction that I refer to the additions which have been made to the present edition of the Animal Œconomy of the hitherto uncollected or unpublished writings of its original author.

These consist of the following essays.

From the *Philosophical Transactions* :

" On the Anatomy of the Siren or Amphibious Bipes (1766)."

" On the Electric Organs of the Torpedo (1773)."

" On the Electric Organs of the Gymnotus (1755)."

" Experiments and Observations on Vegetables with respect to the power of producing Heat (1775)."

" A case of Small-pox communicated by the Mother to the Fœtus (1780)."

" Anatomical Remarks on a New Marine Animal (1785)."

" Observations on the Structure and Œconomy of Whales (1787)."

" On Bees (1792)."

" On the Fibrous Structure of the Crystalline Lens (1793)."

" On the Fossil Bones of the Caverns of Gailenreuth (1794)."

" Six Croonian Lectures read before the Royal Society by Hunter in the years 1776, 1777, 1779, 1780, 1781 and 1782," but withdrawn from publication by the Author.

From the *Medical Commentaries of Dr. Wm. Hunter* :

" Experiments on Absorption by Veins."

From the *Transactions of a Society for the Promotion of Medical and Chirurgical Knowledge*, vol. ii. (1794) :

" Description of the Human Uterus and Ovum in the First Month of Pregnancy."

" Observations on the Growth of Bone."

There is also added,

" An Account of the Anatomy of the Jerboa," contributed by Hunter to the Appendix to Russel's *History of Aleppo.* And, lastly,

" Descriptions of Five Marsupial Quadrupeds," from the Zoological Appendix to White's *Voyage to New South Wales.* (1790.)

In order to bring these different memoirs in juxtaposition with papers on analogous subjects in the original edition of the Animal Œconomy, a slight alteration has been made in the arrangement of the different essays composing that work. Those which relate to generation are brought together at the beginning of the volume; then follow the observations on digestion, animal heat, and other physiological subjects; and lastly, the papers of a descriptive character, which refer more immediately to comparative anatomy and zoology. Thus for the first time are collected into one volume the physiological and anatomical stores, from which, in connexion with the materials composing his museum or destined for its illustration, an adequate idea may be formed of the nature of the great work in which Hunter had purposed to record the sum of his vast experience.

In the year 1786, when Hunter published a collection of his detached memoirs in the first edition of the Animal Œconomy, he observes, with reference to the subject of digestion, " I cannot at present spare sufficient time to give my opinions at large on this subject, with all the experiments and observations I have made upon it, but as soon as I have leisure I shall lay them before the public." And again, in describing the organ of hearing in fishes, he premises that he reserves a more complete investigation of this part of natural history " for a larger work on the structure of animals, which I one day hope to have it in my power to publish," and he states that ever since the year 1760 his researches have been continued in every part of the animal œconomy. Hence instead of regarding the uncommon structures which he discovered in his dissections of different animals as individual peculiarities, he was enabled to advance beyond the anatomists of his own times, and view them from the same eminence to which subsequent induction has raised the observers of the present day: and referring to the

series of preparations in his museum, he boldly states with reference to the structure of the organ of hearing in fish, that it is
" only a link in the chain of varieties displayed in the formation
of this organ of sense in different animals, descending from
the most perfect to the most imperfect in a regular progression."

The importance of these views, and the nature and amount
of the knowledge which they indicated, could not be appreciated by the contemporaries of Hunter in the absence of a
detailed exposition of the evidences on which they were
founded.   It is no wonder, therefore, that we find his earlier
eulogists sometimes founding his claims to scientific eminence
on insecure grounds; some, for example, lauding him as the
author of a theory of the organizing energy, which may be
traced to the time of Aristotle, or as the originator of the
doctrine of the vitality of the blood, which is supported with
so much eloquence by Harvey and his immediate successors;
while others, taking more definite grounds, have often unfortunately selected as his discoveries precisely those' subjects
of Hunter's special researches in which he had but revived
and extended the ideas of his predecessors.   Of this we have
a striking example in the introductory observations on the
character of Hunter contained in Sir Everard Home's Lectures on Comparative Anatomy, vol. i. p. 6, in which the independent function of the vesiculæ seminales and the determination of the organ of hearing in fishes are adduced as Hunterian
discoveries.

The true originators of· these and of other ideas and ,facts
which Hunter may have regarded as his discoveries, and which
he doubtless did discover so far as independent and original
research constitutes a claim to that honour, I have been careful
to point out in every case where my reading has led me to detect in an older author a clear anticipation of Hunter.

It cannot be doubted, however, that the ascription to Hunter,
by his friends and admirers, of facts and opinions to which he
had no title as the original discoverer, must have contributed
to lower his character in the estimation of continental anatomists; whose acquaintance with the vast accumulation of facts
in comparative anatomy due to the labours of the numerous

cultivators of that science in the sixteenth and seventeenth centuries, easily enabled them to detect the weakness of such claims, without perhaps their possessing such a knowledge of Hunter's labours as to justly appreciate their scope and tendency, and to view them, as they deserve to be viewed, in the light of a first great attempt to arrange in one concatenated system the diversified facts in comparative anatomy.

Cuvier, for example, in his review of the progress of science in the latter half of the eighteenth century, a period which may be regarded as a second revival of comparative anatomy and physiology, places Hunter in an inferior category of contributors to those sciences. After eulogizing the share which the erudite Haller took in demonstrating the importance of comparative anatomy to the advancement of physiology, and the corresponding effects which the labours of Daubenton and Pallas produced in establishing sounder ideas of the classification of animals, the historian of the natural sciences goes on to state: " John Hunter in England, the two Monros in Scotland, Camper in Holland, and Vicq D'Azyr in France were the first who followed their footsteps. Camper," he observes, " cast, so to say, a passing glance of the eye of genius on a number of interesting objects, yet almost all his labours were but sketches. Vicq D'Azyr, with more assiduity, was arrested by a premature death in the midst of a brilliant career; but their works inspired a general interest, which has ever since been on the increase."

With reference to the nature or influence of the labours of Hunter, Cuvier is silent; he limits himself to an indication in a marginal note of the Treatise on the Teeth and " les autres écrits de Hunter insérés en partie dans les *Transactions Philosophiques**."

This was meting out but scanty justice to the author of the Treatise on the Blood and of the Observations on the Animal Œconomy, which abound with so many general propositions in comparative anatomy and physiology. If, however, this opinion of Cuvier be excusable under the circumstances under which it was written, it would be unpardonable not to appeal against it upon the evidence of the higher claims of Hunter afforded by

Histoire des Progrès des Sciences Naturelles, depuis 1789, tom. i. p. 302.

the present edition of his works and by those manuscripts which
have already appeared in the catalogue of his Physiological
collection published by the Royal College of Surgeons.   Had
these manuscripts, explanatory of the design of the Hunterian
collection, been published before Cuvier wrote the work from
which we have just quoted, that astonishing result of Hunter's
labours might perhaps have claimed a passing notice from one
whose statements all Europe now receives and all posterity
will regard with confidence and respect.

"*Les autres écrits*," the "other writings" of Hunter to which
Cuvier alludes, are indeed devoted rather to the development
of general principles in physiology than to the detail of the
anatomical observations upon which he founded them.   Many
of the facts ascertained in the course of his higher and more
comprehensive inquiries, and incidentally alluded to in the narration, are however fully as interesting and important as those
which other anatomists have sometimes thought worthy of
being made the subjects of express monographs.

But Hunter had higher aims than the reputation of a mere
collector of facts in comparative anatomy; and this he not only
felt but had expressed in an early period of his career.   In a
manuscript, copied by Mr. Clift, relating to a dissection of a
turtle, he says, "The late Sir John Pringle, knowing of this
dissection, often desired me to collect all my dissections of this
animal, and send them to the Royal Society; but the publishing of a description of a single animal, more especially a common one, has never been my wish."

Howsoever we may regret this feeling, which has undoubtedly deprived the world of the results of much inestimable labour, and has operated in various ways disadvantageously to
Hunter's own reputation, yet it indicates the expanded views
of the man who entertained it.

Had Hunter published *seriatim* his notes of the structures
of the animals which he dissected, these contributions to comparative anatomy would not only have vied with the labours of
Daubenton as recorded in the *Histoire Naturelle* of Buffon,
or with the Comparative Dissections of Vicq d'Azyr which
are inserted in the early volumes of the *Encyclopédie Métho-
dique* and in the *Mémoires de l'Académie Royale de France*,
but they would have exceeded them both together.

It would be tedious to enumerate, name by name, the different species of animals whose organization was investigated and recorded by Hunter. Mr. Clift has evidence* that he left written descriptions, from autopsy, of the anatomy of the following Mammalia:

Of Quadrumana	.	21 Species.
Carnivora	. .	51
Rodentia	. .	20
Edentata	. .	5
Ruminantia	. .	15
Pachydermata	.	10
Cetacea	. .	6
Marsupiata	. .	10
Of Birds	. .	84 Species.
Reptiles	. .	25
Fishes	. . .	19
Of Insects	. . .	29 Species.

Of other invertebrate animals, as mollusca, red-blooded worms, and radiata, upwards of twenty. From the titles of manuscripts, therefore, it appears that Hunter possessed, at the period of his decease, original records of the dissections of three hundred and fifteen different species of animals.

In addition to these, Hunter's preparations testify that he had dissected twenty-three species of mammalia, sixteen species of birds, fourteen species of reptiles, forty species of fishes, forty-two different mollusca, and about sixty species of articulate and radiate animals; all species of animals of whose anatomy we have no evidence that he left written descriptions. So that by adding these undescribed dissections to those of which we derive the evidence from the list of the manuscripts, and of which described dissections his anatomical collection in like manner contains evidences in the dissected and preserved organs, there is proof that Hunter anatomized at least five hundred different species of animals, exclusive of repeated dissections of different individuals of the same species, besides the dissections of plants to a considerable amount.

* See " Evidence before the Medical Committee of the House of Commons."

With respect to the rarer and less known invertebrate animals, Hunter was not content with merely recording their
structure, and displaying its leading peculiarities in preparations; but he caused most elaborate and accurate drawings to
be made from the recent dissections; for which purpose he retained in his family many years an accomplished draughtsman,
Mr. William Bell, better known as the author of two papers in
the Philosophical Transactions, descriptive of the Sumatran
Rhinoceros and the Ecan Bonna (*Platax arthriticus*, Cuv.).
Several examples of these beautiful designs have already been
published by the Council of the Royal College of Surgeons in
the illustrated catalogue of the Hunterian Museum: they relate to the anatomy of the Sepia and Solen, of the Ascidia and
Salpa; they illustrate the circulation of the blood in the Crustacea and Anellida; and the figure which Mr. Hunter has given
of the circulation in the Chlocia capillata, a red-blooded worm,
far surpasses in beauty and detail any of those with which Cuvier
illustrates the memoir * dedicated to what he regarded to his
latest breath as one of his most interesting discoveries.

Hunter had also minutely investigated the anatomy of the
cirripeds†; but of his dissections of these, as of many other
animals, it is to be lamented that the preparations and drawings are now the sole evidences. The illustrations of the anatomy of the Echinodermata, both of the spiny species and of
the unarmed Holothuria, have never been surpassed either as
to minuteness or accuracy; and, excepting the disputed article of the nervous system, little is added in the elaborate and
well-known monograph of Tiedemann, to the anatomy of the
Holothuria as it is displayed by Hunter‡.

Now the anatomical labours of Daubenton were confined to
that class of animals whose structure most nearly resembles
man; he describes the position and length and breadth and
number of parts with most praiseworthy zoological precision,
but never appears to raise his thoughts to the relations of the
structures he detected with the habits of the species, or their
adaptation to function. Hence he has been said to have made

* *Bulletin de la Soc. Philomath.*, 1791, p. 146.
† See Physiological Catalogue of the Hunterian Collection, vol. i. p. 255.
pl. IV.
‡ Ibid., p. 251, pl. III.

more discoveries of which he was unconscious than any other cultivator of comparative anatomy.

Vicq·d'Azyr, on the contrary, adorns his descriptions with many beautiful and philosophical views, but he did not carry his scalpel beyond the vertebrate series; while Hunter explored every modification of animal structure, from man down to the polype.

If Hunter surpassed his contemporaries in the value and amount of the materials which he collected in comparative anatomy, he rises far above them in the application of his facts.

By a profound and unremitting meditation on the diversities of structure presented to his view, he derived more accurate notions than were current amongst his contemporaries of the parts essential to the performance of the different functions, and every idea or doubt thus suggested he tested by the most varied, ingenious, and accurate experiments.

" Many things," he observes, " arise out of investigation which were not at first conceived; and even misfortunes in experiments have brought things to our knowledge that were not, and probably could not have been, previously conceived. On the other hand, I have often devised experiments by the fireside or in my carriage, and have also conceived the result; but when I tried the experiment the result was different, or I found the experiment could not be attended with all the circumstances that were suggested*." Few physiologists indeed, if any, have made more numerous, various, and conclusive experiments than Hunter. Yet he says, " I think it may be set down as an axiom that experiments should not be often repeated which merely tend to establish a principle already known and admitted, but that the next step should be the application of that principle to useful purposes†."

By this series of labours of mind and hand, prosecuted uninterruptedly from year to year, Hunter at length came to establish a body of physiological doctrines, to the happy influence of which on the treatment of the various " ills that flesh is heir to," every cultivator of the healing science now bears grateful testimony.

---

* Animal Œconomy, p. 124 (the pages throughout refer to the present edition).
† Ibid, p. 86.

Most of the enlightened physiologists of this country have acknowledged the high merit and beneficial influence of Hunter's labours; but the general terms in which his merits have been expressed have not availed in raising him from the secondary category of contributors to comparative anatomy, in which he has been classed by Cuvier, and from which some continental writers have lately been disposed to degrade him *.

The present seems, therefore, to be a fitting opportunity to attempt to define the grounds for assigning a higher station to Hunter, considered as a physiologist and comparative anatomist. In this endeavour, however, to prove what Hunter was as a discoverer, we must also fairly state what he was not.

He has been spoken of as the originator of the idea of a subtle imponderable principle operating in the fluids and solids of the organism, and causing the phænomena of life. But such a principle, under various names and with various attributes, has been assigned as the cause of organization by Aristotle, Harvey, Willis, Cudworth, Grew, Van Helmont, and Stahl.

As both Harvey and Hunter had spent laborious lives in earnest inquiries and repeated dissections and experiments, to ascertain relations between structure and function; as both had studied the changes which take place in the form and structure of animals from their embryo state to that of maturity; and as both had carefully traced the successive phænomena which occur in the egg during incubation,—the similarity of their opinions on the nature and powers of the vital principle is correspondingly close.

Both arrived at the conclusion, that an animating principle exists and operates in the ovum prior to the formation of any organ of the future animal. Both attributed the power by which the fecund egg resists putrefaction, while the unprolific one decomposes, to a principle of life, which Harvey more precisely terms the "anima vegetiva†."

---

* See the *Esquisse Historique sur l'Anatomie Comparée*, prefixed to the French translation of the second edition of Carus' Comparative Anatomy, vol. i. p. xxx.

† "Plurimum itaque mecum ipse reputavi, quî fieret, ut ova improlifica gallinæ supposita, ab eodem calore extraneo corrumpantur, putrescant, et fœtida evadant; ovis autem fœcundis idem non contingat." Harveii *De Generatione Animalium Exercitatio* 22.

Hunter, however, carries his researches a step further; he submits the fecund egg to a low temperature, and ascertains a new property, of which Harvey was ignorant, a power, viz. of resisting cold : he also shows that when once frozen, and killed by cold, the dead impregnated egg yields to putrefaction like the unimpregnated one.

Both physiologists observed that if the phænomena of a vital principle were manifested in one part of the organization more than in another, it was in the blood. "For the blood," says Harvey, "is the first formed, and is the primary animate particle of the embryo; it is generated prior to the *punctum saliens*, before the first rudiment of the heart, and is endowed with the vital heat or principle before it begins to move, and from it does pulsation commence. For the thing containing is made to be serviceable to the thing contained.

"Nor is the blood therefore to be called the primogenial part, because that in and from it the organ of pulsation is derived, but also because the animal heat and vital principle are first implanted therein; and in it does life consist. For where heat and motion first begin, there also life doth first arise and last expire."—Harvey, On Generation, pp. 274, 275.

This explicit and beautiful enunciation of the pre-existence of the blood to the machine by which it is mainly circulated, and of its endowment of life, fell barren from the pen of Harvey (if we except the brief practice of transfusion to which it gave rise), and was forgotten, when Hunter resumed the inquiry. And why, it may be asked, was the doctrine of the vitality of the blood inoperative, as taught by Harvey? Because instead of establishing that doctrine by observations and experiments, from which alone it was susceptible of deriving further proof,— instead of applying the principle to the explanation of the phæ-nomena of disease, and to a modification and improvement of

---

"Ovum itaque est corpus naturale virtute animali præditum; principio nempe motus, transmutationis, quietis, et conservationis." *Exercit.* 26.

"Cum enim in ovo macula prius dilatetur, colliquamentum concoquatur et præparetur, plurimaque alia (non sine providentia) ad pulli formationem et incrementum instituantur, antequam quidpiam pulli vel ipsa primogenita ejus particula appareat; quidni utique credamus calorem innatum animamque pulli vegetativam ante pullum ipsum exsistere?" *Exercit.* 57.

remedial measures, Harvey obscures and forgets the conclusions
of his cooler moments of observation, and, as the learned Bar-
clay well observes, excited by the discovery which had extended
his fame so widely over Europe, and had reflected such lustre
on his name and country, he expatiates on the blood as something divine; he has recourse to hyperbole, and describes its
properties in the extravagant language of romance.

Hunter, on the contrary, carries a series of calm and philosophical investigations on the vital properties of the blood to
an extent which has never been surpassed; he examines it under every condition, both in the vessels and out of the vessels,
during circulation and at rest, in health and in disease. He
aims to establish the period in its formation at which it manifests the vital properties; and he fully details the changes which
it undergoes, and the phænomena which supervene in the rest
of the organism when these properties are lost. Lastly, he
tells us how the blood, by means of its vital properties, assists
in the restoration of parts when injured or diseased.

Hunter subjects the blood to both mechanical and chemical
analysis, and endeavours to determine the characteristic properties of its different constituents. It was not known in his
time upon which of these constituents the act of coagulation
depended. Hunter took advantage of a case in which the
red globules subsided, as in some cases they do, more rapidly
than usual, and skimming off the superincumbent colourless
fluid, found that the fibrine, as it is now termed, immediately
coagulated and formed a colourless clot*. A subsequent erroneous theory, which attributed the act of coagulation to the red
globules, has recently been set aside by the application of an
ingenious process for artificially separating the fibrine from the
blood disks before coagulation takes place, and the opinions of
Hunter on this point have been fully established by the experiments of Müller. With respect to the serum, Hunter instituted a number of experiments and made many ingenious observations to determine the relative quantity of the coagulable
to the uncoagulable part. His deductions as to the amount of
nutrient albumen in the blood of animals of different ages, and
under different circumstances, as regards exercise or rest, &c.
formed, from observing the quantity of gravy or uncoagulable

serosity which different roasted meats afforded, is highly characteristic of his original and ever active mind. In seeking
to determine the respective importance of the different constituents of the blood, by the philosophical and most difficult inquiry into their respective periods of formation in the development of the embryo, Hunter made the interesting discovery
that the vessels of the embryo of a red-blooded animal circulated in the first instance colourless blood, as in the invertebrate animals.

" The red globules," he observes, " seem to be formed later
in life than the other two constituents, for we see while the
chick is in the egg the heart beating, and it then contains a
transparent fluid before any red globules are formed, which
fluid we may suppose to be the serum and the lymph *."

I well remember the feelings of surprise with which I listened
while at Paris in 1832 to a memoir read before the Academy of
Sciences by MM. Delpech and Coste, the object of which was
the announcement of the same fact as a novel and important
discovery. The statement of the French observers was received with all the consideration which its importance justly
merited, without its being suspected that our great physiologist
had half a century before embraced it, with all its legitimate
deductions, in the extended circle of his investigations.

In the same spirit in which he investigated the nature of the
blood he also pursued his researches on the properties of the
solids; he endeavours to determine the specific powers and
vital phænomena of the nervous system and of the stomach;
he compares these important parts of the animal body, with
reference to the degree of energy with which their functions
are manifested; he considers the influence which they reciprocally exert in maintaining the vitality of the blood, and the
relative dependence of the whole organism on the integrity of
their vital powers. He also dwells at great length on the sympathies resulting from these mutual relations and dependencies.

In all his physiological researches we may see that instead
of dogmatising on the powers and virtues of an abstract essence,
Hunter endeavours to analyse the vital forces peculiar to each

* Vol. III. p. 66.

organic element, and to classify, as it were, the phænomena of which life consists.

If we turn from Hunter's researches on life to his investigations on another equally difficult and recondite subject in general physiology, viz. Animal, or rather, Organic Heat, we see the same exercise of the powers of the same great and original mind.

He first determines the relative extent to which the power of generating heat or resisting cold is enjoyed in the two grand divisions of organic nature, plants and animals : he next investigates the degree in which that power is possessed by different classes of animals ; then the relation subsisting between that degree and the perfection and complexity of the organization with which the power is associated.   He anticipates some modern physiologists in determining the different power of generating heat manifested by the same species at different periods of life, and advances a step further by considering the different powers of resisting cold which different parts of the same organized body possess in relation to their respective ages and periods of formation*.   He lastly analyses, so to say, the different functions, to determine in what degree the production of heat depends on their exercise; and reciprocally, the influence of the temperature of the body upon the active and healthy maintenance of their functions.

Throughout all this beautiful and justly celebrated inquiry we see the philosopher conscious of the extent of his powers, and of the kind of knowledge which the right exercise of those powers was adapted to acquire.   We nowhere perceive a trace of a desire to establish a theory of the nature of animal heat in the abstract.

Let any one compare the language of Harvey or of Willis, while expatiating on the *calidum innatum*, with the following just remark : " I shall not," says Hunter, " attempt to settle whether heat is a body or matter, or only a property of matter, which appears to me to be merely a difference in terms, for a property must belong to something †."

It is precisely in the same spirit that he conducts his re-

searches on life ; and I would say, after a very careful study of
the writings of Hunter, that of all physiologists he is one to
whom a dogmatic theory of abstract life can least be attributed.
But by those whose notions of Hunter's doctrines are founded
solely on a perusal of the posthumous " Treatise on the Blood"
he is liable to be misconceived, and in opinions expressed from
that limited acquaintance with his writings to be misrepresented.

With the just ideas which Hunter had acquired of the laws
of vitality and organic heat he was enabled to explain many of
the phænomena of digestion more satisfactorily than had been
done by his predecessors Spallanzani and Reaumur.

The following is a fair example of the different views and
kinds of knowledge which these experimenters brought to the
inquiry.

Spallanzani had observed that digestion did not go on in reptiles below a certain temperature, he thought therefore that heat
was necessary to assist in the dissolving processes of the stomach ; Hunter, in reference to the same fact, shows that the
influence here is not merely chemical, but that the heat operates by first raising the sensitive powers, these then transmit
the stimulus to the respiratory and circulating functions, and
lastly to the motive and other actions and faculties, and that the
digestive organs are necessarily excited to corresponding actions, in order to supply the waste occasioned by the working
of the machine, which the heat has thus called into play.

Hunter more accurately determined, and first applied and
rendered fruitful, the fact which Grew incidentally mentions,
viz. That it is the property of a living body or part to resist the
action of the gastric juice; and his celebrated paper " On the
Digestion of the Stomach after Death," is a beautiful example
of the application of his general views in physiology to the explanation of particular phænomena.

Of all his published writings, the papers on Digestion convey
perhaps the best idea of the extent of Hunter's researches
in Comparative Anatomy, and of the soundness of his reason-
ings in general physiology.

Hunter's claims to the originality of observations which have
been reproduced as new by later physiologists, I have pointed
out in the notes to these and other memoirs; and have parti-

cularly endeavoured to define the merits of Hunter as a discoverer in reference to the absorbent system.

Hunter's published writings on the N vous System bear but
a small proportion to the extent of his anatomical investigations
on this subject, especially as they are manifested in the philosophical series of preparations in the Gallery of his collection, in
which the nervous system is traced through its progressive
stags of complication, from the simple filaments of the entozoon
and echinoderm, to the aggregated masses which distinguish the
organization of man. The *fibrous structure* of the brain, the
discovery of which, though due to Coiter as early as 1573, has
sometimes been attributed to Reil and Gall, is displayed by
Hunter in preparations made to show the fact (Nos. 1335, 1336),
and is expressly mentioned in the description of the Anatomy
of the Whale Tribe*.

In treating of the comparative anatomy of the nervous system
in his introductory observations to this division of his Collec-
tion†, Hunter rises to the following generalizations. He divides the animals which have brains, or visible aggregations of
the nervous substance, into six classes, each characterized by a
peculiar modification of the brain.

The '*first class*' has a brain in the form of a ring, through
which passes the œsophagus, and from which the nerves arise,
like radii from a centre. It consists of a pulpy substance, somewhat transparent, which is easily squeezed out when the brain
is cut into.   It is not inclosed in hard parts, and is not defended
from pressure or injuries more than any other internal part.

The examples of this type in his Museum are selected from
the gastropodous class of Mollusca. The same condition of
the nervous system we now know, from the researches of Cuvier, to characterize the whole of a vast division of invertebrate
animals, including, amongst the highest organized of that division, certain species,—the dibranchiate Cephalopods,—in which
the character, as expressed by Hunter, is affected by the development of a cartilaginous cranium for the protection of the cerebral ring; but ulterior researches have not led to any modification of Hunter's description of the typical form of the brain
in the Molluscous sub-kingdom.

* p. 373.   † Physiological Catalogue, vol. iii. p. 4.

In the '*second class*' the brain lies in the head of the animal; it is a pulpy substance, somewhat transparent, which gives it a bluish cast; from its lower part go out two large nerves, one passes on each side of the œsophagus, and they then unite into one, forming a knot at their union; they disunite again, and so unite and disunite alternately through the whole length of the animal, at every union giving off the nerves as from the brain. This structure, Hunter says, he suspects to answer both the use of a medulla spinalis and the great intercostal nerve.

The examples of the class of animals adduced by Hunter as being characterized by this essential form of the nervous system are the leech, earthworm, aphrodita, centipede, caterpillar, scorpion, and lobster. Subsequent researches have shown that it exists in the barnacles, or Cirripedia, which most zoologists now rank in the same primary division with the Anellides, Insects, Arachnidans, and Crustaceans.

In the first class of animals in this neurological arrangement (for in enunciating general propositions respecting any given organ the comparative anatomist becomes involuntarily, as it were, a classificator of animals as well as organs,) Hunter observes, " we had the brain surrounded by soft parts only. In the second it was closely surrounded by soft parts, but these were surrounded by hard. In the '*third class*' the brain has a case of hard parts for itself, called the skull."

Now when Hunter made a brain relatively larger than in his first two classes—protected by a skull,—and continuous with a medulla spinalis extended down the back, and an endowment of the five senses,—the essential neurological characters of his third class of animals,—he erred in not applying them to his fourth, fifth, and sixth classes, as an attribute common to all, and one which distinguished each alike from the two lower classes. The appreciation of the great natural group characterized by a brain and spinal chord, situated on the dorsal aspect of the body, and protected by a vertebral case, was reserved for the sagacious penetration of Cuvier.

However, in so far as Hunter limits his generalizations to the brain alone, he is consistent with himself, and exact in the differential characters which he points out. The brain in fish, for example, or his '*third class*,' is a very irregular mass, inconstant in its form and in the number of its parts; still the "several parts which are similar to those in a superior class may be picked out;" the skull, moreover, is too large for the brain, and the interspace is filled by a cellular membrane, which Hunter compares to the arachnoid.

In the '*fourth class*,' the parts composing the brain "do not lie one upon another, but are very much detached and follow one another," in short, are characterized by their linear arrangement; a character, the accuracy of which, as applied to the Reptilia, has been confirmed by all subsequent experience. It is interesting to observe how Hunter determines the nature of these different detached masses. He says, " The two anterior consist of the cerebrum; the two middle, I should suppose, of the nates and testes, which I take to be the middle lobes detached, because in the bird they are more underneath, not so much between the cerebrum and cerebellum; the posterior is the cerebellum, consisting of one body entirely."* Every eminence, Hunter further observes, has a cavity or ventricle in it. The linear arrangement of the masses of the brain is common both to fishes and reptiles; but the relation of those masses to the skull, and their variable number and proportions, according to Hunter, distinguish the brain in fish. He further observes that in the crocodile the parts of the brain are more closely connected, and that the skull is more in contact with it, in which respect it comes nearer the bird than do any of the other amphibia.

The brain in the '*fifth class*,' or fowl, Hunter characterizes by its greater relative size, and the superposition of its component masses.

In the ' *sixth class*,' or quadrupeds, the brain is in general larger than in the preceding, and the parts more compacted, the whole mass being brought into nearly a globular figure. " The nates and testes are four small bodies, with no visible cavities; are not seen externally, but lie at the posterior end of the third ventricle."†

In the observations printed in the present volume on the branches of the fifth pair which are distributed to the nose and ear, we cannot fail to observe that Hunter had entered on that

* Physiological Catalogue, vol. iii. p. 7. † Ibid., p. 10.

track of inquiry, and perceived the governing principle or idea, which, more clearly appreciated and steadily retained by Sir Charles Bell, has since led to such important improvements in this department of physiology.

Hunter premises his description of the nerves which supply the organ of smelling by calling attention to the constancy which pervades the anatomical conditions of the nerves, and states in general his belief that particular nerves have particular functions, in relation to their differences of origin, union, and distribution*; but this simple enunciation, without the proofs and illustrations of which it was susceptible, became unproductive of its proper results, and appears to have been subsequently lost sight of by Hunter himself, when speculating on the nerves as internuntiate conductors of a *materia vitæ diffusâ*.

A knowledge of Hunter's opinions on the nervous system, derived only from the observations on that subject which occur in the Treatise on the Blood, might lead to the belief that he attributed to all the different nerves one common function; but after perusing the distinct exposition of his views on this branch of physiology as recorded in the Animal Œconomy, it appears to me that Hunter needed only to have resorted to experiment in this, as he did so successfully in other fields of physiological inquiry, to have established the nature and degree of the functional differences of these nerves, of which he describes the anatomical conditions giving rise, as he supposes, to those differences.

He limits himself, however, in his illustration of the grand proposition, by anatomical examples only. He shows that organs like the eye and nose, which are endowed by means of one nerve with a special sense, derive their ordinary sensation from a second nerve having a different origin. This nerve he determines, in the case of the eye and nose, to be the fifth pair. He says the same mode of reasoning is equally applicable to the organ of taste, and he traces the corresponding superadded nerve to the ear.

Hunter further distinguishes the sensations of the stomach

* pp. 187, 188.

b 2

and of the glans penis as being peculiar, and shows that as
these peculiar sensations reside in particular nerves, so at whatever part of the nerve the impression is made it always gives
the same sensation as if affected at the common seat of the sensation of that peculiar nerve.

In another place Hunter makes the ingenious remark that
the nerves which are specially designed to receive peculiar
impressions convey the ideas of such impressions to the brain,
in whatever way they may be affected or stimulated. Thus
he says, " A mechanical impression on the retina produces an
impression of light ; a blow on the ear the sensation of sound*."
And later experiments have only extended this principle, by
showing that whether the nerve be affected by mechanical, chemical, or electrical stimuli, it conveys the same sensation.

Much importance has been attributed to these observations,
on the supposition that they were new, and I have been induced
to dwell thus long upon Hunter's contributions to the physiology of the nervous system, because in most of the recent
works upon that subject he does not receive the credit which
is due to him for having made them.

The physiological discoveries of Bell, Majendie, Mayo, and
Müller have resulted from the combination of experiment with
a philosophical consideration of the anatomical peculiarities of
the nervous system. It was the neglect of experiment in this
department of physiology which rendered Hunter unable to
account for the peculiarities which equally struck his mind
as being connected in an intimate degree with the functions of
the nerves.

Had Hunter combined experiment with dissection when he
traced the lateral branch of the *nervus vagus* in the cod, the
eel, and the, gymnotus, and wondered " that a nerve should
arise from the brain to be lost in common parts, while there was
a *medulla spinalis* giving nerves to the same parts," this probably would not have remained to him, as he expresses it, " one
of the inexplicable circumstances of the nervous system†."

Having been induced to dwell on the improved views which.

* Vol. i. p. 263, of the present edition, and Parkinson's Hunterian Remi-
niscences, p. 12.
† Animal Œconomy, p. 419.

Hunter either established or suggested in different branches of physiology, I proceed next to advance a few instances of his discoveries in comparative anatomy, which, on the supposition that they were original, have contributed to add to the reputation of subsequent anatomists.

1. The organ of hearing in the sepia. The fact that this cephalopod possesses the organ in question is stated at p. 294 of the present edition of the Animal Œconomy, and it is said to differ from that of fishes. The discovery is attributed by Cuvier to Scarpa.

2. The semicircular canals of the Cetacea, described by Hunter in the paper on whales, a structure which Cuvier rightly states that Camper overlooked, but incorrectly claims the discovery as his own.

3. In the latest sketch of the history of comparative anatomy, prefixed to the French translation of Carus's Zootomie, John Hunter is introduced as the impudent self-appropriator of Camper's discovery of the air cells in the bones of birds; and the historian of the science does not honour him with any further notice.

Now the facts with reference to this subject are as follows: Camper's account of the air cells in the bones of Birds was first published in the Dutch language in the year 1774, the same year in which Mr. Hunter's discovery was published in the Philosophical Transactions. The French memoir of Camper was not published till the year 1776, in the seventh volume of the *Memoires Etrang. de l'Academie des Sciences de Paris.* Hunter gives the date of his discovery as being in 1758; Camper his, in the year 1771.

The numerous observations and experiments which their respective memoirs detail are not such as could hastily be got up for an unworthy purpose; but as both memoirs (which differ materially in their general scope and the mode in which the subject is treated) were published in the same year, the honour of the discovery may fairly be attributed to both their authors.

I might dwell on the philosophical comparison which Hunter makes between the abdominal air-cells of the bird and those of reptiles and fishes had he not in this instance been anticipated by Harvey. Harvey, however, was not aware that the respiratory system was extended into the muscular interstices and the cavities of the bones ; the honour of which discovery must be assigned to Hunter and Camper, without the necessity of supposing that either had borrowed from the other.

The preparations in the Hunterian Collection and the Manuscript Catalogues show that Mr. Hunter had discovered the peritoneal canals or openings in the eel, salmon, and the cartilaginous fishes, in the crocodile, and the continuation of the same peritoneal canals into the corpus cavernosum penis in the tortoise and turtle. The latter have been recently re-discovered by MM. Isidore St. Hilaire and Martin St. Ange.

Hunter's printed works, preparations, manuscripts and drawings contain proofs of his discovery of the circulation of the blood in insects, and of the peculiar diffused irregular and extended venous receptacles in these and the crustaceous animals, in the latter of which their existence remains unnoticed, even in the latest works on the subject.

In the Treatise on the Blood* we have an opportunity of judging, by the accuracy of the general propositions which he enumerates on this subject, of the extent of Hunter's researches on the comparative anatomy of the circulating system, and of the spirit in which he prosecuted the induction of particular facts. I cannot resist the quotation of the following passages which relate to the circulation in insects. " In the winged insects which have but one heart, as also but one circulation, there is this heart answering both purposes" (viz. the corporeal and the pulmonary circulations), p. 174.

" Many of those which have one ventricle only have no auricle, such as insects ; but there are others which have both a ventricle and auricle, such as fish, the snail, and many shellfish ; some of the last class have indeed two auricles, with only one ventricle.

" The heart is placed in what is called the chest in the quadruped, bird, amphibia, fish, and the aquatic and terrestrial insect, but not in what may be called the chest in the flying insect.

" The chest in the aquatic insect seems best suited to contain the lungs and branchiæ, and therefore the heart is placed there ; but as the lungs of the flying insect are placed through the whole body the heart is more diffused, extending through the whole length of the animal."

* § 5, p. 173 of the present edition.

" When the veins entering into the heart are small in comparison to the quantity of blood which is wanted in the ventricles, then we have an auricle; but when the veins near to the heart are large, there is no auricle, as in the lobster and generally in insects.

" In all animals which have an auricle and a ventricle, so far as I know, there is a bag (unattached) in which they are placed, called a pericardium; but the insect tribe, whether aerial, aquatic, or terrestrial, have none, their hearts being attached to the surrounding parts by the cellular membrane or some other mode of attachment.

" The heart gives to the blood its motion in most animals, and in all it sends the blood to the organs of respiration; in the flying insect it sends the blood both to those organs and to the body at large, but in fish to those organs only, the body at large in them having no heart. In the amphibia there is an attempt towards a heart both for the lungs and body, but not two distinct hearts. In the bird and quadruped there is a distinct heart for each." And again, " With respect to its use, it is in the most simple kind of heart to propel the blood through the body immediately from the veins, which blood is to receive its purification in this passage when the lungs are disposed throughout the body as in the flying insect."

The researches of Cuvier led him to conceive that there was a generally diffused, but passive, or non-circulated condition of the blood, coexisting in insects with the distribution of the breathing organs through the whole body. Hunter, on the contrary, while he rightly appreciated that condition of the circulating system in insects which related to their peculiar respiration, viz. that the venous blood was diffused apparently through the cellular membrane, in the interstices of the fat, air-cells, and muscles, and that the veins in insects might be called in some measure the cellular membrane of the parts *; yet he well knew the relations of these diffused receptacles of the venous blood to the dorsal heart, and the circulatory movement which was impressed upon the vital fluid by that organ. It is this remarkable error of Cuvier, with reference to the circulation in insects, that has given to the direct observations of

* See Physiological Catalogue, ii. p. 31; also the note at p. 221, vol. iii. of the present edition.

the blood's motion by means of the microscope in the hands of
Carus, Bowerbank, and other excellent observers, the character
of a new discovery.

Hunter first determined the bi-auricular structure of the
heart in the batrachian caducibranchiate reptiles, which he included in the class *Tricoilia* of his classification of animals according to the structure of the heart.

Hunter first discovered, by means of retrograde injections of
the *tubuli uriniferi*, that these essential parts of the kidney
extended to the superficies of that gland, and were not confined
to the medullary substance.   Meckel, who saw while in London the beautiful preparations establishing this fact (Nos. 1202,
1203, 1214, 1215, 1235), described them on his return to Germany to Müller*, who, in his recent elaborate work on the glands,
acknowledges how important this observation was in establishing true notions of the structure of glands.

Hunter extended his researches on the renal organ to the
intervertebrate classes, and shows " the kidney of the snail;"
and the correctness of this ascription to the so-called mucus
gland has been recently established by the observations of Professors Jacobson and de Blainville.

I have selected a few facts from amongst the multitude which
Hunter ascertained in the progress of those investigations, by
which he sought in the simpler modifications of the structures
in the lower animals the true uses of the different organs which
are combined to form the complex frame of man.

I might lastly allude to the extraordinary nature and extent
of Hunter's labours in another track of physiological inquiry,
viz. that which unfolds the laws of generation and animal development; but as the work confided to me by the Council of
the Royal College of Surgeons, viz. the description of the series of preparations on these subjects, which include nearly one
half of Hunter's grand Physiological Collection, is still in progress, I defer the comparison of Hunter's labours in this field
with those of his contemporaries until the whole body of the
evidence of his discoveries can be laid before the public.

The papers, however, which Hunter published in his lifetime, and which form the first part of the present volume, convey a most favourable idea of his views respecting this recon-

* De penitiori structurâ Glandularum, fol. p. 95.

dite branch of physiology. It is here that we find an attempt
to explain congenital defects by reference to the transitory
structures or metamorphoses of fœtal life.

It was a question in the time of Hunter how it happened that
the gut in the hernia congenita came to be in contact with the
testes. Hunter solved the question, by directing attention to
the position of the testis in the abdomen, and to its relations
to the other abdominal viscera, and to the peritoneum, a few
months before the expiration of the term of fœtal development.
He watched the progress of the gland to the scrotum; saw it
carrying along with it a peritoneal pouch like the sac of an intestine, and thus demonstrated, that if the closure of that sac
was prevented by the contemporaneous passage of a loop of intestine, it must remain a common receptacle, both of the part
which had naturally, and the part which had preternaturally,
escaped from the abdomen.

Hunter then goes on to show how the early and transitory
condition of the tunica vaginalis in the human fœtus, and also
the still earlier abdominal position of the testes, are permanent
structures in the lower mammalia.

With respect to monstrosities in general, Hunter had drawn
out a scheme for their classification, and had produced them
by experiment. In the "Account of an extraordinary Pheasant"
he states that every species of animal, and every part of an
animal body, is subject to congenital malformation; but he
knew that such appearances were not attributable to a freak of
Nature, or a matter of mere chance; for he observes that every
species has a disposition to deviate from Nature in a manner
peculiar to itself. It is this principle which forms the basis of the
latest and most elaborate treatise on monsters*, a work which
its author describes as being "the result of his having established, by a great number of researches, that monsters are,
like the beings called normal, subject to constant rules."

With respect to the cause or origin of monsters, Hunter referred it to a condition of the original germ, or, as he expresses
it, "each part of each species seems to have its monstrous form
originally impressed upon it." In the introductory observations to his extensive collection of malformed fœtuses and parts,

---

* *Histoire des Anomalies de l'Organization chez l'Homme et les Animaux, ou
Traité de Tératologie,* par Isid. Geoffroy St. Hilaire: Paris, 8vo. 1832.

he assigns the grounds for this hypothesis, and at the same time enunciates one of the most remarkable laws of aberrant formations. "I should imagine," he writes, "that monsters were formed monsters from their very first formation, for this reason, that all supernumerary parts are joined to their similar parts, as a head to a head, &c. &c." In proof of the important general principles, at a knowledge of which Hunter had arrived, I have elsewhere quoted this passage, together with the following remarkable one from Hunter's descriptions of his drawings illustrative of the development of the chick. "If we were capable of following the progress of increase of the number of the parts of the most perfect animal, as they first formed in succession from the very first, to its state of full perfection, we should probably be able to compare it with some one of the incomplete animals themselves, of every order of animals in the creation, being at no stage different from some of those inferior orders; or in other words, if we were to take a series of animals from the more imperfect to the perfect, we should probably find an imperfect animal corresponding with some stage of the most perfect."*

We may, I think, perceive, from the evident difficulty with which Hunter expresses the idea, that his mind was oppressed with both its novelty and vastness. Men's thoughts require to be familiarized with propositions of such generality before their exact limits and full application can be appreciated.

Sufficient, however, has been adduced to prove the tendency of Hunter's labours, and that he possessed the highest qualifications as an investigator of Nature; unwearied in induction, sagacious in grouping together analogous phænomena, and ever striving to ascend from propositions of less to those of greater generality.

Had the means and time been granted to Hunter to have made public the results of all his labours, or had his manuscripts enunciating, or indicative of, so many general principles been fairly appreciated and given to the world, our teachers of anatomy would not now, after a lapse of half a century, have but begun to explain to their students those beautiful laws of animal development, for the knowledge of which they are indebted to the labours of the professors in the noble schools of

* See preface to the Physiological Catalogue, vol. i. p. ii.

physiology in Continental Europe, where the spirit of Hunterian inquiries seems to have so long exclusively resided. But the period which has elapsed before those general laws began to be appreciated in the country where they were first detected, affords, perhaps, one of the strongest indications of the great advance which Hunter had made in physiological science.

It would be a strange exception to the usual result of an extensive knowledge of comparative anatomy, combined with a tendency to express in general propositions new physiological and structural truths, if the possession and application of that knowledge with that tendency had not led to some corresponding advance towards a natural system of zoological classification. Accordingly we find the contemporaries of Hunter ascribing to him the highest accomplishment which the zoologist can aspire to, that of discerning the natural affinities of a nondescript object; and this in terms and on occasions which seem to imply a general admission of his possession of such attainments. When the rare quadrupeds of Australia were first brought to England, presenting, as they did, to the eye of the zoologist anomalies and peculiarities not less striking than those which perplexed the botanist in the plants from the same part of the world, it was to Hunter that they were referred.

"There was no person," says Dr. Shaw, "to whom they could be given with so much propriety, he perhaps being most capable of examining accurately their structure, and making out their place in the scale of animals*."

It may not be uninteresting to contrast the sketches of systems of zoological arrangement which Hunter has left, with the Linnæan method which prevailed in his time, and which continued to prevail until superseded by the labours of Cuvier, specially and unremittingly directed to that end. We have already seen that Hunter's attempts to enunciate general propositions respecting the nervous system led him to detect the condition characteristic of the molluscous subkingdom, and to speak of the animals with "the brain in the form of a ring," &c. as a class. In still more definite terms he describes the condition of the nervous system which characterizes the articulate Invertebrata.

With respect to that higher type of the nervous system, which

* Zoological Appendix to White's Voyage to New South Wales, p. 481 of the present work.

is manifested in its aggregation into spinal and cerebral masses, we have seen that Hunter alludes to it as distinguishing only the class of fishes from his first and second classes, or the Molluscous and Articulate divisions as they are now termed; and that he failed to perceive that all the other vertebrate classes were equally characterized by it. To Hunter, however, we must award the merit of having first obtained a perception of the distinct group formed by the higher organized vermes of Linnæus, and their essential organical character. Hunter had also investigated the structure of zoophytes, in which no annular brain can be detected; he had conceived the idea of animals in which the nervous matter, or something analogous to it, a *materia vitæ diffusa*, was dispersed throughout the system. And we find another learned contemporary of Hunter, in ascribing a diffused condition of the nervous matter to the Tæniæ, bearing testimony that Hunter had entertained a similar opinion, and had applied that character of the nervous system to many of the lower tribes of animals *.

The distribution of animals according to the nervous element of their organization, is, however, but one of several attempts at classification which Hunter made. The next scheme which we shall quote is one founded upon modifications of the generative function †. Hunter's *first class*, or *Vivipara*, corresponds with the *Zootoka* of Aristotle, and the *Mammalia* of Linnæus; these animals develop their young in the uterus, he says, from a mixture of male and female influence, and bring forth a living offspring.

The *second class*, or *Ovovivipara*, is a subdivision of the *Ootoka* or *Ovipara* of Aristotle, and "hatch their young from an egg in the oviduct, as vipers, slow-worms, some lizards, newts, and the dog-fish."

The *third class* includes the *Ovipara*, or "such animals as exclude their eggs, which are afterwards hatched out of the body;" but this character, as Hunter justly observes, "takes in a wide field."

Fourthly, he says, "We have animals which propagate by slips, and that in two different ways, one by a piece cut off,

---

* See Carlisle, On the Structure and Œconomy of Tæniæ, Linnæan Transactions, vol. ii. p. 253, and vol. iii. p. 116, of the present edition.

† See Introduction to the Physiological Catalogue, vol. iii. p. vi.

the other by branches growing, and these falling off, and producing a distinct animal." Hunter here rightly regards the fissiparous and gemmiparous modes of generation as modifications of the same reproductive process which is characteristic of that lowest group of animals previously indicated by the molecular condition of the nervous system, and "where every other principle of the animal is diffused through the whole," a condition which in the animal kingdom seems essential to the possession of the property of fissiparous reproduction, or to a division of the whole body with a continuance of the vital properties in the parts. Hunter seems, however, to have felt how unsatisfactory and artificial was the classification founded on modes of generation, for he adds in the manuscript in which the above sketch is given, "Animals of any particular class have not one way only of propagating their species, excepting the more perfect, or first class according to hearts, for we have the second and even the third class aping the first, and attempting to be viviparous, as vipers, lizards, and some fishes, as the skate." He might have added examples of ovoviviparous animals, from the molluscous, articulate and radiate classes,—classes which in every other respect are most dissimilar. This idea of an arrangement of the animal kingdom from modifications of the generative function was afterwards carried out by Sir Everard Home*, and applied by him to the definition of the narrower or subordinate groups. But as of all single characters the generative system affords the most arbitrary and unnatural distinctions, and corresponds least with the modifications of the rest of the organization, a classification of animals based upon it is least adapted to afford any of the conveniences of even an artificial system.

In the *Systema Naturæ* of Linnæus the first of the characters by which the six classes of animals are distinguished is derived from modifications of the structure of the heart, as follows :

"*Mammalia*, Cor biloculare, biauritum ;
Aves, Cor biloculare, biauritum ;
Amphibia, Cor uniloculare, uniauritum ;
Pisces, Cor uniloculare, uniauritum ;

---

*. See his *Systema Regni Animalis nunc primum ex ovi modificationibus propositum*, Lectures on Comparative Anatomy, vol. iii. p. 535.

Insecta, Cor uniloculare, inauritum ;
Vermes, Cor uniloculare, inauritum."

But Linnæus combines the cardiac character with others derived from the nature of the blood, the condition of the respiratory organs, the structure of the mouth and generative organs,
the nature of the integuments, &c., and thus makes an approach to a natural system of arrangement.

Hunter, in his distribution of animals into different classes
according to the structure of the heart, uses the cardiac character singly, and produces a purely artificial arrangement; but
his superior anatomical knowledge manifests itself in the accuracy with which he defines the condition of the circulating organ characteristic of the different groups.

His *first class* includes the *Mammalia* and *Aves* of Linnæus,
and he proposes to call it *Tetracoilia,* the heart having four
cavities, viz. two ventricles and two auricles.

The *second class, Tricoilia,* includes those animals which
have a heart with three cavities, viz. one ventricle and two auricles, and corresponds with the *Amphibia* of Linnæus. The
anatomical inaccuracy in the Linnæan character, although so
early corrected by Hunter, long retained its ground in the systematic works of continental naturalists, and continued to be
erroneously applied to the Batrachian section of the Linnean
Amphibia until a very recent period *.

---

* The two auricles were after the time of Linnæus successively assigned in
systematic works to the *Chelonia* and *Sauria.* Blumenbach long continued to
assert that serpents, at least those of Germany, had but one auricle ; Cuvier allowed them two, but denied this higher structure of the heart to the *Batrachia*:
" Ils n'ont au cœur qu'une seule oreillette et un seul ventricule." *Règne Animal,*
ii. p. 101, edit. 1829. Meckel also ascribes this structure to the generality of
the *Batrachia*: " Die Batrachier haben die einfachste Herzform. Das Herz
besteht sehr allgemein nur aus einer Vorkammer und einer Kammer." *Vergl.
Anat.,* band v. p. 215. The more complicated structure of the heart was, however, truly described in the anourous *Batrachia* by Dr. John Davy in 1825 ; his
observations were confirmed by Prof. Weber in 1832 ; and in April, 1834, I
communicated to the Zoological Society the result of a series of examinations
of the hearts of the *Batrachia,* which proved that the whole order, including the
perennibranchiate species, had distinct auricles for the pulmonic and systemic
blood, since which time the tripartite structure of the heart has been universally assigned to the *Batrachia.*

The *third class*, or *Dicoilia*, includes those which have two cavities in the heart, or one ventricle and one auricle, and consists of the gill-fish. The sharks and rays were included by Hunter in this class, but the dicœlous or bipartite structure of their heart presented no obstacle to their junction with the *Amphibia* in the Linnæan arrangement.

Hunter's *fourth class*, or *Monocoilia*, characterized by a heart with but one cavity or ventricle, without an auricle, is restricted to insects of all kinds, i. e. to the articulate animals included by Hunter in his second class according to brains.

By Linnæus the character is applied to all invertebrate animals without exception. Hunter, with more truth, defines a *fifth class* of animals, by the name of *Acardia*, " whose stomach and heart are the same body, as in the blubber (*Medusa*) and polypus." But even with this improvement, the Cardiac arrangement of animals, as proposed by Hunter, is very incomplete. The whole division of the molluscous animals is left out of the system. This did not, however, arise from a want of the knowledge of the structure of the heart in those animals. Hunter well knew the complex condition of the circulating organ in the cuttle-fish, a condition which, had he rigorously carried out his scheme of classification according to hearts, would have indicated a class above the mammalia, and to which the name of *Heptacoilia* might have been applied, since there are three distinct ventricles, one systemic and two pulmonic, and four auricles or venous sinuses in this and other dibranchiate cephalopods. In the snail and other gastropods Hunter had recognised a structure of the heart as complex and perfect as in fish, but having a different relation, both as regards function and position, to the respiratory organ*. In still lower *Mollusca* Hunter had detected the existence of two distinct auricles, with one ventricle †; but his perception of the physiological relations of these different cavities prevented him from associating the mussel with the tortoise, on account of this tricœlous structure of the heart. We may thus perceive amidst the defects of this system of arrangement an evident advance towards a more natural distribution of animals, especially of the

---

* On the Blood, vol. iii. p. 174.   † Ibid., p. 175.

invertebrata, than that which was generally accepted at the period when Hunter wrote. We associate this progress with
Hunter's superior knowledge of the organization and œconomy
of animals as its just and natural cause, and we proceed to adduce additional evidences of Hunter's attempts to frame a natural arrangement of animals.

Perceiving that the modifications of the heart alone were inadequate to the formation of a natural and symmetrical classification of animals, he next tested the efficiency of characters
taken from conditions of the respiratory system, and proposed
the following scheme :

" The *first class* includes all those animals which have lungs
with cells through the whole, and a diaphragm.

" The *second class*, all those which have their lungs attached to the ribs, so as to confine them to their place.

" The *third class*, all those whose lungs come into the belly
and are loose.

" The *fourth class*, all those whose lungs are in their necks,
called gills.

" The *fifth class*, all those whose lungs are in their sides *."

In this scheme we have most exact and concise characters
of the four classes of vertebrate animals, as afforded by the
breathing organs ; and in this case Hunter was enabled by his
profound anatomical knowledge to rise far above Linnæus.

In the *Systema Naturæ*, the *Mammalia* and *Aves*, which
correspond with Hunter's first and second classes, according to
the organs of respiration, have both the same characters assigned to them, " pulmones respirantes reciproce," while the
Amphibia, to which Hunter's third class corresponds, are said
by Linnæus to have " pulmones spirantes arbitrarie."   Neither
Hunter nor Linnæus, however, arrived at the perception of that
condition of the respiratory organs which characterizes their
first four classes in common, viz. that the breathing organs communicate with the mouth ; nor am I aware that the Vertebrata,
have ever been distinguished in any system as *oral breathers*,
in contradistinction to the Mollusca, which may be termed
anal breathers, and to the Articulata, which respire by aper-

---

* Physiological Catalogue, Introduction to the Third Volume, p. v.

turcs or branchial organs arranged symmetrically *at the sides* of the body.

We have thus traced Hunter in his character as a systematic zoologist through a series of attempts at the arrangement of the animal kingdom, in which, like the indefatigable Adanson in a sister science, considering each organ by itself, he formed, by pursuing its various modifications, a series of groups characterized by that organ alone; and doing the same for another organ and another, thus constructed a collection of systems of arrangement, each artificial, because each was founded upon the variations of a single assumed organ.

It would, however, be doing injustice to Hunter to adduce the evidences of these attempts only. In that division of the animal kingdom where he had pushed his researches furthest, he aims to establish a more natural classification, by tracing the variations of all the important organs, and keeping in view the different value of each character; and thus he enunciates several general anatomical and physiological truths. The following are the characters which he assigns to the different classes of the animals now called Vertebrate.

" The properties of the *First Class,* which includes both sea and land animals, are

" *Heart,* made up of four cavities, essential.

" *Lungs,* divided into small cells, and confined to a proper cavity, the enlargement of which is the cause of respiration; essential. Respiration quick (and I believe this is the only class in which it is so); essential.

" *Give suck*; essential.

" *Parts of generation,* made up of testes and one penis in the male; the testes sometimes within and sometimes without the abdomen, but pass forwards. Clitoris, vagina, uterus or uteri, Fallopian tubes, and ovaria, in the female; all essential.

" *Kidneys,* high up in the abdomen; circumstantial.

" *Organ of hearing,* an external canal to the ear, membrana tympani concave externally *, a cochlea; circumstantial.

* This appears to have been written before Mr. Hunter had dissected the organ of hearing in the whale. See p. 381, and note ᵃ.

" The animals of this class are by much the most perfect,
whether sea or land. There is a gradation from the land
to the sea animals, viz. otter, seal, hippopotamus, whale.

" The *Second Class* is confined to the Birds entirely. I do
not know of any animal of this class but what has all the characteristics of the bird. They vary less in any of their parts
than the first class*.

" *Lungs,* attached to the ribs, that they may move with them;
lungs perforated; membranous bags in the abdomen
that receive air in respiration; something like a diaphragm.

" *Parts of generation,* ova crustaceous; one oviduct; one
penis, and that grooved; no bladder. Oviduct in the
female, and penis with the vasa deferentia in the male,
all open in the same cavity with the anus.

" *Liver,* divided into two lobes; cyst-hepatic ducts.

" *Organ of hearing,* little external passage to the ear; membrana tympani convex externally, but one bone (ossiculum auditûs); no cochlea.

" Feathers; wings; two legs; long neck; bill; membrana
nictitans; bursa Fabricii.

" There is none of this class that belong entirely to sea animals; but this class may be said to possess in some
measure three elements, viz. air, earth, and water; but
they *live* no more in the air than other animals, for it is
only for their progressive motion.

" In the *Third Class* we shall find some parts similar to the
second. The third class may be divided into two, for they are
not exactly alike, but one seems to partake of the second and
third; as it were, made up of both. The first division of the
third class, then, is the Lizard and Serpent kind. They have

" *Heart,* two auricles, one ventricle, two aortas which unite
in the abdomen.

" *Lungs,* loose bags, which lie in the thorax and abdomen,
only partially divided. No diaphragm.

---

* So also Cuvier: " De toutes les classes d'animaux, celle des oiseaux est la
mieux characterisée, celle dont les espèces se ressemblent le plus."—*Règne
Anim.,* i. p. 310.

" *Kidneys,* in the lower part of the abdomen. No bladder*.

" *Parts of generation,* two penises, grooved †, which are in the tail. Some oviparous, eggs without shells ; others viviparous, but not as the First Class.

" Some have legs, others none ; some a membrana tympani, which is convex outwardly, as the lizard ; others none, as the snake.

" The other part of this class, which may be termed the *Fourth,* or the Amphibious, are more closely allied to Fish than what the fish of the first class are ‡. These are the common amphibious animals, viz. frogs, turtles, efts, &c. This is also very similar to the two former, and is nearly, as it were, a mixture of both, yet the most essential parts belong, or are similar to the last.

" *Heart,* two auricles, as in the Third ; one ventricle, as in the Third ; aorta, as in the Third.

" *Lungs,* as in the Third.

" *Kidneys,* as in the Third.

" *Parts of generation,* one penis, as in the Second Class ; penis grooved, as in the Second and Third. Some oviparous, as the frog ; others viviparous, as the salamander.

" *Organ of hearing,* some have a membrana tympani, as the frog ; others none, as the tortoise §.

" The *Fourth* or *Fifth Class* (according as the two preceding are regarded as subdivisions of one class, or as two distinct classes) consists of Fishes, and is very distinct from the former so far as I know."

The manuscript from which the preceding remarkable passages are quoted, and which is printed entire in my Prefatory Observations to the Third Volume of the Physiological Catalogue, contains no characters of the Class of Fishes, nor any

* This character is not applicable to the lizards; but the crocodile agrees with the serpents in having no urinary bladder.

† The crocodile has but one.

‡ i. e. Those of the first class which are shaped like fish, and live in water, as the Cetacea.

§ The turtles and tortoises, or Chelonian reptiles, as they are now termed, have a closer affinity to the lizards than to the Batrachia, or frogs and salamanders.

relating to the Invertebrate Classes. It is in the definition of these latter classes, and in the determination of the wider divisions of the Invertebrata, which were equivalent to the entire vertebrate group, that Cuvier chiefly surpassed Hunter as a systematic zoologist. Yet, as I have before observed, Hunter rises above Linnæus even in this department: he had seized the great character of the molluscous sub-kingdom afforded by the nervous system, and had well defined some of the subordinate groups, more especially that which Lamarck afterwards termed *Tunicata*, and which Cuvier denominates " *Acéphales sans Coquilles*," but which Hunter, more correctly, termed " soft-shelled," having perceived the analogy of their external elastic tunic to shell; and having detected, with admirable skill, the relations subsisting between the Ascidiæ and Salpæ in different individuals dissected by him, of which dissections there remain not only the preparations, but several beautiful designs, with the original descriptions*

Of Hunter's appreciation of the progression of affinities we have an example in his sketch of the transition from the terrestrial to the aquatic Mammalia; and I do not doubt that ere long zoologists will uniformly agree in the propriety of passing from the hippopotamus and its pachydermatous congeners to the dugong and the true Cetacea, instead of interposing the Ruminantia between the Pachydermata and Cetacea, as in the Cuvierian system.

Of his mode of considering the affinities of two great and equal groups, Hunter has left the following specimen, which he quaintly designates " Of the similarity of the Fowl with the three-cavity-hearted gentry, called Amphibia:"

" The lungs of the fowl open into their air-cells or bags that are in the cavity of the belly. The lungs in the Amphibia are continued into the belly, are cellular at the upper part, but in most, as the snake, become smooth bags at the lower end, as it were, answering the same purpose as the abdominal bags in the fowl. The cells of the lung-part are large.

" No proper *Diaphragm* in either; but fowls have something similar to one †.

* See Plates 5, 6, and 7, vol. i. Physiological Catalogue.
† See p. 177.

" The *Gall* is green in both.

" The *Kidneys* are placed in what may be called the pelvis ; in both are conglomerated in a particular manner; have the ureter ramifying through their whole substance, and entering into the rectum. The urine is a chalky substance in many of both, and a kind of slime in others.

" The *Testes* are situated in the abdomen in the male of both.

" The *Vasa deferentia* enter the rectum in both.

" The *Penis* is grooved in both.

" Both *oviparous.*

" Structure of *Ear* similar in both.

" *Heart* very different."

These writings fully attest the enlarged views which Hunter entertained of comparative anatomy, and of its application not only to the establishment of sound theories of the functions and relative influences of the different organic systems in the animal body, but also of a natural distribution of different animals into classes arranged according to their affinities. It is in this respect that he has more especially surpassed those of his countrymen who have immediately succeeded him in the same field of inquiry, and whose labours in comparative anatomy have not been productive of adequate results, chiefly from being restricted to the narrower channel of their physiological application.

The museum of Hunter is the chief, but not the sole depository of the dissections by which he established the general principles to which we have alluded.

Hunter had passed his thirtieth year before he had collected a single preparation for himself. All that he had made before that time were added to his brother's collection, which is now the ornament of the University of Glasgow. In commencing his independent labours in anatomy, he conceived the idea of a collection, in which the illustrations of the human or anization should form a part only of a general display of all the types and modifications of animal structure, and practically he was the first who reduced the scattered facts of comparative anatomy to a connected system.

When Hunter had brought his museum to an approximate

degree of perfection*, he then set apart certain days, in which
he exhibited and explained to some chosen minds which could
respond to the conceptions of his own, his great scheme, embracing the demonstration of all the leading modifications of
every organ of the animal body, and of the different stages
which each organ undergoes in its development, to fulfil the
functions it is required to perform in the highest organisms.

Amongst the enlightened men who enjoyed the inestimable
advantage of listening to the explanations which the founder
of the collection gave of his own labours, and of their scope and
tendency, were Camper, Poli, Scarpa, and the now venerable
Blumenbach.

Camper, as a contemporary, and in some respects a rival
of Hunter, may have been less influenced in the general tenor
and success of his investigations in comparative anatomy, by
this circumstance, than the last named and younger naturalists
and physiologists.

We cannot but suppose that the spectacle of the organization of so many rare marine animals, beautifully displayed by so
consummate a practical anatomist as Hunter, must have had a
lasting influence on the mind of Poli; and it is not, perhaps,
assuming too much to trace to this source the taste for anatomy
and the stimulus to the indefatigable and minute dissections of
the Mediterranean mollusca, and the magnificent illustrations of
their organization, which have justly immortalized their author.

In contemplating the gradational and connected series of the
organs of animals, which Blumenbach must have witnessed for
the first time in the museum of Hunter, that learned and accomplished physiologist was doubtless led vividly to appreciate the cumulative force with which comparative anatomy
urges the onward progress of physiological science when all its
scattered facts are concentrated into one orderly system.   In
his subsequent publications of the first systematic treatise of
comparative anatomy the erudition of Blumenbach supplied
many of those links in the series of animal structures which
Hunter derived from Nature's original sources.

In estimating, therefore, the share which Hunter had in ad-

* In the year 1787. See Home's Lectures on Comparative Anatomy, vol. i.
p. 7. and vol. i. p. 107 of the present edition of Hunter's Works.

vancing comparative anatomy and physiology, his annual demonstrations of his collection to such individuals as we have
instanced must not be overlooked. We may admit that while
so vast a proportion of the stores of his experience lay buried
in unpublished manuscripts, his true station in the temple of
Science could hardly be discerned ; but, independently of these
manuscripts, we cannot hesitate in allowing that his published
works, full of profound and original views, combined with the
spectacle of his wonderful dissections, must have effected more
than had been done by any previous author towards raising the
science of comparative anatomy in the scale of human knowledge.

Now, however, we have to estimate the scientific character
of Hunter from more extended grounds.

Enjoying the same privilege of consulting his museum, which
the contemporaries of Hunter so highly esteemed, we also possess the advantage of studying it with the aid of those explanations of its scope and nature which its great founder had left
with a view to ulterior publication.

Thanks to the devotion of the last of Hunter's pupils to the
memory of his great master, the evidences of Hunter's discoveries and labours, as recorded in his collections, are in a better
state of preservation at this moment than they were nearly fifty
years ago, when they first fell to the care and charge of Mr.
Clift. And here I embrace with pleasure the opportunity of
expressing my grateful thanks to that gentleman for the kind
aid which I have on every needful occasion received from him
during the impression of the present work, and of recording
my deep sense of the advantages which I have derived from a
long intercourse with one whom I shall ever regard as the best
of friends and worthiest of men.

It is to the zeal and industry which induced Mr. Clift to
transcribe portions of the Hunterian manuscripts, at a period
when he little suspected their ultimate fate, that we owe our
additional knowledge of the philosophical views which Hunter
entertained of the application of anatomical facts, and of the
general principles which he had deduced from them. As such
of these extracts from the Hunterian Manuscripts as have been
quoted in the present work have already been printed in the

Catalogues of the Hunterian Collections published under the auspices of the Council of the Royal College of Surgeons, it is competent for any one to judge of the grounds on which I have endeavoured to show that Hunter, as a comparative anatomist, merits a higher and altogether different station in science than has been awarded to him by Cuvier.

Instead of viewing Hunter as one who had merely contributed a secondary proportion of detached facts to the general but unarranged stock of materials in comparative anatomy, it appears to me that he marks a new epoch in its history, and that the historian of the natural sciences has just and sufficient grounds for regarding Hunter as the first of the moderns who treated of the organs of the animal body under their most general relations, and who pointed out the anatomical conditions which were characteristic of great groups or classes of animals; as one, in short, throughout whose works we meet with general propositions in comparative anatomy, the like of which exist not in the writings of any of his contemporaries or predecessors, save in those of Aristotle.

RICHARD OWEN.

November 15th, 1837.

N.B. The Editor's Notes are distinguished from the Author's by being placed below the line, within brackets, and by having initial letters prefixed instead of the usual marks of reference.

A

TREATISE

ON THE

ANIMAL ŒCONOMY.

A DESCRIPTION OF THE SITUATION OF THE TESTIS IN THE FŒTUS, WITH ITS DESCENT INTO THE SCROTUM.

A DISCOVERY in any art not only enriches that with which it is immediately connected, but elucidates all those to which it has any relation. The knowledge of the construction of a human body is essential to medicine, therefore every improvement in anatomy must throw additional light on that branch of science. These improvements strike more forcibly if they are on subjects quite new or little understood; and this effect is well illustrated by the advantages which pathology has derived from the discovery of the lymphatics being the absorbent system; and likewise by that case of hernia, where the intestine lies in contact with the testicle; which has been perfectly explained by the discovery of the original seat of the testicle being in the abdomen.

Several years before Haller's Opuscula Pathologica were published, my brother informed me, that in examining the contents of the abdomen of a child, stillborn, about the seventh or eighth month, he found both the testicles lying in that cavity, and mentioned the observation with some degree of surprise. By this we are enabled to account for a circumstance that sometimes happens in the scrotal hernia, as depending on the discovery that the testis is formed in the abdomen, and which we could never explain to our satisfaction till the publication of the Opuscula, to which Dr. Hunter alludes, (Commentaries, page 72,) in the following words:

"In the latter end of the year 1755, when I first had the pleasure of reading Baron Haller's observations On the Hernia Congenita*, it struck my imagination[a] that the state of the testis in the fœtus, and its descent from the abdomen into the scrotum, would explain several things concerning ruptures and the hydrocele, particularly that observation which Mr. Sharp had communicated to me, viz. that in ruptures the intestine is sometimes in contact with the testis.   I communicated my ideas upon this subject to my brother, and desired that he would take every opportunity of learning exactly the state of the testis before and after birth, and the state of ruptures in children.   We were both convinced that the examination of those facts would answer our expectation, and both recollected having seen appearances in children that agreed with our supposition, but saw now that we had neglected making the proper use of them.

" In the course of the winter my brother had several opportunities of dissecting fœtuses of different ages, and of making some drawings of the parts; and all his observations agreed with the ideas I had formed of the nature of ruptures, and of the origin of the tunica vaginalis propria in the fœtus.   But till those observations were repeated to his satisfaction, and were sufficiently ascertained, he desired me not to mention the opinion in my lecture ; and therefore, when treating of the coats of the testis, and of the situation of the hernial sac, &c., I only put in this temporary caution, that I was then speaking of those things as they are commonly in adult bodies, and not as they are in the fœtus : and at last, when I was concluding my lectures for that season, in the end of April 1756, with a course of the chirurgical operations, I gave a very general account of my brother's observations, and showed both the drawing of fig. 2, which was then finished, and the subject from which it was made."

The following observations on this subject were taken from my notes,

* *Alberti Halleri Opuscul. Patholog.*, Lausan. 1755, 8vo, page 53, &c.

---

[a] [Although Haller was in doubt as to the exact period of the descent of the testis, and in error as to the cause of that phenomenon, yet he accurately describes, in the original paper here alluded to, the original relations of the gland to the peritoneum and abdominal viscera, and the formation of the tunica vaginalis, and thus applies the facts which he had discovered to the explanation of the disease he was considering. "Herniarum, ni fallor, congenitarum modus hinc elucescit, quo generantur.   Patulus est processus peritonæi sub renibus positus, qui expectat testem invitatque aperto ostio, atque eo deorsum ex solita lege pulso urgetur, inque scrotum una descendit.   Cum autem his in corporibus testes eodem cum intestinis sacco omnino contineantur, nihil est singularis sive inexpeetati, si ea in apertum saccum a levi vi depressa fuerint." (*Opusc. Patholog.*, p. 56.)   In this paper there are references to the older authors who had noticed the abdominal position of the testes in the fœtus.]

and published by Dr. Hunter in his Commentaries, to which I have added some practical remarks.

" Until the approach of birth, the testes of the fœtus are lodged within the cavity of the abdomen, and may therefore be reckoned among the abdominal viscera.   They are situated immediately below the kidneys, on the fore part of the psoæ muscles, and by the side of the rectum, where this intestine is passing down into the cavity of the pelvis; for in the fœtus, the rectum, which is much larger in proportion to the capacity of the pelvis than in the full-grown subject, lies before the vertebræ lumborum as well as before the os sacrum.   Indeed the case is pretty much the same with regard to all the contents of the pelvis; that is, their situation is much higher in the fœtus than in the adult.   The sigmoid flexure of the colon, part of the rectum, the greatest part of the bladder, the fundus uteri, the Fallopian tubes, &c. being placed in the fœtus above the hollow of the pelvis in the common or great abdominal cavity.

" While the testis remains in the abdomen its shape or figure is much the same as in the adult, and its position or attitude the same as when it is in the scrotum; that is, one end is placed upwards, the other downwards; one flat side is to the right, the other to the left; and one edge is turned backwards, the other forwards; and the vessels enter the posterior edge alike in both the fœtus and adult.   As the testis is not so immediately inclosed in the surrounding parts while it is in the loins, its position may be a little variable, and the most natural seems to be when the anterior edge is turned directly forwards; but as the least touch of anything will throw that edge either to the right side or to the left, then the flat side of the testis will be turned forwards.   It is attached to the psoas muscle all along its posterior edge, except just at its upper extremity; and this attachment is formed by the peritoneum, which covers the testis and gives it a smooth surface, in the same manner as it envelopes the other loose abdominal viscera.

" The epididymis lies along the outside of the posterior edge of the testis, as when in the scrotum, but is larger in proportion, and adheres backwards to the psoas.   When the fœtus is very young, the adhesion of the testis and epididymis to the psoas is very narrow, and then the testis is more loose, and more projecting; but as the fœtus advances in months, the adhesion of the testis to the psoas becomes broader and tighter.

" The vessels of the testis, like those of most parts of the body, commonly rise from the nearest larger trunks, viz. from the aorta and cava, or from the emulgents.

" The artery generally rises from the fore part of the aorta, a little

below the emulgent artery, and often from the emulgent itself, especially in the right side of the body, which may happen the rather, because the trunk of the aorta is more distant from the right testis than
from the left.   Sometimes, but much more rarely, the spermatic artery
springs from the phrenic, or from that of the capsula renalis.   Besides
the artery which rises from the aorta, or emulgent, &c., the testis receives one from the hypogastric artery, which is sometimes as large as
the other.   It runs upwards from its origin, passing close to the vas
deferens in its way to the testis.   The superior spermatic artery sometimes passes before the lower end of the kidney ; and both these arteries
run in a serpentine direction, making pretty large but gentle turnings.
They are situated behind the peritoneum, and both run into the posterior edge of the testis, between the two reflected laminæ of that membrane, much in the same manner as the vessels pass to the intestines
between the two reflected laminæ of the mesocolon or mesentery.

" The veins of the testis are analogous to its arteries, but commonly
change sides with the arteries respecting their origins from the emulgents.   The superior spermatic vein, to begin with its trunk, rises
commonly in the following manner: on the right side, from the trunk
of the vena cava, a little below the emulgent; and on the left side, from
the left emulgent vein.   The reason of this difference between the right
and left spermatic vein, no doubt, is because the cava is not placed in
the middle of the body; so that by the rule of ramification which is
observed in most parts of the body, the cava is the nearest large vein of
the right side, and the emulgent is the nearest large vein of the left
side.   But the difference is inconsiderable; and accordingly we sometimes find the right spermatic vein coming from the right emulgent
vein; and several other varieties are produced, which, so far as I can
observe, follow no precise rule.   There is likewise a spermatic vein,
which rises from the internal iliac, and runs up to the testis with the
inferior spermatic artery.   Both the spermatic veins run behind the
peritoneum with their corresponding arteries, and go into the posterior
edge of the testis, where they are lost in small branches.

" The nerves of the testis, like its blood-vessels, come from the nearest
source ; that is, from the abdominal plexuses of the intercostal, especially
the inferior mesenteric plexus.   They run to the testis, accompanying
its blood-vessels, and are dispersed with them through its substance.
The testis, therefore, with respect to its nerves, may be reckoned an
abdominal viscus ; and this observation will hold good when applied to
the full-grown subject, as well as to the fœtus ; for those branches of
the lumbar nerves which are commonly said to be sent to the testis,
passing through the tendon of the external oblique muscle, in reality

go not to the testis itself, but to its exterior coverings, and to the scrotum."—p. 75.

The testicle receiving its nerves from the plexuses of the intercostal, accounts for the stomach and intestines sympathizing so readily with it and its particular sensation, and for the effects arising in the constitution upon its being injured.

" The epididymis begins at the outer and posterior part of the upper end of the testis, immediately above the entrance of the blood-vessels, where it is thick, round, and united to the testis. As it passes down it becomes a little smaller and more flat, and is only attached backwards to the testis, or rather indeed to its vessels ; for its anterior edge lies loose against the side of the testis forwards; and at its lower end it is again more firmly attached to the body of the testis, so that in the fœtus there is a cavity or pouch formed between the middle part of the testis and the middle part ot the epididymis, more considerable than is commonly observed in full-grown subjects. As the body grows, the epididymis adheres more closely to the side of the testis ; and its greatest part is made up of one convoluted canal, which becomes larger in size and less convoluted towards the lower end, and at last is manifestly a single tube running a little serpentine. That change happens at the lower end of the testis, and there the canal takes the name of vas deferens.

" The vas deferens is a little convoluted or serpentine in its whole course, but is less so as it comes nearer to the bladder ; instead of running upwards from the lower end of the testis, as it does when the testicle is in the scrotum, while that remains in the abdomen, it runs downwards and inwards in its whole course, so that it goes on almost in the direction of the epididymis, of which it is a continuation. It turns inwards from the lower end of the epididymis, under the lower end of the testis, and behind the upper end of a ligament or gubernaculum testis (which I shall presently describe) ; then it passes over the iliac vessels, and over the inside of the psoas muscle, somewhat higher than in adult bodies, and at last goes between the ureter and bladder towards the basis of the prostate gland."—p. 77.

In those animals where the testicles change their situation the cremaster muscle, which should be named *musculus testis*, has two very different positions in the fœtus and in the adult, the first being the same as in those animals whose testicles remain through life in the cavity of the abdomen ; we must therefore conclude that the same purposes are answered by this muscle in the fœtus as in those animals.

The use of this muscle, when the testicle is in the scrotum, appears to be evidently that of a suspensory ; for I find this muscle is strong in proportion to the size of the testicle and pendulous situation in other animals. But what purpose it answers in the fœtus, or in animals whose testicles remain in the abdomen, is not easily imagined, there being no apparent reason why such a muscle should exist[a].

The cremaster, or musculus testis, appears to be composed of the lower fibres of the obliquus internus and transversalis muscles in the fœtus, turning upwards, and spreading upon the anterior surface of the gubernaculum, immediately under the peritoneum ; it appears to be lost on the peritoneum, a little way from the testicle. This, although now inverted, is more evidently seen in adult subjects who have had a hydrocele or rupture ; in such cases the muscle becomes stronger than usual, and its fibres can be traced spreading on the tunica vaginalis, and seem at last to be lost upon it, near to the lower end of the body of the testicle.

The nerves which supply this muscle are probably branches from the nerves of the obliquus internus and transversalis muscles[b] ; for the same cause which throws the abdominal muscles into action produces a similar effect on the musculus testis ; which circumstance appears to be most remarkable in the young subject. When we cough or act with the abdominal muscles, we find the testicles to be drawn up ; the musculus testis and abdominal muscles taking on the same action from the same cause[c].

" At this time of life the testis is connected in a very particular manner with the parietes of the abdomen, at that place where in adult bodies the spermatic vessels pass out, and likewise with the scrotum. This connexion is by means of a substance which runs down from the lower

[a] [The cremaster does not in fact exist in the true *testiconda*, as the elephant, hyrax, seal, walrus, the Cetaceous and Monotrematous Mammalia; in these the testes are merely supported by their vessels and a fold of peritoneum analogous to the broad ligaments of the uterus and ovaries; but when the cremaster is met with in apparent *testicauda* it is always in relation to a partial or temporary escape of the testis from the abdomen, as in bats and most insectivorous Feræ, and in many of the Glires, as the rats, squirrels, beaver, porcupine, &c.]

[b] [The first lumbar nerve, which gives many small branches to the transversalis abdominis, sends off a branch which, in conjunction with smaller branches from the second lumbar nerve, forms the 'external spermatic nerve' from which the cremaster is supplied.]

[c] [As the cremaster is supplied from common or spinal nerves, it is not surprising that it should in some cases, like the occipito-frontalis muscle, be under the control of the will. Mr. Marshall observes, in his work On Recruits, " Some individuals have the voluntary power of contracting and relaxing the cremaster muscle ; others can elevate the testicle on one side but not on the other; and I have seen a few persons who could voluntarily raise a testicle, but had not the power of letting it return into the scrotum."]

end of the testis to the scrotum, and which at present I shall call the ligament, or gubernaculum testis, because it connects the testis with the scrotum, and seems to direct its course through the rings of the abdominal muscles.   It is of a pyramidal form; its large bulbous head is upwards, and fixed to the lower end of the testis and epididymis, and its lower and slender extremity is lost in the cellular membrane of the scrotum.   The upper part of this ligament is within the abdomen, before the psoas, reaching from the testis to the groin, or to where the testicle is to pass out of the abdomen; whence the ligament runs down into the scrotum, precisely in the same manner as the spermatic vessels pass down in adult bodies, and is there lost.   The lower part of the round ligament of the uterus in a fœtus very much resembles this ligament of the testis, and may be plainly traced down into the labium, where it is imperceptibly lost.   That part of the ligamentum testis which is within the abdomen is covered by the peritoneum all round except at its posterior part, which is contiguous to the psoas, and connected with it by the reflected peritoneum and by the cellular membrane.   It is hard to say what is the structure or composition of this ligament; it is certainly vascular and fibrous, and the fibres run in the direction of the ligament itself, which is covered by the fibres of the cremaster or musculus testis, placed immediately behind the peritoneum.   This circumstance is not easily ascertained in the human subject; but is very evident in other animals, more especially in those whose testicles remain in the cavity of the abdomen after the animal is full grown.

  " In the hedgehog the testes continue through life to be lodged within the abdomen, in the same situation as in the human fœtus; and they are fastened by the same kind of ligament to the inside of the parietes of the abdomen at the groin.   Now in that animal I find that the lowermost fibres of the internal oblique muscle, which constitute the cremaster, are turned inwards at the place where the spermatic vessels come out in other animals, making a smooth edge or lip by their inversion, and that then they mount up on the ligament to the lower end of the testis[a].   Sometimes in the human body, and in many other animals, and very often in sheep, the testes do not descend from the cavity of

---

  [a] [The apparent anomaly of this, as of almost every other natural structure, disappears when we attain the requisite amount of knowledge respecting the conditions under which it exists.   The testes of the hedgehog, like those of the mole, (see p. 29,) are subject to remarkable periodical enlargement at the season of copulation, when they are drawn down by the cremaster to the external ring.   In this situation they are favourably placed to be affected by the expulsive actions of the diaphragm and abdominal muscles, by which they are eventually protruded and the cremasteric pouch is inverted. As the testes diminish in size their muscular covering contracts upon them and returns them into the abdomen.]

the abdomen till late in life, or never at all. In the ram, when the testis is come down into the scrotum, the cremaster is a very strong muscle; and, though it be placed more inwards at its beginning, it passes down pretty much as it does in the human body, and is lost on the outside of the tunica vaginalis; but in the ram, whose testis still remains suspended in the abdominal cavity, I find that the cremaster still exists, though it is a weaker muscle; and instead of passing downwards, as in the former case, it turns inwards and upwards, and is lost in the peritoneum that covers the ligament which attaches the testis to the parietes of the abdomen, which in this state of the animal is about an inch and a half in length. In the human fœtus, while the testis is retained in the cavity of the abdomen, the cremaster is so slender that I cannot trace it to my own satisfaction, either turning up towards the testis or turning down towards the scrotum. Yet, from analogy, we may conclude that it passes up to the testicle; since in the adult we find it inserted or lost on the lower part of the tunica vaginalis, in the same manner as in the adult quadruped[a].

" The peritoneum, which covers the testis and its ligament or gubernaculum, is firmly united to the surfaces of these two bodies; but all around, to wit on the kidney, the psoas, the iliacus internus, and the lower part of the abdominal muscles, that membrane adheres very loosely to all the surfaces which it covers. Where the peritoneum is continued or reflected from the abdominal muscles to the ligament of the testis it passes first downwards a little way, as if going out of the abdomen, and then upwards, so as to cover more of the ligament than is within the cavity of the abdomen. At this place the peritoneum is very loose, thin in its substance, and of a tender gelatinous texture; but all around the passage of that ligament the peritoneum is considerably tighter, thicker, and of a more firm texture. When the abdominal muscles are pulled up so as to tighten and stretch the peritoneum this membrane remains loose at the passage of the ligament while it is braced or tight all around; and in that case the tight part forms a kind of border or edge around

---

[a] [By such a pre-arrangement of the relations of the cremaster to the testis the necessity for the latter to overcome in its passage outwards the resistance of the inferior fibres of the transversalis abdominis and obliquus internus is obviated. It cannot reasonably be doubted that the cremaster exists, as such, in the human fœtus prior to the descent of the testis, since it is indubitably present and attached to an abdominal testis in animals where no mechanical cause could have operated to produce this disposition of the muscular fibres. Besides, the use of the cremaster as a supporter and compressor of the testis is obviously too important for such a connexion to have been allowed to result from the gland accidentally, as it were, pushing before it some opposing fibres of the abdominal muscles in its progress outwards, as Carus imagines. See his Comparative Anatomy, by Gore, vol. ii. p. 347.]

the loose double part of the peritoneum, where the testis is afterwards to pass. This loose part of the peritoneum, like the intro-suscepted gut, may, by drawing the testis upwards, be pulled up into the abdomen, and made tight, and then there is no appearance of an aperture or passage down towards the scrotum; but when the scrotum and ligament are drawn downwards, the loose doubled part of the peritoneum descends with the ligament, and then there is an aperture from the cavity of the abdomen all around the fore part of the ligament, which seems ready to receive the testis. This aperture becomes larger when the testis descends lower, as if the pyramidal or wedge-like ligament was first drawn down in order not only to direct but to make room for the testis which must follow it. In some fœtuses I have found the aperture so large that I could push the testis into it as far as the tendon of the external oblique muscle.

" From this original situation within the abdomen the testis afterwards descends to its destined station in the scrotum; but it becomes difficult to ascertain the precise time of this descent, as we hardly ever know the exact age of our subject. According to the observations which I have made, it seems to happen sooner in some instances than in others; but generally about the eighth month. In the seventh month I have commonly found the testis in the abdomen; and in the ninth I have as commonly found it in the upper part of the scrotum. The descent being thus early, and the passage being almost immediately closed, are the principal means of preventing the hernia congenita.

" At the before-mentioned period the testis moves downwards till its lower extremity comes into contact with the lower part of the abdominal parietes: when the upper part of the ligament, which hitherto was within the abdomen, has sunk downwards, it lies in the passage from the abdomen to the scrotum, and in that which is afterwards to receive the testis. As the testicle passes out it in some degree inverts the situation of the ligament passing down beyond it; what was the anterior surface of the ligament while in the abdomen, now becoming posterior and composing the lower and anterior part of the tunica vaginalis, on which the musculus testis is lost. This is more evident in those animals whose testicles can readily be made to pass up from the scrotum to the abdomen. The place where the ligament is most confined, and where the testis meets with most obstruction in its descent, is the ring in the tendon of the external oblique muscle; and accordingly I think we see more men with one testis or both lodged immediately within the tendon of that muscle than who have one or both still included in the cavity of the abdomen, which I shall take notice of hereafter.

" After the testis has got quite through the tendon of the external

oblique muscle it may be considered as now in a way easily to acquire
its determined station, though it commonly remains for some time by
the side of the penis*, and only by degrees descends to the bottom of
the scrotum; and when the testis has descended entirely into the scrotum its ligament is still connected with it, and lies immediately under
it, but is shortened and compressed.

" Having now given an account of the original situation of the testes,
of the time of their descent from the abdomen, and of the route'which
they take in their passage to the scrotum, I shall in the next place describe the manner in which they carry down the peritoneum with them,
and then explain how that membrane forms the tunica vaginalis propria
in common, and the sac of the hernia congenita in some bodies.

" While the testis is descending, and even when it has passed into
the scrotum, it is still covered by the peritoneum, exactly in the same
manner as when within the abdomen, the spermatic vessels running
down behind the peritoneum there as they did when the testis lay before the psoas muscle : that lamella of the peritoneum is united behind
with the testis, the epididymis, and the spermatic vessels, as it was in
the loins, and likewise with the vas deferens; but the testis is fixed posteriorly to the parts against which it rests, being unconnected and loose
forwards, as while it remained in the abdomen. In coming down, the
testis brings the peritoneum with it; and the elongation of that membrane, though in some circumstances it be like a common hernial sac,
yet in others is very different. If we can imagine a common hernial
sac reaching to the bottom of the scrotum, covered by the cremaster
muscle; and that the posterior half of the sac covers and is united with
the testis, epididymis, spermatic vessels, and vas deferens; and that the
anterior half of the sac lies loose before all those parts, it will give a
perfect idea of the state of the peritoneum, and of the testis when it
comes first down into the scrotum. The testis therefore, in its descent,
does not fall loose, like the intestine or epiploon, into the elongation of
the peritoneum, but slides down from the loins, carrying the peritoneum
with it; and both that and the peritoneum continue to adhere, by the
cellular membrane, to the parts behind them, as they did when in the
loins. This is a circumstance which I think may be easily understood,
and yet that does not appear to be the case; for I find students very
generally puzzled with it, imagining that when the testis comes first
down it should be loose all round, like a piece of the gut or epiploon in

---

* [This is the permanent situation of the testis in the Quadrumana, in which also, as
in the human fœtus at the period above mentioned, the tunica vaginalis communicates
with the abdominal cavity.]

a common hernia.   The ductility of the peritoneum, and its very loose
connexion by a slight cellular membrane to the psoas muscle, and all
the other parts around the testis, are circumstances which favour its
elongation and descent into the scrotum with the testis."

" This peculiarity of descent often takes place in some of the intestines ; but can only happen in those which have adhesions to the loins.
This I suspect is only to be met with in old ruptures, never happening
at the first formation of the hernial sac, in which the intestine lies ; and,
I should suppose, could only form very gradually.   The cæcum has
sometimes been found to have descended into the scrotum, and to have
brought along with it the adhesions through its whole course.   The
same thing has happened to the sigmoid flexure of the colon ; and I
have found the whole of it in the left side of the scrotum, with its adhesions brought down from the loins.   Such herniæ cannot be reduced ;
and in case of strangulation, which may be brought on by a fresh portion of intestine coming down, are not to be treated in the common way :
the sac should not be opened, but the stricture divided, and the newly
protruded part reduced.

" It is plain, from this description, that the cavity of the bag, or of
the elongation of the peritoneum, which contains the testis in the scrotum, must at first communicate with the general cavity of the abdomen
by an aperture at the inside of the groin.   That aperture has exactly
the appearance of a common hernial sac ; the spermatic vessels and vas
deferens lie immediately behind it, and a probe passes readily through
it from the general cavity of the abdomen down to the bottom of the
scrotum.   And if this process of the peritoneum be laid open through
its whole length on the fore part, it will be plainly seen to be a continuation of the peritoneum : the testis and epididymis will appear at the
lower part of it, and the spermatic vessels and the vas deferens will be
found covered by the posterior part of the bag in their whole course
from the groin to the testis.

" Thus it is in the human body when the testis is recently come down ;
and thus it is, and continues to be through life, in every quadruped which
I have examined where the testis is in the scrotum ; but in the human
body the communication between the sac and the cavity of the abdomen
is soon cut off.   Indeed I believe that the upper part of the sac naturally begins to contract as soon as the testis has passed through the
muscles ; which opinion is grounded on the following observation.   In
an instance where, from the age of the fœtus and from every other mark,
it was probable that the testis was very recently come down, and yet
the upper part of the sac was very narrow, I pushed the testis upwards,
in order to see if it could be returned.   The attachments of the testis

easily admitted of its ascent, and so did the aperture in the tendon of the external oblique muscle; but the orifice and upper end of the sac would not by any means admit of the testis being passed quite up into the abdomen. However this may be, the upper end of the sac certainly contracts and unites first, and is quite closed in a very short space of time, for it is seldom that any aperture remains in a child born at its full time; and this contraction and union is continued downwards till it comes near the testicle, where this disposition does not exist, leaving the lower part of the sac open or loose through life even in the human subject, and forming the tunica testis vaginalis propria, the common seat of a hydrocele. Many cases of hydrocele in children seem to prove that the progress of this contraction and union is downwards; for in them the water commonly extends higher up the chord than in the adult, except in those of a considerable size; yet in some children this union seems not to take place regularly, being interrupted in the middle, and producing a hydrocele of the chord which neither communicates with the abdomen nor tunica vaginalis testis. The contraction and obliteration of the passage appears to be a peculiar operation of Nature, depending upon steady and uniform principles, and not the consequence of inflammation nor of anything that is accidental; and therefore, if it is not accomplished at the proper time, the difficulty of bringing about a union of the parts is much greater, as is seen in children who have had the sac kept open by a turn of the intestine falling down into the scrotum immediately after the testis. This looks as if Nature, from being balked when she was in the humour to do her work, would not or could not so easily do it afterwards. I shall readily grant that what has been advanced here as a proof of the doctrine may be explained upon other principles; but this at least is certain, that the closing of the mouth and of the neck of the sac is peculiar to the human species[a]; and we must suppose the final intention to be the prevention of ruptures, to which men are so much more liable than beasts from their erect state of body."

---

[a] [The chimpanzee, or African orang-utan (*Simia Troglodytes*, Blum.), which of all mammalia approximates most closely to the human structure, resembles man in the early obliteration of the canal which leads from the peritoneal cavity to the tunica vaginalis. In the Indian orang (*Simia Satyrus*, Linn.), on the contrary, the canal of communication is free. This difference of structure relates doubtless to the different conditions of the lower extremities in these otherwise closely allied quadrumana: in the chimpanzee they are proportionally larger and stronger, the leg can be more extended on the thigh, and the hip-joint is strengthened by a ligamentum teres; in the orang, on the contrary, the lower limbs are feebly developed as organs of support, but have great extent of motion, the hip-joint being, like the shoulder-joint, without a round ligament.]

In some cases the aperture of the sac is not entirely closed, allowing a fluid to pass down and form a hydrocele; which fluid, upon pressure, can be squeezed back into the belly; and instances of this kind sometimes giving the idea of a gut being protruded, make it difficult to determine the exact nature of the case.

" What is the immediate cause of the descent of the testis from the loins to the scrotum? It is evident that it cannot be the compressive force of respiration; because the testis is commonly in the scrotum before the child has breathed, that is, the effect has been produced before the supposed cause has existed. Is the testis pulled down by the cremaster muscle? I can hardly suppose that it is; because, if that was the case, I see no reason why it should not take place in the hedgehog, as well as in other quadrupeds; and if the musculus testis had this power it could not bring it lower than the ring of the muscle.

" Why do the testes take their blood-vessels from such distant trunks? Those physiologists who have puzzled themselves about the solution of this question have not considered that in the first formation of the body the testes are situated not in the scrotum but immediately below the kidneys; and that therefore it was very natural that their blood-vessels should rise nearly in the same manner as those of the kidneys, but a little lower[a]. The great length of the spermatic vessels in the adult body will no doubt occasion a more languid circulation, which we may suppose was the intention of nature.

" The situation of the testis in the fœtus may likewise account for the contrary directions of the epididymis and of the vas deferens in adult bodies, though these two in reality make only one excretory canal. In

---

[a] [The singular course of the recurrent nerves results from a similar mechanical cause. At the period when the rudimentary larynx first derives its nerves from the par vagum, the head and trunk are not separated by a neck, the trachea is not formed, the heart is situated near the base of the cranium, and the branchial arteries given off from the bulb of the then single artery pass above the nerves in question. As the anterior extremities bud forth, the brachial plexuses are developed and the neck begins to elongate; then the rings of the trachea are successively added, and the larynx which before was close to the heart, is carried upward, and the recurrent nerves, restrained by their relations to the arteries, which are now converted into the subclavian on the right side and aortic arch on the left, become proportionately elongated. The recurrent course of the branch of the dental nerve which supplies the pulp of the incisor in the porcupine and other Rodentia is explicable on a similar principle, the relative position of the pulp to the origin of its nerve being gradually changed by the growth of the jaw and extension of the tooth. See the preparation illustrating this fact in the Gallery of the Hunterian Museum, No. 357 B.

It is scarcely necessary to observe that the above mechanical explanation of the course of the recurrent nerves leaves the question of the final cause as open as before. Mr. Hunter, after giving the physical cause of the course of the spermatic artery, next proceeds to inquire into the intention of Nature with reference to that peculiarity.]

the fœtus the epididymis begins at the upper end of the testis; and it is natural, considering it is an excretory tube, that it should run downwards. And it is as natural that the rest of the tube, which is called vas deferens, should turn inwards at the lower end of the testis, because that is its most direct course to the neck of the bladder. Thus we see that in the fœtus the excretory duct is always passing downwards. But the testis is directed in its descent by the gubernaculum, which is firmly fixed to the lower parts of the testis and epididymis, and to the beginning of the vas deferens, and thence must keep those parts invariably in their situation with respect to one another: and therefore in proportion as the testis descends the vas deferens must ascend from the lower end of the testis; and it must, from the passage through the abdominal muscles down to the testis, run parallel with the spermatic vessels.

" The testis, its coats, and the spermatic chord are so often concerned in some of the most important diseases and operations of surgery, particularly in the bubonocele and hydrocele, that their structure has been examined and described by the surgeons, as well as by the anatomists, of every age. Yet the descriptions of the clearest and best writers upon the subject differ so much from one another, and many of them differ so much from what is obvious and demonstrable by dissection, as to render it difficult to account for such a variety of opinions. The very different state of the parts in the quadruped and in the human body, no doubt, must have occasioned error and confusion among the writers of more ancient times, when the parts of the human body were described from dissections and observations made principally upon brutes: and the structure of parts, which are peculiar to the fœtus, having been imperfectly understood, we may suppose, has likewise contributed to cause perplexity and contradiction among authors.

" Baron Haller, in his Opuscula Pathologica, has observed that in infants the intestine sometimes falls down into the scrotum after the testis, or along with it, and occasions what he calls the hernia congenita. In such a case the hernial sac is formed before the intestine falls down, as that ingenious anatomist has observed. There are, besides, two circumstances peculiar to a rupture of this kind, the intestine being always in immediate contact with the testis, and there being no tunica vaginalis propria testis. The structure of the parts in a fœtus explains in the most satisfactory manner both these circumstances, however extraordinary they must appear to a man who has only been accustomed to view the parts in subjects of a more advanced age; and indeed it is so clear that it needs no illustration. It should be observed, however, that the hernia congenita may happen not only by the intestine falling down to the testis before the aperture of the sac be shut up, but perhaps afterwards; for when the sac has been but recently closed it seems possible enough that violence may open it again.

" It must likewise be obvious to every anatomist, who examines the state of the testis in children of different ages, that the mouth and neck only of the sac close up, and that the lower part of the sac remains loose around the testis, and makes the tunica vaginalis propria. Whence it is plain that this tunic was originally a part of the elongated peritoneum; and, as it is undoubtedly the seat of the true hydrocele, it is also plain that the hernia congenita and the true hydrocele cannot exist together in the same side of the scrotum. For when there is a hernia congenita there is no other cavity than that of the hernial sac; and that cavity communicates with the general cavity of the abdomen.

" The observations contained in the two last paragraphs occurred to my brother upon reading Baron Haller's Opuscula Pathologica, and gave rise to my inquiries upon this subject."—*Medical Commentaries,* part i. p. 83.

Having explained the situation of the testicles in the fœtus, and their descent, with the circumstances attending it, I shall next consider the cases in which the change takes place, in one or both testicles, later than the usual or natural time. And having remarked the consequences of this descent at so late a period, I shall take notice of those instances in which the testicles never pass out of the abdomen.

I have said that the early descent of the testicles, and closing of the mouth of the sac, by usually happening before birth, prevent likewise the descent of any part of the abdominal viscera; but when the testicles remain in their first situation beyond this period these advantages are lost; a part of the intestines or epiploon being, under these circumstances, liable to descend along with them.

The first or natural process, in some instances, not having been begun, or having been interrupted before birth, it becomes afterwards very uncertain when the descent will be completed; yet I think the completion most frequently happens between the years of two and ten, while the person is young and growing, being seldom delayed beyond the age of puberty.

It is not easy to ascertain the cause of this failure in the descent of the testicle; but I am inclined to suspect that the fault originates in the testicles themselves. This however is certain, that the testicle which has completed its descent is the largest, which is more evident in the quadruped than in the human subject; as in these we can have an optunity of examining the parts when we please, and can determine how small in comparison with the other that testicle is which has exceeded the usual time of coming down : it never descends so low as the other.

The descent of that testicle is very slow which is not completed before birth, often requiring years for that purpose; and it sometimes never reaches the scrotum, especially the lower part of it. There is oftener I believe an inequality in the situation of the two testicles than is commonly imagined, being seldom equally low in the scrotum; and I am of opinion that the lowest is the most vigorous, having taken the lead readily, and come to its place at once. The part where it meets with the greatest difficulty in its descent is in the division of the tendon of the external oblique muscle called the ring.

How far an erect position of body, the action of the abdominal muscles, and the effect produced upon the contents of the abdomen in breathing may contribute mechanically to the descent of the testicles when the natural operations of the animal economy have failed, I will not pretend to decide; but when we see these combined actions producing an unnatural descent of a portion of intestine, we may conceive that they are likewise capable of contributing to the descent of the testicle.

When the testicle has remained in the cavity of the abdomen beyond the usual time, it is impossible to say whether the disposition for closing up the passage, after it has passed out, is in any degree lost or not; but when it comes down after birth, we can easily suppose a portion of intestine or epiploon is more likely to descend and prevent the closing of the mouth of the sac, than before the child was born, when certain actions had not taken place. We should therefore watch this descent of the testicle, and endeavour, by art, to procure that union which the natural powers are either not disposed to perform, or are prevented from completing by the descent of other parts: but art should not be used too soon, nor till the testicle has got a little way below the ring. As this progress is very slow, especially when the testicle is creeping through the ring, a doubt often arises whether it is better entirely to prevent its passage, or to assist it by exercise or other means; and it would certainly be the best practice to assist it, if that could be done effectually and safely. When it has got upon the outside of the tendon it can in general be easily pushed up again into the abdomen; and in these two situations it will sometimes play backwards and forwards for several years, without ever coming low enough to allow of the use of artificial means to hinder its descent, or to prevent a rupture. In this case it becomes difficult to determine what should be done; but, from what I have seen, I should be inclined to wait the descent, giving it every assistance in my power. Indeed, in all cases I would advise waiting with patience, for in most of those which I have seen, years have elapsed from the first appearance of the testicle under the ring of the abdominal muscle before it has reached that situation in which we may safely apply a truss. I never have perceived that any inconvenience has arisen from waiting, and the danger, if there is any, may be in some degree avoided. I have always recommended moderate, not violent exercise.

When the testicle has got some way below the ring, then the case is to be treated as an inguinal hernia, and a truss applied upon the ring; taking care that the testicle is not injured by it: but as this generally happens at too early a period for the patients themselves to be capable of attending to it, the surgeon who is employed should be very attentive, and those in whose immediate care they are, particularly watchful, that no inconvenience is produced by the truss. I have, however, known a rupture happen in a man thirty years old, where the testicle had not even got into the ring. In such a case I think a truss should be immediately applied; for if it is thought advisable to prevent the testicle from coming down, a truss is equally adapted for that purpose, as for hindering the descent of an intestine where there is an hernial sac.

It sometimes happens that one of the testicles remains in the cavity of the abdomen through life, never acquiring the disposition to change its situation; therefore the person naturally concludes that he has only one testicle; and it can only be known that he had two by an examination of these parts after death; it is, however, possible that in some instances one may be wanting; but, if we are to reason from analogy, we must suppose this to be a very rare case; for it is a very common circumstance, that many quadrupeds have only one testicle in the scrotum; and in such as are killed for food, and from that circumstance come more particularly under observation, if this peculiarity has been noticed, we in general find the other testicle in the cavity of the abdomen; though in some instances they are both found lying in that cavity.

When one or both testicles remain through life in the belly, I believe that they are exceedingly imperfect, and probably incapable of performing their natural functions, and that this imperfection prevents the disposition for descent from taking place. That they are more defective than even those which are late in passing to the scrotum, is to be inferred from what is very evident in quadrupeds, the testicle that has reached the scrotum being in them considerably larger than the one which remains in the abdomen. It is probable that this peculiarity is a step towards the hermaphrodite, the testicle being seldom well formed. I have only seen one case in the human subject where both testicles continued in the abdomen; this proved an exception to the above observation, since we are led to conclude that they were perfectly formed, as the person had all the powers and passions of a man[a]. In such cases nothing is to be done by art, as it is not possible to give the testicles the stimulus of perfection, which I believe is necessary to make them assume the disposition requisite for their descent[b]; and the ring of the external oblique muscle is perhaps less liable, in such instances, to allow a portion of intestine to push down, than where the testicles have passed through it; and such persons may probably be more secure from accidents of this kind than if they had been more perfectly formed.

The testicle, in changing its situation, does not always preserve a proper course towards the scrotum, there being instances of its taking another direction, and descending into the perinæum. How this is brought about is difficult to say; it may possibly be occasioned by something unusual in the construction of the scrotum; or, more probably, by a peculiarity in that of the perinæum itself; for it is not easy to imagine how the testicle could make its way to the parts about the perinæum if these were in a perfectly natural state.

The first instance of this kind that occurred to me was the child of a shopkeeper in Oxford-street, which I visited, in company with Dr. Garthshore, about the year 1775; but what became of the patient afterwards I do not know. I have lately been consulted, in a similar case, by Mr. Hunt, a surgeon, at Burford in Oxfordshire, whose apprehensions of what may be the consequences of a testicle remaining in the perinæum appear to be well founded. The most effectual method of obviating these will probably be to support the testicle in a situation near the groin, by the application of a bandage that may hinder its descent into the perinæum, by which the parts may be in time so consolidated as to retain it by the side of the scrotum.

" DEAR SIR,

" I take the liberty of writing to you, in consequence of having met

---

[a] [It seems remarkable, that with this experience Mr. Hunter should have formed, from inconclusive analogy, and promulgated an opinion tending to occasion so much unhappiness as that which attributes exceeding imperfection, and probable incapacity of performing their natural functions, to testes which in the human subject are retained within the abdomen. That there is nothing in such a situation which necessarily tends to impair their efficiency, is evident, from the number of animals in which they constantly form part of the abdominal viscera. And in those in which the testes naturally pass into a scrotum, their continuance in the abdomen, according to our author's own observation, is accompanied only with a difference of size or shape: now we may readily suppose that this may influence the quantity, but not necessarily the quality of the secretion.]

[b] [The case described in the paper on the vesiculæ seminales, p. 23, seems to offer an exception to this rule; the right testicle had passed through the external ring, although the vas deferens was impervious.]

with a lusus naturæ of a peculiar kind, in the son of a man in this neighbourhood.

" The boy is about twelve months old : his right testicle is situated about an inch below the termination of the scrotum, and half an inch on the right side of the centre of the rapha perinæi, where a kind of pouch is formed of the common integuments, without the least rugous or scrotal appearance on its surface.   It is perfectly detached from the scrotum ; nor can the testis or spermatic process be at any time felt in any part of the scrotum, though I can readily make the testis pass from its situation quite up into the groin ; but immediately upon removing my hand the testis falls down into its pouch ; and I can trace the spermatic chord from the body of the testis up to the ring, running about a fourth of an inch on the right side of the scrotum. The scrotum on each side appears perfectly formed, and the left testis is *in situ naturali*. Now, Sir, as I conceive this peculiar conformation may be attended with great inconvenience to the child when he comes to ride on horseback, and on many other occasions, I beg leave to request your opinion upon it, with respect to what ought to be done to prevent accidents, which must, if left in its present situation, often occur.

" *Burford, Oxfordshire*.   [Signed]   Thomas Hunt."

To illustrate the descriptions which I have given, I have annexed three figures that were carefully taken from nature. [See Plates XXV. and XXVI.]

OBSERVATIONS ON THE GLANDS SITUATED BETWEEN THE RECTUM AND BLADDER, CALLED VESICULÆ SEMINALES.

THOSE bags, in the male of some animals, which are situated between the bladder and rectum, and commonly called ' vesiculæ seminales', have been considered as reservoirs of the semen secreted by the testicles, in the same manner as the gall-bladder is supposed to be a reservoir of the bile. Physiologists must have been led to form this opinion from observing that in the human subject their ducts communicate with the vasa deferentia before their termination in the urethra. This communication was supposed to allow the semen, when not immediately wanted, to pass into the bags from the vasa deferentia by a species of regurgitation. But more accurate observations respecting their structure and contents in the human subject, and on corresponding parts in other animals supposed to answer a similar purpose, joined to the circumstance of their not being found in every class, induced me to conclude that this opinion was erroneous. To throw as much light upon this subject as possible I made a number of experiments, and availed myself of every opportunity which offered of examining whatever could in any way elucidate the point; and, from what I have been able to collect, I think it will appear that they cannot be considered as reservoirs of the semen.

To proceed regularly with my investigation, I shall begin by comparing the contents of these vesiculæ with the semen as it is emitted from the penis of a living man. From which comparison it will appear that the two secretions are very different in their sensible properties of colour and smell; and although the semen which constitutes the first part of the emission is evidently different from the last, yet every part of it is unlike the mucus found in these vesiculæ.

The semen first discharged from the living body is of a bluish white colour, in consistence like cream, and similar to what is found in the vasa deferentia after death; while that which follows is somewhat like the common mucus of the nose, but less viscid. The semen becomes more fluid upon exposure to the air, particularly that first thrown out; which is the very reverse of what happens to secretions in general. The smell of the semen is mawkish and unpleasant, exactly resembling that of the farina of the Spanish chestnut; and to the taste, though at first insipid, it has so much pungency as, after some little time, to stimulate and excite a degree of heat in the mouth. But the fluid contained in these vesiculæ in a dead body is of a brownish colour, and often varies in consistence in different parts of the bag, as if not well mixed. Its smell does not resemble that of the semen, neither does it become more fluid by being exposed to the air.

It may, however, be answered to this that the contents of the vesiculæ are generally found in a putrid state, and have by that means undergone a change in their sensible properties. But the objection is readily obviated by comparing this fluid with that in the vasa deferentia as it comes from the testicles of the same dead body, between which there appears to be no resemblance.

To be still more certain of the nature of what these vesiculæ contain than was possible from the examination of bodies which had been dead some time, I took an opportunity of opening a man, immediately after his death, who had been killed by a cannon-ball. The fluid in the vesiculæ was of a lighter colour than has usually been found in men who have been dead a considerable time; but it was not by any means like the semen either in colour or smell. In another man who died instantaneously, in consequence of falling from a considerable height, whose body I inspected soon after the accident, the contents of the vesiculæ were of a lightish whey colour, having nothing of the smell of semen, and in so fluid a state as to run out on cutting into them.

I have likewise examined with attention a mucus which some men discharge upon straining hard while at stool, or after throwing out the last drops of urine, an action which requires a considerable exertion of the parts. This discharge is generally called a seminal weakness, and is I believe commonly supposed to be the semen*; but in all the cases of this kind in which I have been consulted it nearly resembled the contents of the vesiculæ in the dead body, though perhaps not quite of so deep a colour. I endeavoured in vain to persuade a gentleman who had this complaint that the discharge was not seminal, till by examining his own semen and comparing it with that mucus he was convinced of the difference. This gentleman had the power of emitting the semen in the same quantity as usual immediately after the mucus had been discharged, which is a further proof that this fluid is not semen†.

In this country eunuchs seldom come under our examination; but we have sometimes opportunities of opening the bodies of those who

* Vide Treatise on the Venereal Disease, edit. 1st and 2nd, p. 197. [vol. ii, p. 303 of the present edition.]

† The discharge was truly supposed to be the contents of the vesiculæ; and, it being imagined that these contained semen, according to this reasoning the discharge must be seminal.

have, in consequence of disease or accident, lost one or both testicles; and several subjects of this kind I have inspected after death. Persons who have had one testicle taken away will better illustrate the point in dispute than those who have been deprived of both. For it is to be presumed that such men have afterwards had connexion with women, and consequently had the action of emission, which must have emptied the vesicula of the castrated side, if this had contained semen ; and, as it could not be replenished, it should have been found empty after death. We have also in such cases an opportunity of making comparative observations between the vesicula of the perfect and that of the imperfect side. In the eunuch such emissions never can happen, for the testicles being gone the natural and leading stimulus is lost; therefore, if in them the vesiculæ were found full after death, it might be supposed to be the semen which they had received from the testicles before castration that had remained there from the time of the operation; but castration being, in such cases, usually performed on children, this circumstance should rather be considered as a proof that they secrete their own mucus. Yet it is probable the vesiculæ will neither be so large nor so full in eunuchs as in the perfect man ; for I am of opinion that they are connected with generation, and that if the constitution is deprived of that power these bags will not grow to the full size. But where only one testicle is removed its loss does not in the least affect generation, therefore does not produce any change in the vesicula of that side from which the testicle is taken; because the vesicula does not depend upon the testicle for its secretion, but upon the constitution, and on the person being capable of the act of generation : therefore as one testicle is sufficient to preserve manhood, it is of course capable of keeping up the action of both those glands.

A man who had been under my care, in St. George's Hospital, for a venereal complaint, died there, and was discovered to have lost his right testicle. From the cicatrix being hardly observable it must have been removed some considerable time before his death; and the complaint for which he was received into the hospital is a convincing proof that he had connexion with women after that period.

I inspected the body in the presence of Mr. Hodges, the house-surgeon, and several of the pupils of the hospital. Upon dissecting out and examining the contents of the pelvis, with the penis and scrotum, I found that the vas deferens of the right side was smaller and firmer in its texture than the other, especially at that end next to the abdominal rings, near to the part which had been cut through in the operation. The cellular membrane surrounding the duct, on the right side, was not so loose as on the left; neither were the vessels which ramified on the right vesicula so full of blood. But upon opening the vesiculæ, both appeared to be filled with the same kind of mucus, and similar to that which is found in other dead bodies; the vesicula of the right side being rather larger than that on the left. Whatever, therefore, may be the real use of these vesiculæ, we have a proof from this dissection that in the human subject they do not contain the semen.

In a man who died in St. George's Hospital with a very large bubonocele, the testicle of the diseased side was discovered to have almost lost its natural texture, from the pressure of the hernial sac; and upon examining the testicle with attention there was no appearance of vas deferens till we came near the bladder, where it was almost as large as usual. The vesicula of that side was found to be as full as the other, and to contain the same kind of mucus.

I extirpated the left testicle of a Frenchman, who was a married man, and died about a year afterwards, having been extremely ill for several months before his death. On examining the body, the vesiculæ were both found nearly full, more especially that on the left side, which might be accidental; but the vas deferens of the left side, where it lies along this bag, and where it has a similar structure with the vesiculæ, was likewise filled with the same kind of mucus; which I believe is always the case, whether the testicle has been removed or not.

A young man, a coachman, with his left testicle much diseased, had it removed, at St. George's Hospital, by Mr. Walker, in August 1785; and in February 1786 he returned again to the hospital, on account of uncommon pains all over him. For these he requested to be put into the warm bath; but as he was going from the ward for that purpose, he dropped down and died almost immediately. The body was inspected, with a view to discover the cause of his death; and, upon examination of the vesiculæ, the bag of the left side was as full as that on the right, and the contents in both were exactly similar. In the winter 1788 another case occurred nearly resembling the above.

In dissecting a male subject, in the year 1755, for a side view of the contents of the pelvis, I found a bag on the left side, lying contiguous to the peritonæum, just on the side of the pelvis where the internal iliac vessels divide above the angle of reflection of the peritonæum at the union of the bladder and rectum. The left vas deferens was seen passing on to this bag; and what is very singular, that of the right, or opposite side, crossed the bladder, near its union with the rectum, to join it. I traced the left vas deferens down to the testicle; but, on following the right through the ring of the external oblique muscle, I discovered that it terminated at once, about an inch from its passage out of the abdomen, in a blunt point, which was impervious. On examining the spermatic chord from this point to the testicle, I could not find any vas deferens; but, by beginning at the testicle, and tracing the epididymis from its origin, about half-way along where it lies upon the body of the testicle, I perceived that it at first became straight, and soon after seemed to terminate in a point. The canal at this part was so large as to allow of being filled with quicksilver; which, however, did not pass far, so that a portion of the epididymis was wanting, and likewise the vas deferens for nearly the whole length of the spermatic chord of the right side*. On the left side the vas deferens began where the epididymis commonly terminates, and there was a deficiency of nearly an inch of the extremity of the epididymis†. I then dissected the bag above mentioned, which proved to be the two vesiculæ; for, by blowing air from one vas deferens, I could only inflate half of it, and from the other vas deferens the other half. They contained the mucus commonly found in these bags; but, upon the most accurate examination, I could neither discover any duct leading from them to the prostate gland, nor the remains of one‡.

It was evident in this subject that there was no communication between the vas deferens and epididymis, nor between these bags and the urethra. The caput gallinaginis had the common appearance, but there were no orifices to be found. The testicles were very sound, and the ducts from them to the epididymis were very manifest and contained semen§.

From these circumstances we have a presumptive proof that the semen

* Vide Plate XXVII. fig. 1.   † Vide Plate XXVII. fig. 2.   ‡ Vide Plate XXVIII.

§ As the semen, in consequence of this preternatural formation of parts, could not be conveyed to the urethra in the usual way, I conceived it possible that there might be another unnatural construction to make up for the deficiency in the vas deferens, and therefore examined it very carefully to see if there were no supernumerary vasa deferentia. I was led to do this more particularly from often finding parts resembling them where they could answer no kind of purpose. By a supernumerary vas deferens I mean a small duct which sometimes arises from the epididymis, and passes up the spermatic chord along with the vas deferens, commonly terminating in a blind end, near to which it is sometimes a little enlarged. I never found this duct go on to the urethra; but, in some instances, have seen it accompany the vas deferens as far as the brim of the pelvis. There is no absolute proof that this is a supernumerary vas deferens; but as we find the ducts of glands in general very subject to singularities, and that there are frequently supernumerary ducts; that there are often two ureters to one kidney, sometimes distinct from beginning to end; at other times both arising from one pelvis. These ducts, arising from the epididymis, I am inclined from analogy to believe are of a nature similar to the double ureters. They resemble the vas deferens, as being continuations of some of the tubes of the epididymis; are convoluted where they come off from it; afterwards become a straight canal, and passing along with it for some way, they are then most commonly obliterated.

The idea of their being for the purpose of returning the superfluous semen to the circulation must certainly be erroneous, from their being so seldom met with, and so very seldom continued further than the brim of the pelvis.

can be absorbed in the body of the testicle and in the epididymis, and that the vesiculæ secrete a mucus which they are capable of absorbing when it cannot be made use of. We may likewise infer from what has been said that the semen is not retained in reservoirs after it is secreted, and kept there till it is used, but that it is secreted at the time in consequence of certain affections of the mind stimulating the testicles to this action; for we find that if lascivious ideas are excited in the mind, and the paroxysm is afterwards prevented from coming on, the testicles become painful and swelled from, we may suppose, the quantity of semen secreted, and the increased action of the vessels, which pain and swelling is removed immediately upon the paroxysm being brought on and the semen evacuated; but if that does not take place, the action of the vessels will still be kept up, and the pain in the testicles in general continue till the paroxysm and evacuation of the semen is brought on to render the act complete, without which a stop cannot be so quickly put to the action of the vessels that produce the secretion, nor the parts be allowed so easily to resume their natural state. There is at this time no sensation of any kind felt in the seat of the vesiculæ seminales, which shows that the action is in the testicles, and in them alone. The pain in the testicles, in consequence of being filled with semen and of the action being incomplete, is sometimes so considerable as to make it necessary to produce an evacuation of the semen to relieve the patient.

It may be observed, in support of this opinion, that these bags are as full of mucus in bodies much emaciated, where the person has died from a lingering disease, as in those of the strong and robust, whose death has been occasioned by violence or acute diseases; and they are nearly as full in the old as in the young; which, most probably, would not be the case if they contained semen. These facts, taken from the human subject, are, I think, sufficient to establish the opinion which I have laid down; but, for the satisfaction of others, I shall give such facts and observations as have occurred in my dissection of different animals as tend to clear up the point in question.

These vesiculæ are not similar either in shape or contents in any two genera of animals which I have dissected; and they differ more in size, according to the bulk of the animal, than any other parts whose uses in different animals are supposed to correspond; while the semen in most of those which I have examined may be said to be similar.

ᵃ [This term is here used in a more extended sense than in the present systems of natural history; but even as applied to the Linnæan genera the rule is affected by numerous exceptions of which a comparison of the vesiculæ seminales of the ape with those of the human subject affords a striking example.]

The resemblance which obtains between these bags and the gall-bladder in the human subject by no means holds equally good when applied to other animals.   In the horse they are like two[a] small urinary bladders, almost loose and pendulous, with a partial coat from the peritonæum, under which there are two layers of muscular fibres; they are thicker in their coats at the fundus than any other part, and appear there to be glandular.   Their openings into the urethra are very large, and although they open close to the vasa deferentia do not communicate with them.   The septum between the two ducts is not continued on quite to the urethra, so that they cannot, in strict language, be said to enter that passage separately; but there is not length of common duct sufficient to admit of regurgitation from the vasa deferentia into these bags.   They are not of the same size in the gelding and in the stone-horse, being large in the last.   Their contents in both are exactly similar, and nearly equal in quantity; but in no way resembling the semen emitted by the stone-horse in the coitus, or what is found in the vas deferens after death.

In the boar these bags are extremely large, and divided into cells of a considerable size; or they may more properly be said to form ramifications closely connected with one another, and having a large canal or duct common to the whole.   The ducts contain a whitish fluid, very unlike what is found in the vasa deferentia of the same animal, with which they have not the least communication[b].

In the rat the bags are large and flat, with serrated edges, and lie some way within the abdomen, containing a thick ash-coloured mucus, nearly of the consistence of soft cheese; very different from what is found in the vasa deferentia of the same animal, with which they do not communicate.

---

[a] [There is also in the horse a third vesicula seminalis, of a similar structure to the two lateral ones, between which it is situated, and having, like them, no communication with the vasa deferentia.   This want of correspondence therefore between the number of the vesiculæ and that of the testes affords another argument against their having the relations to each other which exist between the gall-bladder and liver.]

[b] [Tyson particularly notices the glandular structure of the vesiculæ seminales in the peccari and boar, and was led by this circumstance to the same opinion respecting their nature and use as Mr. Hunter is endeavouring to establish by a more extensive and various induction in the present paper. " John van Horn," says Tyson, " would have a threefold matter of the seed: one from the testes, the second from the vesiculæ seminales, and a third from the prostates.   But this De Graaf strongly opposes; and will admit only that from the testes, which is transmitted to the vesiculæ seminales, but not at all bred there. But in our subject, and so in some others, they being glandulous, they must therefore secrete some juice; which, in all likelihood, is some way serviceable, though not principally, in generation."—*Anatomy of the Mexico Musk-hog*, Phil. Trans., vol. xiii. p. 370, 1683.]

In the beaver the bags are convoluted; their ducts have no communication with the vasa deferentia, but both the one and the other open on the verumontanum.

In the Guinea-pig they are composed of long cylindrical tubes, and lie in the cavity of the belly, are smooth on their external surface, and do not communicate with the vasa deferentia. They contain a thick bluish transparent substance, which is softest near the fundus, and becomes firmer towards the openings into the urethra, where it is as solid as common cheese. From this circumstance, and what is observed in the horse, the fundus appears to be the part that secretes this substance, which is very different in colour and consistence from the contents of the vasa deferentia, and is often found in broken pieces in the urethra.

To be more certain that the substance contained in these bags was not the secretion of the testicle, I extracted one of the testicles of a Guinea-pig; and six months afterwards gave it the female. As soon as the action of copulation was over (in which all the parts containing semen should naturally have emptied themselves) I killed the animal, and upon examination found the vesicula of the perfect side, and that of the side from which the testicle had been removed, both filled with a substance in every respect similar. It will scarcely be alleged that this substance had been contained in the bag before the extirpation of the testicle; nor could it be semen, which must have been all thrown out in the previous connexion with the female.

To ascertain that the contents of the vesiculæ are not discharged into the vagina of the female with the semen in the act of emission, I killed a female Guinea-pig as soon as the male had left her, and examined with attention what was contained in the vagina and uterus; in neither could I find any of the mucus of the vesiculæ, which from its firmness must have been easily detected.

In the hedgehog these bags are very large, being more than twice the size of the vesiculæ in the human subject.

Many animals have no such bags; and I believe they are wanting in the greater part of that class which live chiefly upon animal food: they are, however, to be found in some of them, and the hedgehog is an example[a]. There is no apparent difference in the testicles, vasa deferentia, or semen of the animals which have vesiculæ and of those which have none; and the mode of copulation, as far as these bags can be concerned, is very similar in both.

In birds, as far as I have yet observed, there is nothing analogous to

---

[a] [The vesiculæ seminales are wanting in all the Feræ with the exception of the Insectivora; also in the Ruminants, in the carnivorous Cetacea, and in all the Marsupiata; they are equally wanting in the insectivorous Monotremata, which of all mammiferous animals approximate most closely to the oviparous Vertebrata.]

these bags; and yet there appears to be no difference between the mode of copulation of the drake and the bull or ram. It is very natural to suppose that if the vesiculæ were reservoirs of semen they would be more necessary in birds, who have the power of repeating the act of copulation in an infinitely greater degree than quadrupeds; and indeed we find that in birds there are reservoirs, which may account for this power; the vasa deferentia being enlarged just before they open into the rectum, probably to answer that intention. As birds have no urethra, some having merely a groove, as the drake and gander[a], and many being even without a groove, as the common fowl, it was absolutely necessary there should be such a reservoir somewhere; and the necessity of this will appear more evidently by and by.

What I have observed of the reservoir of birds is equally applicable to amphibious animals, and to that order of fish called rays.

From the above observations I think we may fairly conclude that these vesiculæ are not for the purpose of containing semen: the single circumstance of their ducts being united to those of the testicles in the human subject not appearing sufficient to set aside the many facts which are contradictory to such an opinion.

Having endeavoured to show that the function of these vesiculæ has hitherto been misunderstood, the following observations will tend to prove that they are subservient to generation, though their particular use is not yet discovered; and, for the better understanding this part of the subject, I shall premise the following facts.

Animals have their natural feelings raised or increased according to the perfection of the parts connected with such feelings; and the disposition for action is also in proportion to the state of the parts and the excitement of such feelings. But, that these feelings may be duly excited, it is necessary that the animal and the parts should be healthy, in good condition, and in a certain degree of warmth suitable to that class to which the animal belongs. In the greatest part of the globe there is a difference in the warmth of the same district at different periods, constituting the seasons; and the cold in some of them is so considerable as to prevent those feelings or dispositions in animals from taking place, and to render them, for the time, unfit for the purposes of generation*. This is owing to the testicles becoming at this season

---

* It is not required that the season for the copulation of different animals should be equally warm; for the frog copulates in very cold weather, while the snake and lizard, which are also cold, sleeping animals, do not copulate till the season is warm.

---

[a] [After repeated examination, we find the structure of the urethra in the drake to be as here described, viz. a groove, and not a complete canal, as represented by Sir Everard Home. See Phil. Trans. 1802, p. 361. pl. xii.]

small, and being therefore unfit to give such dispositions, as is the case in very young animals. This fact is very obvious in birds, of which the sparrow may be produced as a proof. For if a cock-sparrow is killed in the winter, before the days have begun to lengthen, the testicle will be found very small*; but if that organ is examined at different times in other sparrows, as the warmth of the weather increases, and if this examination is continued to the breeding-season, the difference in the size of the testicle will be very striking†. This circumstance is not peculiar to birds, but is common, as far as I yet know, to all animals which have their seasons of copulation. In the buck we find the testicles are reduced to a very small size in the winter; and in the land-mouse, mole, &c. this diminution is still more remarkable. Animals, on the contrary, which are not in a state of nature have no such change taking place in their testicles; and, not being much affected by seasons, are consequently always in good condition, or in a state to which other animals that are left to themselves can only attain in the warmer season. Therefore in man, who is in the state we have last described, the testicles are nearly of the same size in winter as in summer; and nearly, though not exactly, the same thing may be observed in the horse, ram, &c., these animals having their seasons in a certain degree.

The variation above taken notice of is not confined to the testicles, but also extends to the parts which are connected with them. For in those animals that have their seasons for propagation the most distinctly marked, as the land-mouse, mole, &c., the vesiculæ are hardly discernible in the winter, but in the spring are very large, varying in size in a manner similar to the testicle. It may, however, be alleged that the change in these bags might naturally be supposed to take place, even admitting them to be seminal reservoirs; but what happens to the prostate gland, which has never been supposed to contain semen, will take off the force of this objection, since in all the animals which have such a gland (and which have their season for propagation) it undergoes a similar change. In the mole the prostate gland in winter is hardly discernible, but in the spring becomes very large and is filled with mucus.

From these observations it is reasonable to infer that the use of the vesiculæ in the animal œconomy must, in common with many other parts, be dependent upon the testicles. For the penis, urethra, and all the parts connected with them, are so far subservient to the testicles that I am persuaded few of them would have existed if there had been no testicles in the original construction of the body[a]; and these would

---

* Vide Plate XXIX. fig. 1.   † Vide Plate XXIX. fig. 5.

[a] [The construction and functions of the penis in reptiles and those birds which possess the organ prove the correctness of this view; and very striking evidence of the

have been so formed as merely to assist in the expulsion of the urine. To illustrate this opinion, let us observe what is the difference between these parts in the perfect male and in a male that has been deprived of the testicles when very young, at an age in which they have had no such influence upon the animal œconomy as to affect the growth of the other parts.   In the perfect male the penis is large; the corpora cavernosa* being capable of dilatation.   The corpus spongiosum is very vascular†; that part of the canal which is called the bulb is considerably enlarged, forming a cavity; and the musculi acceleratores urinæ, as they are termed, are strong and healthy.   In many animals which have a long penis, the muscular fibres are continued forwards to the end of it; and in others, though not extended so far, they are very large.

On the contrary, in the castrated animal the penis is small, and not capable of much dilatation; the corpus spongiosum is less vascular; the cavity at the bulb is little larger than the canal of the urethra; and the muscles are white, small, and have a ligamentous appearance.   The same observations are true, if applied to the erectores penis.

The penis of the perfect male is of a sufficient length, when erected, to reach to the further end of the vagina of the female.   In the castrated animal it is much shorter, and erections having then become unnecessary, the parts which should project often adhere to the inside of the prepuce.   The erectores muscles in the perfect male are strong enough

* The cells of the corpora cavernosa are muscular, although no such appearance is to be observed in men; for the penis in erection is not at all times equally distended. The penis in a cold day is not so large in erection as in a warm one; which, probably, arises from a kind of spasm that could not act upon it if it were not muscular.

In the horse the parts composing the cells of the penis appear evidently muscular to the eye; and in a horse just killed they contract upon being stimulated[a].

† It may not be improper to observe, that the corpus spongiosum urethræ and glans penis are not spongy or cellular, but made up of a plexus of veins.   This structure is discernible in the human subject, but much more distinctly seen in many animals, as the horse, &c.

exclusive relation of the penis to the functions of the testes is afforded by the discoveries in natural history which have been made since the time of Hunter.   Thus, in those remarkable Australian quadrupeds the Ornithorhynchus and Echidna, which form the passage from the mammiferous to the oviparous vertebrates, the penis, although perforated through its whole extent, does not carry off the urine, which escapes by the cloaca, but the urethra is destined solely for the passage of the fecundating fluid during the time of the coitus.]

[a] [The disposition of the muscular fasciculi of this part is chiefly longitudinal, interlacing in an undulating manner with the transverse tendinous fibres.   They are most numerous near the termination of the corpora cavernosa, and gradually diminish as they approach the origin.   When examined with a high magnifying power the ultimate fibres of these fasciculi exhibit, but in a fainter degree, the transverse striæ characteristic of the voluntary muscular fibre.]

to squeeze at once the blood out of the crura into the body of the penis, so as to straighten and contract the urethra instantaneously, and the acceleratores urinæ* have sufficient power to throw out the semen that is gradually accumulated at the bulb for ejection.

The prostate gland†, Cowper's glands, and the glands along the urethra (of which the lacunæ are the excretory ducts), are in the perfect male large and pulpy, secreting a considerable quantity of slimy mucus, which is salt to the taste; it is most probably for the purpose of lubricating those parts, and is only thrown out when in vigour for copulation: while in the castrated animal these are small, flabby, tough, and ligamentous, and have little secretion. From this account there appears to be an essential difference between the parts connected with generation of the perfect male, and those which remain in one that has been castrated, more especially if that operation had been performed while the animal was young.

If it is objected that the same changes did not take place in the men from whom one testicle had been removed, it may be answered, that the operation was performed late in life; and one testicle being left, that was sufficient to carry on the necessary actions, and consequently to preserve the powers; therefore whatever parts had a connexion with these powers, would still have the stimulus of perfection given to them.

The different appearance of the bulb and the muscles would seem to point out, in the perfect male, the enlargement of the bulb to be for the purpose of a receptacle for the semen; for although I have denied the

* I shall call these muscles 'expulsores seminis,' as I apprehend their real use to be for the expulsion of that secretion: these muscles, likewise, throw out those drops of urine which are collected in the bulb from the last contractions of the bladder, and they have been, from this circumstance, named acceleratores urinæ; but if a receptacle had not been necessary for the semen, those muscles had probably never existed, and the last drops of urine would have been thrown out by the action of the bladder and urethra, as in some measure is the case in the castrated animal. That the urethra has the power of contraction is evident upon the application of any stimulus, for I have seen the urethra refuse to allow an injection to pass on; and in that part where the injection stopped, a fulness was felt, which terminated at once: this contraction is most probably in the internal membrane; it also will often refuse the passage of a bougie.

† The prostate gland is not common to all animals. It is wanting in the bull, buck, and most probably, I believe, in all ruminating animals. In this class the coats of the vesiculæ are much thicker and more glandular, than in those which have prostate glands; it is therefore natural to suppose that the vesiculæ answer nearly the same purposes as the prostate gland [a].

The prostate gland, and Cowper's glands, as well as the vesiculæ, are wanting in birds, in the amphibious animals, and in those fish which have testicles, as all of the ray kind.

[a] [The glands in the Ruminants here termed 'vesiculæ,' are now regarded as a bifid prostate.]

vesiculæ to be reservoirs, yet, as it was necessary that the semen should be accumulated somewhere before ejection, I shall endeavour to prove, from the mode of copulation in the animals we are best acquainted with, that the bulb is intended for that purpose.   Let us, therefore, give a short account of the different parts concerned in coition; and by observing the dependence which they have upon one another, see how this proof will come out.

The erection of the penis is produced by a stop being put to the returning blood, and this stoppage is so complete, that no mechanical pressure applied to the body of the penis can force the blood on into the veins.   This erection answers two purposes; it gives size and strength to the penis, and it renders the canal of the urethra smaller. The corpus spongiosum of the urethra and the glans, which is only a continuation of it, are filled with blood from the same cause, but not so completely as the body of the penis, since from them it can be forced out into the veins by pressure*.   This accumulation of blood in the corpus spongiosum diminishes the canal of the urethra so much, that any pressure upon one part of it will have a considerable effect upon the other; not only by lessening its capacity at the part pressed, but by forcing the blood forward, the parts beyond will be still more distended, and consequently the canal of the urethra be in that proportion diminished.   The semen, in the time of copulation, in such animals as remain long in that act, is gradually squeezed along the vasa deferentia (as it is secreted) into the bulb; and when the testicles cease to secrete, the paroxysm, which is to finish the whole operation, comes on.   The se-

---

* In April 1760, in the presence of Mr. Blount, I laid bare the penis of a dog, almost through its whole length; traced the two veins that came from the glans (which in this animal makes the largest part of the penis), and separated them from the arteries by dissection, that I might be able to compress them at pleasure without affecting the arteries.   I then compressed the two veins, and found that the glans and large bulb became full and extended; but when I irritated the veins, in order to see if there was any power of contraction in them which might occasionally stop the return of the blood, no such appearance could be observed[a].

---

* [From this experiment, it is obvious that Hunter regarded the stoppage of the circulation through the veins as being produced by external compression.   Douglas (*Myographiæ Comparatæ Specimen*, p. 9,) had previously described the muscles which compress the vena dorsalis penis in the dog; and Cowper had more fully and particularly detailed the structure and actions of the muscles which have a corresponding office in the opossum, observing that " the muscles of the cavernous bodies of the penis of this creature, having no connexion with the os pubis, cannot apply the dorsum penis to the last-named bone, and compress the vein of the penis, whereby to retard the refluent blood and cause an erection, as we have observed in other creatures; but some large veins of the penis here take a different course, and pass through the middle parts of the

men acting as a stimulus to the cavity of the bulb of the urethra, the muscles of that part of the canal are thrown into action; the fibres nearest the bladder, probably, act first, and those more forward in quick succession; the semen is projected with some force; the blood in the bulb of the urethra is by the same action squeezed forward, but requiring a greater impulse to propel it, is rather later than the semen, on which it presses from behind; the corpus spongiosum being full of blood, acts almost as quick as undulation, in which it is assisted by the corresponding constriction of the urethra, and the semen is hurried along with a considerable velocity[a].

From the facts which I have stated respecting the organs of generation, the observations which I have made, and the series of actions which I have considered as taking place in the copulation of animals, I think the following inferences may be fairly drawn:

That the bags, called vesiculæ seminales, are not seminal reservoirs, but glands secreting a peculiar mucus; and that the bulb of the urethra is, properly speaking, the receptacle in which the semen is accumulated previous to ejection.

Although it seems to have been proved that the vesiculæ do not contain the semen, I have not been able to ascertain their particular use; we may, however, be allowed upon the whole to conclude that they are, together with other parts, subservient to the purposes of generation.

---

bulb, and are only liable to compression made by the intumescence of the muscles C C (muscles of the bulb) that inclose them. "But the chief agent in continuing the erection of the penis in this animal is the sphincter muscle of its anus, or rather cloaca; and not only the sphincter muscle of the cloaca of the male oppossum, but that of the female also closely embraces the penis in coition, and effectually retard the refluent blood from its corpora cavernosa, by compressing the veins of the penis." (*Phil. Trans.*, vol. xxiv. 1704, p. 1584.)]

[a] [Besides the functions here assigned to the bulb of the urethra, in relation to the reception and propulsion of the semen, we may also notice its uses in reference to the distention of the glans penis, of which Cowper, in his description of the male organs of the opossum above quoted, gives a remarkable example. He observes: "As the bulb of the urethra in man is framed for the use of the glans, to keep it sufficiently distended when required, so it seems it is necessary to have *two* of these bulbs inclosed with their particular muscles in this animal, to maintain the turgescence of its *double* or forked glans when the penis is erected." (*Phil. Trans.*, vol. xxiv., 1704, p. 1585.)]

ACCOUNT OF THE FREE-MARTIN.

GENERATION, from a seed, requires the concurrence of two causes to give it perfection : the one to form the seed, the other to give it the principle of action*.

The cause forming the seed is called the female, the other the male; but those two causes in general make only a part of a whole animal, or are rather parts superadded to an animal. Probably these characteristics were first observed in such animals as had the female parts complete in one, and the male in the other; therefore the terms female and male have been applied to the whole animal, dividing them into two distinct sexes, and the parts which formed the one sex or the other were called the female or the male parts of generation. But, upon a more accurate knowledge of animals and of their parts of generation, these were found in many of the inferior tribes to be united in the same animal, which from possessing both has got the name of hermaphrodite.

As the distinction of male or female parts is natural to most animals, as the union of them in the same animal is also natural to many, and as the separation of them is only a circumstance making no essential difference in the structure of the parts themselves, it becomes no great effort or uncommon play in Nature sometimes to unite them in those animals in which they are commonly separated; a circumstance we really find takes place in many animals of those orders in which such an union is unnatural. From this state of the case hermaphrodites may be divided into two kinds, the natural and unnatural.

The natural hermaphrodite belongs to the inferior and more simple genera of animals, of which there is a much greater number than of the

* It may be necessary for some of my readers to have explained to them what I mean by a seed. I do suppose that the word seed was first applied to grain, or that which is always called seed in the vegetable; which seed is the part of such vegetables in which the matter of the young vegetable exists or is formed. The principle of arrangement in the farina, or male part, fitting the seed for action, being at first not known, a false analogy between the vegetable and animal was established, and the matter secreted by the testes was called the seed; but, from the knowledge of the distinct sexes in the vegetable, it is well known that the seed is the female production in them, and that the principle of arrangement for action is from the male. The same operation and principles take place in many orders of animals, the female producing a seed in which is the matter fitted for the first arrangement of the organs of the animal, and which receives the principle of arrangement fitting them for action from the male.

more perfect; and as animals become more complicated, have more parts, and each part is more confined to its particular use, a separation of the two necessary powers for generation seems also to take place[a].

The unnatural hermaphrodite[b], I believe, now and then occurs in every tribe of animals having distinct sexes, but is more common in some than

[a] [The animals in which the organs of the two sexes are naturally combined in the same individual are confined to the invertebrate division, and are most common in the molluscous and radiate classes. If the term hermaphrodite may be applied to those species which propagate without the concourse of the sexes, but in which no distinct male organ can be detected, as well as to those in which both male and female organs are present in the same body, then there may be distinguished three kinds of hermaphroditism.

First, the *cryptandrous*, or in which the female or productive organs are alone developed. Ex. the acephalous mollusks, as the oyster, lamp-cockle, and ascidia; the cystic entozoa, echinoderms, acalephes, polyps, and sponges.

Second, the *heautandrous*, or in which the male organs are developed, but so disposed as to fecundate the ova of the same individual. Ex. the cirripeds, the rotifers, the trematode and cestoid entozoa.

Third, the *allotriandrous*, or in which the male organs are so disposed as not to fecundate the ova of the same body, but where the concourse of two individuals is required, notwithstanding the co-existence in each of the organs of the two sexes. Ex. the gastropodous mollusks, with the exception of the pectinibranchiate order, the class Annellida.

All the other invertebrates, as the cephalopods and pectinibranchiate gastropods, the insects, arachnidans and crustaceans, the epizoa, and the nematoid entozoa, are, like the vertebrate classes, diœcious, or composed of male and female individuals.]

[b] [The unnatural hermaphrodites may be divided into those in which the parts peculiar to the two sexes are blended together in different proportions, and the whole body participates of a neutral character, tending towards the male and female as the respective organs predominate, and into those in which the male and female organs occupy respectively separative halves of the body, and impress on each lateral moiety the characteristics of the sex. This latter and very singular kind of hermaphroditism has hitherto been found only in insects and crustaceans. In the Extracts from the Minute-Book of the Linnean Society, printed in the 14th Vol. of their Transactions, it is stated that Alex. MacLeay, Esq., Sec. L.S., exhibited a curious specimen showing that two Papiliones, referred to distinct families by Fabricius, are in reality the male and female of the same species. This specimen presented the forms and colours of both sexes, divided by a longitudinal line on the body: the right wings and side of the body being as in the male (*Papilio Polycaon*, Fabr.), and the left as in the female (*Papilio Laodocus*, Fabr.). In Loudon's Magazine of Natural History, (vol. iv. p. 434,) an experienced entomologist, Mr. J. O. Westwood, has given descriptions and figures, not only of dimidiate hermaphrodites, (the example is the *Bombyx Penii*) but also of quartered hermaphrodites: the latter singular condition is exemplified in a specimen of the *Bombyx castrensis*, in which the right wing, left antenna, and left side of the abdomen are male; the left wing, right antenna, and right side of the abdomen are female: and again in a specimen of the stag-beetle (*Lucanus Cervus*), in which the left jaw and right elytrum are masculine, and the right jaw and left elytrum feminine. In most dimidiate hermaphrodites the left side is masculine; but an example of the contrary has been observed in *Sphinx Populi*. It is to be regretted that the condition of the internal organs of generation cannot be ascertained in the above singular examples; but this deficiency is in some degree supplied by the results of Dr. Nicholl's dissection of a hermaphrodite

in others*; and is to be met with, in all its gradations, from the distinct
sex to the most exact combination of male and female organs. This,
I fancy, happens most rarely in the human species, never having seen
an instance. I can say the same of dogs[a] and cats, with which last, however, I am less acquainted; but in the horse, ass, sheep, and black cattle
it is very frequent.

There is one part common to both the male and female organs of generation in all animals which have the sexes distinct: in the one sex it
is called the penis, in the other the clitoris; its specific use in both is
to continue, by its sensibility, the action excited in coition till the paroxysm alters the sensation. In the female it probably answers no other
purpose; but in the male it is more complicated, to adapt it for the purpose of conducting and expelling the semen that has been secreted in
consequence of the actions so excited.

Though the unnatural hermaphrodite be a mixture of both sexes, and
may possess the parts peculiar to each in perfection, yet it cannot possess in perfection that part which is common to both. For as this common part is different in one sex from what it is in the other, and it is
impossible for one animal to have both a penis and clitoris, the common
part must of course partake of both sexes, and consequently render the
hermaphrodite so far incomplete; but these parts peculiar to each sex
may be perfectly joined in the same animal, which will convey an idea
of the truest hermaphrodite[b]. Although it may not be necessary, to con-

* Quere: Is there ever, in the genera of animals that are natural hermaphrodites, a
separation of the two parts forming distinct sexes? If there is, it may account for the
distinction of sexes ever having happened[c].

---

lobster, (*Phil. Trans.*, xxxvi. p. 290,) in which a testis was found on that side of the body
which exhibited externally the male characteristics, and an ovarium on the opposite side.].

   [a] [For an example of hermaphroditism in a dog, see *Phil. Trans.*, lxxxix. p. 157.]

   [b] [In a recent work on hermaphroditism, by Geoffroy St. Hilaire, a mechanical reason
is assigned for the non-existence of a penis and clitoris in the same individual, viz.
because both parts arise from the same points of the pelvis; but in many animals
neither the one nor the other has any bony attachment, and the explanation above given,
founded on the similarity of their functions, is more philosophical and satisfactory.]

   [c] [The separation of the two sexual organs from one another in the same body occurs
in many of that class of natural hermaphrodites which we have termed 'allotriandrous';
and there are many examples in the Hunterian collection showing the fact. What, therefore, Mr. Hunter seems here to refer to is a spontaneous fission of the body in the inter-
val separating the two sexual parts, so that one portion of the body shall contain the
male and the other the female organs. Some annellides, as the Naïs, exhibit the phenomenon of spontaneous fission, but the separation never occurs so as to divide the two
sexual organs from one another, and appropriate one to each division; and were even
such an occurrence to be supposed ever to take place, the application of the fact to explain the occurrence of the distinct sexes in the naturally diœcious classes seems more
worthy of a speculatist of the Lamarckian school than of a sober observer of Nature.]

stitute an hermaphrodite, that the parts peculiar to the one sex should be blended with those of the other, in the same way that the penis is with the clitoris, yet this sometimes takes place in parts whose use in the distinct sexes is somewhat similar, the testicle and ovarium sometimes forming one body, without the properties of either. This compounded part in those animals that have the testicle and ovarium differently situated is generally found in the place allotted for the ovarium; but in such animals as have the testicle and ovarium in the same situation, as the bird tribe, the compound of the two, when it occurs, will also be found in that common situation.

The parts of the female appropriated for the purpose of supplying the young with nourishment are variously placed in different animals. In the horse, black cattle, sheep, and other graminivorous animals, their situation is between the hind legs; and this being also the place allotted for the testicles of the male of this tribe, and probably of all those in which the testicles come out of the cavity of the belly; in the hermaphrodite therefore, which has both these parts, the testicles must to a certain degree descend into the udder, though that cannot receive them so readily as the scrotum.

The hermaphrodites which I have seen have always appeared externally and at first view to be females, from the penis being the part principally deficient, and there being an opening behind like the bearing in the female; and as the testicles in such hermaphrodites seldom come down, the udder is left to occupy its proper place. In animals the female of which is preserved for breeding only, as sheep, goats, pigs, &c., these are generally kept, from their being supposed to be females.

Among horses such hermaphrodites are very frequent: I have seen several, but never dissected any. The most complete was one in which the testicles had come down out of the abdomen into the place where the udder should have been (viz. more forward than the scrotum), and, though not so pendulous as the scrotum in the perfect male of such animals, had all the appearance of an udder. There were also two distinct nipples, which, although they exist in the male, have no perfect form, being blended with the sheath or prepuce, of which there was none here. The external female parts were exactly similar to those of the perfect female; but instead of a common-sized clitoris, there was one about five or six inches long, which when erect pointed almost directly backwards.

I procured a foal-ass, very similar in external appearance to the horse above mentioned, and killed it to examine the parts. It had two nipples, but the testicles were not come down as in the above, owing perhaps to the animal's being yet too young.   There was no penis passing round the pubis to the belly, as in the perfect male ass.

The external female parts were similar to those of the she-ass. Within the entrance of the vagina was placed the clitoris; but much longer than that of a true female, it measuring about five inches.   The vagina was pervious a little beyond the opening of the urethra into it, and from thence up to the fundus of the uterus there was no canal. The uterus was hollow at the fundus, or had a cavity in it, and then divided into two horns, which were also pervious.   Beyond the termi- nation of the two horns were placed the ovaria as in the true female; but I could not find the Fallopian tubes.   From the broad ligaments, to the edges of which the horns of the uterus and ovaria are attached, there passed towards each groin a part similar to the round ligaments in the female, which were continued into the rings of the abdominal muscles; but with this difference, that there accompanied them a process or theca of the peritoneum, similar to the tunica vaginalis communis in the male ass; and in these thecæ were found the testicles, but I could not ob- serve any vasa deferentia passing from them.

Here then were found, in the same animal, the parts peculiar to each sex (although very imperfect), and that part which is common to both, but different in each, was a kind of medium of that difference.

Something similar to the above I have seen in sheep, goats, &c.; but I shall not at present trouble the reader with a description of herma- phrodites in general, as it is a very extensive subject, admitting of great variety, which would make them appear a production of chance; whereas the intention of this account is to point out a circumstance which takes place in the production of hermaphrodites in black cattle that appears to be almost an established principle in their propagation, and is per- haps peculiar to that species of animal.

It is a fact known, and I believe almost universally understood, that when a cow brings forth two calves, and one of them a bull-calf and the other to appearance a cow, that the cow-calf is unfit for propagation, but the bull-calf grows up into a very proper bull.   Such a cow-calf is called in this country a FREE-MARTIN, and is commonly as well known among the farmers as either cow or bull.   Although it will appear, from the description of this animal, that it is an hermaphrodite (being in no respect different from other hermaphrodites), yet I shall retain the term, free-martin, to distinguish the hermaphrodite produced in this way from those which resemble the hermaphrodite of other animals; for I know that in black cattle such a deviation may be produced without the cir cumstance of twins: and even where there are twins, the one a male the other a female, they may both have the organs of generation perfectly formed. But when I speak of those which are not twins, I shall call them hermaphrodites : the only circumstance worth our notice being a singularity in the mode of production of the Free-martin, and its being, as far as I yet know, peculiar to black cattle.

This calf has all the external marks of a cow-calf, similar to what was mentioned in the unnatural hermaphrodite, viz. the teats and the external female parts called by farmers the bearing; and when they are preserved, by those who know the above fact, it is not for propagation, but for all the purposes of an ox or spayed heifer, viz. to yoke with the oxen and to fatten for the table*.

It is known that they do not breed; they do not show the least inclination of the bull, nor does the bull ever take the least notice of them†. They very much resemble, in form, the ox or spayed heifer, being considerably larger than either the bull or the cow, having the horns very similar to the horns of an ox.

The bellow of the free-martin is similar to that of an ox, having more resemblance to that of the cow than of the bull. Free-martins are very much disposed to grow fat with good food. The flesh, like that of the ox or spayed heifer, is generally much finer in the fibre than either the bull or cow, is supposed to exceed that of the ox and heifer in delicacy of flavour, and bears a higher price at market.

However, it seems that this is not universal, for I was lately informed by Charles Palmer, Esq., of Luckley in Berkshire, that a free-martin having been killed in his neighbourhood, from the general idea of its being better meat than common, every neighbour bespoke a piece, which turned out nearly as bad as bull-beef; worse, at least, than that of a cow. It is probable that circumstance might arise from this animal having more the properties of a bull than the cow, as we shall see hereafter that they are sometimes more the one than the other‡.

Although what I have advanced with respect to the production of

---

* I need hardly observe here, that if a cow has twins, and they are both bull-calves, that they are in every respect perfect bulls; or if they are both cow-calves, they are perfect cows.

† Vide Leslie on Husbandry, pp. 98, 99.

‡ The Romans called the bull, taurus; they, however, talked of tauræ in the feminine gender. And Stephen observes, that it was thought the Romans meant by tauræ, barren cows, and called them by this name because they did not conceive. He also quotes a passage from Columella, lib. vi. cap. 22, "and like the tauræ, which occupy the place of fertile cows, should be rejected, or sent away." He likewise quotes Varro, De Re Rustica, lib. ii. cap. 5, "The cow which is barren is called taura." From which we may reasonably conjecture that the Romans had not the idea of the circumstances of their production.

free-martins be in general true, yet, by the assistance of Benjamin Way, Esq., of Denham, near Uxbridge, who knew my anxiety to ascertain this point, I was lately furnished with an instance which proves that it does not invariably hold good.

One of his cows having produced twins, which were to appearance male and female, upon a supposition that the cow-calf was a free-martin, he obligingly offered either to give it me, or to keep it till it grew up, that we might determine the fact: as I conceived it to be a free-martin, and was to have the liberty of examining it after death, I desired that he would keep it; but, unfortunately, it died at about a month old. Upon examining the organs of generation, they appeared to be those of the female, and perfectly formed; but to make this more certain, I procured those of a common cow-calf, and comparing them together, found them exactly alike. This made us regret that the animal had not lived to an age that might have determined if it was capable of breeding; for the construction of the parts being to appearance perfect, is not sufficient of itself to stamp it a true or perfect female; as I can suppose that the parts being perfectly formed, but without the power of propagation, may constitute the most simple kind of hermaphrodite. It is, however, most probable that this was a perfect female, which is an exception to the common rule; and I have been informed there are instances of such twins breeding[a]. If there are such deviations, as of twins being perfect male and female, why should there not be, on the other hand, an hermaphrodite produced singly, as in other animals? I had the examination of one which seemed, upon the strictest inquiry, to have been a single calf; and I am the more inclined to think this true, from having found a number of hermaphrodites among black cattle, without the circumstances of their birth being ascertained.

Hermaphrodites are to be met with in sheep; but, from the account given of them, I should suppose that they are not free-martins. I have seen several which were supposed to be hermaphrodites, but which were imperfect males, having the penis terminating in the perinæum, the orifice of which appeared like the bearing in the female. Such are not naturally stimulated to put themselves in the position of the female when they void their urine, so that when it passes the surrounding parts

---

[a] [An instance of this nature is recorded in the fifth volume of Loudon's Magazine of Natural History, p. 765. "Jos. Holroyd, Esq., of Withers, near Leeds, had a cow which calved twins, a bull-calf and a cow-calf. As popular opinion was against the cow-calf breeding, it being considered a free-martin, Mr. Holroyd was determined to make an experiment of them, and reared them together. They copulated, and in due time the heifer brought forth a bull-calf, and she regularly had calves for six or seven years afterwards."]

are wetted by it, and being covered with wool, and retaining the urine, keeps them continually moist, and gives the animal a strong smell. They are mentioned as both male and female.

I believe it had never been even conjectured, notwithstanding all these peculiarities, what was the true nature of the free-martin; and from the singularity of the animal, and the account of its production, I was almost tempted to suppose the whole a vulgar error. Yet by the universality of the testimony in its favour, it appearing to have some foundation, I eagerly sought for an opportunity to see and examine them. I have succeeded in this inquiry, and have seen several, the first of which was one belonging to John Arbuthnot, Esq. of Mitcham, and was calved in his own farm. He was so obliging as to allow me to satisfy myself, first by permitting a drawing to be made of the animal while alive, which was executed by Mr. Gilpin, and afterwards to examine the parts when the animal died. At the time the drawing was made of Mr. Arbuthnot's free-martin, John Wells, Esq. of Bickley Farm, near Bromley in Kent, was present, and informed us that a cow of his had calved two calves, one of which was a bull-calf, and the other a cow-calf. I desired Mr. Arbuthnot to request Mr. Wells to keep them, or let me buy them of him; but, from his great desire of natural knowledge, he very readily consented to preserve both till the bull showed all the signs of a good bull; and when the free-martin was killed, he allowed me to inspect the parts.

Of all the specimens which I have dissected, I shall only give the descriptions of the three which point out most distinctly the complete free-martin, with the gradations towards the male and female.

THE DESCRIPTION OF THE THREE FREE-MARTINS.

Mr. Wright's Free-Martin, five years old.

This animal had more the appearance and general character of the ox, or spayed heifer, than of either the bull or cow. The vagina terminated in a blind end, a little way beyond the opening of the urethra, from which the vagina and uterus were impervious. The uterus, at its extreme part, divided into two horns. At the termination of the horns were placed the testicles, instead of the ovaria, as is the case in the female. The reasons why I call these bodies testicles are the following. First, they were above twenty times larger than the ovaria of the cow, and nearly the size of the testicles of the bull, or rather of those of the ridgil, the bull whose testicles never come down. Secondly, the spermatic arteries were similar to those of the bull, especially of the ridgil.

Thirdly, the cremaster muscle passed up from the rings of the abdominal muscles to the testicles, as it does in the ridgil*.

There were the two bags placed behind, between the bladder and the uterus. Their ducts opened into the vagina, a very little way beyond the opening of the urethra; but there was nothing similar to the vasa deferentia.

As the external parts had more of the cow than the bull, the clitoris, which may be reckoned an external part, was also similar to that of the cow, not at all in a middle state, between the penis of the bull and the clitoris of the cow, as I have described in the hermaphrodite horse. There were four teats: the glandular part of the udder was but small.

This animal cannot be said to have been a mixture of all the parts of both sexes, for the clitoris had nothing similar to the penis in the male, and it was deficient in the female parts, by having nothing similar to the ovaria; neither had the uterus a cavity.

Mr. Arbuthnot's Free-Martin†.

The external parts were rather smaller than in the cow. The vagina passed on, as in the cow, to the opening of the urethra, and then it began to contract into a small canal, which passed on to the division of the uterus into the two horns, each horn passing along the edge of the broad ligament laterally towards the ovaria.

At the termination of these horns were placed both the ovaria and the testicles; they were nearly of the same size, and about as large as a small nutmeg.

To the ovariaª I could not find any Fallopian tube.

To the testicles were vasa deferentia, but they were imperfect. The left one did not reach near to the testicle; the right only came close to it, but did not terminate in a body called the epididymis. They were both pervious, and opened into the vagina near the opening of the urethra.

---

* Although I call these bodies testicles, for the reason given, yet they were only imitations of them, for when cut into they had nothing of the structure of the testicle; not being similar to anything in Nature, they had more the appearance of disease. From the seeming imperfection of the animal itself, it was not to be supposed that they should be testicles; for then the animal should have partaken of the bull, which it certainly did not.

† This animal was seven years old; had been often yoked with the oxen; at other times went with the cows and bull; but never showed any desires for either the one or the other.

ª [It is probable that these bodies were, as in the case previously noted, remains of the corpora Wolffiana.]

On the posterior surface of the bladder, or between the uterus and bladder, were the two bags, called vesiculæ seminales in the male, but much smaller than what they are in the bull; the ducts opened along with the vasa deferentia. This was more entitled to the name of hermaphrodite than the first or third, for it had a mixture of all the parts, though all were imperfect.

Mr. Wells's Free-Martin.

This animal was between three and four years old when killed; and had never been observed to show any signs of desire for the male, although it went constantly with one; and looked more like a heifer than free-martins usually do.

The teats and udder were small compared with those of a heifer, but rather larger than in either of the former examples; the beginning of the vagina was similar to that of the cow, but soon terminated a little beyond the opening of the urethra, as in the first-described. The vagina and uterus, to external appearance, were continued, although not pervious, and the uterine part divided into two horns, at the end of which were the ovaria.

I could not observe in this animal any other body which I could suppose to be the testicle.

There was on the side of the uterus an interrupted vas deferens broken off in several places.

Behind the bladder, or between that and the vagina, were the bags called vesiculæ seminales, between which were the terminations of the two vasa deferentia.

The ducts of the bags, and the vasa deferentia, opened as in the last instance.

This could not be called an exact mixture of all the parts of both sexes, for here was no appearance of testicles.

The female parts were imperfect, and there was the addition of part of the vasa deferentia, and the bags called vesiculæ seminales.

This circumstance of having no testicles, perhaps, was the reason why it had more the external appearance of a heifer than what they commonly have, and more than either of the two former.

AN ACCOUNT OF AN EXTRAORDINARY PHEASANT.

EVERY deviation from that original form and structure which gives the distinguishing character to the productions of Nature, may not improperly be called monstrous. According to this acceptation of the term, the variety of monsters will be almost infinite[a]; and, as far as my knowledge has extended, there is not a species of animal, nay, there is not a single part of an animal body, which is not subject to an extraordinary formation.

Neither does this appear to be a matter of mere chance; for it may

---

[a] [Mr. Hunter attempted, notwithstanding, to reduce this variety of monsters to definite groups, and left the following outline of a classification of monsters, in an explanatory introduction to the extensive series of those objects in his collection:

"1. Monsters from preternatural situation of parts.

"2. ————— addition of parts.

"3. ————— deficiency of parts

"4. ————— combined addition and deficiency of parts, as in hermaphroditical malformation."

Licetus[1], Huber[2], and Malacarne[3] had proposed classifications of monsters prior to the time of Hunter, all of which are more or less tinctured with the superstitions of the times; thus, the *tenth* class in the system of Licetus is appropriated to the offspring of the illicit intercourse of demons with women: the *fifteenth* of Malacarne contains the brutes with human members, &c. Blumenbach, towards the end of the eighteenth century, published an arrangement of monsters which closely resembles that of Hunter; he, however, distinguishes, but without sufficient reason, unnatural hermaphrodites from monsters, and divides the latter into

"1. Monsters by an unnatural conformation of certain parts of the body,—*Fabrica aliena.*

"2. ————— transposition of parts,—*Situs mutatus.*

"3. ————— a deficiency of parts,—*Monstra per defectum.*

"4. ————— supernumerary parts,—*Monstra per excessum.*"

The study of the various congenital aberrations from the specific form presented in the different classes of the animal kingdom, has since been ably and successfully pursued by Meckel, Geoffroy St. Hilaire, Otto, Breschet, Charuet, &c., the general results of whose labours may be found in the *Histoire Générale et Particulière des Anomalies de l'Organization chez l'Homme et les Animaux, ou Traité de Tératologie*, by Isid. Geoffroy Saint-Hilaire; 8vo, 1832.]

---

[1] Fortunius Licetus, *De Monstris*, ex recensione G. Blasii: Amstelodami, 1665, 4to.

[2] *Observationes nonnullæ de Monstris*: 4to, Cassel, 1748.

[3] " De' Mostri umani de' Caretteri fondamentali su cui ne se portrebbe stabilire la Classificazione," *Mem. della Soc. Ital.*, tom. ix. 4.

be observed that every species has a disposition to deviate from Nature in a manner peculiar to itself[a]. It is likewise worthy of remark, that each species of animals is disposed to have nearly the same sort of defects, and to have certain supernumerary parts of the same kind : yet every part is not alike disposed to take on a great variety of forms; but each part of each species seems to have its monstrous form originally impressed upon it[b].

It is well known that many orders of animals have the two parts designed for the purpose of generation different in individuals of the same species, by which they are distinguished into male and female; but this is not the only mark of distinction, in the greatest part the male being distinguished from the female by various other marks. The varieties which are found in the parts of generation themselves I shall call the first or principal marks, being originally formed in them, and belonging equally to both sexes; all others depending upon these I shall call secondary, as not taking place till the first are becoming of use, and being principally, although not entirely, in the male.

One of the most general marks is, the superior strength of make in the male ; and another circumstance, perhaps equally so, is this strength being directed to one part more than another, which part is that most immediately employed in fighting. This difference in external form is more particularly remarkable in the animals whose females are of a peaceable nature, as are the greatest number of those which feed on vegetables, and the marks to discriminate the sexes are in them very nu-

---

[a] [The value of the principle here enunciated will be appreciated, when it is stated that it is the basis of the latest and most elaborate work on the subject of monsters. It is claimed for Geoffroy St. Hilaire as the most important of his deductions in Teratology, and the chief point in which his system differs from, and is superior to, those of his predecessors. "C'est de principes precisement inverses que mon père a pris sur point de départ; et c'est aussi, comme cela devait être à des résultats inversés qu'il est parvenu. Etablissant, par un grand nombre de recherches, que les monstres sont, comme les êtres dits normaux, soumis à des règles constantes, il est conduit à admettre que la méthode de classification que les naturalistes emploient pour les seconds, peut être appliquée avec succès aux premiers." Isid. Geoffroy St.-Hilaire, *loc. cit.*, p. 99.]

[b] [In this principle Mr. Hunter is opposed to Geoffroy St.-Hilaire, who attributed the production (*l'ordonnée*) of monstrosities to the operation of exterior or mechanical causes at some period of fœtal development. Defective formation in parts of a fœtus has indeed been produced by destroying a portion of the respiratory surface of an egg during incubation; but this result by no means affords adequate grounds for assigning as the sole cause of every malformation accidental adhesions between the fœtus and its coverings. Mr. Hunter also made experiments with reference to monstrosities, and succeeded in effecting what, at first sight, seems the most difficult to produce, viz. the monsters by excess, of which several specimens of *Lacerta*, with a double tail (No. 2219—2223), afford examples. It is evident, however, from the expression in the concluding paragraph of the text, that he regarded the cause of congenital malformation as existing in the primordial germ.]

merous. The males of almost every class of animals are probably disposed to fight, being, as I have observed, stronger than the females;
and in many of these there are parts destined solely for that purpose, as
the spurs in the cock, and the horns in the bull; and on that account
the strength of the bull lies principally in his neck; that of the cock in
his limbs.

In carnivorous animals, whose prey is often of a kind which requires
strength to kill, we do not find such a difference in the form of the male
and female, very little being discernible in the dog and bitch, in the he
or she cat, or in the cock and hen of the eagle [a]. A difference, however,
is often perceivable in the whole or in some part of their external
covering; the mane of the lion distinguishing him from the lioness; and
the males of such animals as neither fight nor feed on flesh, being only
distinguishable from the female by some peculiarity in the covering of
their bodies, as the cock and hen in many birds. The male of the human species is distinguished from the female both by his general strength
and his covering, as also by a difference of voice.

In these orders of animals whose sexes are distinct, we may not only
observe the genital organs to be subject to mal-conformation, as in any
other part of the animal, but that an attempt is sometimes made to
unite the two organs in the same animal body, making what may be
called an unnatural hermaphrodite. In producing the unnatural hermaphrodite the same laws seem to operate as in the mal-conformation
of other parts of animals; it being observable, that these deviations obtain through a whole species precisely in the same manner. I have
already given an account of the free-martin, which exhibits a mixture
of the two parts of generation in the same animal.

It is my intention at present to extend my inquiry on this subject no
further than what relates to the resemblance which one sex bears to
another in those distinguishing properties which I term secondary; for
we find that there is often a change of the natural properties of the
female sex into those of the secondary of the male; the female, in such
cases, now and then assuming the secondary peculiarities of the male.
It is to be observed, that some classes are more liable than others to this
change, a singular example of which is to be the subject of the following
pages.

To bring the foregoing observations into one point of view, I here
beg leave to remark, that in animals just born, or very young, there are
no peculiarities to distinguish one sex from the other, exclusive of what

---

[The difference in the size of the two sexes is sufficiently marked in most of the
Raptorial birds; but it is the female which has the advantage in this respect.]

relates to the organs of generation, which can only be in those who have external parts; and that towards the age of maturity the discriminating changes before mentioned begin to appear; the male then losing that resemblance he had to the female in various secondary properties*; but that in all animals which are not of any distinct sex, called hermaphrodites, there is no such alteration taking place in their form when they arrive at that age. It is evidently the male which at this time in such respects recedes from the female, every female being at the age of maturity more like the young of the same species than the male is observed to be; and if the male is deprived of his testes when young, he retains more of the original youthful form, and therefore more resembles the female.

From hence it might be supposed that the female character contains more truly the specific properties of the animal than the male; but the character of every animal is that which is marked by the properties common to both sexes, which are found in a natural hermaphrodite, as in a snail, or in animals of neither sex, as the castrated male or spayed female.

But where the sexes are separate, and the animals have two characters, the one cannot more than the other be called the true, as the real distinguishing marks of each particular species, as has been mentioned above, are those common to both sexes, and which are likewise in the unnatural hermaphrodite. That these properties give the distinct character of such animals is evident, for the castrated male and the spayed female have both the same common properties; and when I treated of the free-martin, which is a monstrous hermaphrodite, I observed that it was more like the ox than the cow or bull; so that the marks characteristic of the species which are found in the animal of a double sex are imitated by depriving the individual of certain sexual parts, in consequence of which it retains only the true properties of the species.

They are curious facts in the natural history of animals, that by depriving either sex of the true parts of generation, they shall seem to approach each other in appearances, and acquire a resemblance to the unnatural hermaphrodite.

In some species of animals that have the secondary properties we have mentioned, there is a deviation from the general rules, by the perfect female, with respect to the parts of generation, assuming more or less the secondary character of the male

This change does not appear to arise from any action produced at the first formation of the animal, and in this respect is similar to what takes

* This is not common to all animals of distinct sexes, for in fishes there is no great difference; nor in many insects; nor in dogs, as has been already observed: however, it is considerable in many quadrupeds, but appears to be most so in birds.

place in the male; neither does it grow up with the animal as it does to
a certain degree in the male, but seems to be one of those changes which
happen at a particular period, similar to many common and natural
phenomena; like to what is observed of the horns of the stag, which
differ at different ages; or to the mane of the lion, which does not grow
till after his fifth year, &c.[a]

This change has been observed in some of the bird tribe, but principally in the common pheasant; and it has been observed by those who
are conversant with this bird, when wild, that there every now and then
appears a hen pheasant with the feathers of a cock: all, however, that
they have described on the subject is, that this animal does not breed,
and that its spurs do not grow. Some years ago one of these was sent
to the late Dr. William Hunter, which I examined, and found it to have
all the parts peculiar to the female of that bird. This specimen is still
preserved in Dr. Hunter's museum.

Dr. Pitcairn having received a pheasant of this kind from Sir Thomas
Harris, showed it as a curiosity to Sir Joseph Banks and Dr. Solander.
I happening to be then present, was desired to examine the bird, and
the following was the result of my examination.

I found the parts of generation to be truly female, they being as perfect as in any hen pheasant that is not in the least prepared for laying
eggs, and having both the ovary and oviduct.

As the observations hitherto made have been principally upon birds
found wild, little of their history can be known; but from what took
place in a hen pheasant, in the possession of a friend of Sir Joseph Banks,
it appears probable that this change of character takes place at an advanced period of the animal's life, and does not grow up with it from
the beginning. This lady, who had for some time bred pheasants, and
paid particular attention to them, observed that one of the hens, after
having produced several broods, moulted, when the succeeding feathers
were those of a cock, and that this animal was never afterwards impregnated. Hence it is most probable that all the hen pheasants found wild,
having the feathers of a cock, were formerly perfect hens, but have been
changed by age, or perhaps by certain constitutional circumstances[b].

---

[a] [We have observed in the young African lions at the Zoological Gardens, that the
mane began to be distinctly developed at the third year, and was completed at the fourth.]

[b] [The cause of the change in the plumage which Mr. Hunter here alludes to, has
been proved by subsequent dissections to be effective and not uncommon. See the
paper entitled 'On the Change in the Plumage of some Hen-Pheasants,' by Wm. Yarrell,
Esq., Phil. Trans. 1827, in which the author states, that "certain constitutional circumstances producing this change may, and do occur, at any period during the life of
the fowl, and that they can be produced by artificial means."]

Having bought some pheasants from a dealer in birds, among which were several hens, I perceived, the year after, that one of the hens did not lay, and that she began to change her feathers. The year following she had nearly the plumage of the cock, but less brilliant, especially on the head; and it is more than probable that this was an old hen, nearly under circumstances similar to those before described.

Lady Tynte had a favourite pied pea-hen which had produced chickens eight several times; having moulted when about eleven years old, the lady and family were astonished by her displaying the feathers peculiar to the other sex, and appeared like a pied peacock. In this process the tail, which became like that of the cock, first made its appearance after moulting; and in the following year, having moulted again, produced similar feathers. In the third year she did the same, and, in addition, had spurs resembling those of a cock. She never bred after this change in her plumage, and died in the following winter during the hard frost in the year 1775–6. This bird is now preserved in the museum of the late Sir Ashton Lever*.

From what has been related of these three birds, we may conclude, that this change is merely the effect of age, and obtains to a certain degree in every class of animals. We find something similar taking place even in the human species; for that increase of hair observable on the faces of many women in advanced life is an approach towards the beard, which is one of the most distinguishing secondary properties of man.

Thus we see the sexes which, at an early period, had little to distinguish them from each other, acquiring about the time of puberty secondary properties, which clearly characterize the male and female, the male at this time receding from the female, and assuming the secondary properties of his sex.

The female, at a much later time of life, when the powers of propagation cease, loses many of her peculiar properties, and may be said, except from mere structure of parts, to be of no sex, even receding from the original character of the animal, and approaching, in appearance, towards the male, or perhaps more properly towards the hermaphrodite.

---

* It might be supposed that this bird was really a cock which had been substituted for the hen; but the following facts put this matter beyond a doubt. First, there was no other pied pea-fowl in the county. Secondly, the hen had nobs on her toes, which were the same after her change. Thirdly, she was as small after the change as before, therefore too small for a cock. Fourthly, she was a favourite bird, and was generally fed by the lady, and used to come for her food, which she still continued to do after the change in the feathers.

AN EXPERIMENT TO DETERMINE THE EFFECT OF EXTIR-
PATING ONE OVARIUM UPON THE NUMBER OF YOUNG
PRODUCED[a].

IN all animals of distinct sex, the females, those of the Bird-kind
excepted, have, I believe, two ovaria, and of course the oviducts are
in pairs.

By distinct sex I mean when the parts destined to the purposes of
generation are of two kinds, each kind appropriated to an individual of
each species, distinguished by the appellation of male and female, and
equally necessary to the propagation of the animal. The testicles, with
their appendages, constitute the male; the ovaria, and their appendages,
the female sex.

As the ovaria are the organs which, on the part of the female, furnish
what is necessary towards the production of the third, or young animal, and as females appear to have a limited portion of the middle stage
of life allotted for that purpose, it becomes a question, whether those
organs are worn out by repeated acts of propagation; or whether there
is not a natural and constitutional period to that power on their part,
even if such power has never been exerted? If we consider this subject in every view, taking the human species as an example, we shall
discover that circumstances, either local or constitutional, may be capable of extinguishing in the female the faculty of propagation. Thus
we may observe when a woman begins to breed at an early period, as
at fifteen, and has her children fast, that she seldom breeds longer than
the age of thirty or thirty-five; therefore we may suppose either that
the parts are then worn out, or that the breeding constitution is over:
If a woman begins later, as at twenty or twenty-five, she may continue
to breed to the age of forty or more; and there are, now and then, instances of women who, not having conceived before, have had children
as late in life as at fifty years or upwards. After that period few women
breed, even though they should not have bred before; therefore there
must be a natural period to the power of conception. A similar stop to
propagation may likewise take place in other classes of animals, probably in the female of every class, the period varying according to cir-

---

[a] [Originally published in the Philosophical Transactions, vol. lxxvii. p. 233; read,
March 22, 1787.]

cumstances. But still we are not enabled to determine how far it depends on any particular property of the constitution, or of the ovarium alone.

As the female, in most classes of animals, has two ovaria, I imagined that by removing one it might be possible to determine how far their actions were reciprocally influenced by each other, from the changes which by comparison might be observed to take place, either by the breeding-period being shortened, or perhaps, in those animals whose nature it is to bring forth more than one at a time, by the number produced at each birth being diminished.

There are two views in which this subject may be considered. The first, that the ovaria, when properly employed, may be bodies determined and unalterable respecting the number of young to be produced. In this case we can readily imagine that, when one ovarium is removed, the other may be capable of producing its determined number in two different ways: one, when the remaining ovarium, not influenced by the loss of the other, will produce its allotted number, and in the same time; the other, when affected by the loss, yet the constitution demanding the same number of young each time of breeding, as if there were still two ovaria; it must furnish double the number it would have been required to supply had both been allowed to remain, but must consequently cease from the performance of its function in half the time. The second view of the subject is, by supposing that there is not originally any fixed number which the ovarium must produce, but that the number is increased or diminished according to circumstances; that it is rather the constitution at large that determines the number; and that if one ovarium is removed, the other will be called upon by the constitution to perform the operations of both, by which means the animal should produce with one ovarium the same number of young as would have been produced if both had remained.

With an intention to ascertain those points as far as I could, I was led to make the following experiment; and for that purpose gave pigs a preference to any other animal, as being easily managed, producing several at a litter, and breeding perfectly well under the confinement necessary for experiments. I selected two females of the same colour and size, and likewise a boar-pig, all of the same farrow; and, having removed an ovarium from one of the females, I cut a slit in one ear to distinguish it from the other. They were well fed and kept warm, that there might be no impediment to their breeding; and whenever they farrowed, their pigs were taken away exactly at the same age:

About the beginning of the year 1779 they both took the boar; the one which had been spayed earlier than the perfect female. The distance of time, however, was not great, and they continued breeding at nearly the same times. The spayed animal continued to breed till September 1783, when she was six years' old, which was a space of more than four years. In that time she had eight farrows; but did not take the boar afterwards, and had in all seventy-six pigs. The perfect one continued breeding till December 1785, when she was about eight years old, a period of almost six years, in which time she had thirteen farrows, and had in all one hundred and sixty-two pigs; after this time she did not breed: I kept her till November 1786.

I have here annexed a table of the different times of each farrow, with the number of pigs produced.

Spayed Sow.

Farrows.	Number of young.	Time.
1	6	Dec. 1779.
2	8	July 1780.
3	6	Jan. 1781.
4	10	Aug. 1781.
5	10	Mar. 1782.
6	9	Sept. 1782.
7	14	May 1783.
8	13	Sept. 1783.
	76	

November following she was put to the boar, but brought no pigs. April 1784, she was again put to the boar, without effect, and never was observed to take the boar afterwards, although often with him. November 1784, she was killed.

Perfect Sow.

Farrows.	Number of young.	Time.
1	9	
2	6	
3	8	
4	13	Dec. 1781.
5	10	June 1782.
6	16	Dec. 1782.
7	13	June 1783.
8	12	Oct. 1783.
	87	

Eleven pigs more than were produced by the spayed sow in her eight farrows.

Farrows.	Number of young.	Time.
9	12	Feb. 1784.
10	16	June 1784.
11	12	Dec. 1784.
12	16	May 1785.
13	19	Dec. 1785.
	75	

After which she bred no more.

The first eight farrows were................. 87
The last five farrows were 75

Total.. 162
The number from the spayed one.... 76

More than farrowed by the imperfect animal 86

It is observable that both sows rather increased in their number each time as they grew older, although not uniformly; the difference between the first and last in both animals being considerable.

From the above table we find that the sow with only one ovarium bred till she was six years old, from the latter end of 1779 till September 1783, about four years, and in that time brought forth seventy-six pigs. The perfect animal bred till she was eight years of age; and if conception depended on the ovaria, we might have expected that she would bring forth double the number at each birth; or, if not, that she would continue breeding for double the time. We indeed find her producing ten more than double the number of the imperfect animal, although she had not double the number of farrows; but this may perhaps be explained by observing that the number of young increased as the female grew older, and the perfect sow continued to breed much longer than the other.

From a circumstance mentioned in the course of this experiment it appears that the desire for the male continues after the power of breeding is exhausted in the female; and therefore does not altogether depend on the powers of the ovaria to propagate, although it may probably be influenced by the existence of such parts.

If these observations should be considered as depending on a single experiment, from which alone it is not justifiable to draw conclusions, I have only to add that the difference in the number of pigs produced by each was greater than can be justly imputed to accident, and is a circumstance certainly in favour of the universality of the principle I wished to ascertain *.

From this experiment it seems most probable that the ovaria are from the beginning destined to produce a fixed number, beyond which they cannot go, although circumstances may tend to diminish that number; but that the constitution at large has no power of giving to one ovarium the power of propagating equal to both; for in the present experiment the animal with one ovarium produced ten pigs less than half the number brought forth by the sow with both ovaria. But that the constitution has so far a power of influencing one ovarium as to make it produce its number in a less time than would probably have been the case if both ovaria had been preserved, is to be inferred from the above-recited experiment.

* It may be thought by some that I should have repeated this experiment; but an annual expense of twenty pounds for ten years, and the necessary attention to make the experiment complete, will be a sufficient reason for my not having done it.

THE CASE OF A YOUNG WOMAN WHO POISONED HER-SELF IN THE FIRST MONTH OF HER PREGNANCY:

BY THOMAS OGLE, SURGEON, GREAT RUSSELL-STREET, BLOOMSBURY.

To which is added, an Account of the Appearances after Death; by the late John Hunter[a].

MARY HUNT, servant to a gentleman in Charlotte-street, Bedford-square, twenty-five years of age, had for some time shown a partiality for one of the footmen in the same family. She became all at once exceedingly dejected, which was supposed to proceed from his neglecting her; and on Thursday, the 19th of April, at twelve o'clock at night, took half an ounce of white arsenic, and immediately afterwards drank a quart of wine; about one o'clock she had so much pain in her stomach as to be obliged to call for assistance.

The symptoms were excruciating pain in the stomach, sickness, vomiting, excessive thirst, and a small tremulous pulse; these were followed by pain in the bowels, and several purging stools.

She drank brandy and water, wine and water, and several quarts of plain water, to relieve the thirst and ease the pain. Some hours after taking the arsenic she became easier, expressed a desire to be left alone, being inclined to sleep, and remained several hours in a dosing or comatose state, from which she did not recover, and died about one o'clock on Friday, thirteen hours after taking the arsenic.

Upon inspecting the body after death there were found the following appearances.

In the cavity of the abdomen there was an appearance of the effects of slight inflammation on the peritoneal coat of the small intestines.

The stomach contained a greenish fluid, with a curdy substance in it, in all amounting to about twelve ounces.

On the internal surface of the great curvature near the cardia a portion of the villous coat, about the size of a crown-piece, was partly destroyed, and of a dark red colour, with a regularly defined edge, and some of the arsenic adhering to different parts of its surface. The rest of the stomach was in a natural state. This appearance in the stomach was an effect produced by the arsenic.

---

a [Originally published in the Transactions of a Society for the Improvement of Medical and Chirurgical Knowledge, vol. ii. p. 63. Communicated to the Society by Everard Home, and read August 5, 1794.]

The uterus was a little enlarged, and had the vessels unusually loaded with red blood.

There was an uncommon quantity of blood in the vessels of the ovaria and Fallopian tubes, but principally in those of the ovarium, and morsus diaboli of the left side.

The organs of generation being carefully removed, and both ovaria being slit open, there was found in the left a corpus luteum.

It was evident, from this circumstance, that conception had taken place; which led to an inquiry respecting the last appearance of her menses, which appeared by the evidence of the family to have been little more than a month before her death.

With the dread upon her mind of being with child, the usual period of menstruation had hardly elapsed without its appearing, which confirmed her suspicions, before she, in a fit of despair, put an end to her life.

From this evidence, the period of conception could not exceed a month, and probably was much within that time.

As it was interesting to have the parts accurately examined, to see what information might be acquired respecting the fœtus at so early a period, they were given to Mr. Hunter for that purpose, whose observations upon them are contained in the following account.

The arteries of the uterus were injected, and the smaller vessels were filled to so great a degree of minuteness that the whole surface became extremely red.

The cervix uteri and os tincæ were of their natural size; but the body, or that portion of the uterus next the fundus, was a little enlarged, and more prominent externally in the middle. The spermatic vessels were also enlarged.

On cutting into the substance of the uterus, it had more of a laminated structure than in the unimpregnated state: this appearance of lamellæ appeared upon examination to be formed by veins somewhat enlarged, compressed and transversely divided. The uterus was unusually soft in texture, and terminated on the internal surface in a pulpy substance.

The blood-vessels of the uterus passed into and ramified upon this pulpy substance, which was continued across at the cervix uteri, so as to make the cavity of the uterus a circumscribed bag; and at this part the pulpy substance was so thin as to resemble the retina.

This cavity had a smooth but irregular internal surface, and the pulpy substance upon which it was formed was evidently blood coagulated and varied in its thickness in different parts. Upon a longitudinal section of the uterus, the posterior part of the coagulum, which was the thickest, was nearly half an inch; where it terminated towards the cervix it was pendulous and unattached. There were also several loose processes, all turned towards the cervix, one of them very thin, as broad as a silver penny, and only attached by one edge to the fundus near the opening of the right Fallopian tube.

On slitting open the Fallopian tubes, the coagulum was found to pass some way into them, and to extend more than half an inch on the left side, which had the corpus luteum. The coagulum was thickest at the orifice of the tube, and there adhered to the inner surface for the eighth part of an inch; beyond which it became smaller and terminated in a point. In the left tube the coagulum was in two places coiled or folded upon itself, as if thrown back by the action of the tube. The portions of the coagulum at the orifices of the tubes were hollow.

When the inner surface of the cavity of the uterus was examined with a magnifying glass it was found extremely vascular, and dotted with innumerable whitish spots too small to be seen by the naked eye.

In the examination of this uterus and Fallopian tubes, as Mr. Hunter's chief object was the detection of the embryo, no precaution was omitted which could be devised to prevent it being overlooked or destroyed.

The uterus was opened in a bason of clear water, the incision was conducted with great circumspection, and very slowly continued, till the whole of the cavity was exposed. Every part of the internal surface was minutely examined with magnifying glasses; but in no situation was there anything resembling an embryo to be found.

The presence of a corpus luteum, the enlargement of the uterus, the newly-formed vascular membrane, or decidua, lining the cavity, and the history of the case, sufficiently prove conception to have taken place; and the embryo being nowhere detected by an examination so accurate, and conducted by an anatomist so skilful in minute investigation, would induce a belief that the fœtus had not been sufficiently advanced to take on a regular form.

The appearances in the uterus, here described, the late Dr. Hunter, in his lectures, mentioned to have seen at a very early period after impregnation: so far they are not entirely new. The accuracy of the examination renders this case valuable, as it seems to enable us to decide a point hitherto not at all understood—that certain changes in the uterus not only take place previous to the reception of the fœtus, but that the fœtus does not acquire a visible form for some time after these changes have been made[a].

---

[a] [The positive conclusions deduced from this case, viz. that certain changes take place in the uterus within one month after conception, have been confirmed by all those

anatomists who have enjoyed similar opportunities of examining the uterine organs within the same period.   These changes consist essentially in the effusion of fibrine or coagulable lymph from the villi of the lining membrane of the uterus, which villi also become much elongated and highly vascular; and minute vessels are continued from them into the effused lymph, forming loops or arches in that substance.   This process is compared by Hunter, in the following paper, to the effusion of lymph consequent on the introduction of an extraneous living part into any of the cavities of the body: and Professor von Baer, in a recent elaborate description of the uterus of a female who drowned herself eight days after impregnation, makes the same comparison.   Professor Weber, in an examination of the uterus seven days after conception, also speaks of the great vascularity of its inner surface, and describes the villi as consisting of small cylinders placed perpendicularly to the inner surface of the uterus, united by a slimy membrane, and forming together a layer of a pale soft substance, from half a line to a line in thickness; whilst in some places the cylinder presented the length of from two to three lines.

With respect to the negative results of Mr. Hunter's examination relative to the reception of the foetus in the uterus, and "its acquisition of a visible form," I suppose that the word 'foetus' is here used to express the product of generation, or ovum, especially as it is stated, that "in the examination of the uterus and Fallopian tubes Mr. Hunter's chief object was the detection of the 'embryo.'"   Now if the product of generation were really expected to have been seen in that state of development which we understand by the terms embryo and foetus, its presence was most likely overlooked; since, from the analogy of the dog and rabbit, it most probably would have existed merely as a small pellucid vesicle or ovum, supposing that it had escaped from the ovarium; and it is to be regretted that the expression " there was found in the left 'ovarium' a corpus luteum" is all the evidence on that point which the present case affords.

In the bitch, Von Baer has shown that the ova pass into the Fallopian tubes on the eighth day after impregnation, and that when they reach the uterus they lie quite free in its cavity, are perfectly transparent, of a somewhat elongated form, and extremely delicate texture, and are from half a line to a third of a line in diameter.

In the rabbit, the observations of De Graaf, of Prevost and Dumas, and of Coste, prove that the ova pass into the tubes the third (or, according to Coste, the second) day after impregnation; they reach the horns of the uterus on the fourth day, and are then about a line in diameter, in the form of pellucid bubbles, free and moveable.

According to Home, the human ovum has reached the uterus on the eighth day after impregnation, when it is described as presenting an elliptical form, rather more than a line ($\frac{19}{200}$ parts of an inch) in length, and $\frac{9}{200}$ parts of an inch in breadth.   It is composed of two membranes, of which the external is of considerable thickness and consistence, very little transparent, quite smooth, and milk-white: the internal membrane or bag consists 'of a seemingly very thin, perfectly smooth, and glossy membrane, which seemed to have considerable strength.'   This internal membrane contained a thick slimy matter, like honey, and "two round corpuscles, apparently more opake, and of a yellowish tint," regarded as "the probable seat of the future heart and brain."

On comparing the preceding account with the observations that have been made on the mammiferous ovum, it will be found that the nearest resemblance to the supposed human ovum obtains in that of the ornithorhynchus, at least in the texture of the two membranes described, of which the external must be regarded as the chorion, the internal as the membrana vitelli.   In the ornithorhynchus, as in the ovo-viviparous reptiles, the chorion is dense and unyielding; but in the specimens which we examined, and which, as in Sir Everard Home's case, had been subjected to the action of spirit, the chorion was semitransparent.   In those mammalia, however, which approximate the human species in the placental development of the foetus, the ovum, when it has been detected un-

attached in the uterus, has invariably presented a translucency and delicacy of its membranes, with which the structure of the human ovum, as described by Home, is totally
at variance; and, from the tenour of the whole account, we believe the object to have
been what Mr. Bauer, to whom its description and delineation were confided[1], declared
it to resemble, viz. the egg of an insect.

Rejecting, then, the description we have just been considering,—and its apocryphal
character is rightly admitted by all physiologists of the present day, who have investigated the nature of the mammiferous ovum,—the determination of the period of the
passage of the human ovum into the uterus after impregnation, and its condition and
structure when first received into that cavity, still remain open to the researches of the
physiologist.]

----

[1] "As the ovum was so extremely small as to admit of dispute whether it was one
or not, I carried it immediately to Kew, to Mr. Bauer, who, after examining it, said it
looked like the egg of an insect."—*Phil. Trans.*, p. 255.

Mr. Clift, who laid open the uterus in question, and patiently scrutinized the whole
of its cavity without perceiving any trace of an ovum, has always been of opinion that
the one afterwards detected by Home was dropped from one of the numerous flesh-flies
which were buzzing about at the time of the examination.

ON THE STRUCTURE OF THE PLACENTA.

THE connexion between the mother and fœtus in the human subject, has in every age, in which science has been cultivated, called forth the attention of the anatomist, the physiologist, and even the philosopher; but both that connexion, and the structure of the parts which form the connexion, were unknown till about the year 1754. The subject is certainly most interesting, and the discovery important; and it is my intention, in the following pages, to give such an account of it as I hope may be acceptable to the public*; while, at the same time, I establish my own claim to the discovery. But that I may not seem to arrogate to myself more merit than I am entitled to, let me, in justice to another person, relate what follows.

The late indefatigable Dr. MacKenzie, about the month of May, 1754, when assistant to Dr. Smellie, having procured the body of a pregnant woman, who died undelivered at the full term, had injected both the veins and arteries with particular success, the veins being filled with yellow, the arteries with red †.

Having opened the abdomen, and exposed the uterus, he made an incision into the fore part, quite through its substance, and came to what seemed to be an irregular mass of injected matter. The appearance being new he proceeded no further, and greatly obliged me, by desiring my attendance to examine parts, in which the appearances were so uncommon. The examination was made in his presence, and in the presence of several other gentlemen, whose names I have now forgotten; but I have reason to believe that some are settled in this country, who I hope will have an opportunity of perusing this publication‡.

* This paper was read at the Royal Society, but as the facts had before that time been given to the public, it was not published in the Philosophical Transactions.

† Dr. MacKenzie being then an assistant to the late Dr. Smellie, the procuring and dissecting this woman without Dr. Smellie's knowledge was the cause of a separation between them, for the leading steps to such a discovery could not be kept a secret. The winter following Dr. MacKenzie began to teach midwifery in the Borough of Southwark.

‡ If I should be so fortunate as to have this publication fall into any of those gentlemen's hands, I hope they will favour me with their opinion of my state of the facts, which led to the discovery.

It may be suspected by some (but none I hope to whom I have the pleasure of being known,) that I am not doing Dr. MacKenzie justice, and am perhaps suppressing some part of that share of the discovery to which he is entitled. This idea (if ever it should

I first raised, with great care, a part of the uterus from the irregular mass, and in doing this observed regular pieces of wax passing obliquely between it and the uterus, which broke off, leaving part attached to that mass; and on attentively examining the portions towards the uterus, they plainly appeared to be a continuation of the veins passing from it to this substance, which proved to be placenta.

I likewise observed other vessels, about the size of a crow-quill, passing in the same manner, although not so obliquely; these also broke upon separating the placenta and uterus, leaving a small portion on the surface of the placenta; and on examination they were discovered to be continuations of the arteries of the uterus. My next step was to trace these vessels into the substance of what appeared placenta, which was first attempted in a vein; but that soon lost the regularity of a vessel, by terminating at once upon the surface of the placenta in a very fine spongy substance, the interstices of which were filled with the yellow injected matter. This termination being new, I repeated the same kind of examination on other veins, which always led me to the same terminations, never entering the substance of the placenta in the form of a vessel. I then examined the arteries, tracing them in the same manner towards the placenta, and found that, having made a twist, or close spiral turn upon themselves, they were lost on its surface. On a more attentive view, I perceived that they terminated in the same way as the veins; for opposite to the mouth of the artery the spongy substance of the placenta was readily distinguished with the red injection intermixed.

Upon cutting into the placenta I discovered, in many places of its substance, yellow injection, in others red, and in many others these two colours mixed. The substance of the placenta, now filled with injection, had nothing of the vascular appearance, nor that of extravasation, but had a regularity in its form which showed it to be naturally of a cellular structure, fitted to be a reservoir for blood.

I perceived, likewise, that the red injection of the arteries (which had been first injected,) had passed out of the substance of the placenta into some of the veins leading from the placenta to the uterus, mixing itself with the yellow injection; and that the spongy chorion, called the de-

arise,) I may probably not be able to remove; but I hope it will also be seen that I myself have given rise to it; believing, if I had been so inclined, that I might have suppressed Dr. MacKenzie's name altogether without ever running the hazard of being detected. I was indeed so tenacious of my claim to the discovery, that I wrote this account in Dr. MacKenzie's lifetime, with a design to publish it; and often communicated my intentions to Dr. George Fordyce, who I knew was very intimate with the Doctor, in consequence of both teaching in the same place, and making many experiments together; therefore he is a kind of collateral witness, that what I now publish is the same account which I gave in Dr. MacKenzie's lifetime.

cidua by Dr. Hunter, was very vascular, its vessels going to and from the uterus, being filled with the different coloured injections.

After having considered these appearances, it was not difficult for me to determine the real structure of the placenta and course of the blood in these parts: but the company, prejudiced in favour of former theories, combated my opinion; and it was even disputed whether or not these curling arteries could carry red blood. After having dissected the uterus, with the placenta and membranes, and made the whole into preparations, tending to show the above facts, I returned home in the evening, and communicating what I had discovered to my brother, Dr. Hunter, who at first treated it and me with good-humoured raillery; but on going with me to Dr. MacKenzie's he was soon convinced of the fact. Some of the parts were given to him, which he afterwards showed at his lectures, and probably they still remain in his collection.

Soon after this time Dr. Hunter and I procured several placentæ, to discover if, after delivery, the termination of the veins and the curling arteries could be observed: they were discernible almost in every one; and by pushing a pipe into the placenta we could fill not only its whole substance, but also the vessels on that surface which was attached to the uterus, with injection.

The facts being now ascertained and universally acknowledged, I consider myself as having a just claim to the discovery of the structure of the placenta, and its communication with the uterus, together with the use arising from such structure and communication, and of having first demonstrated the vascularity of the spongy chorion.

It is not necessary at present to enter into the various opinions which have been formed on this subject; because, whatever they were, they could not be just, the structure of the parts not being known: neither shall I endeavour to give a complete description of all the parts immediately connected with uterine gestation, but content myself with describing the structure of the placenta, as far as it has any relation to the uterus and child; and with explaining the connexion between the two; leaving the reader to examine what has been said upon this subject by others, especially by Dr. Hunter, in that very accurate and elaborate work which he has published on the Gravid Uterus, in which he has minutely described and accurately delineated the parts, without mentioning the mode of discovery.

The necessary connexion subsisting in all animals between the mother and fœtus, for the nourishment of the latter, as far as I know, takes place in two ways. In some it is continued, and subsists through the whole term of gestation; in others the union is soon dissolved; but an apparatus is provided, which at once furnishes what is sufficient for the support of the animal till it comes forth.

The first of these are the viviparous, the second the oviparous animals, both of which admit of great variety in the mode by which the same effect is produced*. In the first division is included the human species, which alone will engage our present attention. But before I describe this connexion, it may be necessary that the reader should understand my idea of generation: I shall therefore refer him to what I have said upon that subject in my account of the free-martin†.

In the human species, the anatomical structure of the mother and embryo, relative to fœtation, being well known, it will only be necessary fully to describe the nature of the connexion between them, which is formed by the intermediate substance called placenta. For this purpose we must first consider the placenta as a common part; next, the uterus as belonging to the mother, yet having an immediate connexion with the placenta, from which the nourishment of the fœtus is to be derived, which will lead us lastly to a consideration of those peculiarities of structure by means of which the fœtus is to receive its nourishment, and which likewise constitutes its immediate communication with the placenta. It is the structure of this intermediate substance, and its connexion with the child and the uterus of the mother, which have hitherto been so little understood, and without an accurate knowledge of which it was impossible any just idea could be formed of its functions.

The placenta is a mass lying nearly in contact with the uterus; indeed it may in some degree be said to be in continuity with a part of its internal surface. On the side applied to the uterus the placenta is lobulated, having deep irregular fissures. It is probable, from this structure of the placenta, that the uterus has an intestine motion while in the time of uterine gestation, not an expulsive one; which those lobes of the placenta allow of; but all these lobes are united into one uniform surface on that surface next to the child, where its umbilical vessels ramify. When we cut into the placenta its whole substance appears to be little else than a network, or spongy mass, through which the blood-vessels of the fœtus ramify, and indeed seems to be principally formed by the ramifications of those vessels; it exhibits

---

* It may be remarked here, that the oviparous admit of being distinguished into two classes, one where the egg is hatched in the belly, as in the viper, which has been commonly called viviparous; the others, where the eggs have been first laid and then hatched, which is the class commonly called oviparous, such as all the bird tribe; and many others, as snakes, lizards, &c.

† See page 34.

hardly any appearance of connecting membrane; but we cannot readily suppose it to be without such a membrane, as there is so much regularity in its texture. The cells, or interstices of each lobe, communicate with one another, even much more freely than those of the cellular membrane in any other part of the body; so that whatever fluid will pass in at one part, readily diffuses itself through the whole mass of lobe; and all the cells of each lobe have a communication at the common base.

This structure of the placenta, and its reciprocal communication with the two bodies with which it is immediately connected, form the union between the mother and fœtus for the support of the latter. Prior to the time I have mentioned above, anatomists seem to have been wholly unacquainted with the true structure of placenta. By notes taken from Dr. Hunter's lectures, in the winter 1755-6, it appears that he expressed himself in the following manner*. "The substance of the placenta is a fleshy mass, which seems to be formed entirely of the vessels of the umbilical rope." In another part, mentioning the appearances when injected, he says: "and upon a slight putrefaction coming on, you will find the whole appearing like a mass of vessels": then says, "there is always a white uninjected substance between the vessels; but whether lymphatics or what I cannot tell." This uninjected substance, mentioned by Dr. Hunter, is what forms the cellular structure.

The placenta seems to be principally composed of the ramifications of the vessels of the embryo, and may have been originally formed in consequence of those next to the uterus laying hold by a species of animal attraction of the coagulable lymph which lines the uterus. It might take place in a manner resembling what happens when the root of a plant spreads on the surface of moist bodies, with this difference, that in the present instance the vessels form the substance through which they ramify, as in the case of granulations.

At the time, or perhaps before, the female seed enters the uterus, coagulable lymph, from the blood of the mother, is thrown out everywhere on its inner surface, either from the stimulus of impregnation taking place in the ovarium, or in consequence of the seed being expelled from it. But I think the first the most probable supposition; for we find in extra-uterine cases that the decidua is formed in the uterus, although the ovum never enters it, which is a proof that it is produced by the stimulus of impregnation in the ovarium, and that it is prior to the entrance of the ovum into the uterus. When it has en-

---

* These quotations were taken from Mr. Galhie's MS. of Dr. Hunter's lectures, who is one of the gentlemen that favoured Dr. Hunter, upon a former occasion, with the use of his notes. See Dr. Hunter's Commentaries.

tered the uterus it attaches itself to that coagulable lymph, by which, being covered and immediately surrounded*, there is formed a soft pulpy membrane, the decidua, which I believe is peculiar to the human species and to monkeys, I never having found it in any other animal. That part which covers the seed or fœtus, where it is not immediately attached to the uterus, and likewise forms a membrane, was discovered by Dr. Hunter, and is by him called decidua reflexa†. The whole of this coagulable lymph continues to be a living part for the time; the vessels of the uterus ramify upon it; and where the vessels of the fœtus form the placenta there the vessels of the uterus, after passing through the decidua, open into the cellular substance of the placenta, as before described. As this membrane lines the uterus and covers the seed, it is stretched out, and becomes thinner and thinner, as the uterus is distended by the fœtus growing larger, especially that part of it, called decidua reflexa, which covers the fœtus; as there it cannot possibly acquire any new matter, except we could suppose that the fœtus assisted in the formation of it. This membrane is most distinct where it covers the chorion; for where it covers the placenta it is blended with coagula in the great veins that pass obliquely through it, more especially all round the edge, where innumerable large veins come out; but the chorion and decidua can be easily distinguished from one another, the decidua being less elastic.

From the description now given, I think we are justified in supposing the placenta to be formed entirely by the fœtus, which is further confirmed by extra-uterine cases, and by the formation of the membrane in the egg, there being no living organic part to furnish them; and the decidua we must suppose to be a production of the mother: of both which the circumstance of the decidua passing between the placenta and uterus may be considered as an additional proof. For if the vessels of the fœtus branched into a part of the decidua, we might conceive the whole placenta to be formed from that exudation; the portion of it, where the vessels had ramified like the roots of a plant, becoming thicker than the rest, and forming the placenta. If that were the case, this

---

* This is somewhat similar to another operation in the animal œconomy. If an extraneous living part is introduced into any cavity it will be immediately inclosed with coagulable lymph. Thus we find worms inclosed, and hydatids, that have been detached, afterwards inclosed; but in those cases this is a consequence of the pressure of the extraneous body, whereas in the uterus it is preparatory.

† The placenta is certainly a fœtal part, and is formed on the inside of the spongy chorion, or decidua. How far the decidua reflexa is a uterine part I do not yet know; if it is, then the ovum must be placed in a doubling of the coagulum, which forms the decidua: but if the ovum is attached to the inside of the decidua, then the decidua reflexa is belonging to the fœtus.

membrana decidua, when traced from the parts distinct, and at a distance from the placenta, should be plainly seen passing into its substance all round at the edges, as a continuation of it. But the fact is quite otherwise; for the decidua can be distinctly traced between the placenta and uterus, hardly ever passing between the lobuli, the vessels of the fœtus never entering into it, and of course none of them ever coming in absolute contact with the uterus. But what may be considered as still a stronger proof that the decidua is furnished by the uterus is, that in cases of extra-uterine conception, where the fœtus is wholly in the ovarium or Fallopian tube, we find the uterus lined with the decidua, having taken on the uterine action; but no placenta, that being formed by the fœtus, and therefore in the part which contained it.

The vessels of the fœtus adhering, by the intervention of the decidua, to a certain portion of the uterus when both are yet small, as the uterus increases in every part of its surface during the time of uterine gestation, we must suppose that this surface of adhesion increases also; and that by the elongation of those vessels of the fœtus in every direction this substance should likewise be increased in every direction. This is in some degree the case, yet the placenta does not occupy so much of the enlarged surface of the uterus as one at first would expect.

The vessels of the uterus in the time of the gestation are increased in size nearly in a proportion equal to the increased circumference of the uterus, and consequently in a proportion much greater than the real increase of its substance. But when we reflect that the uterus ought not to be considered as hollow, but as a body nearly solid, on account of its contents, which derive support from this source, and that a much greater quantity of blood must necessarily pass than what is required for the support of the viscus itself, we cannot be at a loss to account for the greatly increased size of its vessels.

The arteries which are not immediately employed in conveying nourishment to the uterus go on towards the placenta, and, proceeding obliquely between it and the uterus, pass through the decidua without ramifying; just before they enter the placenta, after making two or three close spiral turns upon themselves, they open at once into its spongy substance without any diminution of size, and without passing beyond the surface, as above described. The intention of these spiral turns would appear to be that of diminishing the force of the circulation in the vessels as they approach the spongy substance of the placenta, and is a mechanism calculated to lessen the quick motion of the blood in a part where a quick motion was not required. These curling arteries at this termination are in general about half the size of a crow's quill, and sometimes larger.

The veins of the uterus appropriated to bring back the blood from the placenta commence from this spongy substance by such wide beginnings as are more than equal to the size of the veins themselves. These veins pass obliquely through the decidua to the uterus, enter its substance obliquely, and immediately communicate with the proper veins of the uterus. The area of these veins bears no proportion to their circumference, the veins being very much flattened.

This structure of parts points out at once the nature of the blood's motion in the placenta; but as this is a fact but lately ascertained, a just idea may perhaps be conveyed by saying that it is similar, as far as we yet know, to the blood's motion through the cavernous substance of the penis.

The blood, detached from the common circulation of the mother, moves through the placenta of the fœtus; and is then returned back into the course of the circulation of the mother, to pass on to the heart.

This structure of the placenta, and its communication with the uterus, leads us a step further in our knowledge of the connexion between the mother and fœtus. The blood of the mother must pass freely into the substance of the placenta, and the placenta most probably will be constantly filled; the turgidity of which will assist to squeeze the blood into the mouths of the veins of the uterus, that it may again pass into the common circulation of the mother; and as the interstices of the placenta are of much greater extent than the arteries which convey the blood, the motion of the blood in that part must be so much diminished as almost to approach to stagnation. So far and no further does the mother appear to be concerned in this connexion.

The fœtus has a communication with the placenta of another kind. The arteries from the fœtus pass out to a considerable length, under the name of the umbilical arteries, and when they arrive at the placenta ramify upon its surface, sending into its substance branches which pass through it, and divide into smaller and smaller, till at last they terminate in veins; these, uniting, become larger and larger, and end in one, which at last communicates with the proper circulation of the fœtus.

This course of vessels, and the blood's motion in them, is similar to the course of the vessels and the motion of the blood in other parts of the body[a].

---

[a] [It is well known that the accuracy of this description has been disputed by several Continental anatomists, and has especially been called in question in this country by Dr. Robert Lee, F.R.S., who, with a zeal becoming a sincere lover of truth, deemed it his duty to submit to the scientific world the results of a series of investigations, which he considered to be irreconcileable in some respects with the Hunterian descriptions. During the period in which Dr. Lee was examining, at the College of Surgeons

In addition to what I have said about the connexion between the mother and child in natural cases, it is necessary to observe, that though

---

the Hunterian Preparations, illustrative of the structure and connexions of the placenta, his observations on the obscurity produced by apparently extravasated injection, led me to think of some less objectionable mode of demonstrating the vascular communication between the uterus and placenta, if it existed; or of proving, more satisfactorily than the appearances pointed out by him in the Hunterian preparations seemed to do, that there was no such communication.

This I proposed to do by dissecting the parts under water before disturbing them, either by throwing forcibly foreign matter into the vessels, or by separating the placenta from the uterus, to observe the appearances presented by the opposed surfaces; a proceeding which, if done in the air, is liable to the objection of the possibility of having torn the vessels which were passing across, and the coats of which are acknowledged to be extremely delicate.

For this purpose I was furnished by Dr. Lee with sections of an uninjected and naturally connected uterus and placenta, at the sixth month of uterine gestation, which I fixed under water in an apparatus used for dissecting mollusca, and commenced the dissection from the outside, removing successively, and with great care, the layers fibres, and tracing the veins as they passed deeper and deeper in the substance of the uterus in their course to the deciduous membrane; in which situation, as the thinnest pellicle of membrane is rendered distinct by being supported in the ambient fluid, I naturally expected to see the coats of the veins continued into the deciduous membrane and placenta, and to be able to preserve the appearance in a preparation, if it actually existed in nature. Every vein, however, when traced to the inner surface of the uterus, appeared to terminate in an open mouth on that aspect; the peripheral portion of the coat of the vein, or that next the uterus, ending in a well-defined and smooth semicircular margin, the central part adhering to, and being continuous with, the decidua.

In the course of this dissection I observed that where the veins of different planes communicated with each other, in the substance of the walls of the uterus, the central portion of the parietes of the superficial vein invariably projected in a semilunar form into the deeper-seated one : and where (as was frequently the case, and especially at the point of termination on the inner surface,) two, or even three, of these wide venous channels communicated with a deeper sinus at the same point, the semilunar edges decussated each other so as to allow only a very small part of the deep-seated vein to be seen. It need scarcely be observed how admirably this structure is adapted to ensure the arrest of the current of blood through these passages, upon the contraction of the muscular fibres with which they are everywhere immediately surrounded.

On another portion of the same uterus and placenta, I commenced the examination under water by turning off the placenta and deciduous membrane from the inner surface of the uterus. In this way the small tortuous uterine arteries which enter the deciduous membrane were readily distinguishable, though not filled with injected matter ; and, as it was an object to avoid unnecessary force in the process of separation, they were cut through, though they are easily torn from the decidua. But with respect to the veins, they invariably presented the same appearances as were noticed in the first dissection, terminating in open semicircular orifices, which are closed by the apposition of the deciduous membrane and placenta. This membrane is, however, thinner opposite these orifices than elsewhere, and *in some places appeared to be wanting*, or, adhering to the vein, was torn up with it; but in these cases the minute vessels of the placenta only

the uterus is appropriated for the support of the fœtus, as best fitted for that purpose, yet it is not essential to its growth; as any other part

---

appeared, and never any indication of a vascular trunk or cell commensurate with the size of the vein whose terminal aperture had been lifted up from the part.

The above results of my examination of the impregnated uterus, which had been furnished to me by Dr. Lee, I communicated, as I had promised to do, to that gentleman. They appeared decisive of the fact that the veins of the uterus were not continued as such across the decidua, to terminate in visible cells in the substance of the placenta; but whether the terminal orifices of the veins derived no returning blood from the interstices of the decidual laminæ, was by no means certain. For my own part, having satisfied myself of the passage of the tortuous uterine arteries into the decidua, I undoubtedly considered the uterine venous sinuses as the most probable and natural channels by which the blood conveyed from the uterus by the tortuous arteries would return again to that body; although I was unable to determine from this dissection how the blood was returned into the open mouths of the veins.

It must be admitted, that an impregnated uterus at the fifth month, where the vessels, which are very small, had been contracted by the spirit in which the parts had been preserved, was not a very favourable subject for so delicate an investigation; and I accordingly felt extremely desirous of repeating the dissections on gravid uteri at a more advanced period. These opportunities do not, as is well known, frequently occur: about a year after I was, however, favoured by Dr. Lee with a large portion of a gravid uterus of a woman who died about the ninth month of gestation, in which the uterine veins had been gently filled with red size injection. This preparation was submitted to the same mode of dissection. In tracing those veins which passed to the inner surface of the uterus, near the middle of the placenta, the injection was seen to be continued from them into oblique, wide, but shallow channels, leading through the external decidua into the placental decidua, and had thence been diffused through the fine spongy cellular tissue which everywhere surrounds and supports the fœtal capillaries. On comparing these appearances with my first dissection, I perceived that the uterine vein, opposite the mouth of which I had supposed the decidua to be wanting, and whose orifice was in contact with the capillaries of the placenta, was in reality one of the oblique decidual canals, returning the blood from the cellular substance of the placenta into the uterine vein, its continuity with which had been preserved.

The continuation of the uterine veins into decidual canals was much more distinct in those which terminated near the circumference of the placenta; and here the irregular portions of injection, which filled the canals as far as the surface of the placenta, were evidently circumscribed, by distinct parietes, and not the result of confused extravasation: the injection from the decidual canals had passed into the large interlobular spaces, or maternal sinuses of the placenta, and thence had become diffused, generally for the extent of an inch, into the spongy or cellular texture of the placenta.

The uterine arteries in this case had not been injected, but were easily traceable passing through the external and placental decidua, as far as the internal surface of the latter, and apparently opening or being lost on the spongy surface of the placenta.

With reference to preparations of vascular and cellular structures like the placenta, it is not easy to enforce conviction from the appearances they present, in consequence of the difficulty of distinguishing between natural and accidental extravasation.

Having, however, carefully compared the Hunterian preparations with the results of my own examinations of the gravid uterus at the full period, I now believe they all fully bear out Mr. Hunter's general view, viz. that the maternal blood is diffused, by means of the tortuous arteries, into the spongy cellular substance of the placenta, where

in which the child may be situated, is capable of receiving the same provisionary stimulus for supplying it with nourishment as the uterus; and this, I believe, is peculiar to generation. This prompts me to make the following observations upon the different situations of the fœtus in extra-uterine cases, which are extraordinary, happen seldom, and when they do occur are often attended with so many hindrances to critical investigation, as hardly to allow of thorough or satisfactory information.

Such cases are readily distinguished from natural ones by the uterus being found entire and empty; and they may be divided into three different kinds, according to the situation of the fœtus in the ovarium, Fallopian tube, or in the cavity of the abdomen.

From a want of the appearances which usually attend the natural process, the investigation of extra-uterine cases is attended with considerable difficulty. For where uncommon actions have taken place, as, well as in cases of disease, the natural texture of the parts is very much altered, and appears to be lost, not only by the parts themselves being enlarged, but from having a great deal of new matter superadded to them, by which they lose their natural distinctness, and become less fitted for examination than those which only have a relation to them, and which preserve their natural actions peculiar to that state.

From these difficulties, and a want of accuracy in those who made the examination, it is not at present clear, with respect to many of the extra-uterine cases upon record, whether they were ovarian cases, Fallopian tube cases, or abdominal cases; when, if they had been acquainted with the principle in which they differ, nothing could have been more easy than to distinguish them. It is not difficult, perhaps, at the very first view, to distinguish an abdominal case from either of the two first: for if the ovaria and Fallopian tube are entire, natural, and can be well distinguished to be as those parts are when the circumstances are natural, then we may be sure it is an abdominal case. Appearances, however, may not in all cases be distinct; but the parts may adhere, or be otherwise rendered so obscure, that an abdominal case might be con

---

it bathes the capillaries of the fœtal circulation, and is returned by the oblique decidual adventitious sinuses and channels into the orifices of the uterine veins. Thus the placental intercommunication between the fœtus and mother, in the human subject and Quadrumana, is carried on by the contact of the fœtal capillaries with maternal extravasated blood; while in the Ruminants, the mare, and the sow[1], it takes place by the apposition of capillaries to capillaries, and the two parts of the placenta, viz. fœtal and maternal, can be separated. In the Feræ and Rodentia there appears to be an intermediate structure.]

[1] [In the last two examples the placenta may be said to be diffused over nearly the whole surface of the chorion.]

founded with either of the two first; therefore it is essential to have a characteristic difference established between the two first, and the third.

The invariable difference between the two first, and the abdominal cases, will be in the vessels by which the child is nourished: for the arteries and veins belonging to the part in which the child is contained must be enlarged; which, being the increase of a natural part, will be readily ascertained, and the nature of the case as readily determined. We may lay it down as a principle, that when the spermatic artery and veins of either side are enlarged in an extra-uterine case, that the fœtus is in the ovarium or Fallopian tube; since there are no other blood-vessels which supply these parts; and if any other system of vessels, as the mesenteric, are increased in size, while the spermatic are in a natural state, we may with equal certainty conclude the fœtus to be contained in the general cavity of the belly. As this becomes the great criterion, and as the situation and time will not always allow very nice investigation on the spot, where the person employed has an opportunity of taking away the parts concerned, I would advise his taking along with them the aorta and vena cava, cut through above the origins of the spermatic vessels.

OBSERVATIONS ON THE PLACENTA OF THE MONKEY.

Monkeys always copulate backwards: this is performed sometimes when the female is standing on all-fours; and at other times the male brings her between his thighs when he is sitting, holding her with his fore paws.

The female has her regular periods for the male, but she has commonly too much complaisance ever to refuse him. They carry this still further, for they receive the male when with young, even when pretty far gone: at least this was the case with one of which I am going to give an account.

A female monkey, belonging to Mr. Endersbay, in the summer 1782, had frequently taken the male. The keeper observed that after the 21st of June she became less lively than usual, although it was not suspected that she had conceived; but some time after appearing to be bigger in the belly, it created a suspicion of her being with young. Great attention was paid to her, and great care was taken of her. She went on gradually increasing in size; and at last something was observed to move in her belly at particular times, and the motion could even be felt through the abdominal muscles. She became indolent, and

did not like to leap or perform her usual feats of activity. Towards
the latter part of the time they perceived the breast and nipple to have
become rather fuller, and that a kind of water could be squeezed out at
the nipple. Some time before she brought forth, she became red about
the hips and posteriors, which redness extended to the inside of the
thighs. It being now certain that she was with young, I desired that
she might be particularly attended to when there were signs of approaching delivery, both on her own account and that of the young one,
and requested the afterbirth might be carefully preserved, as that part
would assist to ascertain the mode of uterine gestation. These directions were attentively followed; and when in labour it was observed
that she had regular pains, that when the young one was in part come
into the world, she assisted herself with her fore paws, and that it came
with the hind parts first. This happened on the 15th of December 1782,
in all about six months after conception; and when she brought forth
her young one it shewed signs of life, but died immediately, owing probably to the unfavourable mode of its being brought into the world.
When delivered she took the young one up, and although it was dead
clasped it to her breast.

The afterbirth was preserved entire, and was perfectly fit for examination. It consisted of placenta, with the membranes and navel-string,
which all very much resembled the corresponding parts in the human
subject, as will now be described.

The placenta had the appearance of being divided into two oblong
bodies, united by their edges, each terminating in an obtuse point at the
other end, which were of course at some little distance from one another.

It is probable that these two points were placed towards the openings of the Fallopian tubes, where the uterus assumes a form resembling
two obtuse horns.

The two lobes above mentioned were made up of smaller ones, united
closely at their edges, which were more apparent and distinct at some
parts than at others. Some of these lobes were divided by fissures which
seem to be derived from one centre, while there were others near the edges
passing in a different direction, in which fissures are placed veins or sinuses that receive the blood laterally from the lobes. The substance of
the placenta seems to be cellular, as in the human subject: this structure allows a communication to be kept up between different parts of
each lobe, and the sinuses allowing of a communication between the different lobes of which the placenta is composed, the blood passes into
the fissures before it enters the veins; in which respect it differs from
the human placenta.

The arteries from the uterus, on the surface of the placenta, were visible, but too small to be injected : I cannot therefore say how they terminated in the placenta.

The principal veins arose in general from the fissures beginning from the surface, as in the human placenta; but besides these, there were other small ones; all which, we may suppose, pass through the decidua and enter the substance of the uterus, most probably in the same way as in the human subject.

The membranes are the amnios, the chorion, and the membrana decidua. These appear to be much the same as in the human, except that the decidua is considerably thicker, especially where it passes between the uterus and the placenta.

The navel-string in the monkey is not proportionally so long as in the human, and is very much and very regularly twisted.

There is no urachus, and of course no allantois; not even the small ligament that appears to be a drawing-in of the bladder at its attachment to the navel, the bladder here being rounded.

ACCOUNT OF A WOMAN WHO HAD THE SMALLPOX DURING PREGNANCY, AND WHO SEEMED TO HAVE COMMUNICATED THE SAME DISEASE TO THE FŒTUS. BY JOHN HUNTER, ESQ., F.R.S.[a]

Read January 17, 1780.

Mr. Grant's Account.

ON the 5th of December, 1776, Mrs. Ford had been seized with shivering and the other common symptoms of fever, to which were added great difficulty of breathing and a very hard cough. Mr. Grant saw her on the 7th, and he took from her eight ounces of blood, and gave her a composition of the saline mixture with spermaceti and magnesia every six hours.

This had operated by the 8th two or three times very gently, when most of the complaints were relieved; but the cough still shaking her violently, bleeding seemed necessary to be repeated, more particularly as she looked upon herself to be in the sixth month of her pregnancy. The medicine was continued without the magnesia.

In the evening (viz. the 8th) the smallpox appeared, which proved of a mild kind, and moderate in quantity. Its progress was rather slower than might have been expected; but the woman passed through the disease in great spirits, sitting up the greatest part of the day during the whole time, and taking only a paregoric at night, and, as occasion required, a little magnesia; thus the symptoms were mitigated, and the cough at last became very little troublesome.

On the 25th she complained of a pain in her side. Eight ounces of blood were taken away. The next day she was quite free from pain, and thought herself as well on the 27th as her particular situation would admit of; after which she was not visited by Mr. Grant till the 31st, when she was in labour.

Mr. Wastall's Letter on the same subject.

December 30, 1776, I was sent for to Mrs. Ford, a healthy woman, about twenty-two years of age, who was pregnant with her first child. She had come out of the country about three months before. Soon

---

[a] [Originally published in the Philosophical Transactions, vol. lxx. 1780.]

after her arrival in town she was seized with the smallpox, and had been under the care of Messrs. Hawkins and Grant, who have favoured me with the particulars here annexed.

I called upon her in the afternoon; she complained of violent griping pains in her bowels, darting down to the pubes. On examining, I found the os tincæ a little dilated, with other symptoms of approaching labour. I sent her an anodyne spermaceti emulsion, and desired to be called if her pains increased. I was sent for. The labour advanced very slowly; her pains were long and severe: she was delivered of a dead child with some difficulty.

Observing an eruption all over the body of the child, and several of the pustules filled with matter, I examined them more particularly; and recollecting that Dr. Leake, in his Introductory Lecture to the Practice of Midwifery, had observed, that it might be necessary to inquire whether those adults who are said totally to escape the smallpox have not been previously affected with it in the womb, I sent a note to Dr. Leake, and likewise to Dr. Hunter, in hopes of ascertaining a fact hitherto much doubted. Dr. Leake came the same evening, and saw the child. Dr. Hunter came afterwards, with Mr. Cruickshank, and examined it; also Mr. John Hunter and Mr. Falconer; who all concurred with me, that the eruption on the child was the smallpox. Dr. Hunter thought the eruption so like the smallpox that he could hardly doubt; but said, that in all other cases of the same kind that he had met with, the child in utero had escaped the contagion.

From Mr. Grant's Notes.

The eruption appeared on Mrs. Ford in the evening of the 8th of December, and she was delivered the 31st, that is, twenty-three days after the appearance of the eruptions.

Reflections by Mr. John Hunter.

The singularity of the above case, with all its circumstances, has inclined me to consider it with some attention.

There can be no doubt that the mother had the smallpox, and that the eruption began to appear on the 8th of December: also, that it went through its regular stages, and that on the 31st, viz. twenty-three days after the first appearance of the eruption, the woman was delivered of the child, who is the subject of this paper.

Secondly, the distance of time when she had the smallpox before delivery, joined with the stage of the disease in the child when born, which probably was about the sixth or seventh day of the eruption, viz. about

fifteen or sixteen days after the beginning of the eruption on the mother, perfectly agrees with the possibility of the infection's being caught
from the mother.

Thirdly, The external appearance of the pustules in the child was
perfectly that of the smallpox, as must have appeared from the relation
given in Mr. Wastall's letter. Most of the pustules were distinct, but
some were blended or united at their base. The face had the greatest
number, and these were in general the most indistinct. They were
somewhat flattened, with a dent in the middle*.

So far were the leading circumstances and external appearances in
favour of their being the variolous eruption; but although these leading
circumstances and external appearances were incontrovertible, yet they
were not an absolute proof of this being the genuine smallpox; therefore
I must be allowed to consider this subject a little further, and see how
far all the circumstances correspond or are similar to the true smallpox.
In the smallpox we have a previous fever, in place of which, in the present case, we have no information but that of the mother's having had
the smallpox within such a limited time as may favour the possibility
of infection in the womb; yet we may presume that the child must have
had considerable fever preceding such an eruption, of whatsoever kind
it was.

In the smallpox the eruption goes through pretty regular stages in
its progress and declension, which circumstances we know nothing of
in the present case; but even this fever, the eruptions, and their progress, are not absolutely proofs that the disorder is the smallpox when
it is caught in the common and natural way; and in proof of this assertion,
it may be observed, that practitioners every now and then are mistaken.

It may be asked, What is the true characteristic of the smallpox?
That by which it differs from all other eruptions that we are acquainted
with? The most certain character of the smallpox that I know is, the
formation of a slough, or a part becoming dead by the variolous inflammation; a circumstance which hitherto, I believe, has not been taken
notice of.

This was very evident in the arms of those who were inoculated in
the old way, where the wounds were considerable, and were dressed
every day; which mode of treatment kept them from scabbing, by which
means this process was easily observed; but in the present method of
inoculation it is hardly observable: the sore being allowed to scab, the
slough and scab unite and drop off together. The same indistinctness

* I endeavoured to take some matter upon the point of two lancets; but not having
an opportunity of making an experiment myself, I gave them to two gentlemen, who,
I imagine, were afraid of inoculating with them.

attends the eruptions on the skin; and in those patients who die of, or die while in, the disease, where we have an opportunity of examining them while the part is distinct, this slough is very evident.

This slough is the cause of the pit after all is cicatrized; for it is a real loss of substance of the surface of the cutis; and in proportion to this slough is the remaining depression.

The chickenpox comes the nearest in external appearance to the smallpox; but it does not commonly produce a slough.

As there is generally no loss of substance in this case, there can be no pit. But it sometimes happens, although but rarely, that there is a pit in consequence of a chickenpock; then ulceration has taken place on the surface of the cutis, a common thing in sores.

In the present case, besides the leading circumstances mentioned in the case of the mother, corresponding with the appearances on the child, and the external appearances themselves, we have in the fullest sense the third and real or principal character of the smallpox, viz. the slough in every pustule; from all which, I think, we may conclude, that the child had caught the smallpox in the womb; or at least a disease, the effects of which were similar to no other known disease.

In opening the bodies of those who had either died of, or died while under, the smallpox, I always examined carefully to see whether any internal cavity, such as the œsophagus, trachea, stomach, intestines, pleura, peritoneum, &c., had eruptions upon them or not; and never finding any in any of those cavities, I began to suspect that either the skin itself was the only part of the body susceptible of such a stimulus, or that the skin was subject to some influence to which the other parts of the body were not subject, and which made it alone susceptible of the variolous stimulus. If from the first cause, I then concluded it must be an original principle in the animal œconomy. If from the second, I then suspected that external exposure was the cause; and I was the more led into this idea, from finding that these eruptions often attack the mouth and throat, two exposed parts; add to which, that we generally find the eruptions most on the exposed parts of the body, as the face, &c.

With these ideas in my mind, I thought I saw the most favourable opportunity of clearing up this point. I therefore very attentively examined most of the internal cavities of this child; such as the peritoneum, pleura, trachea, inside of the œsophagus, stomach, intestines, &c., but observed nothing uncommon. I have already observed, that in this child the face and extremities were the fullest, similar to what happens in common; from all which I may be allowed to draw this conclusion, that the skin is the principal part which is susceptible of the variolous stimulus, and is not affected by any external influence whatever.

The communication of the smallpox to the child in the womb may be supposed to happen in two ways; one by infection from the mother, as is supposed in the above case; the other, by the mother's having absorbed the smallpox matter from some other person, and the matter being carried to the child from the connexion between the two, which we may suppose done with or without first affecting the mother.

Testimonies and opinions are various with respect to these two facts. Boerhaave seems to have been led by his experience to think that such infection was not communicable; for we find that he attended a lády, who having, in the sixth month of her pregnancy, had the confluent smallpox, brought forth at the regular period a child, who showed not the least vestige of his mother's disease.

His commentator, however, Van Swieten, supports a different opinion (see his Comment. vol. v.). He quotes a case from the Philosophical Transactions, vol. xxviii. No. 337, p. 165, of a woman who, having just gone through a mild sort of smallpox, was, by means of a strong dose of purging physic, thrown into a miscarriage, and brought forth a dead female child, whose whole body was covered with variolous pustules full of ripe matter: but this history is founded only on the relation of a midwife to a clergyman, and therefore not absolutely to be depended upon as accurately stated; however, it is more than probable that there was a case as described, and that there were really eruptions on the skin of the child similar to the smallpox.

Van Swieten likewise mentions what Mauriceau relates of himself. This author testifies that he had often heard his father and mother say that the latter, when big with him, and very near her time of delivery, had a painful attendance on one of her children, who died of the small-pox on the seventh day of the eruption; and that on the day following the death of this child Mauriceau came into the world, bringing with him five or six true pustules of the smallpox.

It does not appear, however, from this recital whether or not Mauriceau passed through life free from any posterior infection; but admitting that this eruption of Mauriceau's was truly the smallpox, yet I should very much doubt his having caught it from the child who died of it: as it should seem that the pustules of Mauriceau were of the same date with those of the child who died. Van Swieten appeals to a more recent case, which had been reported to him by persons of great credit, and is recorded in the Philos. Trans., vol. xlvi. p. 235.

"A woman big with child, having herself long ago had the small-pox, very assiduously nursed a maidservant during the whole process of this disease.. At the proper time she brought forth a healthy female child, in whose skin Dr. Watson asserted that he discovered evident marks of the smallpox, which she must have gone through in the womb; and the same physician pronounced that this child would be free from future infection. After four years her brother was inoculated; and Dr. Watson obtained permission of the parents to try the same experiment on the girl. The operation was performed on both children in the same manner, and the pus used in both cases was taken from the same patient. The event, however, was different: for the boy had the regular eruption, and got well; but the girl's arm did not inflame nor suppurate. On the tenth day from the insertion of the matter she turned pale suddenly, was languid for two days, and afterwards was very well. In the neighbourhood of the incision there appeared a pustule, like those pustules that we sometimes observe in persons who, having had the disease, attend patients ill of the smallpox."

In the Epistles of T. Bartholinus, Cent. II. p. 682, there is the following history: " A poor woman, aged thirty-eight years, pregnant, and now near the time of delivery, was seized with the symptoms of the smallpox, and had a very numerous eruption. In this state she was delivered of a child, as full of variolous pustules as herself. The child died soon after birth; the mother three days afterwards." Van Swieten infers that the mother and the child were in this case infected at the same time; therefore, the child not infected by the mother.

Dr. Mead asserts that when a woman in the smallpox suffers an abortion the fœtus is generally full of the contagion; but that this does not happen always. This variety, he says, depends on the state of the mother's pustules when the child is born; that is, whether they are or are not in a state of purulence. Whence he has observed it sometimes to happen that on the second day from the birth, or the third, or any day before the eighth, the disease caught from the mother shows itself in eruptions on the child.

Dr. Mead here relates the history of a lady of quality, of which this is the substance. A lady, in the seventh month of her pregnancy, had the confluent smallpox, and on the eleventh day of the disease brought forth a son, having no signs of the disease on his body; and she died on the fourteenth day. The infant having lived four days, was seized with convulsions, and, the smallpox appearing, died. The doctor infers from hence that, the suppuration being in some measure completed on the eleventh day, the mother's disease was communicated then to the fœtus, and made its appearance on the child after eight days.

If there be no abortion, Dr. Mead pronounces that the child will ever be free from the disease, unless the birth should happen before the maturation of the pustules. He brings a case to prove that the fœtus in the womb may be infected by the contagion of which the mother does not partake. "A woman, who had long before suffered the smallpox, nursed her husband, under that disease, towards the end of her pregnancy; and was brought to bed at the due time. The child was dead, and covered all over with variolous pustules."

With respect to the case quoted from Mauriceau, it has been proved by Sir George Baker (Med. Transact., vol. ii. p. 275,) that Dr. Mead drew a conclusion from it directly contrary to the author's meaning. The negative opinion appears evidently to be supported by that history.

Sir George Baker mentions in the same paper the case of two pregnant women who were inoculated at Hertford. They both had the smallpox favourably, and afterwards brought forth their children perfectly healthy at the usual time. Both these children, at the age of three years, were inoculated with effect.

Sir George Baker likewise mentions a case which fell under the observation of Dr. Clarke of Epsom. "A woman towards the end of her pregnancy had the smallpox, from which she narrowly escaped. Five weeks after the crisis she was delivered of a healthy female child, who having numerous marks on her skin was judged by all who saw her to have undergone the same distemper before her birth. However, at the end of twelve months she had the smallpox in a very severe manner. Both the mother and child were lately living at Epsom."

Since, then, we see that it is very probable that the smallpox may be caught from the mother when she is infected, it may be asked why does not this happen oftener? In answer to this we may suppose that this is not so ready a way as when the child is exposed to catch it after the birth, as we find too that a difference can be produced after birth; viz. inoculation is a much readier way of catching it than what is called the natural way. It may likewise be said that many women who are with child, and have the smallpox during pregnancy, do not recover; therefore both mother and child die before the disease can have time to produce eruptions upon the child. Finally, in many of those cases where the mother recovers, there is sometimes produced a miscarriage, which also hinders the infection from taking place in the child. However, many women go through the whole disease, and the child shows no marks of the smallpox.

Thus have I stated facts relative to the present subject, with some of the best authorities on both sides of the question; and shall now leave the reader to form his own judgement.

SOME OBSERVATIONS ON DIGESTION.

THE paper which I formerly presented to the Royal Society, " On the Stomach itself being digested after Death, was published in 1772, in the 62nd volume of the Philosophical Transactions, and has attracted the attention of Spallanzani[a] and others. In the course of these my observations I shall make some remarks upon the experiments and opinions of these gentlemen, compare them with those of Reaumur[b], and, having given some general facts of my own upon digestion, shall conclude by adding a copy of the above-mentioned paper, with the hope that others will take up the subject in a more enlarged point of view, and prosecute an inquiry which is of so much consequence in the investigation of the operations of the animal œconomy. I cannot at present spare sufficient time to give my opinions at large on this subject, with all the experiments and observations I have made upon it; but as soon as I have leisure I shall lay them before the public.

To discover new parts has been a principal object in the researches of the young or practical anatomist; but the connexion, arrangement, mode of action, and uses of the whole, or of particular organs, have more commonly been reserved for the consideration of those whose views were extended further, and whose powers of reasoning had been enlarged by habits of observation and inquiry. Curious and speculative men have likewise made attempts in this way, but often without being sufficiently acquainted with the structure of the parts they were about to consider, and consequently ill informed respecting their relations and connexions with one another. Not contented to reason from those which were most obvious, which might have led to useful knowledge, they have been directed by what best suited their fancy, and have principally attempted the most obscure and intricate. Generation, or the mode of continuing the species, and digestion, or the means of preserving the individual, have been with them the great objects of inquiry; yet it does not appear that they have been very successful. Although

---

[a] [Spallanzani's observations on digestion appeared first in his work called *Fisica Animale e Vegetabile*, 12mo, 1782; a translation of which was published in London, with the title ' Dissertations relative to the Natural History of Animals and Vegetables,' in 1784.]

[b] [" Sur la Digestion des Oiseaux," *Mém. de l'Acad. des Sciences de Paris*, 1752, pp. 266—307, and pp. 461—495.]

digestion, as being one of the most important operations of the animal œconomy, and most obvious in its effects, supplies a number of facts to assist in ascertaining its powers, little has been hitherto made out towards investigating the various circumstances under which it is performed.

The mode of dividing the food for the increase of its surface, in some animals, suggested one method of explaining the process of digestion; and the secretion of a juice, which was supposed to have the power of converting vegetable and animal matter into a fluid proper for the purposes of nutrition, furnished another. Both these opinions have had their advocates; and while one party contended for a mechanical power, supposed to exist in the gizzard, the other had recourse to a chemical power, and considered fermentation as the great agent in digestion. They were, however, rather speculative philosophers than practical anatomists, and have frequently been misled with respect to the very facts and observations whose result was to decide the truth of their opinions. What, for instance, does it explain in digestion, that the force of the gizzard of a turkey is found equal to four hundred and seventy-three pounds? Does it afford a better solution of our doubts than we should derive from determining the force of the mill that grinds the wheat into flour? Or, on the other hand, will the most correct idea of fermentation enable us to account for the various phænomena in the operation of digestion? But we can have no very high idea of experiments made by men who, for want of anatomical knowledge, have not been able to pursue their reasoning beyond the simple experiment itself.

The great object should have been an endeavour to discover the universal agent in digestion; for the digestive organ is evidently constructed in a different manner in different animals. The mechanical power for the division of the food is not universal; and those gentlemen who consider this power in the gizzard as the immediate cause of digestion, forgot that the same effect was produced in other classes of animals with a different structure of stomach, by means of the grinding teeth. Thus, while the gizzard favoured the theory of the mechanical reasoner, that idea was again destroyed by the membranous structure of the stomach in many animals, which equally supplied the chemist with arguments in favour of the process of fermentation.

It is more difficult than those gentlemen imagine, to acquire on this subject information sufficiently accurate to be able to explain a process so complicated as that of digestion. There are in Nature's operations always two obvious extremes; and the mind of man eagerly adopts that which accords with some principle to which he is attached, and with which he is best acquainted, the intermediate connexions and gradations, as being less striking, not so forcibly affecting a superficial inquirer.

It happens, unfortunately, that those who from the nature of their education are best qualified to investigate the intricacies, and improve our knowledge of the animal œconomy, are compelled to get their living by the practice of a profession which is constant employment. The only educated men who have leisure are those of the Church, some of whom we frequently find commencing philosophers and physiologists, though they have not had that kind of education which would best direct their pursuits. Experiments, it is true, may be made by men of this description; but these must neither be much complicated, nor have any immediate relation to those branches of knowledge with which they have had few opportunities of being acquainted : at best, they will seldom go further than to explain a single fact. To look through a microscope and examine the red globules of blood, to view animalculæ, and give a candid account of what they see, are points on which such inquirers may be allowed to indulge themselves; but it is presumption in them to affect to reason of a science in which they can have but a very superficial knowledge, or to expect to throw light on subjects that they have not taken the previous steps to understand. It should be remembered that nothing in Nature stands alone; but that every art and science has a relation to some other art or science, and that it requires a knowledge of those others, as far as this connexion takes place, to enable us to become perfect in that which engages our particular attention.

These strictures are applicable to all those who have made experiments to explain digestion. The effect of the mechanical powers being easily understood, those who considered digestion mechanically have in general explained them justly as far as they applied to the gizzard; but their reasoning went no further, and they supposed these effects to be digestion. Those again who took it up chemically, being little acquainted with chemistry and totally ignorant of the principles of the animal œconomy, have erroneously explained the operations of the animal machine as subject to the laws of chemistry.

The first inquirers into digestion, struck only by the extremes of structure, the gizzard, and membranous stomach, paid no regard to the gradations leading from the one to the other; which, if properly examined, would have materially assisted them to explain the functions of the stomach.

Vallisneri, considering the power of the gizzard in one view only, imagined it would be as liable to be affected by the mechanical powers necessary for digestion as the grain which was to be digested; therefore supposed the existence of a solvent. But though Vallisneri is entitled to no merit from this idea, as the premises are false, yet this opinion of his set Reaumur to work, and has been the means of bringing several curious facts to light[a]. The experiments of Reaumur were first made with a view to confute that opinion, and therefore birds having gizzards were adapted to his purpose. In this pursuit he only attended to such parts of the experiments as best accorded with his own opinion, yet carefully guarded against every possible accident that might affect their accuracy. Had trituration been the immediate cause of digestion, his experiments on the gizzards of birds were unnecessary; since it would have been sufficient to have examined the food after it had been masticated by the teeth of animals who have grinders, the teeth and gizzard answering one and the same purpose. But the circumstance of animals which masticate their food in their mouth having also a stomach, should have taught that there was something more in digestion than trituration.

Reaumur's first experiments were made to ascertain the strength of the gizzard, with its effects, to prove that sharp cutting substances when swallowed in no way injured its internal coat, and that the common food of the bird was not dissolved when guarded against its action. Yet, after all these proofs, he seems to doubt, and says, " Are we to conclude that grinding alone is sufficient to convert the grain and other aliment into a matter proper for the nutrition of the animal, without undergoing any other preparation? Several reasons seem to oppose this : trituration alone might reduce the grain into a flour; but flour alone is not chyle." " From the smell of the aliment (taken from the gizzards of birds) are we not led to conclude that it undergoes a fermentation? This smell may be said to arise from the liquor with which the aliment is mixed; but is it likely that juices do not dispose to fermentation substances in which it is so easily excited? Fruit and flour, made into a paste, require little more than heat to make them ferment." From these experiments, made with a view to prove that digestion is carried on by trituration, Reaumur was led to suppose a solvent. But

---

[a] [In this historical sketch, so rare in the writings of Hunter, of the opinions entertained by previous physiologists on the subject of digestion, the suggestion by Tyson of the existence and use of a solvent or corrodent fluid ought to have had a place. In his Anatomy of a Rattlesnake he observes, " The food, before it can prove aliment, must be comminuted, and broken into the smallest particles; which in these membranous stomachs I can't see how it can be performed but by corrosion. A principal menstruum in doing this I take to be that liquor which is discharged by the glands that are seated, in some, at the beginning of the throat, and are called *salival*; or just above the stomach or gizzard of birds, and called the *echinus*; or in others in the stomach itself, and called the glandulous coat, and such I take the inner coat of the stomach of our rattlesnake to be."—*Philos. Trans.*, xiii. 1683, p. 33.]

as there are some birds whose stomachs do not seem sufficiently strong to have the power of trituration, he selected the buzzard as being of that kind, and the fittest for the subject of his experiments, from the circumstance of its throwing up whatever is solid and indigestible; therefore, without killing the bird, he could know the result, and repeat the experiment as often as he thought necessary.

From the stomach in the buzzard being incapable of trituration, he concluded that a solvent was necessary for digestion; but, to preclude all mechanical effects of the stomach, in his experiments he employed tin tubes filled with meat, which, after the tubes had remained twenty-four hours in the stomach of the buzzard, was reduced to three fourths of its size, was like threads, and was neither putrid, sour, nor volatile, but insipid. On this effect he made his remarks, which are very pertinent. In another experiment, which was still more accurate and conclusive, he was convinced of the action of a solvent. He then tried the soft bones of young animals, and found they were digested; and that though the hard bones were not acted on so readily, yet, by returning the same bones several times into the stomach, they were digested at last.

Reaumur was next anxious to know if such birds as were intended by Nature to live upon meat could also digest vegetables; but the result was not so satisfactory. He gave bread to his buzzard, which upon being returned had the appearance of having been chewed. He next tried a piece of ripe pear, which, after having been twenty-four hours in the stomach, had lost some of its weight, and had the appearance of being boiled or baked; and thence he concludes that its powers are too weak to digest vegetables so as to nourish the animal.

To ascertain the nature of the liquor which had such powers, he tasted the jelly to which the meat and bone had been reduced, supposing that it must be well impregnated with this fluid; but he could only distinguish a bitter or a saltish taste. To have an opportunity of more certainly determining the nature of this solvent, he made his buzzard swallow small tubes filled with sponge, which imbibed fifty grains of this liquor, having the same taste as the jelly, and changing blue paper to a red. He tried the effects of this liquor on meat out of the body, with comparative experiments in water; and after twenty-four hours the meat in the water was become putrid; but that in the liquor from the stomach was only softened, not dissolved. To see how far the analogy held good in membranous stomachs, he gave two bones to a dog, which being killed after twenty-six hours, they were found lessened in size, and become as soft as horn. He found that the stomach of the dog did not alter the shape of any of his tubes.

He conveyed grass and hay, inclosed in tubes, into the stomachs of ruminating animals, which substances were not digested, but appeared as if macerated.

Let us enumerate the experiments and facts made out by Reaumur.

The gizzard was not hurt by acting upon glass, which it ground to a powder.

The stomach or gizzard had hardly any visible motion.

The force of the gizzard was ascertained.

The size of the stones found in the gizzard was in proportion to the size of the bird.

The stomach of a buzzard digested bone, from which he concluded the gastric juice had a solvent power; but it did not digest bread, although it acted in a slight degree on fruit.

He made experiments with the gastric juice.

The juice in the ruminating animals' stomachs produced no effect on hay or grass when inclosed in tubes.

Reaumur's experiments, although not complete, paved the way for future investigation; and Spallanzani, proceeding on the same ground, has not only confirmed them by his own, but has established several points not completely made out by Reaumur; for in some instances Reaumur gave up the point too soon, especially in the experiments respecting the buzzard's power of digesting vegetables. Reaumur not possessing general knowledge sufficient to direct him in his pursuits, was necessarily confined to what he was most master of, the mere making experiments. Being neither an anatomist nor a physiologist, he has not been perfectly just in his description of parts, having considered the crop and the œsophagus leading from it to the gizzard as two distinct stomachs; but this, however, is only to be set down as a piece of anatomical ignorance, not affecting the subject in the least. Spallanzani is also deficient in his anatomical knowledge; yet it must be owned that his experiments, as far as they go, are in themselves conclusive; but like all mere experiment-makers, he is not satisfied even with those which are clear and decisive, but multiplies them most unnecessarily, without varying them to elucidate other and essential parts of the same subject. I think we may set it down as an axiom, that experiments should not be often repeated which tend merely to establish a principle already known and admitted; but that the next step should be, the application of that principle to useful purposes. If Spallanzani had employed half his time in this way, and had considered digestion under all the various states of the body and stomach, with all the varieties of food, both natural and artificial, he had employed his time much better than in making experiments without end.

The food of animals in general being composed either of vegetables, animals, or both, and a solvent admitted as an agent in digestion, it only remained to prove, that the effect of the process of digestion was to produce from these various substances an animal matter, similar in all animals who live on such substances. But the application of principles requires more than simply the knowledge of the principle itself, and therefore those who cannot reason from analogy, or draw general conclusions from a few convincing facts, and who require to have every relative conclusion or inference proved by an experiment, must be pleased with Spallanzani; but he must tire even those whom he informs, and much more those who read his works in expectation of something new.

To make comparative experiments upon the digestive power, the different animals destined for that purpose should be under similar circumstances as far as relates to digestion; they should be equal in age, for the growing eat more than the full-grown, and of course digest faster; which point, therefore, can be best ascertained by selecting those in each class of animals which have attained their full growth. They should be equal in fatness, for this makes a very material difference in the powers of digestion in the same animal; and they should be equal in health, a circumstance which, of all others, probably makes the greatest difference in the powers of the stomach. In comparing animals of the same class, the atmosphere should likewise be of the same temperature; for the different classes of animals are variously affected by the same degree of heat. Experiments made upon snakes and lizards in the winter will differ greatly from those made in the summer, while similar experiments made on dogs will have nearly the same result in both seasons. Nor will the powers of the stomach be found always equal in the same class. Sleeping animals of the quadruped kind, as hedgehogs, do not digest in the winter, but in the summer only; therefore the conclusions to be drawn from experiments made respecting the digestive powers in the one, are not at all applicable to those made in the other season.

Spallanzani observed that the snake digested food faster in June, when the heat was at 82° and 83°, than in April, when it was only 60°; from whence he concludes, that heat assists digestion; but this heat is not the immediate, but the remote cause of the increased power; heat having produced in the animal greater necessity for nourishment, and of course greater powers, gastric juice was secreted faster or in greater quantity.

As a proof that heat does not act as an immediate, but only as a remote cause in assisting digestion, I shall mention the effect it produced upon a hedgehog, the subject of Mr. Jenner's third experiment on the heat of that animal, related in another part of this work*.

* Vide page 143.

"The hedgehog, while the heat of the stomach was at 30°, had neither desire for food, nor power of digesting it; but when increased by
inflammation in the abdomen to 93°, the animal seized a toad which
happened to be in the room, and upon being offered some bread and
milk, it immediately ate it. The heat roused up the actions of the
animal œconomy; and the parts being unable to carry on these actions
without being supplied with nourishment, the stomach was stimulated
to digest, to afford them that supply."

Spallanzani also mentions the slowness of digestion in serpents, and
quotes Bomare, who gives an account of a serpent at Martinico, in
whose stomach a chicken had remained for three months without being
completely digested, the feathers still adhering to the skin*. The truth
of this fact I should very much doubt, especially in so warm a climate
as that of Martinico, where I must suppose the digestive powers to be
constantly required; unless there is in Martinico, as in colder climates, a
torpid season[a], where the act of digestion is not necessary; but in that
case the serpent would not have swallowed the chicken.

At Belleisle, in the beginning of the winter 1761–2, I conveyed worms
and pieces of meat down the throats of lizards when they were going
into winter quarters, keeping them afterwards in a cool place.   On
opening them at different periods I always found the substances which
I had introduced entire, and without any alteration : sometimes they
were in the stomach; at other times they had passed into the intestine;
and some of the lizards that were preserved alive voided them towards
the spring, with but very little alteration in their structure.   So that
digestion is regulated by the other actions of the body : warmth requires
action suitable to that warmth; the body requires nourishment suitable
to that action; and the stomach being called upon, performs the office of
digestion.

Nothing can show more clearly that the secretion of the gastric juice is
increased in proportion to the call for nourishment in the body, than what
happened to Admiral Byron and Captains Cheap and Hamilton, when
shipwrecked on the west coast of South America, who, after suffering
months of hunger and fatigue, were reduced to skin and bone; yet when
they came to good living, Byron thus expresses himself[†]: "He (viz. the

---

* Bomare, *Dict. d'Histoire Nat.*   † Page 181.

---

[a] [This conjecture is true; the dry season in some tropical climes is that during which
reptiles and insects retire to their hiding-places and become torpid; they are awakened
and called into activity by the showers of the rainy season.

The tenrec, a mammiferous animal of Madagascar and the Mauritius, resembling the
hedgehog, also sleeps in a state of lethargy from April to November, when the mean
temperature exceeds our summer heat.]

governor) ordered a table to be spread for us, with cold ham and fowls, which only we three sat down to, and in a short time dispatched more than ten men with common appetites would have done. It is amazing that our eating to that excess we had done, from the time we first got among these kind Indians, had not killed us; we were never satisfied, and used to take all opportunities, for some months after, of filling our pockets when we were not seen, that we might get up two or three times in the night to cram ourselves. Captain Cheap used to declare that he was quite ashamed of himself."

Spallanzani has made several attempts to prove what few will subscribe to, that stones in the gizzards of birds are of no use towards the breaking or grinding down the grain; and that they are picked up without design. These stones have long been supposed to answer the purposes of trituration, and have been considered as affording assistance to the stomach, in the manner of teeth, and of course as being necessary to the act of digestion. Spallanzani combats this opinion; but as stones are universally found in gizzards, and it was necessary to account for the mode of their being conveyed there, he attributes it to chance. But we find that the gizzards which have most occasion for them, and are most able to use them, are likewise best supplied with them: to corroborate which facts may be added what we observed before, that in the larger gizzards are found the largest pebbles. In a turkey two hundred were found; in a goose, a thousand; which could not depend entirely upon chance. In trying whether the stones were of service, Spallanzani introduced tubes, needles, and lancets into gizzards in which there were but very few stones, yet found them broken. In this experiment these substances had been forty-eight hours in the gizzards; whereas in the former experiments, with the same kind of tubes, thirty-six hours was the longest time; in another, eighteen hours; and in another, the breaking of them was begun in less than two hours; therefore the experiments were not perfectly fair, as the times were not equal. What he thinks the most conclusive is, that where he had taken care there should be no stones, the hard indigestible substances were acted upon much in the same way as when there were stones; but in this experiment he does not give the time, which is very accurately stated in most of the others.

He discovered that the inner surface of the stomach was not hurt by such substances; and indeed it is scarcely possible for the inner coat of the stomach of a fowl to be pierced by such as are even sharp-pointed, the quantity of its motion being so inconsiderable as hardly to make them pass through its inner coat. But the principal cause of their being harmless arises from the motion being lateral, and not pressing perpendicularly to the axis, one surface sliding in a contrary direction to the other, and that not in a straight, but in a circular direction, as will be explained hereafter.

In considering the strength of the gizzard, and its probable effects when compared with the human stomach, it must appear that the gizzard is in itself very fit for trituration; we are not, however, to conclude that stones are entirely useless; for if we compare the strength of the muscles of the jaws of animals which masticate their food with those of birds which do not, we shall say that the parts are well calculated for the purpose of mastication; yet we are not from thence to infer that the teeth in such jaws are useless, even although we have proof that the gums do the business when the teeth are gone. If stones are of use, which we may reasonably conclude they are, birds have an advantage over animals having teeth, so far as stones are always to be found, while the teeth are not renewed. Spallanzani concludes, " That we have at length a decision of the famous question concerning the use of these pebbles, so long agitated by authors; it appearing that they are not at all necessary for the trituration of the firmest food, &c."; but says, "He will, however, not deny that when put in motion by the gastric muscles, they are capable of producing some effects on the contents of the stomach." Now if we constantly find in an organ substances which can only be subservient to the functions of that organ, should we deny them to be of any use because the part can to a certain degree do its office without them?

To account for pebbles being found in the gizzard, Spallanzani supposes the birds to have picked them up by chance, or not to have distinguished between their food and these stones. But it appears singular that only those which have gizzards should be so stupid; and he owns that Redi and himself found that birds died of hunger, yet without having picked up more stones than usual, which we might suppose they would have done if they had not had a choice, or could not have distinguished stones from the grain on which they feed.

The stones assist in breaking the grain, and by separating its parts in the beginning of the process, and afterwards by rubbing off the surface already digested, allow the gastric juice to come more completely in contact with the whole.

It has been said, that the motion of the gizzard is so small as hardly to be observable, and that it cannot be felt by the hand. But as its cavity is very small, and must be capable of adapting itself to the quantity it contains (or it could not possibly grind), much motion is not necessary for the purposes of trituration: a swelling and collapsing, like the motion of the heart, would have no effect. The extent of motion in grindstones need not be the tenth of an inch, if their motion is alternate and in contrary directions. But although the motion of the gizzard is hardly visible, yet we may be made very sensible of its action by putting the ear to the sides of a fowl while it is grinding its food, when the stones can be heard moving upon one another[a].

It may be remarked, that the motion of the whole intestinal canal, from the fauces to the anus, is naturally so slow, as not to be excited into quick actions. The food passes slowly along the œsophagus; and in a man, fluids which might be expected to act even by their own gravity, descend but slowly: yet I think we may be certain that the œsophagus has always a regular contraction, and that the lower parts must relax in progression as it contracts above; so that no position of the body makes any difference in this action.

Upon exposing the stomach in living animals it does not appear much agitated or affected, even by being handled or otherwise irritated. The same thing may be observed in the whole track of intestines: and we find that when the fæces are expelled by the action of the gut alone, that the expulsion is slow; the stomach and rectum, however, can be emptied at once; but that is done by the abdominal and other muscles. We know that the action of vomiting is performed entirely by the diaphragm and abdominal muscles; and we know that by the same action the contents of the rectum can be expelled. Neither is any other power required to empty the stomach in vomiting, these muscles being often capable of forcing the bowels themselves out of the abdomen, and of producing a rupture. It is not necessary the stomach itself should act violently to produce an evacuation of its contents; nor is it even necessary it should act at all; for the lungs themselves do not act in the least when any extraneous matter is to be thrown up; and coughing is to the lungs what vomiting is to the stomach[b]. The muscles of respiration

---

[a] [Harvey makes a similar observation on birds of prey: "Falconibus, aquilis, aliisque avibus ex præda viventibus, si aurem prope admoveris dum ventriculus jejunus est, manifestos intus strepitus, lapillorum illuc ingestorum, invicemque collisorum percipias."—*Opera Omnia*, 4to, p. 208. These investigations by means of the ear relative to the internal actions of animal bodies deserve a place in the history of auscultation.]

[b] [The conclusion which Hunter deduces from philosophical and just analogies, with respect to the share performed by the stomach in the act of vomiting, has not been considered satisfactory, at least if we may judge from the experiments which have subsequently been made with a view to determine that point. But perhaps M. Majendie was not aware of what our illustrious physiologist had written on the subject, as he introduces his experiments to our notice as if the passive state of the stomach in vomiting had never before been suspected: "On a cru long-temps que le vomissement dépendait de la contraction brusque et convulsive de l'estomac," &c.; and then goes on to detail his notorious experiment on the dog, for whose stomach he substituted a pig's bladder;

arc the active parts in emptying the lungs, and can act both naturally and preternaturally. The muscles of the thorax and abdomen do not act naturally on the contents of the abdomen, but often act preternaturally, producing an evacuation from its viscera.

There is this difference in the action of the parts in coughing and vomiting: the cough is performed by the proper muscles of respiration, which are those of expansion, supported by the abdominal, while the diaphragm is passive.

Vomiting is performed by the abdominal muscles and diaphragm, while those of inspiration are supporting this action.

In coughing the ribs are suddenly depressed, which diminishes the capacity of the thorax ; and that the diaphragm may not be allowed to sink down and increase the capacity of the thorax, which would counteract the depressors of the ribs, the abdominal muscles at the same time act, which supports the diaphragm in its place, and probably may by this action assist in bringing down the ribs. To give as much force to this action as possible, the glottis is shut till the action is begun, and then the glottis opens instantaneously, which obliges the depressors of the ribs to begin the effort with their full action.

The proper muscles of inspiration do not tire so soon in this action as the abdominal, for in violent coughing the muscles of the abdomen become sore.

In vomiting these actions are reversed. The muscles of the cavity of the abdomen act, in which is to be included the diaphragm ; so that the capacity of the abdomen is lessened, and the action of the diaphragm rather raises the ribs; and there is also an attempt to raise them by their proper muscles, to make a kind of vacuum in the thorax, that the œsophagus may be rather opened than shut, while the glottis is shut so as to let no air enter the lungs. The muscles of the throat and fauces act to dilate the fauces, which is easily felt by the hand, making there a vacuum, or what is commonly called a suction ; so that when all these actions take place together, the stomach is immediately emptied.

In violent coughing we find that a kind of mixed action takes place ; for although the diaphragm has not acted, yet the stomach is so much squeezed as to discharge its contents; and it affects the diaphragm,

---

by which he proved, that when filled with fluid and put into a situation to be pressed upon, the contents of the bladder would flow out. By dividing the phrenic nerves, and paralysing the diaphragm, Majendie also proved that the abdominal muscles alone were capable of producing vomiting; and by another experiment, he satisfied himself that the diaphragm alone was sufficient for that act when all the abdominal muscles had been dissected off, and the peritoneum left entire.]

which is often thrown into action, and brings on vomiting at the same time; therefore violent coughing palls the stomach.

There is reason to believe that the natural motion in all stomachs is regular; and I am more inclined to be of this opinion from what takes place in the stomach of animals which are covered with hair, and which lick their own bodies, and of such as feed on whole animals which are likewise covered with hair. In the stomach of the calf, for instance, which licks its skin with its tongue, and swallows whatever is attached to the rough surface of that organ, balls of hair are often found; and on examining their surface the hairs in each hemisphere seem to arise from a centre, and to take the same direction, which is circular, corresponding to what would appear to be the axis of this motion, and resembling what we see in different parts of the skin of animals whose hair takes different turns. This regularity in the direction of the hair, in such balls, could not be produced if there was not a regular motion in the stomach. This motion is also proved in the dog; for I have seen a ball of this kind that had been thrown up from a dog's stomach, where the same regularity in the turns of the hair was very evident and complete. The same motion seems also to take place in the bird kind; and of this the cuckoo is an example, which, in certain seasons living on caterpillars, some of which have hairs of a considerable length on their bodies, the ends of these are found sticking in the inner horny coat of the stomach or gizzard, while the hairs themselves are laid flat on its surface; not in every direction, which would be the case if there was no regular motion, but all one way, arising from a central point placed in the middle of the horny part, and the appearance on the surface of both sides of the gizzard evidently corresponding[a]. These two facts prove, in my opinion, a regular circular motion taking place in the gizzard and membranous stomach, and therefore, most probably, something similar is carried on in stomachs of all the various kinds. Indeed this motion in the stomach is so considerable, that when there is no horny defence, we find the coats sometimes pierced by hard pointed substances. Thus, the cows which feed on the grass of bleaching-grounds have their stomachs, especially the second, stuck full of pins; and fish which prey upon and swallow other fish entire, often have their stomachs pierced by the bones.

Spallanzani calls the inner coat cartilaginous whereas in fact, it is a

---

[a] [The appearance is so regular, that this hairy lining of the gizzard has been mistaken for a natural peculiarity of the cuckoo. In one of these gizzards, which was exhibited at a meeting of the Zoological Society, I found the supposed gastric hairs under the microscope to present the complex structure characteristic of those of the larva of the tiger-moth (*Arctia Caja*). See Proceedings of the Zool. Soc. 1834, p. 9.]

horny substance, forming an inner cuticle, but differing in some respects from the common cuticle; this horny substance not only differs in structure from the common cuticle, but in its attachment, from cuticle, nails, and hoofs. The cutis, where it is covered by such substances, has a vast number of villi on its surface, which pass into corresponding perforations in the cuticle; from this structure of parts, when the cuticle, nails, or hoofs are separated, their inner surface appears to be full of small perforations, and the cutis from which they have been removed is villous; and these villi are more numerous in some parts than in others, where the sense of touch is required to be delicate or acute. But the inner lining of the gizzard is just the reverse, that surface of the horny substance which is in contact with the gizzard being villous, and when separated, the inner surface of the gizzard appearing perforated. These villi are either the last-formed parts of this horny substance, or are the fibres of which the horny coat is composed. It is probable that this horny substance takes the form of villi that it may be more firmly connected with the gizzard, in which acute sensation is not required.

I may remark here, that the experiments made on the digestion of ruminating animals have been very deficient[a], arising from this process in them being more complicated than in the stomachs of other animals, and requiring attention to be paid to certain circumstances, which cannot take place in stomachs of only one cavity.

The circumstance mentioned by Spallanzani, of ruminating animals voiding the tubes by the anus, shows that the whole food is not necessarily returned into the mouth to be chewed a second time; for if it were, the tubes would certainly come up likewise, and would as certainly be thrown out of their mouths as improper to be chewed, a circumstance which often really happened. But it was hardly necessary to make experiments to ascertain whether ruminating animals digested meat, when we know that in some cold countries the cattle are fed on dried fish, and most animals eat their own secundines: indeed the circumstance of animals living upon both animal and vegetable food might have taught us that the mode of digesting both (whatever it is) was the same; therefore all that was wanted must have been to discover that mode; except we could absurdly conceive that two different modes might take place in the same stomach at the same time.

Spallanzani gives the opinion of authors respecting digestion; and so

---

[a] [This deficiency has recently been supplied by M. Flourens, in an elaborate series of experiments made on living sheep, in which fistulous communications had been established between the external surface and the different cavities of the stomach. See *Annales des Sciences Naturelles.*]

anxious is he to combat the idea of its being fermentation, that he will hardly allow that fermentation ever takes place in the stomach. That fermentation can go on in the stomach there is no doubt; but when that happens, it arises from the powers of digestion being defective. Milk, vegetables of all kinds, wine, and whatever has sugar in its composition, become much sooner sour in some stomachs than they would if left to undergo a spontaneous change out of the body; and even spirits in particular stomachs, almost immediately degenerate into a very strong acid. I am inclined to suppose that it is the sugar which is converted into spirit, and the spirit into acid; consequently a glass of brandy, from being much stronger, because less diluted, most probably contains as much matter likely to become acid as half a pint of wine. In other substances, besides those mentioned above, the fermentative process (unless prevented by that of digestion) appears to begin sooner in the stomach than out of the body. All oily substances, particularly butter, very soon become rancid after being taken into the stomach; and this rancidity is the effect of the first process of the fermentation of oil. Mr. Sieffert has been able to restore rancid oils to their original sweetness, by adding to them their due quantity of fixed air*; the loss of which I consider as the first process in this fermentation, similar to what happens in the fermentation of animal and vegetable substances.

Animal food does not so readily ferment in the stomach when combined with vegetables as when it is not; for the vegetables running more quickly into fermentation, preserve the meat from putrefaction. Put a piece of meat and some sugar, or bread, into water, and let them stand in a warm place; the bread and sugar will begin to ferment, the water will become sour, and the meat be preserved; but the acid becoming weaker, as the fermentation advances towards the putrefactive, the meat at last begins to acquire the same putrid disposition†. Yet this last part of the process cannot, I think, take place in the stomach, as a succession of acids will be formed, by which the meat will be preserved sweet till it is digested: the formation of this acid in the stomach, most probably, not preventing the digestion of those substances which are incapable of being rendered acid.

Bread allowed to remain in the stomach of a dog for eight hours is so much changed that it will not run into the vinous fermentation, but when taken out and kept in a warm place becomes putrid; its putrefaction, however, is not so quick as a solution of meat that has been in the stomach for the same length of time. Similar effects are produced when milk and bread are the food administered; and perhaps the gas-

* Physical and Chemical Essays, by Sir Tobern Bergman.
† Of this Sir John Pringle was not aware in making his experiments on this subject.

tric juice, when in sufficient quantity, will always prevent the vinous fermentation.

Spallanzani's next trials were to determine whether the gastric juice had the power of recovering meat already putrid: a fact which might have been proved by one experiment; for if very putrid meat is given to a dog, and the dog killed after some time, the meat will be found sweet, and all putrefaction at an end. Therefore his allowing fresh meat to continue a longer or shorter time in the stomach was immaterial, as it could not become putrid.

It appears from the above facts that the stomach has not so much power in preventing the acetous fermentation in vegetables as in correcting the putrefactive disposition in animal substances. For although this cannot be certainly known in those who eat both animal and vegetable food, yet it does not appear that the putrefaction of animal substances, where nothing else is eaten, takes place so quickly in the stomach as the change which is produced in vegetables; the acetous disposition is therefore either stronger than the putrefactive, or it more readily takes place: and indeed the living body shows this sufficiently; for we very often find an acid thrown up, but seldom or never anything putrefactive.

It may be admitted as an axiom that two processes cannot go on at the same time in the same part of any substance; therefore neither vegetable nor animal substances can undergo their spontaneous changes while in the act of being digested, it being a process superior in power to that of fermentation. But if the digestive power is not perfect, then the vinous and acetous fermentation will take place in the vegetable, and the putrefactive in the food of those animals which live wholly on flesh; although in the last I imagine but very seldom. The gastric juice, therefore, preserves vegetables from running into fermentation, and animal substances from putrefaction; not from any antiseptic quality in the juice, but, by making them go through another process, preventing the spontaneous change from taking place. In the greater number of stomachs there is an acid, even although the animal has lived upon meat for many weeks; but as this is not always the case, we must suppose it is only formed occasionally. Whether the stomach has a power of immediately secreting this acid, or first secretes a sugar which afterwards becomes acid, is not easily ascertained[a]; but I should be in-

---

[a] [The singular case of the man with an external fistulous communication with the stomach, detailed by Mr. Beaumont, who has so ably availed himself of the circumstance to elucidate several obscure points in the process of digestion, has afforded the means of determining this question. The stomach in its empty and inactive state contains no gastric juice; but when mechanically stimulated, as by touching the inner surface with

clined to suppose, from analogy, the last to be the case: animals in health seeming to have the power of secreting sugar; for we find it in the milk, and sometimes in the urine, in consequence of disease. Acid sometimes prevails in the stomach to so great a degree as to become a disease, attended with very disagreeable symptoms; the stomach converting all substances which have a tendency to become acid into that form. To ascertain whether there was an acid naturally in the sto- mach the most satisfactory mode was to examine the contents before the birth, when the digestive organs are perfect, and when no acid could have been produced by disease, or anything that had been swallowed. Accordingly, in the slink-calf, near the full time, there was no acid found in the stomach, although the contents had the same coagulating powers with those of animals who have sucked.

As we find stomachs possessed of a power of dissolving the whole substance of a bone, it is reasonable to suppose that its earth is destroyed by the acid in the stomach.

The stomach appears not only to be capable of generating an acid, but also to have the power of producing air: which last effect, I believe, arises from disease. It is not easy to account for the formation of this air; yet as the stomach is a reservoir for substances disposed to ferment, it might reasonably be supposed to arise from the food going into that process. But this, in my opinion, will not account for the vast quantity of air frequently thrown up from the stomach, even where food has not been swallowed for a considerable time, and where digestion appeared to have been completed. For we must conclude this process to have been completed, if the food was not found to have disagreed with either stomach or bowels, and that the stools were good. When the gout falls on the stomach the quantity of air thrown up is often immense, and the same thing may be observed in some cases commonly called nervous; yet the process of digestion will not account for this formation of air, as no air is to be found in healthy stomachs*: neither is it to be accounted for from a defect in digestion, as that would probably be productive of worse consequences.

I am inclined to believe that the stomach has a power of forming air, or letting it loose, from the blood, by a kind of secretion. We cannot, however, bring any absolute proof of this taking place in the stomach, as it may in all cases be referred to a defect in digestion; but we have

---

the bulb of a thermometer, that secretion is immediately poured out, and manifests the usual acid properties. (Beaumont: "Experiments and Observations on the Gastric Juice, and on the Physiology of Digestion.")

* In all my experiments on digestion, in dogs, I have never been able to detect any air in the cavity of the stomach.

instances of air being found in other cavities, where no secondary cause can be assigned. I have been informed of persons who have had air in the uterus or vagina, without having been sensible of it but by its escaping from them without their being able to prevent it; and who, from this circumstance, have been kept in constant alarm lest it should make a noise in its passage, having no power to retard it as when it is contained in the rectum. This fact being so extraordinary made me somewhat incredulous, but rendered me more inquisitive, in the hope of being enabled to ascertain and account for it; and those of whom I have been led to inquire have always made the natural distinction between air passing from the vagina and by the anus: that from the anus they feel and can retain, but that in the vagina they cannot; nor are they aware of it till it passes. A woman, whom I attended with the late Sir John Pringle, informed us of this fact, but mentioned it only as a disagreeable thing. I was anxious to determine if there were any communication between the vagina and rectum, and was allowed to examine, but discovered nothing uncommon in the structure of these parts. She died some time after; and, being permitted to open the body, I found no disease either in the vagina or uterus. Since that time I have had opportunities of inquiring of a number of women concerning this circumstance, and by three or four have been informed of the same fact, with all the circumstances above mentioned. How far they are to be relied upon I will not pretend to determine. I have likewise found air in the cellular membrane in gunshot wounds, that had passed some way under the skin, without being able to account for its being there by any mechanical effect of the ball.

That air is either formed from the blood, or let loose by some action of the vessels, both naturally and from disease, is an undeniable fact. We find air formed in some fishes, to answer natural purposes; for in those whose air-bladders do not communicate externally (many of which there are) we must suppose it to have been formed there. We also find it in animals after death; and I have a piece of the intestine of a hog which has a number of air-bladders in it*. Mr. Cavendish was so kind as to examine this air, and he found " it contained a little fixed air; and the remainder not at all inflammable, and almost completely phlogisticated." I have often seen such vesicles on the edges of the lungs; but these may be supposed to have been a kind of aneurismal air-cells filled from the trachea, and are circumscribed and impervious, so that in the state we find them they have no communication with the external air. In one instance I have discovered air in an abscess, which could·

* Vide Plate XXXVII.

not have been received from the external air, nor could it have arisen from putrefaction. The case is as follows:

A lady, about forty years of age, had been afflicted with complaints in the bladder and parts connected with it. From the symptoms, her disease was supposed by some to be the stone, though upon examination no stone was found; and she had also an umbilical hernia, for which I had been consulted. She grew gradually worse, and from being lusty, became a thin woman. A small tumour appeared in the groin, and the skin over it became red, similar to an abscess when the matter is beginning to point externally; but before her death this subsided. A few days before she died I was desired to examine a swelling on the lower and right side of the belly, extending nearly from the navel to the spine of the ilium on the right side. It was tense, evidently contained air, and could be made to sound almost like a drum. It had come on within a few weeks, and I was puzzled to account for it, there being clearly no connexion between that tumour and the umbilical hernia. I was inclined to suppose it to be a ventral hernia, containing the cæcum and part of the colon, filled with air; but as she had stools, as there were no symptoms of a strangulated gut nor any uneasiness in the bowels, as I could not make the air recede, but felt it as if confined to that part, I own I could form no conjecture what the case really was. The woman dying in a few days, I was permitted to examine the body. That I might not interfere with the tumour, or umbilical hernia, I made an opening into the abdomen on the right side of the linea alba, and on examining the cavity of the abdomen, found everything natural, except a small portion of the epiploon adhering to the inside of the navel; the parietes of the abdomen corresponding with the tumour being in a natural state. On pressing the tumour by the hand, air was heard to make its escape; whether by the vagina or anus was at first doubtful; but on examining with more attention, it was discovered to come from between the labia. I next opened the tumour externally, and let out the air, which was not in the least putrid, and was contained in a sac tolerably smooth on its inside, made up of compressed cellular membrane, the abdominal muscles and tendons forming the posterior surface, which extended as low as the inferior edge of Poupart's ligament. The contents of the abdomen were tolerably sound; but when I inspected the viscera contained in the pelvis, they were found adhering to each other; the bladder to the body of the uterus; the broad ligaments and ovaria to the uterus; and on examining these adhesions, I discovered a cavity between the bladder, uterus, and vagina, on the right side, something like an abscess. From the right side of this cavity there was a canal ascending to the brim of the pelvis, in the course of the round ligament, as far as to the going out of the iliac vessels, which it seemed to accompany; and this canal, when it passed from behind Poupart's ligament, communicated with the tumour above mentioned. I then endeavoured to discover if there were any communication between the rectum and the abscess, but could find none, the gut appearing to be quite sound. Having removed the whole contents of the pelvis, with the canal leading to Poupart's ligament, and the ligament itself, with such of the abdominal muscles as composed part of the sac, I found both the rectum and vagina perfectly sound. The uterus had a polypus forming on its inside; neither the rectum nor uterus had any connexion with the abscess; but there was a small communication between the abscess and the bladder, that portion of the bladder which made part of the abscess being very much diseased.

From this history of the appearances of the tumour before death, and the particular account I have given of the dissection, the reader may be able to draw his own conclusions relative to the origin of the air. It certainly appeared to have been formed in this bag; and it was only towards the latter end of her life that it could have made its escape into the cavity of the bladder, for it was not possible to squeeze the air out of the tumour when I first saw her; but just before death it became more flaccid. It could not be formed or let loose, in consequence of putrefaction, for the air itself was free from any smell; and although the cavity between the vagina and bladder had on its internal surface the irregular ulcerated appearance of an abscess, yet that on the abdomen had not, was tolerably smooth, and had rather the appearance of having been formed in consequence of some foreign matter accumulating there.

This circumstance, of an animal having the power of forming air, or separating it from the juices by a kind of secretion, appears at first view to be supported by the experiments of Dr. Ingenhousz*.

The Doctor observed, that when we immerse our bodies "in a cold or warm bath," or "by plunging the hand and arm even in cold water," globules of air soon appear upon the skin; and to be certain of the air coming from the body, he took all the necessary precautions to prevent the external air being carried into the water along with the body (which would certainly be a consequence if the body or part were immersed quickly, or when dried). But although his experiments seem to prove this opinion, yet I imagine there is a circumstance the Doctor did not attend to at the time, which renders them very fallacious; for he did not consider that water for the most part contains a great deal of air; therefore the globules of air might as readily come from the water as

* Experiments upon Vegetables, proving their great power of purifying the common air, &c.

from the body, which makes it necessary to ascertain, by experiment, from whence the air comes which is attached to the body when immersed in water.

Water takes up air in proportion to its coldness, until it loses the property of water, and becomes solid: upon this principle we may account for globules of air being found attached to the skin when a part of the body is immersed in water colder than itself; for when we immerse the whole body we increase the heat of the water, especially that next to the skin; and if we immerse only a part, as an arm, it being commonly in a smaller quantity of water, the water immediately surrounding it is also warmed. As a proof that it is the air from the water, and not from the surface of the body*, it matters not what the substance is that is immersed if it is but warmer than the water; for a piece of iron, heated to about 150°, immersed in water about 70°, will warm the water in contact with it so as to make it part with its air. This effect of heat is further proved by making another trial, with only this difference, that the iron be ten degrees colder than the water; in that case little or no air will be separated, and of course no bubbles observed. The bubbles of air do not appear to arise entirely from the degree of warmth of the water, but also in some measure from a solid body being immersed in it, that seems to have a power of attracting the air, whose affinity to the water is now weakened by heat; for simply heating the water to the same degree will not separate the air, as we find that no bubbles are then produced. The power of attracting the air appears therefore in some sort to depend upon the solidity of the body immersed; at least bodies have a greater number of bubbles in proportion to their solidity; for upon making comparative experiments between iron, stone, wood, and cork, the air separated from the water upon the surface of the iron and stone is in considerable quantity; that upon the wood very small, and scarcely any at all upon the cork.

As these observations on the generation (or secretion) of air in cavities

* " Count de Milly, in the Berlin Transactions for the year 1777, published experiments to show that there is an excretion of air, or, as it is termed, 'an aerial transpiration,' from the whole surface of the human body while it remains in warm water; but Dr. Pearson found, on repeating these experiments, that there was no appearance of aerial bubbles on the surface of the cuticle during bathing in warm water that had been previously boiled, so as to expel the air usually mixed and united to river and spring water. The human body, when immersed in the bath at Buxton, and kept at rest in it for some time, was covered with air-like bubbles; but these bubbles appeared in the same manner on any solid body whatever that was placed in it. It is therefore supposed that the attraction to the human body of the air, commonly suspended in water, especially when heated to the temperature of a warm-water bath, has been mistaken for an excretion of air from the cuticle."

seemed to have a connexion with the present inquiry, I thought they might properly enough be introduced here; but I shall content myself with having mentioned the circumstance, and pursue the subject of digestion.

To determine with absolute certainty in what particular portion of the canal this important process of digestion is performed, is perhaps impossible; but there is the greatest reason to believe that it is principally carried on in the stomach, with a little variation in different animals. We may venture to affirm that it does not at all take place in the long and contracted œsophagus of the quadruped, the secretion of that part being a slimy mucus, possessed of no power similar to that of the gastric juice, but only intended to facilitate the passage of the food into the stomach.

Neither has the mucus secreted in certain parts of the œsophagus of birds, as in the crop of those which have one, any digestive power; while, on the contrary, we find the lower end, which is extremely glandular, to be capable of secreting a juice with all the properties of the gastric; and that passing into the cavity of the stomach becomes a substitute in this class of animals for the deficiency of the secretion of the stomach itself, which in some is lined with a horny substance, and in others with a cuticle. Even in birds the seat of digestion is chiefly in the stomach, the juice secreted in the lower part of the œsophagus passing into that cavity; and the mucus secreted by the other parts of the œsophagus, as in the crop of those which have one, has no such power. But if any digestible substance should be retained in the œsophagus, as may happen in many of those which swallow whole animals, digestion may even go on in its inferior portion. In the gull and heron, which take down snakes and fish entire, the tails may remain in the œsophagus till the head is digested in the stomach; and in such cases the tail itself may be acted upon in that situation.

As a further proof that digestion is carried on principally in the stomach, let us observe what happens to the yolk of an egg in the bird newly hatched. The yolk is not in the least consumed in the time of incubation, but appears to be reserved for the nourishment of the chick between the time of hatching, and its either being supplied with food by its parents, or being able to procure it for itself; for we find, that although the yolk passes into the gut at some distance from the stomach, yet it is carried up to the stomach to be digested; and I have even seen it in the crop, being retained there till wanted.

In those animals whose stomach consists of several cavities, the precise place where digestion is carried on has not been ascertained. I think, however, that in the ruminating class, in which it has four cavities, it may be set down as a fact that digestion goes on in the fourth, which is best proved by feeding the animal with a substance that does not require any kind of preparation for digestion, such as milk. If a calf be killed about half an hour after it has sucked its mother, we shall find the whole milk in the fourth cavity firmly coagulated, and formed into a ball, while the first, second, and third cavities contain only such food as requires mastication, or what other preparation is necessary to fit it for digestion. Such animals have the power of conveying the food from the œsophagus, either to the first or fourth cavity, according to the nature of the food; and for this purpose there is a groove leading directly from the œsophagus to the fourth stomach, which I suppose can be converted into a canal when wanted.

It is possible that digestion may likewise be carried on in the duodenum, especially in its upper part, if either the intestine secretes the same juice with the stomach, or that some of the gastric juice and part of the food have passed into the intestine before it has been completely turned into chyle[a].

Although the stomach is the seat of digestion, it is not solely appropriated to that purpose; and in many animals these organs are not to be considered as only a digesting bag or bags, but in part as a reservoir for food. This is most remarkable in the ruminating animals, where the first stomach or bag is merely a reservoir, and in this respect analogous to a crop. It is the same in the porpus, and, I believe, in most animals of this class; although it cannot be supposed that those return the food who have not the power to masticate. In some animals which do not ruminate there is not the same necessity for distinct pouches, the stomach consisting either of one bag singly, or of stomach with appendages, as in the peccari. But the whole organ is not endowed with the property of secreting the gastric juice, there being a part whose structure is very different from that appropriated to digestion, and covered by a cuticle, as in the first, second, and third stomach of the ruminating animals, and in the first stomach of the porpus. The pec-

---

[a] [This conjecture is confirmed by the observations of Tiedemann and Gmelin, who found that when any vegetable fecula passed the pylorus unaltered it was converted in the duodenum, as in the stomach, into sugar and amydine.

Majendie attempted to subject this question to direct experiment, but failed from not having insured the continuance of the substance experimented on in the necessary situation. He found, on introducing a piece of raw flesh into the duodenum of a healthy dog, that in an hour it had been carried to the rectum: its weight was slightly diminished, but there was no other change than a discoloration of its surface. In another experiment he fixed a morsel of flesh in the small intestine with a thread; after the lapse of three hours it had lost about half its weight: the fibrin had been principally acted upon; what was left was entirely cellular, and extremely fœtid. See *Precis Elémentaire de Physiologie*, ii. p. 114.]

cari, the common hog, and the rat are likewise instances of this; and the same circumstance takes place, in a smaller degree, in the horse.

This increase in the cavity of the stomach, beyond what is necessary for digestion alone, is peculiar to the animals that take in more food than is immediately wanted, or whose food is of a nature which requires a certain degree of preparation prior to digestion. The crop of the eagle, and perhaps the first stomach of the porpus, are of the first kind; the crop in the gallinaceous fowls, and the first stomach in ruminating animals, of the second[a]. It is the disposition of such animals to fill these cavities; and the quantity which they are capable of containing makes them seldomer require to be filled; it is probable, likewise, that it is the sensation excited by this fulness which gives satisfaction to the animal, and takes off the further desire for food, an effect similar to what is produced in other animals from filling the stomach itself; and these having no such provision, are longer and oftener employed in pursuit of food.

I should be apt to consider the power of the gastric juice to coagulate milk, and some other animal mucilages*, as a test of the stomach being the seat of digestion; for although milk may be coagulated by other substances, yet when found in that state in the stomach it is probably for the purpose of digestion, milk and many other natural substances requiring to be coagulated before they can be digested. I have found this coagulating power in the stomach of every animal that I have examined for that purpose, from the most perfect down to reptiles[b];

* Milk is the substance commonly known to be coagulated by the gastric juice; but I find that it has also the same power over the white of an egg. Give to a dog some raw egg, and kill him half an hour after he has swallowed it, the egg will be found coagulated in his stomach, as if boiled. The crystalline humour in the stomachs of fishes is likewise found coagulated.

[a] [According to this difference in their functions, we find that the crop of the eagle is relatively smaller than that of the fowl, and the passage of its contents to the stomach is more direct and easy. The first stomach of the porpus is still smaller in comparison with the rumen of the sheep; and besides acting as a storehouse for the food, digestion goes on in it to a considerable extent. This is effected, not by secretion from its own parietes, which, as Hunter observes, are lined with a cuticle, but most probably by the gastric juice regurgitated into it from the second stomach, which is highly glandular. The flesh of fish is found separated from the bones, and these in different stages of softening, in the first stomach; indeed, the construction of the aperture of communication between the first and second stomachs of the porpus is such, that food can pass into the latter only in a very comminuted state.]

[b] [By "reptiles" there is reason to believe Mr. Hunter meant 'creeping things,' as insects and worms. The 'Reptilia' of modern naturalists he invariably calls by the Linnæan name 'Amphibia,' or by his own term, 'Tricoilia.' In the Introduction to

and in the appendages which I have considered as only reservoirs preparatory to digestion, (as the first stomach in the ruminating animal,
and the crop in birds,) I have discovered no such power. Yet it is not
the digestive power which coagulates those substances, complete coagulation taking place even where digestion does not at all go on[a].
This is evident every day in children who suck, and who have diseased
stomachs ; for we see them throw up the milk coagulated, and discharge
it undigested by stool. A very remarkable instance occurred in a child
that had lost entirely the power of digestion, yet the milk taken down
came away strongly coagulated, some even as firm almost as cheese ;
which seems to show that the coagulating power is seldom wanting,
although the other may.

The gastric juice is a fluid somewhat transparent, and a little saltish
or brackish to the taste ; but whether this is essential or only accidental
is not easily determined. Indeed there are very few of our secretions
which have not some salt in them ; it being found in the tears, the saliva, the secretion of the glans penis, of the glands of the urethra, and
in the first and the last milk secreted in the udders of animals.

I am not inclined to suppose that there is any acid in the gastric juice
as a component or essential part of it, although an acid is very commonly discovered, even when no vegetable matter has been introduced
into the stomach*. The acid may be increased in some diseases, and

* The only trial to which I ever put the gastric juice was with the syrup of violets, to
ascertain if it was acid ; and in many of the trials the colour of the mixture was changed

---

the Series of Digestive Organs, (Phys. Catalogue of the Hunterian Collection, vol. i.)
he says, " In some reptiles the teeth are placed in the œsophagus," alluding to preparations of a Nereis; and in a manuscript, published in the same volume of the Physiological Catalogue, there is proof that he experimented on an insect with especial reference to the seat of the digestive power. After detailing the peculiarities of the digestive organs in the flesh-fly (*Musca vomitoria*), he observes :

" The bag belonging to the first-described canal is to be considered a craw or crop,
viz. a reservoir for the food to be ready for digestion; and as the abdomen contains
almost every internal part of the animal, it is obliged to be situated in this cavity. That
it is a reservoir for food I proved by experiment : I kept some of these flies fasting for
some time : I then gave them milk, which they drank readily ; and when I thought
they had filled their bellies, I put them into spirits, which assisted in coagulating the
milk wherever it might be. On opening the abdomen, I found this bag full of curd
and whey, as also some in the stomach. I kept a fly for twelve hours without food,
and then gave it milk, and killed it, and found no milk in the crop, but it had got
through almost the whole tract of intestines : here the animal had immediate occasion
for food, therefore the milk did not go into the crop. This experiment at the same
time shows that, probably, every part of the intestine digests, for the stomach makes
no distinct bag."]

[a] [Or rather the digestive power may be equal to the coagulation, but not to the completion of the digestion of the coagulable substances.]

in others the disposition to form it may be destroyed, which may be the reason why, by a kind of instinctive principle, many girls are fond of eating sour fruit and of drinking vinegar; while others, on the contrary, from a different cause, often eat chalk, lime, and other substances of that sort. But the acid not being always found, it is not yet determined on what occasions it is formed, or in what manner it is destroyed.

The process of digestion differs from every other natural operation in the change it produces on different bodies; yet it is by no means fermentation, though it may somewhat resemble it. For fermentation, a spontaneous process, is that natural succession of changes by which vegetable and animal matter is reduced to earth; therefore must be widely

to red. But it is necessary, for the accuracy of the experiment which is to determine this fact, that the animal should not be fed upon vegetables for some time before the trial is made, these being liable in some degree to become sour; therefore it is hardly fair to make the experiment on the contents of the stomach of animals who live upon vegetables. In many trials of this kind we may be deceived, and led to suppose an alkali; for certain animal secretions being of a yellow cast, when such are mixed with the syrup of violets the mixture is changed to a green. The truth of the experiment may, however, be known by adding a little acid; for if the green has been produced merely by a mechanical mixture, it will become immediately a scarlet, by being then a mixture of red and yellow; but if the secretion is not only of a yellow colour, but of an alkaline nature, it will also continue green; and by adding a little more acid than what saturates the alkali the colour will then become orange[a].

---

[a] [Various opinions have been entertained as to the acidity of the gastric juice. Spallanzani believed it to be a neutral fluid. Carminati could detect no acid in the gastric juice of carnivorous animals and mixed feeders, but found it to exist in that of vegetable feeders. (*Ueber die Natur des Magensaftes*, Wien, 1785.) Helm, who examined the gastric juice in a patient with a fistulous opening in the stomach, also states that it contains no sensible acid. (*Zwei Krankengeschicten*, Wien, 1803.) The same cause of error has probably operated in each of the preceding cases, viz. not making a sufficient distinction between the ordinary mucous secretion of the stomach and the peculiar fluid which is poured out from the stimulus of the contact of food, or any innutritious substances. In the experiments of Tiedemann and Gmelin the ordinary secretion of the stomach in fasting horses and dogs was found to be almost neutral, or very slightly acid; but on stimulating the surface by means of stones, (by which any cause of error from a change of fermentable substances, as alluded to by Hunter, was avoided,) then the secretion manifested unequivocally the presence of acidity. Beaumont has more fully established the acidity of the gastric juice in the work before quoted. He observed in the man with gastric fistula that the gastric juice was poured out from numerous minute clear points or papillæ. It is a clear inodorous fluid, with a somewhat salt and very marked acid taste, like that of thin mucilage which has been soured with muriatic acid. It dissolves in water, wine, and alcohol; slightly effervesces with alkali; decomposes slowly, and retards the decomposition of animal matter. Saliva imparts to the gastric juice a blue colour and a frothy appearance. Chemical analysis shows the gastric juice to contain both the muriatic and acetic acids, alkaline phosphates, muriate of soda, magnesia, and lime, and an animal matter which is soluble in cold but not in hot water.]

different from digestion, which converts both animal and vegetable substances into chyle, in the formation of which there cannot be a decomposition similar to fermentation.

Digestion is likewise very different from chemical solution, which is only a union of bodies by elective attraction. But digestion is an assimilating process; and in this respect is somewhat similar in its action to that excited by morbid poisons. It is a species of generation, two substances making a third; but the curious circumstance is its converting both vegetable and animal matter into the same kind of substance or compound, which no chemical process can effect. The chyle is compounded of the gastric juice and digestible substances when perfectly converted; and it is probable that the quantity of gastric juice may be nearly equal to that part of the food which is really changed into chyle. If so, it demonstrates the necessity of a very quick secretion, to supply a quantity so very considerable; but with this advantage, that it is not lost to the constitution.

The progress of the conversion of food into chyle may be often seen in the stomach of animals at different times after feeding. Fishes are good subjects on which to make observations for this purpose, as they swallow their food whole; and as that food is commonly fish, and often too large to be completely admitted into the stomach. As they do not masticate their food, it is not adapted to the cavity of the stomach; and therefore part of it is often found lying in the œsophagus; a circumstance by which the comparative progress of digestion is rendered more obvious.

It may also be well observed in the stomach of a dog, in which the whole quantity taken has been swallowed at once. In the great end the food will be but little altered; towards the middle, more; and towards the pylorus it will be similar to what is found in the duodenum[a].

From the structure of the stomach in ruminating animals they are badly adapted to assist our inquiries on this subject, because metallic balls, or whatever is swallowed in so hard and solid a form as to be unfit for digestion, requiring to be ruminated, will often be thrown out when returned into the mouth for that purpose; or it may lie a long time in the first stomach without being either thrown up or passed into the fourth, as I have frequently seen; therefore the chance of its getting into the fourth stomach in a proper time to fit it for the object of

[a] [The cardiac and pyloric portions of the stomach possess the digestive power in very different degrees, it being much more energetic in the latter. In the stomachs of Carnivora and Rodentia the two portions are commonly found divided by a constriction; and the same hour-glass contraction of the stomach is occasionally met with in the human subject. See Sir Everard Home, Phil. Trans. 1817, p. 347.]

an experiment being very uncertain, no great light can be derived from trials made on animals of this class.

Live or fresh vegetables, when taken into the stomach, are first killed, by which a flabbiness in their texture is produced, as if they had been boiled; and then they can be acted upon by the gastric juice.

Meat appears to undergo no change as preparatory to digestion, but at once to submit to its union with the gastric juice; for, after having been acted upon, it seems first to lose its texture, then becomes cineritious in colour, next gelatinous, and last chyle. The first change made upon milk and some other secretions, as the yolk and white of an egg, is coagulation; after which the gastric juice begins to acquire a power of uniting with them.

The first change which is produced on animal substances out of the body, either by being exposed to heat or by becoming spontaneously putrid, is similar to the second of the three changes which takes place in digestion; and is only preparatory to the complete change, whether that be digestion or putrefaction.

It appears from many experiments that the digested or animalized part, when carried into the intestine, is attracted by the villous coat, or clings to it as if entangled among the villi; while the excrementitious part, such as bile, is found lying unconnected in the gut, as if separated from the other[a].

The food of animals in general consists of vegetable or animal substances; and vegetables seem intended to support one class, with a view to its being the food of another. Although there are classes of animals intended to subsist on each particular kind of food, yet they do not all invariably keep to the same kind in every stage of life, many being nourished by animal food when young that afterwards live on vegetables; which circumstance will be more fully discussed when treating of the first food of pigeons.

All stomachs do not equally digest the same substance, although it be their natural food. The caterpillar digests the expressed juice, but not the substance; while other animals are capable of dissolving nearly the whole. Some animals, as the common cattle, can feed on a variety of vegetables, although they may have a preference; but there are others

---

[a] [In chylification, the alkaline principles of the bile combine with the acids which the chyme has received in its formation in the stomach, and the albuminous or chylous principles are developed and attracted by the villi; while the resinous parts of the bile, combined with the excrementitious particles of the chyme, are more or less completely separated. The most characteristic change which, according to Prout, takes place in the intestine is the conversion of part of the chyme into albumen, which happens even when no albuminous matter was originally contained in the food or formed in the stomach.]

that will hardly eat of more than one kind. Of this last sort are insects in general, and the silkworm will scarcely touch anything but
mulberry leaves ; but I believe those that live upon animal food are not
so restricted in their choice.

It is probable that all animal and vegetable substances are equally
capable of being digested, if equally soft in their texture ; but some
being much firmer in that respect, and others also united with indigestible matter, as the earth in bones, more strongly resist the powers of
the gastric juice ; therefore mastication and trituration become necessary to bring them to a similar consistence. But substances may be
rendered too soft, for a fluid is difficult of digestion ; and we may observe, that Nature having given us very few fluids as articles of food,
to render these few fitter for the action of the digestive powers, a coagulating principle is provided to give them some degree of solidity *.
It is not easy to assign a reason why fluidity should be unfavourable to
the process of digestion, more especially as it seems essential to those
of fermentation and chemical solution. The requisite degree of solidity
I should suppose to be that of curd, or what is produced by the coagulation of animal mucilages, as of the white of an egg. But this is only
supposition, founded on the idea that Nature's general principles are
right, and all the corresponding parts adapted to one another, except
when monstrous, either in form or action.

Mastication is the effect of a mechanical power, produced by parts
particularly provided for that purpose, which are of various kinds, fitted
for that sort of food on which the animal is by Nature intended to live,
and may be imitated with equal advantage by many other pieces of
mechanism.

The masticating powers are of three kinds. The first is that which
merely fits the substance for deglutition, as in the lion and many other
carnivorous animals ; and which, in the ruminating tribe, renders the
food fit to be swallowed, that it may undergo such preparation in the
first stomach as is necessary before it is further masticated for digestion. The second is that which not only fits the food for deglutition,
but exposes it to the action of the gastric juice, by breaking the shells

* The circumstance of the crystalline humour, which is solid, being coagulated prior
to its being digested, renders it probable that all animal substances go through that process, and that the loss of texture which they undergo arises from coagulation [a].

---

[a] [This coagulation happens to all animal substances which contain albumen ; but it
can hardly be considered, Dr. Prout observes, " to be essential to the subsequent process ; for gelatine, a staminal alimentary principle, nearly resembling albumen in its
composition, undergoes, under similar circumstances, no such solidifying change. (Br.
Tr., p. 494.)]

or husks in which the nourishment is contained, and in which it would
be defended from the powers of digestion. And the third is that which
divides and bruises the food before it is received into the stomach;
which mastication is of considerable service, by producing a saving in
food[a].

The husk of the seeds of plants, although a vegetable substance, appears to be indigestible in its natural state. Whether this arises from
the nature of the husk itself, or from its compactness, I am not quite
certain, but am inclined to suppose the last, as we find the cocoa, which
is only a husk, to be digestible when ground to a powder and well boiled.
We know likewise that cuticle, horn, hair, and feathers, although animal substances, are not affected, in the first instance, by the gastric
juice ; yet if reduced in Papin's digester to a jelly, that jelly can be acted
upon in the stomach : we must therefore suppose that a certain natural
degree of solidity in animal and vegetable substances renders them indigestible. This compactness in the husk seems to be intended to preserve, while under ground, the farinaceous part of the seed, in which
the living principle is placed, the husk having probably no other power
of resisting putrefaction than what arises from its texture; but whatever may be the use of the husk, it must be connected with the vege-
tative process of the plant. The same purpose of preservation is probably
answered by the shells of all ova. Although husks are not capable of
being dissolved in the gastric juice, they allow of transudation, and
that the seed is in some degree affected by it is known by its swelling
in the stomach; yet it can only take up a certain proportion of it, and
that not sufficient to convert it into chyle, the gastric juice having no
power of action upon the husks themselves. Therefore we see grain of
all kinds, when swallowed whole, pass through entire, though swelled ;
and even the kernels of some nuts, as chestnuts, are not digestible when
eaten raw.

The essential oils of vegetables and animals are indigestible; but
being soluble either in the gastric juice or chyle, they become medicinal,
from their stimulating powers. The essential oil of vegetables, but
more particularly that of animals, seems to pervade the very substance
of those animals whose food contains much of this oil. Thus, we find
sea-birds, whose constant food is fish, taste very strongly of fish; and
those who live on that kind of food only during certain times of the
year, as the wild duck, have that taste only at such seasons. This fact
is so well known that it was hardly necessary to put it to the test of an

[a] [Blumenbach has well suggested that the vitality of the seeds is thus destroyed
and they are made subject to the influence of the gastric juice.]

experiment; yet I took two ducks, and fed one with barley, the other with sprats, for about a month, and killed both at the same time : when they were dressed, the one fed wholly with sprats was hardly eatable, it tasted so strongly of fish.

Although bones are in part composed of animal substance, and so far digestible, yet they require stronger powers to digest them than common meat, from the animal substance being guarded by the earth. Thus the animal part of a bone is less easily soluble in an alkali than flesh, or than even the animal part when deprived of its earth by an acid; nor will a bone, being guarded by the calcareous earth, submit to putre-faction so readily as meat; therefore animals which live upon others, and swallow them whole, as the heron, digest bone with more ease than the crow or magpie, that are not accustomed to swallow bones, but commonly pick the flesh only.

The degree of ease or difficulty with which substances are digested, will not only arise from a difference in solidity, but from a difference in the structure of the parts themselves; brain, liver, muscle, and tendon being digestible in the order here put down.

There is not only a difference in the degree of facility with which the various kinds of natural food are digested, but these can also be made to undergo changes by art, which render them still more easy of diges-tion; for it appears from my experiments that boiled and roasted, and even putrid meat, is easier of digestion than raw, which, in the two first, may be supposed to arise from their juices being coagulated; but the same reason will not hold good with regard to the putrid[a]. A raw egg is thought more easy of digestion than an egg hard boiled, although the raw one must be coagulated in the stomach before it can be digested; and it has likewise been observed, that what is easy of digestion in one stomach will not be so in another; but such cases may probably arise from the stomach not being in a healthy state.

In many animals the whole of the food does not appear to be digested, the substance in part being found in the fæces; for if a dog is fed with tallow, his excrements will consist of a somewhat firm unctuous sub-stance, so that the oil is only digested in part. The circumstance of

---

[a] [From the various experiments instituted by Sir Astley Cooper on the digestibility of different substances, it appears that pork is more digestible than mutton, this than veal, while beef is the least digestible of any. In feeding dogs with determinate quan-tities of each, and opening them at the expiration of a given period, it happened that in some instances the pork and mutton had entirely disappeared, while the beef re-mained but little altered. Fish and cheese were also found to be very digestible sub-stances. Potatoes were digestible in a less degree. Boiled veal was found to be two thirds more digested than the same meat roasted, &c. Muscular tissue, skin, gristle, tendons, bone, were digestible in the order here set down.]

some part of the food, though digestible, not being acted upon by the gastric juice, may arise from two causes: first, from many parts of vegetables being too firm in texture to be digested in the same time with the other food, and being therefore carried along in a crude state, together with the chyle, into the duodenum; and secondly, from the stomach at the time being so much disordered as to digest imperfectly. We know that food may lie a considerable time in the stomach when it is diseased without being digested. Food has been retained in the stomach twenty-four hours, and thrown up without being in the least altered, the animal at the time not requiring nourishment: this often arises from disease, and is also the case with those which go to rest in the winter.

The powers of digestion may in some instances be estimated by the appearance of the excrement, in which, if the food appears not to be much altered, we may conclude that digestion has had little or no influence on it. Thus, the excrement of a flea, that has lived on blood, is nearly, to appearance, pure blood, not having even lost its colour.

Animals take food in proportion to the quantity of nourishment contained in it, of which the stomach appears, from instinct, to be capable of judging; and also in proportion to the powers they possess of converting what they eat into chyle. A caterpillar, perhaps, eats more in proportion to its size than any other animal that lives on the same kind of food; for not having the power of dissolving the vegetable, but only of extracting a juice or infusion from it, the bit of leaf comes away entire, coiled up and hardened; but by being put into water, unfolds like tea.

There are few animals that do not eat flesh in some form or other, while there are many who do not eat vegetables at all; and therefore the difficulty to make the herbivorous eat meat is not so great as to make the carnivorous eat vegetables. Where there is an instinctive principle in an animal, directing it either to the one species of food or the other, the animal will certainly die rather than break through of its own accord that natural law; but it may be made to violate every natural principle by artificial means. That the hawk tribe can be made to feed upon bread, I have known these thirty years; for to a tame kite I first gave fat, which it ate very readily; then tallow and butter; and afterwards small balls of bread rolled in fat or butter; and by decreasing the fat gradually it at last ate bread alone, and seemed to thrive as well as when fed with meat. This, however, produced a difference in the consistence of the excrements, for when it ate meat they were thin, and it had the power of throwing them to some distance; but when it ate bread they became firmer in texture, and dropped like the excrement of a common fowl. Spallanzani attempted, in vain, to make an eagle eat bread by itself; but by inclosing the bread in meat, so as to deceive the eagle, the bread was swallowed, and digested in the stomach.

The excrements of animals we may suppose to be that part of the common food which is indigestible; and as food is either animal or vegetable, and each different kind adapted to distinct classes of animals, it is natural to believe that the excrementitious part of each will be different; and where the animal feeds upon both, that the excrement will be of a mixed nature. Although this appears probable, it is only true in a certain degree; for the mode of digestion, and whether the animal has a cæcum and colon, with their peculiar form, have all an influence in the changes which the food undergoes. Vegetable food produces more excrement than animal, and this according to the kind or parts of vegetables that are eaten. The woody parts and husks, which are indigestible, produce the most; the true farinaceous part the least: why there should be any at all from the farinaceous and animal substance, except what has eluded the action of the digestive organs, is not easily accounted for.

All fæces have a tendency to putrefaction, but least in those animals which feed on vegetables. Indeed, the excrement from vegetable food alone could hardly ever become putrid if it was not mixed with the mucus of the intestines, and would even then be kept sweet by the tendency which undigested vegetables have to take on the vinous and acetous fermentation. But the fæces of those which live entirely on animal food in general very soon become putrid; and indeed often before they are voided; but such animals are either without cæcum or colon; or if not, what they have is very short; so that the excrement not being long retained, has less time to become putrid. When the fæces stagnate so as to take on either the vinous or putrefactive fermentation, air is let loose, which will be according to the nature of the fermentation; most probably, from the vegetable it will be fixed, and from the animal, inflammable air.

The fæces of the greatest number of animals are tinged by the bile, which in some gives them a yellowish green colour; in the bird they are generally green, but sometimes white, from being mixed with the urine. The fæces of the maggot appear to be loaded with bile; for besides being yellow, they are extremely bitter, which is known by eating the kernel of a nut that has a maggot in it. Some kinds of food, when not wholly digested, give a tinge to the fæces, as grass to the excrement of cows.

The animals which feed upon vegetables alone commonly have their fæces somewhat solid; but the degree will vary according to the state of the vegetable, whether green or dried; and therefore the particular state of the fæces will depend on the nature of the indigestible part of the food, and must be different according to the digestive powers in different animals. An animal that feeds upon grass has the fæces much softer than when fed on the same kind of grass made into hay ; and therefore the fæces of the herbivorous animals are softer in the summer than the winter; but green vegetable food does not produce soft fæces in all animals, for the caterpillar, which lives upon the leaves of vegetables, has its fæces almost dry; and we find in some ruminating animals, as sheep, that the difference in the fæces during summer and winter is inconsiderable. The quadrupeds and birds that live principally upon vegetables generally have their cæca large and the colon long, as we see in many of the ruminating animals. Some have the colon both long and large, as the horse and those of the rat tribe, which circumstance has considerable effects in allowing the fæces to become dry : in a few of the ruminating animals, and of the rat kind, they are formed into small portions.

The fæces of quadrupeds living upon animal food are commonly soft, and in birds are fluid ; but in such as live on both animals and vegetables, they are in consistence of a mixed nature, and will be more or less soft according to the food. If a dog is fed entirely on animal substance its fæces will be soft; if wholly on vegetable, as on bread, they will become so hard as to be expelled with difficulty [a].

---

[a] [The following differences were found by Dr. Prout in the contents of the rectum of dogs which had been fed on

Vegetable Food.

Of a firm consistence, and of an olive brown colour, inclining to yellow. Smell fœtid and offensive. Did not coagulate milk.

A. Water; quantity not ascertained.

B. Combination or mixture of altered alimentary substances in much greater excess than in the colon, with some mucus; insoluble in acetic acid, and constituting the chief bulk of the fæces.

C. Albuminous matter, none.

D. Biliary principle, partly changed to a perfect resin.

E. Vegetable gluten? none; but contained a principle soluble in acetic acid, and precipitable very copiously by oxalate of ammonia.

F. Insoluble residuum, consisting chiefly of vegetable fibres mixed with hairs.

Animal Food.

Consisted of firm scybala, of a dark brown colour, inclining to chocolate. Smell very fœtid. Milk was coagulated by the water in which it had been diffused.

A. Water; quantity not ascertained.

B. Combination or mixture of altered alimentary matters in much greater excess than in either the colon or cæcum, with some mucus; insoluble in acetic acid, and constituting the chief bulk of the fæces.

C. Albuminous matter, none.

D. Biliary principle more considerable than in the vegetable fæces, and almost entirely changed to a perfectly resinous-like substance.

E. Vegetable gluten? none; but contained a principle soluble in acetic acid, and precipitable very copiously in oxalate of ammonia.

F. Insoluble residuum, consisting chiefly of hairs.]

Spallanzani made some experiments to prove that digestion is carried on after death; but they are not so conducted as to correspond with the appearances met with in the dead body where that process has taken place, and the coats of the stomach itself have been in part digested. An experiment, although it may be very well and accurately made so far as the experiment goes, if a close connexion is not preserved with the purpose for which it was made, the conclusions to be drawn from it cannot correspond with the intention. This is exactly the case with the experiments of Spallanzani, which, although they prove that meat was digested in the stomach after the animal was killed (which no one doubted), yet are not at all calculated to show that the stomach itself may be digested. In fact, the mode in which they were managed rather tended to prevent that effect from taking place, for the gastric juice, by having substances introduced on which it could act, was less likely to affect the coats of the stomach. That the digestion was not carried on merely by the gastric juice secreted before the animal was apparently dead, is evident, from his own account, some of the food which had been introduced and digested being found in the duodenum, a thing that could not have happened if a cessation of the actions of life in the involuntary parts had taken place when visible life terminated. There had been an action, and most probably a secretion, in the stomach. The only experiment that can be made with any probability of a decided result, is to kill the animal while the stomach is empty, and observe what afterwards takes place. There are few stomachs that do not show, when examined after death, some of the inner villous coat destroyed, which may have been done by the gastric juice in the ducts of the glands which secrete it.

Dr. Stevens, in an inaugural dissertation on this subject, published at Edinburgh 1777, gives a number of experiments, some of which are well devised, to ascertain the substances that are easiest of digestion, a thing in fact more wanted than the cause of that process: but many of his experiments, more especially those on ruminating animals, were not made with sufficient accuracy. How the chopped hay and potherbs came to be so much changed in the first stomach of a ruminating animal I cannot conceive, as I have reason to believe it has not the least power of digesting, and should doubt very much that hay was capable of being wholly digested in any stomach. His experiment made on substances out of the body proves that the gastric juice is not able in all cases to prevent the vinous and acetous fermentation in vegetables, and is a circumstance which I believe often takes place in the living body when the stomach is weak. He seems to be in some apprehension for the safety of the stomach itself, from the action of so powerful a solvent as the gastric juice; but though inclined to suppose that the living powers of the animal may guard it against such effects, yet he is still disposed to fear that in all cases they may not be sufficient.

The living power in the stomach must indeed be very weak to admit of its being digested; where that was likely to happen, I imagine the secretion of the gastric juice would be too defective to allow of the stomach being acted upon.

Dr. Stevens gives two cases, with the dissections, to prove that the living stomach has not always the power to resist the action of the gastric juice; but he has not made it clear that those very stomachs might not have been digested after death. The appearance of the edges of the hole should have been more particularly described; for if it took place before death it is probable it was owing to ulceration, which I have sometimes seen. Men should be very accurate in ascertaining the truth of facts before they advance them, especially when they tend either to overturn a received opinion or to establish a new one. As to the possibility of animals swallowed alive being digested, no fresh proofs are necessary, as we eat oysters every day; but this does not prove that they are digested while alive. In his experiments made on ruminating animals and the dog, as the vegetables were not so readily digested as the meat, he concludes, "It is possible every species of animal has its peculiar gastric liquor, capable of dissolving certain substances only" which is certainly not true.

Mr. Senebier relates some experiments made by Mr. Gosse upon himself, but which hardly contain anything except a curious conjecture of Mr. Senebier's, "That distention of the stomach is the cause of the secretion of the gastric liquor." He mentions the substances, both animal and vegetable, which are not digestible; then those difficult of digestion; afterwards, those easily digested; also what substances facilitate digestion, and what retard it. But if we are to judge of the truth of these facts from a detail of the experiments which he made to ascertain them, I am quite inclined to believe that the experiments have not been made with sufficient accuracy to be depended upon.

ON THE DIGESTION OF THE STOMACH AFTER DEATH.

The following account of the stomach being digested after death was drawn up at the desire of the late Sir John Pringle, when he was President of the Royal Society; and the circumstance which led to it was as follows. I had opened, in his presence, the body of a patient who had been under his care, in which the stomach was found to be in part dissolved; a thing that appeared to him very unaccountable, there having been no previous symptom which could have led him to suspect any disease in the stomach. I took that opportunity of explaining to him my ideas respecting it; and that, having long been employed in making experiments on digestion, I had been induced to consider this as one of the facts which proved a converting power in the gastric juice. I mentioned my intention of publishing the whole of my observations on digestion at some future period; but he desired me, in the mean time, to give this fact by itself, with my remarks; as it would prove that there is a solvent power existing in the stomach, and would be of use in the examination of dead bodies[a].

An accurate knowledge of the appearances in animal bodies, where death has been the consequence of some violence while they were otherwise in health, ought certainly to be considered as necessary to qualify us to judge truly of the state of the body in those that die of diseases. An animal body undergoes changes after death; but it has never been sufficiently considered what those changes are, or how soon they may take place; yet till this be done it is impossible we can form an accurate judgement of the appearances which present themselves at the time of inspection. The diseases of an animal body (mortification excepted) are always connected with the living principle, and are not in the least similar to the changes which take place in the dead body: without a knowledge of this, an opinion drawn from dissections must always be very imperfect or very erroneous. Appearances which are in themselves natural may be mistaken for those of disease; we may see diseased parts, and suppose them in a natural state; we may consider a circumstance to have existed before death which was really a consequence of it; or we may imagine it to be a natural change after death, when it was in fact a disease of the living body. It is easy to see, therefore, how a man in this state of ignorance must blunder when he comes to connect the appearances in a dead body with the symptoms that were observed in life; and, indeed, all the advantage to be derived from opening dead bodies depends upon the judgement and sagacity with which this sort of comparison is made.

---

[a] [The original paper is printed in the 62nd volume of the Philosophical Transactions; and was read June 18th, 1772. It begins as follows: " An accurate knowledge of the appearances in animal bodies that die of a violent death, that is, in perfect health, or in a sound state, ought to be considered as a necessary foundation for judging of the state of the body in those that are diseased." The remainder of the essay is given in the 2nd edition of the Animal Œconomy, with verbal alterations of the same kind and degree as are exemplified in the paragraph above quoted; with the omission of one sentence and a note, which are subjoined at the end of the paper.]

There is a case of a mixed nature, which can neither be reckoned a process of the living body nor of the dead: it participates of both, in as much as its cause arises from life, and the effect cannot take place till after death. To render this more intelligible, it will be necessary to state some general ideas concerning this cause and effect.

An animal substance, when joined with the living principle, cannot undergo any change in its properties but as an animal; this principle always acting and preserving the substance possessed of it from dissolution, and from being changed according to the natural changes which other substances undergo.

There are a great many powers in nature which the living principle does not enable the animal matter, with which it is combined, to resist, viz. the mechanical and most of the strongest chemical solvents. It renders it, however, capable of resisting the powers of fermentation, digestion, (and perhaps several others,) which are well known to act on this same matter, and entirely to decompose it, when deprived of the living principle. The number of powers which thus act differently on the living and dead animal substance not being ascertained, we shall only take notice of two, putrefaction and digestion, which do not affect this substance, unless when it is deprived of the living principle. Putrefaction is an effect which arises spontaneously; digestion is an effect of another principle, and shall here be considered a little more particularly.

Animals, or parts of animals, possessed of the living principle, when taken into the stomach, are not in the least affected by the powers of that viscus so long as the animal principle remains. Hence it is that we find animals of various kinds not only can live in the stomach, but are even hatched and bred there; yet the moment that any of these lose the living principle, they become subject to the digestive powers of the stomach. If it were possible for a man's hand, for example, to be introduced into the stomach of a living animal, and kept there for some considerable time, it would be found that the dissolvent powers of the stomach could have no effect upon it; but if the same hand were separated from the body, and introduced into the same stomach, we should then find that the stomach could immediately act upon it. Indeed, if the first were not the case, the stomach itself ought to have been made of indigestible materials; for were not the living principle capable of preserving animal substances from being acted upon by the proces of digestion, the stomach itself would be digested; and accordingly we find that the stomach, which at one instant, that is, while possessed of the living principle, was capable of resisting the digestive powers which it contained, the next moment, viz. when deprived of the living principle, is itself capable of being digested, not only by the digestive powers of other stomachs, but even by the remains of that power which itself had of digesting other things.

These observations lead us to account for an appearance which we often find in the stomachs of dead bodies; and they at the same time throw considerable light upon the nature of digestion. The appearance we allude to is a dissolution of the stomach as its great extremity, in consequence of which there is frequently a considerable aperture made in that viscus. The edges of this opening appear to be half dissolved, very much like that kind of solution which fleshy parts undergo when half digested in a living stomach, or when acted upon by a caustic alkali, viz. pulpy, tender, and ragged.

In these cases the contents of the stomach are generally found loose in the cavity of the abdomen, about the spleen and diaphragm; and in many subjects the influence of this digestive power extends much further than through the stomach. I have often found that, after the stomach had been dissolved at the usual place, its contents let loose had come into contact with the spleen and diaphragm, had dissolved the diaphragm quite through, and had partly affected the adjacent side of the spleen, so that what had been contained in the stomach was found in the cavity of the thorax, and had even affected the lungs to a small degree.

There are very few dead bodies in which the stomach at its great end is not in some degree digested; and one who is acquainted with dissections can easily trace these gradations. To be sensible of this effect nothing more is necessary than to compare the inner surface of the great end of the stomach with any other part of its inner surface: the sound portions will appear soft, spongy, and granulated, and without distinct blood-vessels, opake and thick; while the others will appear smooth, thin, and more transparent; and the vessels will be seen ramifying in its substance, and upon squeezing the blood which they contain from the larger branches to the smaller, it will be found to pass out at the digested ends of the vessels, and to appear like drops on the inner surface.

Though I have often seen such appearances, and supposed that they must have been seen by others, yet I was quite at a loss to account for them. At first I supposed them to have been produced during life, and was therefore inclined to look upon them as the cause of death, only that I never found they had any connexion with the patient's symptoms; but I was still more at a loss to account for them when I discovered they were most frequent in those who died by sudden violence; a circumstance which made me suspect that the true cause was not guessed at*.

---

* The first time that I had occasion to observe this appearance where death had been produced by violence, and where it could not therefore easily be supposed to be the

At this time I was employed in making experiments upon digestion in different animals, all of which were killed at different times, after having been fed with various kinds of food : many of these were not opened immediately after death, and in some of them I found the above-described appearances in the stomach. The better to pursue my inquiry on the subject of digestion, I procured the stomachs of a vast variety of fishes, whose deaths are always violent, and who may be said to die in perfect health, with their stomachs usually full. In them we can observe the progress of digestion most distinctly, the shape of their stomachs being very favourable for that purpose. They likewise swallow their food whole, that is, without mastication, and swallow fish that are much larger than the digesting part of the stomach can contain; therefore in many instances the part swallowed which was lodged in the digesting part of the stomach was found more or less dissolved, while that which remained in the œsophagus was perfectly sound; and in many of these I saw the digesting part of the stomach itself reduced to the same dissolved state as the digested part of the food.

Being employed upon this subject, and therefore enabled to account more readily for appearances which had any connexion with it, and observing that the half-dissolved parts of the stomach were similar to the half-digested food, it immediately struck me that it was the process of digestion going on after death; and that the stomach, being dead, was no longer capable of resisting the powers of that menstruum which itself had formed for the digestion of food[a].

These appearances of the stomach after death throw considerable light on the principles of digestion, and show that it neither depends on

effect of disease, was in a man who had his skull fractured by one blow of a poker. Just before this accident he had been in perfect health, and had taken a hearty supper of cold meat, cheese, bread, and ale. Upon opening the abdomen, I found that the stomach, though it still contained a good deal, was dissolved at its great end, and a considerable part of its contents lay loose in the general cavity of the belly; a circumstance which puzzled me very much. The second instance was in a man who died at St. George's Hospital, a few hours after receiving a blow on his head which fractured his skull. From these two cases, among various conjectures about so strange an appearance, I began to suspect it might be peculiar to cases of fractured skull, and therefore, whenever I had an opportunity, I examined the stomach of every person who died from that accident; but I found many of them which had not this appearance. I afterwards met with the same appearance in a man who had been hanged.

---

[a] [Then follows in the original paper:

"With this idea, I set about making experiments to produce these appearances at pleasure, which would have taught us how long the animal ought to live after feeding, and how long it should remain after death before it is opened; and above all, to find out the method of producing the greatest digestive power in the living stomach: but this pursuit led me into an unbounded field."—*Phil. Trans.* (1772), p. 453.]

a mechanical power, nor contractions of the stomach, nor on heat, but something secreted in the coats of the stomach, and thrown into its cavity, which there animalizes the food, or assimilates it to the nature of the blood[a]. The power of the gastric juice is confined or limited to certain substances, generally of the vegetable and animal kingdoms; and although this menstruum is capable of acting independently of the stomach, yet it is indebted to that viscus for its existence and continuance.

---

[a] [In the original paper the following note here occurs: "In all the animals, whether carnivorous or not, upon which I made observations or experiments to discover whether or not there was an acid in the stomach (and I tried this in a great variety,) I constantly found that there was an acid, but not a strong one, in the juices contained in that viscus in a natural state." The omission of this note both in the 1st and 2nd editions of the Animal Œconomy was probably a consequence of the doubt subsequently entertained by Hunter of the natural presence of an acid in the gastric juice; but as the existence of hydrochloric acid as an essential constituent of the animalizing secretion of the stomach is now satisfactorily determined, we have thought it proper to restore this record of the agreement of a great proportion of Hunter's experience with that of late observers on this subject.]

ON A SECRETION IN THE CROP OF BREEDING PIGEONS, FOR THE NOURISHMENT OF THEIR YOUNG.

THE nourishment of animals admits, perhaps, of as much variety in the mode by which it is to be performed as any circumstance connected with their œconomy, whether we consider their numerous tribes, the different stages through which every animal passes, or the food adapted to the support of each in their distinct conditions and situations. We are likewise to include in this view that endless variety in the means by which this food is procured, according to the class of the animal and the particular stage of its existence. If the food was the same through every period of the life of an animal; if every individual of a tribe lived on the same kind, and procured it by the same mode, our speculations would then admit of a regular arrangement. But when we see that the food adapted to one stage of an animal's life is rejected at another, and that animals of one class in some respects resemble those of another, by hardly having any food peculiar to themselves, the subject becomes so complicated that it is not surprising if we are at a loss to arrange the various modes by which animals are nourished.

Animal life may not improperly be divided into three states or stages. The first comprehends the production of the animal and its growth in the fœtal state; the second commences when it emerges from that state by what is called the birth, yet for a certain time must, either mediately or immediately, depend on the parent for support; the third may be said to take place when the animal is fit and at liberty to act for itself. The first and third stages are perhaps common to all animals; but there are some classes, as fishes, spiders, &c., which seem to have no second stage, but pass directly from the first to what is the third in other animals. Of those requiring a second stage, the polypus and the viviparous animals continue to derive their nourishment immediately from the parent; while the oviparous are for some time supported by a substance originally formed with them, and reserved for that purpose[a].

---

[a] [The species of polypus to which Mr. Hunter here refers is most probably the fresh-water gemmiparous hydra; but the period during which the young polype is growing at the expense of the parent seems rather to correspond to the first or fœtal stage of existence than the second: when, again, the communication with the digestive sac of the parent is obliterated, the young polype derives its nourishment from without by the

There is infinite variety in the means by which Nature provides for the support of the young in the second stage of animal life. In many insects it is effected by the female instinctively depositing the egg, or whatever contains the rudiments of the animal, in such a situation that, when hatched, it may be within reach of proper food; others, as the humble-bee and black-beetle '[*Blatta*],' collect a quantity of peculiar substance, which both serves as a nidus for the egg, and nourishment for the maggot, when the embryo arrives at that state. Most birds, and many of the bee-tribe, collect food for their young; when at a more advanced period the task of feeding them is performed by both male and female, with an exception in the common bee, the young ones of which are not fed by either parent, but by the working-bees, which act the part of the nurse. There is likewise a number of animals capable of supplying immediately from their own bodies the nourishment proper for their offspring during this second stage, a mode of nourishment which has hitherto been supposed to be peculiar to that class of animals which Linnæus calls Mammalia; nor has it, I imagine, been ever suspected to belong to any other.

I have, however, in my inquiries concerning the various modes in which young animals are nourished, discovered that all of the dove kind are endowed with a similar power. The young pigeon, like the young quadruped, till it is capable of digesting the common food of its kind, is fed with a substance secreted for that purpose by the parent animal; not, as in the Mammalia, by the female alone, but also by the male, which, perhaps, furnishes this nutriment in a degree still more abundant. It is a common property of birds, that both male and female are equally employed in hatching, and in feeding their young in the second stage; but this particular mode of nourishment, by means of a substance secreted in their own bodies, is peculiar to certain kinds, and is carried on in the crop.

Besides the dove kind, I have some reason to suppose parrots to be endowed with the same faculty, as they have the power of throwing up the contents of the crop, and feeding one another. I have seen the cock parroquet regularly feed the hen, by first filling his own crop, and then supplying her from his beak. Parrots, maccaws, cockatoos, &c., when they are very fond of the person who feeds them, may likewise

exercise of its tentacles, until it is finally cast off. The viviparous animals are the Mammalia, and the nourishment alluded to is the lacteal secretion. The nutritious substance with which the oviparous animals continue for a short period to be supported after their exclusion from the egg is the yolk, which has then passed into the abdomen, where it is finally absorbed.]

be observed to have the action of throwing up the food; and often do it. The cock pigeon, when he caresses the hen, performs the same kind of action as when he feeds his young; but I do not know if at this time he throws up anything from the crop.

During incubation the coats of the crop in the pigeon are gradually enlarged and thickened, like what happens to the udder of females of the class Mammalia in the term of uterine gestation. On comparing the state of the crop when the bird is not sitting, with its appearance during incubation, the difference is very remarkable. In the first case it is thin and membranous; but by the time the young are about to be hatched, the whole, except what lies on the trachea, becomes thicker, and takes on a glandular appearance, having its internal surface very irregular*. It is likewise evidently more vascular than in its former state, that it may convey a quantity of blood sufficient for the secretion of the substance which is to nourish the young brood for some days after they are hatched.

Whatever may be the consistence of this substance when just secreted, it most probably very soon coagulates into a granulated white curd, for in such form I have always found it in the crop; and if an old pigeon is killed just as the young ones are hatching, the crop will be found as above described, and in its cavity pieces of white curd, mixed with some of the common food of the pigeon, such as barley, beans, &c. If we allow either of the parents to feed the brood, the crop of the young pigeons when examined will be discovered to contain the same kind of curdled substance as that of the old ones, which passes from thence into the stomach, where it is to be digested.

The young pigeon is fed for a little time with this substance only, as about the third day some of the common food is found mingled with it: as the pigeon grows older the proportion of common food is increased; so that by the time it is seven, eight, or nine days old, the secretion of the curd ceases in the old ones, and of course no more will be found in the crop of the young. It is a curious fact that the parent pigeon has at first a power to throw up this curd without any mixture of common food, although afterwards both are thrown up according to the proportion required for the young ones.

I have called this substance curd, not as being literally so, but as resembling that more than anything I know; it may, however, have a greater resemblance to curd than we are perhaps aware of, for neither this secretion, nor curd from which the whey has been pressed, seems to contain any sugar, and do not run into the acetous fermentation. The

---

* Vide Plate XXXIX.

property of coagulating is confined to the substance itself, as it produces no such effect when mixed with milk.

This secretion in the pigeon, like all other animal substances, becomes putrid by standing, though not so readily as either blood or meat, it resisting putrefaction for a considerable time; neither will curd much pressed become putrid so soon as either blood or meat.

OBSERVATIONS ON THE GILLAROO-TROUT, COMMONLY CALLED IN IRELAND THE GIZZARD-TROUT[a].

ONE of the digestive organs of the gillaroo-trout being so very re-markable as to have given name to the fish, and to have been considered as its distinguishing characteristic, it is my intention to inquire whether its resemblance to a gizzard be sufficiently strong to render the term of gizzard-trout a proper appellation, and what place its stomach ought to hold among the corresponding organs of other animals. For this purpose it will be necessary to state certain facts connected with the subject, and take a general view of the varieties which occur in the di-gestive organs in different animals.

The food of animals may be divided into two kinds, what does, and what does not, require mastication to facilitate digestion. The flesh of animals is of the latter kind; but grain, and many other substances which serve for aliment, require a previous grinding or trituration, and therefore animals living on this kind of food are furnished with organs for that purpose. Granivorous quadrupeds have the two powers, for mastication and digestion, separate or distinct from one another; the first being executed by teeth, which serve as so many grindstones for reducing their food to smaller parts, before it is conveyed into the sto-mach for digestion; but the form of these teeth varies very considerably in different animals, although the food be the same. This grinding also fits it for deglutition; for neither grain nor herbs could be swallowed without having first been masticated. When so prepared, it is, with regard to the digestive power, rendered similar to animal food; therefore in many of the granivorous the stomach resembles that of the carnivo-rous animals; and whenever the stomach in the granivorous quadruped departs from this general rule, there is a peculiarity in the operations of digestion. Birds that live upon substances, for the digestion of which trituration is indispensably necessary, have the powers of mastication and digestion united in one part, the gizzard, which is particularly con-structed for that purpose, but is more uniform in its construction than the teeth, varying only by being stronger or weaker in its powers; therefore the genus of birds exhibits less variety, respecting the organs relating to digestion, than the quadruped. In granivorous birds, there-

[a] [Originally published in the Philosophical Transactions, vol. lxiv. (1774.)]

fore, one single organ answers both to the teeth and stomach of granivorous quadrupeds, and consequently the gizzard alone of birds will
as clearly point out the food of the species as both teeth and stomach
together, in those animals in which the two offices of mastication and
digestion are not performed together in the same part.

As it appears to be the difference of stomachs only that fits birds for
their different kinds of food, as there is little difference in construction,
excepting only in strength; and as the food of the different species is
of every kind, from the hardest grain to the softest animal matter, we
may conclude that every gradation of the stomach is to be found among
them, from the true gizzard, which is one extreme, to the mere membranous stomach, which is the other. In consequence of this, it must
be as difficult to determine the exact limits of the two different modes
of construction to which the names of gizzard and stomach specifically
belong, as, in any other case, to distinguish proximate steps in the slow
and imperceptible gradations of Nature.

The two extremes of true gizzard and membranous stomach are easily
defined; but they run so into each other, that the end of one and the
beginning of the other is quite imperceptible. Similar gradations are
observable in the food: the kinds suited to the two extremes mixing
together in different proportions adapted to the intermediate states of
stomach.

A true gizzard is composed of two strong muscles, placed opposite
and acting upon each other, like two broad grindstones. These muscles
are joined together at their sides by a middle tendon, into which the
muscular fibres are inserted, and which forms the narrow anterior and
posterior sides of the flat quadrangular cavity in which the grinding is
performed. The upper end of this cavity is occupied by the termination of the œsophagus, and the beginning of the intestine. The lower
end consists of a thin muscular bag connecting the edges of the two
muscles together.

By these two more soft and flexible substances being thus interposed
between the two strong grinding muscles a double advantage is gained;
for, whilst one gives an easy passage to the œsophagus and gut, when
both act together they serve in some degree as a hinge, on which the
two muscles may be said to move, by the middle tendon allowing of a
free motion of the grinding surfaces on each other, which is necessary
for the comminution of food.

The two flat lateral sides of the grinding cavity are lined with a thick
horny substance, similar to a hard and thick cuticle; the narrow anterior and posterior tendinous parts are also lined with a cuticle, but not
so strong as the former; this horny substance is gradually lost at one

end in a very thin cuticle, which lines the passages of the œsophagus
and intestine for a little way, and at the other end is lost in the same
manner in the membranous bag.

The two large muscles may be considered as a pair of jaws, whose
teeth are occasionally supplied, being small rough stones or pebbles
which the animal swallows, which from the feeling of the tongue can
distinguish such as are proper from those which are not, instantly dropping out of its mouth such as are smooth and otherwise unfit for the
purpose.

Some birds with gizzards have also a craw or crop, which serves as
a reservoir, and for softening the grain ; but as all of them have not
this organ, it is not to our present purpose.

There are other animals, besides this class of birds, which masticate
their food in the stomach ; but teeth are placed there by Nature : of this
kind are crabs and lobsters.

The gradation from gizzard to stomach is made by the muscular sides
becoming weaker and weaker, and the food keeps pace with this change,
varying gradually from vegetable to animal[a]. In one point of view, therefore, food may be considered as a first principle, with respect to which
the digestive organs with their appendages act but as secondary parts,
being adapted to and determined by the food as the primary object.

We find then that in all granivorous animals there is an apparatus for
the mastication of the food, although often differing in construction and
situation ; but in true carnivorous animals, of whatever tribe, mastication not being so necessary, they have no apparatus for that purpose.
The teeth of such quadrupeds as are carnivorous serve chiefly to procure food and prepare it for deglutition ; the same thing is performed
in the true carnivorous birds by their beak and talons, whose office it is
to procure the aliment and fit it for deglutition, corresponding in this
respect with the teeth of the others. Applying this reasoning to fish,
it seems, at first sight, as if there were no occasion in them for that
variety of structure in the digestive organs as is found in the before-
mentioned quadrupeds and birds, the food of fish being principally of
one sort, namely animal ; which, however, with regard to the digestive
powers, is to be distinguished into two kinds, viz. common soft fish and
shell-fish. Such fish as live on the first kind have, like the carnivorous
quadrupeds and birds, no apparatus for mastication, their teeth being
intended merely for catching the food and fitting it to be swallowed.
But the shells of the second kind of food render some degree of masti-

---

[a] [The gizzards of birds which live on hard-coated coleopterous insects are stronger
than those which have to digest soft pulpy fruits.]

cating power necessary to fit it for its passage either into the stomach or through the intestines; and accordingly we find in certain fish a structure suited to the purpose.

Thus the mouth of the wolf-fish is almost paved with teeth, by means of which it can break shells to pieces and fit them for the œsophagus of the fish, and so effectually disengage the food from them, that though it lives upon such hard food, the stomach does not differ from that of other fish; the organs of mastication and digestion, therefore, in this animal, exactly correspond to those of many granivorous quadrupeds.

Other fish, on the contrary, approach nearer to the structure of birds by having their stomach furnished to a certain degree with a masticating power, which in many is very imperfect compared with the gizzards of fowls. Perhaps the difference is only what the difference of food will properly allow; as in fish which have this power, the food being still animal, and in general but imperfectly covered with the shell, it probably requires only to be broken, perhaps hardly that, for the mere purposes of digestion, as food is digested when introduced into the stomach in silver balls with only a few small holes, but it may be necessary to fit the shells for passing along the intestines after the fish is digested. In the *Bulla lignaria* of Linnæus this apparatus is more perfect, consisting of two bones, which we must suppose capable of grinding hard shells; but the food of granivorous birds requires to be ground into a kind of meal.

Of all the fish I have seen, the mullet is the most complete instance of this structure, its strong muscular stomach being evidently adapted, like the gizzard of birds, to the two offices of mastication and digestion. The stomach of the fish now before us holds the second place.

But still neither of these stomachs can be justly ranked as gizzards, since they want some of the most essential characters, viz. a power and motion fitted for grinding, and the horny cuticle[a]. The stomach of the Gillaroo-trout is, however, more globular than that of most fish, better adapted for small food, and endued with sufficient strength to break the shells of small shell-fish; which will probably be best done by having more than one in the stomach at a time, and also by taking pretty large and smooth stones into the stomach, which will answer the purpose of breaking, but not so well that of grinding, nor will they hurt the stomach, as they are smooth, when swallowed; but this stomach can scarcely possess any power of grinding, as the whole cavity is lined with a fine villous coat, the internal surface of which appears everywhere to be digestive, and by no means fitted for mastication.

---

[a] [We have examined the gizzard of the mullet (*Mugil Capito*, Cuv.), and find that it is lined by a distinct layer of rough and easily separable cuticle.]

The stomach of the common stream-trout is exactly of the same structure with that of the gillaroo; but its coat not so thick by two thirds*. How far this difference in thickness of stomach is sufficient to form a distinct species, or barely a variety of the same, is only to be determined by experiment†.

The œsophagus in the trout is considerably longer and smaller than in many other classes of fish.

The intestines are similar to those of the salmon, herring, sprat, &c.

The pancreas is appendiculated.

The teeth show them to be fish of prey.

So far as we are led to determine by analogy, we must not consider the stomach of this fish as a gizzard, but as a true stomach.

* The common stream-trout swallows shell-fish, and also pretty large smooth stones, which serve as a kind of shell-breakers.

† Viz. take some gillaroo-trout, male and female, and put them into water in which there are no trout, to see if they continue the same[a].

[a] [They are considered to be varieties of the *Salmo Fario*, Linn., by the best modern naturalists: see Yarrell's 'British Fishes,' vol. ii. p. 57.]

EXPERIMENTS AND OBSERVATIONS ON ANIMALS, WITH RESPECT TO THE POWER OF PRODUCING HEAT[a].

SOME late ingenious experiments and observations, published in the Philosophical Transactions[b], upon a power which animals seem to possess of generating cold, induced me to look over my notes, containing some which I had made in the year 1766, indicating an opposite power in animals, whereby they are capable of resisting any external cold while alive, by generating within themselves a degree of heat sufficient to counteract it. Those experiments were not originally instituted with any expectation of the event which resulted from them, but for the purpose of satisfying myself whether an animal could retain life after being frozen, as has been confidently asserted both of fishes and snakes. For that these, after being frozen, still retain so much of life as when thawed to resume their vital actions, is a fact so well attested that we are bound to believe it; and had my experiment succeeded, it was my intention to have tried the effects of freezing on living animals to a much greater degree than can ever happen accidentally.

I mention these circumstances to account for what might otherwise be attributed to negligence and inattention, namely, the little nicety that was observed in measuring the precise degree of cold applied in the experiments. Accuracy in this particular was not aimed at, being of no consequence in the inquiry more immediately before me. The cold was first produced by means of ice and snow with sal ammoniac or sea-salt, to about the 10° of Fahrenheit's thermometer: ice was then mixed with spirit of nitre; but what degree of cold was thus produced I did not examine. This cold mixture was made in a tub surrounded with woollen cloths, and covered with the same, to prevent the effects of the heat of the atmosphere upon the mixture itself, and to preserve, as much as possible, a cold atmosphere within the vessel. Animal juices, as the blood, freeze at 25°, so that a piece of dead flesh could be frozen in an atmosphere cooled to that point.

---

[a] [This Essay includes the greater part of two papers, one published with the title 'Experiments on Animals and Vegetables, with respect to the Power of producing Heat,' in the Philosophical Transactions, vol. lxv. (read June 22, 1775); the other, 'On the Heat, &c. of Animals and Vegetables,' in the Philosophical Transactions, vol. lxviii. (read June 19, and Nov. 13, 1777.)]

[b] ['Experiments and Observations in a heated Room,' by Charles Blagden, M.D., F.R.S., vol. lxv. p. 111.]

EXPERIMENTS.

Experiment I. was made on two carp.   These were put into a glass vessel with common river water, which was placed in the freezing mixture.   The water not freezing fast enough, to hasten that effect as much cooled snow was added as to render the whole thick.   The snow round the carp melting, we put in more fresh snow, which, melting also, was repeated several times, till we grew tired, and at last left them covered up in the yard to freeze by the joint operation of the surrounding mixture and the natural cold of the atmosphere[a].   They were frozen at last, after having exhausted the whole powers of life in the production of heat.   That this was really the case, could not be known till I had completed that part of the experiment for which the whole was begun, viz. the thawing of the animals.   It was done very gradually; but the animals did not, with flexibility, recover life; and while in this cold, showed signs of great uneasiness by their violent motions. N.B. In some of these experiments, where air was made the conductor of the cold and heat, that the heat might be more readily carried off from the animal, a leaden vessel was used.   It was small for the same reason; and as it was necessary for the animal's respiration that the mouth of the vessel should communicate with the open air, it was made deep, that the cold of the atmosphere round the animal might not be diminished too quickly by the warmth of the open air, which would have spoiled it as a conductor.

Experiment II. was upon a dormouse, the vessel in which it was confined being sunk in the cold mixture almost to its edge.   The atmosphere round the animal soon cooled; its breath froze as it came from the mouth; a hoar-frost gathered on its whiskers, and on all the inside of the vessel, and the external points of the hair became covered with the same.   While this was going on the animal showed signs of great uneasiness; sometimes it would coil itself into a round form, to preserve its extremities and confine its heat; and finding that ineffectual, would then endeavour to make its escape*.   Its motions became less violent

---

* This shows that cold carried to a great degree rather rouses than depresses the animal action; but it appears, from many circumstances and observations, that a certain degree of cold produces inactivity both in the living and sensative principle, which will be further illustrated hereafter.

---

[a] [This experiment is alluded to by Dr. Blagden, who observes, " The power of generating heat seems to attend life very universally.   Not to mention other well-known experiments, Mr. Hunter found a carp preserve a coat of fluid water round him long after all the rest of the water in the vessel had been congealed by a very strong freezing mixture."—*Phil. Trans.*, lxv. p. 122.]

by the sinking of the vital powers: its feet were at last frozen; but we were not able to keep up the cold a sufficient time to freeze the whole animal, the hair being so bad a conductor of heat that the consumption was not more than the animal powers were capable of supporting*.

Experiment III. was made with another dormouse; and taught by the failure of the last experiment, I took care that the hair should not a second time be an obstruction to our success. Having, therefore, first made the animal wet all over, that its heat might be more rapidly carried off, it was put into a leaden vessel, and the whole placed in the cold mixture as before. The animal soon gave signs of feeling the cold, by repeated attempts to make its escape; and the breath and water evaporating from its body being soon frozen, appeared like a hoar-frost on the sides of the vessel and on its whiskers; but while the vigour of life lasted it defied the approach of the cold. However, from the hair being wet, and thereby rendered a good conductor, there was a much greater consumption of heat than in the former experiment, which hastened on the diminution of the power of producing it. The animal dying, soon became stiff, and, upon being thawed, was found quite dead.

Experiment IV. A toad being put into a vessel with water, at such a depth as not to cover its mouth, was placed in the mixture cooled to between 10° and 15°. The water froze so near to the body of the animal as quite to inclose it, but without destroying life; yet, though not frozen, it hardly ever recovered the use of its limbs.

Experiment V. was with a snail, which froze very soon, in a cold between 10° and 13°. These two last experiments were made in the winter, when the living powers of the animals selected for the trial are very weak; they might have resisted the cold more strongly in the summer. Why the animals mentioned in the above experiments died before they were frozen, while those which are exposed to the atmosphere in very cold climates do not, is a point I shall not pretend to determine, not knowing the difference between the effects of a natural and an artificial cold. It may be accounted for by supposing that the natural cold in climates in which animals are found frozen is so intense as to produce congelation immediately, before the powers of life are exhausted; at least whether it is so or not is worthy of inquiry.

It appears from the above experiments, first, That most probably the animals were deprived of life before they were frozen; secondly, That there was an exertion or expense of animal power in resisting the effects of cold, proportioned to the necessity; thirdly, That this exertion was

* These experiments were made in presence of Dr. George Fordyce and Dr. Erwin, teacher of Chemistry at Glasgow, the latter of whom came in accidentally in the middle of our operations.

in proportion to the perfection of the animal, and the natural heat proper to each species and to each age. This exertion might also perhaps depend in some degree on other circumstances not hitherto observed; for from Experiments II. and III. upon dormice, I find that in the animals which are of a constitution to retain nearly the same heat in all temperatures of the air, it required the greatest cold I could produce to overcome this resisting power; while by Experiments IV. and V. on the toad and snail, whose natural heat is not always the same, but is altered very materially according to the external heat or cold, this power was exhausted in a degree of cold not exceeding 10° or 15°; and the snail being the most imperfect of the two, its powers of generating heat appeared to be much the weakest.

That the imperfect animals will allow of a considerable variation in their temperature of heat and cold, is proved by the following experiments. The thermometer being at 45°, the ball was introduced by the mouth into the stomach of a frog, which had been exposed to the same cold. It rose to 49°. I then placed the frog in an atmosphere made warm by heated water, where I allowed it to stay twenty minutes; and upon introducing the thermometer into the stomach, it raised the quicksilver to 64°. To what degree the more imperfect animals are capable of being rendered hotter and colder at one time than another, I have not yet ascertained[a]; but the torpidity of these animals in our winter is probably owing to the great change wrought in their temperature by the external heat and cold. The cold in their bodies is to such a degree as in a great measure to put a stop, while it lasts, to the vital functions; while in warmer climates no such effect is produced[b].

This variety (in the power of producing heat) not only takes place in animals of different orders, but in some degree in the same animal at different ages, even according to the different age of the parts in the same animal: a young animal requires more warmth than one full-grown; and although an animal is equally old in all its original parts, yet there are often new ones formed in consequence of diseases; and we find that these new or young parts in animals are not so able to support life as the old, at least for some time: but as animals are of different

---

[a] [The snail (*Cyclostomum thermale*) which lives in the hot springs of Abano feeds, moves about with great activity, and propagates in water of the temperature of 100° Fahrenheit. The Entozoa of warm-blooded animals become in a certain degree torpid in cold water, but revive and exhibit lively motions when placed in warm water of 95° Fahrenheit.]

[b] [The Reptiles and many of the Invertebrate animals of tropical climates seek their hiding-places and fall into a state of lethargy during the dry season, when the heat is most intense. A quadruped of Madagascar, the tenrec, which is nearly allied to our hedgehog, becomes lethargic at the dry season, when its insect food is inaccessible.]

ages, and the same animal is always growing older, and of course more and more perfect, they then become more capable of generating heat than when they were younger[a]. This, however, has its limitations, for after a certain period they again lose this power, and therefore require a less strongly conducting medium, or warm atmosphere.

This power of generating heat seems to be a property in an animal while alive. In the more perfect animals it is to preserve a standard heat; and as they are most commonly in an atmosphere colder than themselves, they have most commonly occasion to exert it, and it is therefore a power only of opposition and resistance; for it is not found to exert itself spontaneously and unprovoked, but must always be excited by the energy of some external frigorific agent, or disease; yet it is natural to such animals that this power should be called forth, as will be observed by and by. It does not depend on the motion of the blood, as some have supposed, because it likewise belongs to animals which have no circulation[b]: and the nose of a dog, which is always nearly of the same heat in all temperatures of the air, is well supplied with blood[c]; although we must allow, where this power is greatest the circulation is the quickest. Neither can it be said to depend upon the nervous system, for it is found in animals that have no brain or nerves. However, it must be allowed that all that class which possess this power in the highest degree have the largest brain, although this power is not in the

[a] [Young animals consume, in proportion, less oxygen than adults; consequently, a less proportion of carbonic acid is formed in the change of the arterial into the venous blood, and a less amount of heat is extricated. When exposed to cold they become torpid, lose their heat, and also their sensibility, in which latter circumstance, and in some other points, they differ considerably from the hybernating animal in its state of lethargy.]

[b] [An argument of this importance deserved to be stated with more circumstance. Mr. Hunter does not say what the animals are which have no circulation. It is possible, however, that he was alluding to bees. But these insects we know enjoy a circulation, governed, as his own dissections show, by a dorsal heart. And insects manifest the power of generating heat above that of other invertebrate animals precisely in consequence of the greater activity of their locomotive, respiratory, and sanguiferous functions. It is true, however, that mere motion of the blood is not a cause of animal heat, because the circulation goes on in the hybernating animal when in its cold and lethargic state; but the blood's motion is here inoperative as a cause of heat, because in torpidity no chemical change takes place in the blood during its passage through the capillaries, either of the systemic or pulmonic systems of vessels; it is only venous blood that is moving.]

[c] [The temperature of the nose of a dog is lowered by the constant evaporation of the moisture excreted from its surface; when this secretion is checked in consequence of internal disease, then the nose soon grows hot; and the dryness and heat of this part, both in the dog and other animals, form a common symptom of loss of health, as we have frequently had occasion to observe in the animals in the Zoological Gardens.]

least in proportion to the quantity of brain in that class[a]. It is most probable that it arises from some other principle ; a principle so connected with life that it can, and does, act independently of circulation, sensation, and volition, and is that power which preserves and regulates the internal machine. This power of generating heat is in the highest perfection when the body is in health; and in many deviations from that state we find that its action is extremely uncertain and irregular, sometimes rising higher than the standard, and at other times falling much below it. Instances of this we have in different diseases, and even in the same disease, within very short intervals of time. A very remarkable one fell under my own observation, in a gentleman who was seized with an apoplectic fit; and while he lay insensible in bed, covered with blankets, I found that his whole body would, in an instant, become extremely cold in every part, continuing so for some time; and, as suddenly, would become extremely hot. While this was going on alternately there was no sensible alteration in his pulse for several hours[b].

Being satisfied of the foregoing fact, that animals had a power of generating heat, I pursued the subject still further; not so much with a view to account for animal heat, as to observe the different phenomena, with the variations or difference in the heat in different animals. In the course of my experiments, having found variations in the degree of heat and cold in the same experiment, for which I could not account, I suspected that this might arise from some imperfection in the construction of the thermometer. I mentioned to Mr. Ramsden my objections to the common construction of that instrument, and my ideas of one more perfect in its nature, and better adapted to the experiments in which I was engaged. He accordingly made me some very small thermometers, six or seven inches long, not above two twelfths of an inch thick in the stem, having the external diameter of the ball very little larger than that of the stem, on which was marked the freezing point.

---

[a] [Although, from the experiments on vegetables subsequently given, it appears that vital heat is not dependent on a nervous system ; yet it has been shown that the production of heat in warm-blooded animals is modified by the nervous influence. See the Physiological Researches, ' On the Influence of the Brain on the action of the Heart, and on the generation of Animal Heat,' by B. C. Brodie, F.R.S., Phil. Trans., vol. ci. p. 36; vol. cii. p. 380; also the experiments of Home and Mayo, Phil. Trans., vol. cxv. p. 7; and by Legallois, *Annales de Chimie*, t. iv. 1817.]

[b] [Here ends the first paper in the 65th vol. of the Phil. Trans. The second communication commences as follows: " In the course of a variety of experiments on animals and vegetables, I have frequently observed that the result of experiments in the one has explained the œconomy of the other, and pointed out some principle common to both; I have therefore collected some experiments which relate to the heat and cold of those substances;" and then proceeds as in the text.]

The stem was embraced by a small ivory scale, so as to slide upon it easily, and retain any position. Upon the hollow surface of this scale were marked the degrees, which were seen through the stem[a]. By these means the size of the thermometer was very much reduced, and it could be applied to soft bodies with much more ease and certainty, and in many cases in which the former ones could not be conveniently used; I therefore repeated with it such of my former experiments as had not at first proved satisfactory, and found the degrees of heat very different, not only from what I had expected, but also from what I had found by my former experiments with thermometers of the common construction.

I have observed above, and find it supported by every experiment I have made on the heat and cold of animals, that the more perfect have the greater power of retaining a certain degree of heat, which may be called their standard heat, and allow of much less variation than the more imperfect animals: however, it will appear from the three experiments which I am now going to relate, that many, if not all of the more perfect, are still incapable of keeping constantly to one degree, but may be altered from their standard heat either by external applications or disease. These variations are much greater below that standard than above it, the perfect animals having a greater power of resisting heat than cold, so that they are commonly near their ultimate heat. Indeed we do not want any other proof of a variation than our own feelings, being all sensible of heat and of cold, which sensations could not be produced without an alteration really taking place in the parts affected; and that alteration could not take place if they did not become actually warmer or colder. I have often cooled my hands to such a degree that I could warm them by immersing them in water just pumped; therefore my hands were really colder than the pump-water.

An increase of absolute heat must alter the texture or position of the

parts, so as to produce the sensation which we call heat; and as that heat is diminished, the texture or position of the parts is altered in a contrary way, and, when carried to a certain degree, becomes the cause of the sensation of cold. Now these effects could not take place in either case without an increase or decrease of absolute heat in the part; heat, therefore, in some one of its different degrees, must be present. I shall not in this place attempt to settle whether heat is a body or matter, or only a property of matter, which appears to me to be merely a difference in terms; for a property must belong to something. When heat is applied to the surface of the body the skin becomes in some degree heated according to the application, which may be carried so far as actually to burn the living parts: on the contrary, in a cold atmosphere

---

[a] [Plate XL.]

a man's hand may become so cold as to lose that sensation altogether, and change it for pain. Absolute heat and cold may be carried so far as even to alter the structure of the parts upon which the actions of life depend.

As animals being subject to variations in the degrees of heat and cold from external applications are of course, in this respect, affected in some measure like inanimate matter; and therefore, as parts are elongated or recede from the common mass, these effects more readily take place; for instance, all projecting parts and extremities, more especially toes, fingers, noses, ears, combs of fowls, particularly of the cock, are more readily cooled, and are therefore most subject to be affected by cold. Animals are not only subject to an increase and decrease of heat, similar to inanimate matter, but the transition from one to the other (as far as they admit of it) is nearly as quick. I shall not, however, confine myself to sensation alone, as that is in some degree regulated by habit; for a habit of uniformity in the application of heat and cold to an animal body renders it more sensible of the smallest variation in either; while by the habit of variety it will become, in a proportional degree, less susceptible of all such sensations. This is proved every day, in cold weather, by people who are accustomed to clothe themselves warm. In them the least exposure to cold air, although the effect produced in the skin is perhaps not the hundredth part of a degree, immediately gives the sensation of cold, even through the thickest covering: those, on the contrary, who have been used to go thinly clothed, can bear the variation of some degrees without being sensible of it; of this the hands and feet afford an instance in point, exciting the sensation of cold when applied to another part of the body, without having before given to the mind an impression of cold existing in these parts themselves. The projecting parts and the extremities are those which admit of the greatest change in their degrees of heat and cold without materially affecting the animal or even its sensations. I find that by heat or cold externally applied to such parts, the thermometer may be made to rise or fall; but not in an equal proportion as when applied to inanimate matter. Nor are the living parts cooled or heated in the same proportion, as appears from the application of the thermometer to the skin; for the cuticle is to be considered as a dead covering, capable of receiving greater degrees of heat and cold than the living parts underneath; and as it might be suspected that the whole of the variation was in this covering, to remove any such doubt I made the following experiments.

Experiment I. I placed the ball of the thermometer under my tongue, where it was perfectly covered by all the surrounding parts; and having kept it there for some minutes, I found that it rose to 97°; yet it rose no higher by being continued there. I then took several pieces of ice, about the size of walnuts, and put them in the same situation, allowing them only to melt in part, that the application of cold might be better kept up, occasionally spitting out the water arising from the solution. Having continued this for ten minutes, I found, on introducing my thermometer, that it fell to 77°; so that the mouth at this part had lost 20° of heat. The thermometer gradually rose to 97° again; but did not in this experiment sink so low as it would have done in the hand, if a piece of ice had been held in it for the same length of time. Perhaps the surface under the tongue being surrounded with warm parts renders it next to an impossibility to cool it below that degree; but I rather suspect that such parts as the hand will allow of greater latitude in this respect, from having insensibly acquired the habit of varying the degree of cold, and becoming of course less susceptible of its impressions, and therefore less easily excited.

As a further proof that the more perfect animals are capable of varying their heat in some measure according to the external heat applied, I shall adduce the following experiments made on the human subject.

The mouth being a part so frequently in contact with the external atmosphere in the action of breathing, whatever is put into it may be supposed to be influenced by that atmosphere; this will always render an experiment made in that part, relative to heat and cold, somewhat uncertain. I imagined that the urethra would answer better, because, being an internal cavity, it can only be influenced by heat and cold applied to the external skin of the parts. I imagined also that, whatever effects the application of heat and cold might have, they would sooner take place in the urethra, as being a projecting part, than in any other part of the body; and therefore, if living animal substance was in any degree subject to the common laws of matter in this respect, the urethra would be readily affected. To determine this I procured a person who allowed me to make such experiments as I thought necessary.

Experiment II. I introduced the ball of my thermometer into the urethra about an inch; which having remained there about a minute, the quicksilver rose to 92°; at two inches it rose to 93°; at four inches to 94°; and when the ball had got as far as the bulb of the urethra, where it was surrounded by warm parts, the quicksilver rose to 97°.

Experiment III. These parts being immersed for one minute in water, heated only to 65°, and the thermometer introduced about an inch and a half into the urethra, the quicksilver rose to 79°; which was repeated several times with the same result. To discover if there were any difference in the quickness of the transition of heat and cold in living and dead parts, and to determine if the extent to which each would go were likewise different, I procured a dead penis, for the purpose of making the comparative experiments that follow; being clearly of opinion that all such trials should be as similar as possible, except in those points where the difference (if there is any) makes the essential part of the experiment.

Experiment IV. The heat of the penis of a living person, an inch and a half within the urethra, being found exactly 92°; and the dead one being heated to the same degree, I had both immersed in the same vessel, with the water at 50°, when, by introducing the thermometers several different times, I was able to note the comparative quickness with which they cooled from 92°, and observed that the dead cooled sooner by two or three minutes; the living sunk the quicksilver to 58°, and the dead to 50°: the thermometer, although continued there some time longer, fell no lower. I repeated this experiment several times, with the same result; although at one time there was a small difference in the degrees of heat of the penis and also of the water; but the difference in the result was nearly proportional in all the three different trials, therefore the same conclusions may be drawn from them. In these last experiments very little difference was observed between the cooling of a dead and of a living part; a circumstance which we cannot suppose to take place uniformly through the whole body, as in that case living animals would always be of the same degree of heat with the atmosphere in which they live. The subject of these experiments not choosing to have the part cooled lower than 53° or 54°, prevented my observing if the powers of generating heat were exerted to a greater degree when the heat was brought so low as to threaten destruction; but by some experiments on mice, which will be related hereafter, it will appear that the animal powers are roused to exert themselves in this respect when necessary.

Having found, from the above experiments, that parts of an animal were capable of being cooled below the common or natural heat, I proceeded to make others, with a view to ascertain if the same parts were capable of being made much hotter than the standard heat of animals. The experiments were made in the same manner as the former, only the water was now hotter than the natural heat of the animal.

Experiment V. The natural heat of the parts being 92°, they were immersed for two minutes in water heated to 113°, and, the thermometer being introduced as before, the quicksilver rose to 100° and a half. This experiment I also repeated several times, but could not raise the heat of the penis beyond $100\frac{1}{2}$°: this was probably owing to the person not being able at the time to bear the application of water warmer than 113°. By way of comparison, I made

Experiment VI. The living and dead parts being both immersed in water, gradually made warmer and warmer from 100° to 118°, and continued in that heat for some minutes, the dead part raised the thermometer to 114°, while the living raised it no higher than 102¼°. It was observed, by the person on whom the experiment was made, that after the parts had been in the water about a minute, the water did not feel hot; but on its being agitated it felt so hot that he could hardly bear it. Upon applying the thermometer to the sides of the living glans, the quicksilver immediately fell from 118° to about 104°, while it did not fall more than a degree when put close to the dead; so that the living glans cooled the surrounding water to a certain distance*.

Experiment VII. The heat of the rectum in the same man was 98° and a half exactly.

In the second, third, fourth, fifth, and sixth experiments, an internal cavity, which is both very vascular and sensible, was evidently influenced by external heat and cold, though only applied to the skin of the part; while in the seventh experiment another part of the same body, where external heat and cold could make little or no impression, was of the standard heat. Although it will appear, from experiment, that the rectum is not the warmest part of an animal, yet, in order to determine how far the heat could be increased by stimulating the constitution to a degree sufficient to quicken the pulse, I repeated the seventh experiment after the man had eaten a hearty supper and drank a bottle of wine, which increased the pulse from 73° to 87°, and yet the thermometer only rose to 98° and a half.

Having formerly made experiments upon dormice during the sleeping season, with a view to see if there were any alteration in the animal œconomy at that time, I found among my notes an account of some which appear to our present purpose; but to be more certain of the accuracy of the former experiments, I repeated them with my new thermometer.

Experiment VIII. In a room, in which the temperature of the air was between 50° and 60°, a small opening was made in the belly of a dormouse, of a sufficient size to admit the ball of my thermometer, which, being introduced into the belly at about the middle of that cavity, rose to 80°, and no higher.

Experiment IX. The mouse was put into a cold atmosphere of 15°

---

* This might furnish an useful hint respecting bathing in water, whether colder or warmer than the heat of the body: for if intended to be either colder or hotter, it will soon be of the same temperature with that of the body; therefore in a large bath the patient should move from place to place, and in a small one there should be a constant succession of water of the intended heat.

above 0, and left there for fifteen minutes; after which, the thermometer being introduced a second time, it rose to 85°.

Experiment X. The mouse was again put into a cold atmosphere for fifteen minutes; and the thermometer being introduced, the quicksilver at first rose to 72° only, but gradually came up to 83°, 84°, and 85°.

Experiment XI. It was put a third time into the cold atmosphere, and allowed to stay there for thirty minutes: the lower part of the mouse, at the bottom of the dish, was almost frozen; the whole of the animal was numbed, and a good deal weakened. The thermometer being introduced, the heat was found to vary in different parts of the belly: in the pelvis, near the parts most exposed to the cold, it was as low as 62°; in the middle, among the intestines, about 70; but near the diaphragm it rose to 80°, 82°, 84°, and 85°; so that in the middle of the body the heat had decreased 10°. Finding a variation in different parts of the same cavity in the same animal, I repeated the same experiments upon another dormouse.

Experiment XII. Having brought a healthy dormouse, which had been asleep from the coldness of the atmosphere, into a room in which there was a fire (the atmosphere at 64°), I introduced the thermometer into its belly, nearly at the middle, between the thorax and pubis, and the quicksilver rose to 74° or 75°; turning the ball towards the diaphragm, it rose to 80°; and when I applied it to the liver, it rose to 81+°.

Experiment XIII. The mouse being placed in an atmosphere at 20°, and left there half an hour, when taken out was very lively, even much more so than when put in. Introducing the thermometer into the lower part of the belly, the quicksilver rose to 91°; and upon turning it up to the liver to 93°.

Experiment XIV. The animal being replaced in the cold atmosphere at 30° for an hour, the thermometer was again introduced into the belly; at the liver it rose to 93°; in the pelvis to 92°; the mouse continuing very lively.

Experiment XV. It was again put back into an atmosphere, cooled to 19°, and left there an hour; the thermometer at the diaphragm was 87°; in the pelvis 83°; but the animal was now less lively.

Experiment XVI. Having been put into its cage, the thermometer being placed at the diaphragm, in two hours afterwards was at 93°.

As I was unable to procure hedgehogs in the torpid state, to ascertain their heat during that period, I got my friend Mr. Jenner[a], surgeon, at Berkeley, to make the same experiments on that animal, that I

---

[a] [Afterwards Dr. Jenner, the discoverer of Vaccination.]

might compare them with those in the dormouse; and his account is as follows:

" Experiment I. In the winter, the atmosphere at 44°, the heat of a torpid hedgehog, in the pelvis, was 45°, and at the diaphragm 48½°.

" Experiment II. The atmosphere 26°, the heat of a torpid hedgehog, in the cavity of the abdomen, was reduced so low as 30°.

" Experiment III. The same hedgehog was exposed to the cold atmosphere of 26° for two days, and the heat of the rectum was found to be 93°; the wound in the abdomen being now so small that it would not admit the thermometer.

" A comparative experiment was made with a puppy, the atmosphere at 50°; the heat in the pelvis, as also at the diaphragm, was 102°.

" In summer, the atmosphere at 78°, the heat of the hedgehog, in an active state, in the cavity of the abdomen, towards the pelvis, was 95°; at the diaphragm 97°."

We find, from these experiments, that the heat of an animal is increased under the circumstances of cold, whenever there are actions to be carried on for which heat is necessary.

In the experiments on the first dormouse the heat of the animal was 80°, which is below the standard heat of the actions of that animal; and after being put into the cold mixture its heat was raised to 85°. In the second dormouse the heat was raised, by repeated experiments, from 75° to 93°. This question naturally occurs here: Was the increase of heat in the animals generated to resist the artificial cold produced by placing them in a cold atmosphere? or was it owing to a wound having been made into the cavity of the abdomen, and an exertion of the animal powers being required to repair the injury, which exertion could not take place without the increased degree of heat? That it was in consequence of the wound, appears evident from the experiment made upon the second hedgehog; for in an atmosphere of 26° of heat it was in a very torpid state, and did not raise the thermometer higher than 30°; but after being wounded and put back into the cold, and kept there for two days, its heat in the rectum was 93°, and so far from being torpid, it was lively, and the bed in which it lay felt warm*.

Why the heat of the dormouse should be so low as 80°, in an atmosphere of between 50° and 60°, is not easily accounted for, except as the effect of sleep. But I should very much suspect that sleep, simply considered, is out of the question, it being an effect that takes place in all degrees of heat and cold. In animals whose voluntary actions are

---

* It is found, from experiments, that the heat of an inflamed part is nearly the greatest or standard heat of the animal, it appearing to be a part of the process of inflammation to raise the heat up to the standard.

suspended by cold, that appears to produce its effect by acting in a certain degree as a sedative, in consequence of which the animal faculties are proportionably weakened, though they still retain, even under such circumstances, the power of carrying on all the functions of life. Beyond this point cold seems to act as a stimulant, and rouses the animal powers to action for self-preservation. It is more than probable that most animals are in this predicament, and that there is a degree of cold corresponding with every particular order of animals, by which, when applied, the voluntary actions must be suspended.

When a man is asleep he is colder than when awake; and I find in general that the difference is about one degree and a half; sometimes less. But this difference in the degree of cold between sleeping and waking is not a cause of sleep, but an effect; for many diseases produce a much greater degree of cold in the animal without giving the least tendency to sleep; therefore the inactivity of animals from cold must be different from sleep. Besides, all the operations of perfect life, as digestion, sensation, &c., are going on in the time of natural sleep, at least in the perfect animals; but none of these operations are performed in the torpid state of animals[a].

To see if the result of these experiments upon dormice was peculiar to that species, I wished to repeat the same experiments upon common mice, for which purpose, in

---

[a] [Some recent experiments of Dr. Marshall Hall confirm the accuracy of the distinction here drawn between sleep and torpidity, and also show that the ordinary sleep of hybernating warm-blooded animals differs from that of non-hybernating species, by inducing a more impaired state of the respiration, and a diminution of the power of evolving of heat. Although consciousness or sensibility be lost, automatic susceptibility of impressions is remarkably perfect during torpidity.   Dr. Hall states that the slightest touch applied to one of the spines of the torpid hedgehog immediately rouses it to draw a deep sonorous inspiration, which is its characteristic response to such disturbance while in that state.   The merest shake induces few respirations in the hybernating bat. (Phil. Trans., 1832, p. 15.) So also with respect to circulation, this vital operation appears to be performed uninterruptedly, though slowly, during hybernation. M. Prunelle (*Annales du Muséum*, tom. xviii. p. 28.) found that the pulsations of the heart of a bat, which, while it is awake and active amount to 200 in a minute, are reduced to 50 or 55 when it is torpid. Dr. M. Hall, who succeeded, by an ingenious contrivance, in subjecting the wing of a torpid bat to microscopical examination, found the circulation to be slow in the minute arteries and veins; but the beat of the heart was regular, and generally about twenty-eight times in a minute. (*Ibid.* p. 17.)   The blood which is thus circulated is venous, the respiration being nearly, if not totally, suspended; and its propulsion in this state is explained on the augmented irritability of the muscular system, which is manifested by the double heart of the torpid mammal being stimulated to contract by carbonized blood, like the heart of the cold-blooded and slow-breathing batrachian reptile.]

Experiment XVII: I made use of one strong and vigorous; and the atmosphere being at 60°, I introduced the thermometer into the abdomen : the ball being at the diaphragm the quicksilver was raised to 99°, but at the pelvis only to 96¾°.

Here there was a real difference of about 9° between the dormouse and the common, the dormouse only raising it to 80°, in two animals of the same size, in some degree of the same genus, and at the same season of the year, and the atmosphere of nearly the same temperature.

Experiment XVIII. The same mouse was put into a cold atmosphere of 13° for an hour, and then the thermometer was introduced as before ; but the animal had lost heat, for the quicksilver at the diaphragm was raised only to 83°, in the pelvis to 78°.

Here the real heat of the animal was diminished 16° at the diaphragm, and 18° in the pelvis, while in the dormouse it gained 5°, but lost upon a repetition.

Experiment XIX. In order to determine whether an animal that is weakened has the same powers, with respect to preserving heat and cold, as one that is vigorous and strong, I weakened a mouse by fasting, and then introduced the ball of the thermometer into its belly : the ball being at the diaphragm, the quicksilver rose to 97° ; in the pelvis to 95°, being two degrees colder than the strong mouse. The mouse being put into an atmosphere as cold as the other, and the thermometer again introduced, the quicksilver stood at 79° at the diaphragm, and 74° in the pelvis.

In this experiment the heat at the diaphragm was diminished 18°, in the pelvis 21°.

This greater diminution of heat in the second than in the first we may suppose proportional to the decreased power of the animal, arising from want of food.

To determine how far different parts of other animals than those already mentioned were of different degrees of heat, I made the following experiments upon a healthy dog.

Experiment XX. The ball of the thermometer being introduced two inches within the rectum, the quicksilver rose to 100½°. The chest of the dog was then opened, and a wound made into the right ventricle of the heart; and immediately on the ball being introduced, the quicksilver rose to 101° exactly. A wound was next made some way into the substance of the liver, and the ball being introduced, the quicksilver rose to 100½°. It was next introduced into the cavity of the stomach, where it stood exactly at 101°. All these experiments were made within a few minutes.

Experiment XXI. The thermometer was introduced into the rectum of an ox, and the quicksilver rose exactly to 99½°.

Experiment XXII. This was also repeated upon a rabbit, and the quicksilver rose to 99½°.

From experiments on mice and upon the dog, it plainly appears that every part of an animal is not of the same degree of heat; and hence we may reasonably infer, that the heat of the vital parts of man is greater than either the mouth, rectum, or the urethra.

To determine how far my idea was just, that the heat of animals varied in proportion to their degree of perfection, I made the following experiments upon fowls, which I considered as one remove below what are commonly called quadrupeds.

Experiment XXIII. I introduced the ball of the thermometer successively into the intestinum rectum of several hens, and found that the quicksilver rose as high as 103°, 103½°, and in one of them to 104°.

Experiment XXIV. I made the same experiments on several cocks, and the result was the same.

Experiment XXV. To determine if the heat of the hen was increased when she was prepared for incubation, I repeated the twenty-third experiment upon several sitting or clucking hens; in one the quicksilver rose to 104°, in another to 103½°, in a third to 103°, as in the twenty-third experiment.

Experiment XXVI. I placed the ball of the thermometer under the same hen, in whose rectum the quicksilver was raised to 104°, and found the heat as great as in the rectum.

Experiment XXVII. Having taken some of the eggs from under the same hen, where the chick was about three parts formed, I broke a hole in the shell, and introducing the ball of the thermometer, found that the quicksilver rose to 99½°. In some that were addled I found the heat not so high by two degrees; so that the life in the living egg assisted in some degree to support its own heat.

Is the increase of three or four degrees of heat, which is the difference found between the fowl and the quadruped, for the purpose of incubation? The heat in the eggs, which was caused and supported by that of the fowls, was not above the standard of the quadrupeds; and it would probably have been less if the heat of the hen had not been so great.

Finding, from the above experiments, that fowls were some degrees warmer than that class commonly called quadrupeds (although certainly less perfect animals), I chose to continue the experiments upon the same principle, and made the following upon those of a still inferior order.

The next remove from the fowl being what is commonly called the Amphibia.

Experiment XXVIII. I introduced the thermometer into the stomach, and afterwards into the anus of a healthy viper, and the quicksilver rose from 58° (the heat of the atmosphere in which it was) to 68°; so that it was ten degrees warmer than the common atmosphere[a].

Experiment XXIX. Having ascertained the heat of the water in a pond, in which there were carp, to be 65½°, I took a carp out of this water, and having introduced the thermometer into its stomach, the quicksilver rose to 69°; so that the difference between the water and the fish was only 3½°.[b]

Experiment XXX. The heat of the atmosphere at 56°; some earthworms were put into a glass vessel, and a thermometer being immersed among them, the quicksilver stood at 58½°.

This experiment was repeated; the atmosphere at 55°; and the worms were found to be 57°.

Experiment XXXI. The atmosphere at 54°; four black slugs were put into a small vessel, and a thermometer immersed among them stood at 55¼°.

Experiment XXXII. The atmosphere at 56°; three leeches were put into a small glass vessel, and a thermometer immersed among them stood at 57°.

This experiment was repeated; the atmosphere at 54°; when the thermometer stood at 55½°.

To see how far the colder animals had a power of preserving their standard heat when exposed to severe cold, I made the following experiments.

Experiment XXXIII. A viper, whose heat was 68°, was put into a pan, and the pan into a cold mixture of about 10°; after remaining there

---

[a] [The observations of Czermack correspond with the above experiment. He found that the difference between the temperature of the animal and that of the surrounding medium was greater in serpents and lizards than in other reptiles. The temperature of a turtle (*Chelonia Mydas*) was 82° when the surrounding atmosphere was 84°. That of a frog was 48° when the surrounding water was 44°. That of a Proteus was 64°, the surrounding water being 56°.]

[b] [Certain saltwater fishes, as the bonito and thunny, which have the gills supplied with nerves of unusual magnitude, and therefore probably enjoy a more energetic respiration, which have also a very powerful heart, and the quantity of red blood such as to give the muscles a dark red colour, manifest a higher degree of temperature than the white fishes of fresh water, on which Mr. Hunter experimented. Dr. John Davy found that the bonito had a temperature of 99° Fahrenheit when the surrounding medium was 80°·5. See Philos. Trans. 1835.]

about ten minutes had its heat reduced to 37°. Being allowed to stay ten minutes longer, the mixture at 13°, its heat was reduced to 35°. It was continued ten minutes more in the mixture at 20°, and its heat was reduced to 31°; nor did it sink lower, its tail beginning to freeze, and the animal now becoming very weak. It may be remarked, that it cooled much slower than many of the animals mentioned in the following experiments.

The frog being in its structure more similar to the viper than to either the fowl or fish, I made the following experiments on that animal.

Experiment XXXIV. I introduced the ball of the thermometer into its stomach, and the quicksilver stood at 44°. I then put the frog into a cold mixture, and the quicksilver sunk to 31°; the animal appeared almost dead, but recovered very soon : beyond this point it was not possible to lessen the heat without destroying the animal. But its decrease of heat was quicker than in the viper, although the mixture was nearly the same.

The next experiments were made on fishes.

Experiment XXXV. In an eel, the heat in the stomach, which at first was at 37°, sunk, after it had been some time in the cold mixture, to 31°. The animal at that time appeared dead, but was found to be alive the next day.

Experiment XXXVI. In a snail, whose heat was at 44°, it sunk, after it had been put into the cold mixture, to 31°, and then the animal froze.

Experiment XXXVII. Several leeches having been put into a bottle, and the bottle immersed in the cold mixture, the ball of the thermometer being placed in the middle of them, the quicksilver sunk to 31°; and by continuing the immersion for a sufficient time to destroy life, the quicksilver rose to 32°, and then the leeches froze. In all these experiments the animals when thawed were found dead.

Finding that animals of the imperfect classes will, without life being totally extinguished, admit of their heat being reduced to that point at which the dead solids and fluids freeze, but if sunk much below that, death must be the consequence, I wished therefore to be able to determine to what degree the heat of the animal could be raised.

Experiment XXXVIII. A healthy viper was placed in an atmosphere heated to 108°, and allowed to stay seven minutes; when the heat of the animal in the stomach and anus was found to be 92½°; beyond which it could not be raised in the above state of the atmosphere. The same experiment was made upon frogs, with nearly the same result.

Experiment XXXIX. An eel, very weak, its heat at 44°, which was nearly that of the atmosphere, was put into water heated to 65°, for fifteen minutes; and, upon examination, it was found of the same degree of heat with the water.

Experiment XL. A tench, whose heat was 41°, was put into water at 65°, and left there ten minutes; the ball of the thermometer being introduced both into the stomach and rectum, the quicksilver rose to 55°. These experiments were repeated with nearly the same result.

To determine whether life had any power of resisting heat and cold in inferior classes of animals, I made comparative trials between living and dead ones.

Experiment XLI. I took a living and a dead tench, and a living and a dead eel, and put them into warm water; they all received heat equally fast: and when they were exposed to cold, both the living and the dead admitted the cold likewise with equal quickness.

I had long suspected that the principle of life was not wholly confined to animals, or animal substance endowed with visible organization and spontaneous motion; but supposed that the same principle might exist in animal substances, devoid of apparent organization and motion, when the power of preservation was simply required.

I was led to this opinion about twenty years ago, when busied in making drawings of the growth of the chick in the process of incubation. I then observed, that whenever an egg was hatched, the yolk (which is not diminished in the time of incubation) was always perfectly sweet to the very last; and that the part of the albumen, which has not been expended on the growth of the animal, some days before hatching, was also perfectly sweet, although both were kept in a heat of 103° in the hen's egg for three weeks, and in the duck's for four; but I observed that if an egg was not hatched, that egg became putrid in nearly the same time with any other dead animal matter.

To determine from other tests how far eggs possessed a living principle, I made the following experiments.

Experiment XLII. After having placed an egg in a cold about 0, till it froze, I allowed it to thaw; by which process it was to be supposed the preserving powers of the egg must be destroyed. I then put this egg into the cold mixture, and with it one newly laid, and found the difference in freezing was seven minutes and a half, the fresh one so much longer time resisting the powers of cold.

Experiment XLIII. A new laid egg being put into a cold atmosphere, fluctuating between 17° and 15°, took above half an hour to freeze; but when thawed and put into an atmosphere at 25°, it froze in half the time. This experiment was repeated frequently with nearly the same result.

To ascertain the comparative degree of heat between a living and a dead egg, and also to determine whether a living egg be subject to the same laws with the more imperfect animals, I made the following experiments.

Experiment XLIV. A fresh egg, and one which had been frozen and thawed, were put into the cold mixture at 15°: the thawed one soon came to 32°, and began to swell and congeal; the fresh one sunk to 29¼°, and in twenty-five minutes later than the dead one it rose to 32°, and began to swell and freeze.

In this experiment the effect on the fresh egg was similar to that produced on the frog, eel, snail, &c., where life allowing the heat to be diminished two or three degrees below the freezing point, afterwards resisted all further decrease; but the powers of life being expended by this exertion, the parts froze like any other dead animal matter.

From these experiments it appears that a fresh egg has the power of resisting heat, cold, and putrefaction in a degree equal to many of the more imperfect animals; and it is more than probable this power arises from the same principle in both.

From the circumstance of those imperfect animals (upon which I made my experiments) varying their heat so readily, we may conclude that heat is not so very essential to life in them as in the more perfect; although it be essential to many of the operations, or what may be called the secondary actions of life, such as digesting food* and propagating the species, both which, especially the last, requiring the greatest powers an animal can exert. The animals which we call imperfect being chiefly employed in the act of digestion, we may suppose their degree of heat to be only what that action requires; it not being essentially necessary for the life of the animal that heat should ever rise so high in them as to call forth the powers necessary for the propagation of the species†. Whenever therefore these imperfect animals are

* How far this idea holds good with fishes, I am not certain.

† The hedgehog may be called a truly torpid animal; and we find that its actual heat is diminished when the actions are not vigorous [a]. From a general review of this

---

[a] [The experiments by which this important fact was established are those numbered I. and II., page 143. They were made after the publication of the original memoir in the Philosophical Transactions, in which the note consequently commences thus: "How far the animal heat is lowered in the more perfect animals, when these secondary actions are not necessary, as in the bat, hedgehog, bear, &c., I have not been able to determine, not having the opportunities of examining these animals. Dormice are in a mixed state, between the voluntary and involuntary, and we find the heat diminished when the actions are not vigorous; and, from a general review of this whole subject, it would appear that a certain degree of heat in the animal is necessary for digestion, and that necessary heat will be according to the nature of the animal."—*Phil. Trans.* 1778, p. 91.

exposed to a cold so great as to weaken their powers, and disable them from performing the first of these secondary actions, they in some measure cease to be voluntary agents, and remain in a torpid state during that extreme degree of cold which always occurs during some part of the winter in the countries they inhabit; and the food of such animals not being in general produced in the cold season is a reason why this torpidity becomes in some measure necessary[a].

From the heat of such animals sinking to the freezing point, or even lower, and then becoming stationary, and the animal not being able to support life in a much greater degree of cold for any length of time, we see a reason why they should always endeavour to procure places of abode in the winter where the cold seldom sinks to that point. We find toads burrowing, frogs living under large stones, snails seeking shelter under stones and in holes, and fishes having recourse to deep water; the heat of all those places being generally above the freezing point even in our hardest frosts; which are however sometimes so severe as to kill many whose habitations are not well chosen.

When the frost is more intense and of longer standing than common, or in countries where the winters are always severe, there is generally snow on the ground, and the water freezes: the advantage arising from these two circumstances is great; the snow serving as a blanket to the earth, and the ice to the water*.

whole subject it would appear that a certain degree of heat in the animal is necessary for its various œconomical operations, among which is digestion; and that necessary heat will be according to the nature of the animal, and, probably, the nature of the operations to be performed. A frog will digest food when its heat is at 60°, but not when at 35° or 40°; and it is very probable that, when the heat of the bear, hedgehog, dormouse, bat, &c. is reduced to 70°, 75°, or 80°, they lose their power of digestion; or rather that the body, in such a degree of cold, has no call upon the stomach. That animals in a certain degree of heat must always have food is further illustrated by the instance of bees. The construction of a bee is very similar to that of a fly, a wasp, &c. A fly and a wasp can allow their heat to diminish, as in the fish, snake, &c. without losing life, but a bee cannot; therefore a bee is obliged to keep up its heat as high as what we call its digestive heat, but not its propagating; for which purpose they provide against such cold as would deprive them even of their digestive heat, if they had not food to preserve it.

* Snow and ice are perhaps the worst conductors of heat of any substance yet known. In the first place, they never allow their own heat to rise above the freezing point, so that no heat can pass through ice or snow when at 32°, by which means they become

---

[a] [The torpidity induced by cold in hybernating animals is unlike that which is similarly induced in non-hybernating animals; in the former it is an action of preservation, in the latter one of destruction. See the paper before quoted, by Dr. Marshall Hall.]

As all the experiments I ever made upon the freezing of animals (with a view to see if it were possible to restore the actions of life when thawed) were tried upon whole ones; as I never saw life return by thawing*, and wished to see how far parts were similar to the whole in this respect, it being asserted, and with some authority, that parts of a man may be frozen, and afterwards recover,—I made, for this purpose the following experiments upon an animal of the same class as ourselves.

In January 1777, I mixed salt and ice till the cold was about 0; in the side of the vessel was a hole, through which I introduced the ear of a rabbit; and, to carry off the heat as fast as possible, it was held between two flat pieces of iron that went further into the mixture. That part of the ear projecting into the vessel became stiff, and when cut did not bleed; the part divided by the scissors flying from between the blades like a hard chip.

The ear having remained in the mixture nearly an hour, soon thawed when taken out, began to bleed, and became so very flaccid, as to double upon itself, from losing its natural elasticity. When out of the mixture nearly an hour, it became warm; and this warmth increasing to a considerable degree, it also began to thicken, in consequence of inflamma-

an absolute barrier to all heat that is at or above that degree; hence the heat of the earth, or whatever substance they cover, is retained; but they are conductors of heat below 32°. Perhaps that power decreases in proportion as the heat decreases under that point.

In the winter 1776, a frost coming on, the surface of the ground was frozen; but a considerable fall of snow fell, and continued several weeks: the heat of the atmosphere during the time was often at 15°; but so little did the frost affect the ground underneath that the surface of the ground thawed, and the earth retained the heat of 34°, in which beans and pease will grow.

The same thing took place in a pond where the water was frozen on the surface to a considerable thickness: a large quantity of snow having fallen, and covered the ice, the heat of the water was preserved; the ice thawed, and the snow, at its under surface, was found mixed with the water.

The heat of the water under the snow was at 35°, in which fishes lived very well.

It would be an attempt worthy the attention of the philosopher to investigate the cause of the heat of the earth, upon what principle it is preserved, &c.

* Vide Phil. Trans. for the year 1775, vol. lxv. part ii. p. 446 ª.

ª [That animals, lower in the scale than any which Hunter experimented on with this view, may, after having been frozen, recover life by thawing, is rendered at least highly probable from the following statement by Rudolphi. In his description of the *Filaria capsularia* he observes, " Vermis vitæ satis tenax est, ut per octiduum in frigida conservaverim, et Filarias in Harengis congelatis rigidas et glacie tectas frigidâ affusâ reviviscere viderim." (*Hist. Entoz.*, vol. ii. p. 62.)

tion, while the other ear continued in its usual degree of cold. The day following the frozen ear was still warm; and even two days after retained its heat and thickness, which continued for many days after.

About a week after this, the mixture being the same as in the former experiment, I introduced the ears of the same rabbit through the hole, and froze them both: the sound one however froze first, probably from its being considerably colder at the beginning. When withdrawn they soon thawed, both soon became warm, and the fresh ear thickened as the other had done before.

Such a change in the parts does not always take place so quickly; for on repeating the experiment on the ear of another rabbit till it became as hard as a board, it was found to be longer in thawing than in the former experiment, and much longer before it became warm; in two hours, however, it had acquired some degree of warmth, and on the day following was hot and thickened.

In the spring, 1776, I perceived that my cocks in the country had their combs smooth, with an even edge, and not so broad as formerly, appearing as if near one half of them had been cut off. Having inquired into the cause of this, my servant told me that it had happened in that winter during the hard frost, he having then observed that the combs had in part dropped off, also that the comb of one cock had entirely separated; but this I did not see, as by accident he was burnt to death. I naturally imputed this effect to the combs having been frozen to so great a degree during the severe weather as to have the life of the part destroyed. To determine therefore, by experiment, the solidity of this reasoning, I made the following experiment.

I selected for the purpose a very large young cock, having a comb of considerable breadth, with deep serrated edges, the processes of which were full half an inch long. My attempts to freeze the substance of the comb did not succeed; for that, being thick and warm, resisted the effects of the cold, and only the serrated edges were frozen. The frozen parts became white and hard, and when I cut off a little bit did not bleed, nor did the animal show any signs of pain. I next immersed in the cold mixture one of his wattles, which was very broad and thin; it froze very readily; and upon thawing both the comb and wattle they became warm, but of a purple colour, having lost that transparency which remained in the other parts of the comb and in the other wattle. The wound in the comb now bled freely.

Both comb and wattle recovered perfectly in about a month. The natural colour returned first nearest to the sound parts, increasing gradually till the whole had acquired a healthy appearance.

There was a very material difference in the effect between those fowls, the serrated edges of whose combs I suspected to have been frozen in the winter of 1775–6, for they must have dropped off. The only way in which I can account for this difference is, that in those fowls the parts were kept so long frozen that the unfrozen or active parts had time to inflame, and had brought about a separation of the frozen parts, treating them exactly as dead, similar to a mortified part; and that before they thawed, the separation was so far completed as to deprive them of further support.

As it is confidently asserted that fishes are often frozen, and again return to motion, and as I had never succeeded in any of my trials of the kind upon whole fishes, I made some experiments upon particular parts, to which I was led by having found a material difference in the result of experiments made upon the whole, and on parts of the more perfect animals.

I froze the tail of a tench, as high as the anus, which became as hard as a board; when thawed, that part was whiter than common; and when it moved, the whole tail moved as one piece, and the termination of the frozen part appeared like the joint on which it moved.

On the same day I froze the tails of two gold fishes till they became as solid as a piece of wood. They were put into cold water to thaw, and appeared for some days to be very well; but that part of the tails which had been frozen had not the natural colour, and the fins of the tails became ragged. About three weeks after, a fur came all over the frozen parts; their tails became lighter, so that the fishes were suspended in the water perpendicularly; they had almost lost the power of motion; and at last died. The water in which they were kept was New River water, shifted every day, and in quantity about ten gallons.

I made similar experiments upon an order of animals still inferior, viz. common earth-worms.

I first froze the whole of an earth-worm as a standard; when thawed it was perfectly dead.

I then froze the anterior half of another earth-worm; but the whole died.

I next froze the posterior half of an earth-worm; the anterior half continued alive, and separated itself from the dead part.

From some of these experiments it appears that the more imperfect animals are capable of having their heat and cold varied very considerably, but not according to the degree of heat or cold of the surrounding medium in which they can support life; for they can live in a cold considerably below the freezing point, and yet the living powers of the animal will not allow their heat to be diminished much beyond 32°. Whenever the surrounding cold brings them so low, the power of generating heat takes place; and if the cold is continued, the animals exert this power till life is destroyed; after which they freeze, and are immediately capable of admitting any degree of cold.

EXPERIMENTS AND OBSERVATIONS ON VEGETABLES,
WITH RESPECT TO THE POWER OF PRODUCING HEAT[a].

To ascertain whether vegetables could be frozen, and afterwards retain all their properties when thawed, or had the same power of generating heat with animals, I made several experiments. Vegetable juices
when squeezed out of a green plant, such as cabbage and spinage,
froze in a cold of about 29°; and between 29° and 30° thawed again,
which is about 4° above the point at which the animal juices freeze
and thaw.

Experiment I. I took a young growing bean, about three inches long
in the stalk, and put it into the leaden vessel with common water, and
then immersed the whole into the cold mixture. The water very
soon froze all round it; however, the bean itself took up a longer time
in freezing than the same quantity of water would have done; yet it
did freeze, and was afterwards thawed and planted in the ground, but
it soon withered. The same experiment was made upon the bulbous
roots of tulips, and with the same success.

Experiment II. A young Scotch fir, which had two complete shoots
and a third growing, and which consequently was in its third year, was
put into the cold mixture, which was between 15° and 17°. The last
shoot froze with great difficulty, which appeared to be owing in some
measure to the repulsion between the plant and the water. When
thawed, the young shoot was found flaccid. It was planted; the first
and second shoot we found retained life, while the third, or growing
shoot, withered.

Experiment III. A young shoot of growing oats, with three leaves,
had one of the leaves put into the cold mixture at 22°, and it soon
was frozen. The roots were next put in, but did not freeze; and when
put into the ground the whole grew, excepting the leaf which had been
frozen. The same experiment was made upon the leaves and roots of a
young bean, and attended with the same success.

Experiment IV. A leaf taken from a growing bean was put into the
cold mixture and frozen, and afterwards thawed, which served as a

---

[a] [This paper includes those portions of the two communications to the Royal Society, On the Heat of Animals and Vegetables, which were omitted by Hunter in the
'Animal Œconomy.' See Phil. Trans., lxv., 1775, p. 450.]

standard. Another fresh leaf was taken and bent in the middle upon itself; a small shallow leaden vessel was put upon the top of the cold mixture, and the two leaves put upon its bottom; but one half of each leaf was not allowed to touch the vessel by the bend: the cold mixture was between 17° and 15°, and the atmosphere at 22°. The surfaces of the two leaves which were in contact with the lead were soon frozen in both; but those surfaces which rose at right angles, and were therefore only in contact with the cold atmosphere, did not freeze in equal times; the one that had gone through this process before froze much sooner than the fresh one. The above experiment was repeated when the cold mixture was at 25°, 24°, and the atmosphere nearly the same, and with the same success; only the leaves were longer in freezing, especially the fresh leaf.

Experiment V. The vegetable juices above mentioned being frozen in the leaden vessel, the cold mixture at 28°, and the atmosphere the same, a growing fir-shoot was laid upon the surface, also a bean-leaf; and upon remaining there some minutes, they were found to have thawed the surface on which they lay. This I thought might arise from the greater warmth of these substances at the time of application; but by moving the fir-shoot to another part, we had the same effect produced.

Experiment VI. A fresh leaf of a bean was exactly weighed; it was then put into the cold atmosphere and frozen. In this state it was put back into the same scale, and allowed to thaw. No alteration in the weight was produced.

From the foregoing experiments it appears, first, that plants, when in a state of actual vegetation, or even in such a state as to be capable of vegetating under certain circumstances, must be deprived of their principle of vegetation before they can be frozen. Secondly, vegetables have a power within themselves of producing or generating heat; but not always in proportion to the diminution of heat by application of cold, so as to retain at all times an uniform degree of heat; for the internal temperature of vegetables is susceptible of variations to a much greater extent indeed than that of the more imperfect animals, but still within certain limits: beyond these limits the principle of vegetable, as of animal life, resists any further change. Thirdly, the heat of vegetables varies according to the temperature of the medium in which they are, which we discover by varying that temperature, and observing the heat of the vegetable. Fourthly, the expense of the vegetating powers in this case is proportioned to the necessity, and the whole vegetable powers may be exhausted in this way. Fifthly, this power is most probably in proportion to the perfection of the plant, the natural heat proper to each species, and the age of each individual. It may also perhaps depend, in some degree, on other circumstances not hitherto observed; for in Experiment II. the old shoot did not lose its powers, while that which was young or growing did; and in Experiments II. and III. we found that the young growing shoot of the fir was with great difficulty frozen at 15°, while a bean-leaf was easily frozen at 22°; and in Experiment V. the young shoot of the fir thawed the ice at 28° much faster than the leaf of the bean. Sixthly, it is probably by means of this principle that vegetables are adapted to different climates. Seventhly, that suspension of the functions of vegetable life, which takes place during the winter season, is probably owing to their being susceptible of such a great variation of internal temperature. Eighthly, the roots of vegetables are capable of resisting cold more than the stem or leaf; therefore, though the stem be killed by cold, the root may be preserved, as daily experience evinces. The texture of vegetables alters very much by the loss of life, especially those which are watery and young; from being brittle and crisp, they become tough and flexible. The leaf of a bean when in full health is thick and mossy, repels water as if greasy, and will often break before it is considerably bent; but if it is killed slowly by cold, it will lose all these properties, becoming then pliable and flaccid: deprived of its power of repelling water, it is easily made wet, and appears like boiled greens. If killed quickly by being frozen immediately, it will remain in the same state as when alive; but upon thawing, will immediately lose all its former texture. This is so remarkable, that it would induce one to believe that it lost considerably of its substance; but from Experiment VI. it is evident that it does not. The same thing happens to a plant when killed by electricity*. If a growing juicy plant receives a stroke of electricity sufficient to kill it, its leaves droop, and the whole becomes flexible.

So far animal and vegetable life appear to be the same; yet an animal and a vegetable differ in one very material circumstance, which it may be proper to take particular notice of in this place, as it shows itself with remarkable evidence in these experiments. An animal is equally old in all its parts, excepting where new parts are formed in consequence of diseases; and we find that these new or young parts in animals, like the young shoots of vegetables, are not able to support life equally with the old; but every plant has in it a series of ages. According to its years, it has parts of all the successive ages from its first formation; each part having power equal to its age, and each part, in this respect, being

* To kill a whole plant by electricity, it is necessary to apply the conductor, or give a shock to every projecting part; for any part that is out of the line of direction will still retain life.

similar to animals of so many different ages. Youth, in all cases, is a state of imperfection; for we find that few animals that come into the world in winter live, unless they are particularly taken care of; and we may observe the same of vegetables. I found that a young plant was more easily killed than an old one; as also the youngest part of the same plant.

[a] As I had formerly, in making my experiments upon animals relative to heat and cold, made similar ones on vegetables, and had generally found a great similarity between them in these respects, I was led to pursue the subject on the same plan; but I was still further induced to continue my experiments upon vegetables, as I imagined I saw a material difference between them in their power of supporting cold.

From observations and the foregoing experiments, it plainly appears that the living principle will not allow the heat of such animals to sink much lower than the freezing point, although the surrounding atmosphere be much colder, and that in such a state they cannot support life long; but it may be observed, that most vegetables of every country can sustain the cold of their climate. In very cold regions, as in the more northern parts of America, where the thermometer is often 50° below 0, where people's feet are known to freeze and their noses to drop off if great care be not taken, yet the spruce-fir, birch, juniper, &c. are not affected.

Yet, that vegetables can be affected by cold, daily experience evinces; for the vegetables of every country are affected if the season be more than ordinarily cold for that country, and some more than others; for in the cold climates above mentioned the life of the vegetable is often obliged to give way to the cold of the country: a tree shall die by the cold; then freeze and split into a great number of pieces; and in so doing produce considerable noise, giving loud cracks, which are often heard at a great distance.

In this country the same thing sometimes happens to exotics from warmer climates. A remarkable instance of this kind happened this winter in His Majesty's garden at Kew. The *Erica arborea*, or tree-heath, a native of Spain and Portugal, which had kept its health extremely well against a garden wall for four or five years, though covered with a mat, was killed by the cold, and then, being frozen, split into innumerable pieces[*]. But the question is, Is every tree dead that is

---

[*] This must be owing to the sap in the tree freezing, and occupying a larger space when frozen than in a fluid state, similar to water; and that there is a sufficient quantity of sap in a tree newly killed, is proved by the vast quantity that flows out on

frozen? I can only say, that in all the experiments I ever made upon trees and shrubs, whether in the growing or active state, or in the passive, that whole or part which was frozen was dead when thawed.

The winter 1775–6 afforded a very favourable opportunity for making experiments relative to cold, which I carefully availed myself of. However, previous to that winter, I had made many experiments upon vegetables respecting their temperature, comparatively with that of the atmosphere, and when they were in their different states of activity: I therefore examined them in different seasons, with a view to see what powers vegetables have. I shall relate these experiments in the order in which they were made.

They were begun in the spring, the actions of life upon which growth depends being then upon the increase; and they were continued till those actions were upon the decline, and also when all actions were at an end, but whilst the passive powers of life were still retained.

The first were made on a walnut-tree, nine feet high in the stem, and seven feet in circumference in the middle.

A hole was bored into it on the north side, five feet above the surface of the ground, eleven inches deep towards the centre of the tree, but obliquely upwards, to allow any sap which might ooze through the wounded surface to run out.

I then fitted to this part a box, about eight inches wide and five deep, and fastened it to the tree: the bottom of the box opened like a door with a hinge. I stuffed the box with wool, excepting the middle, opposite to the hole in the tree; for this part I had a plug of wool to stuff in, which, when the door was shut, inclosed the whole. The intention of this was to keep off, as much as possible, all immediate external influence either of heat or cold.

The same thermometer with which I made my former experiments, seven inches and a half long, was sunk into a long feather of a peacock's tail, with a slit upon one side to show the degrees; by this means the ball of the thermometer could be introduced into the bottom of the hole.

Experiment I. March 29. I began my experiments at six in the morning, the atmosphere at 57¼°, the thermometer in the tree at 55°; when it was withdrawn the quicksilver sunk to 53°, but soon rose to 57¼°*.

---

wounding a tree. But what appeared most remarkable to me was, that in a walnut-tree, on which I made many of my experiments, I observed that more sap issued out in the winter than in the summer. In the summer, a hole being bored, scarcely any came out, but in the winter it flowed out abundantly.

    * The sinking of the quicksilver upon being withdrawn I imputed to the evaporating of the moisture of the fluid upon the ball.

This experiment was repeated three times with the same success. Here the tree was cooler than the atmosphere, when one should rather have expected to find it warmer, since it could not be supposed to have as yet lost its former day's heat.

Exp. II. April 4th, half-past five in the evening. The tree at 56°, the atmosphere at 62°; the tree therefore still cooler than the atmosphere.

Exp. III. April 5th. Wind in the north, a coldish day, six o'clock in the evening; the thermometer in the tree was at 55°, the atmosphere at 47°; the tree warmer than the atmosphere.

Exp. IV. April 7th, a cold day, wind in the north, cloudy. At three in the afternoon the thermometer in the tree was at 42°, the atmosphere at 42° also.

Exp. V. April 9th, a cold day, with snow, hail, and wind in the north-east. At six in the evening the thermometer in the tree at 45°, the atmosphere at 39°.

Here the tree was warmer than the atmosphere, just as might have been expected. If these experiments prove anything, it is that there is no standard; and probably these variations arose from some circumstance which had no immediate connexion with the internal powers of the tree; but it may also be supposed to have arisen from a power in the tree to produce or diminish heat, as some of them were in opposition to the atmosphere.

After having endeavoured to find out the comparative heat between vegetables and the atmosphere when the vegetables were in action, I next made my experiments upon them when they were in the passive life.

As the difference was very little when in their most active state, I could expect but very little when the powers of the plant were at rest.

From experiment upon the more imperfect classes of animals it plainly appears, that although they do not resist the effects of extreme cold till they are brought to the freezing point, they then appear to have the power of resisting it, and of not allowing their cold to be brought much lower.

To see how far vegetables are similar to those animals in this respect, I made several experiments: I however suspected them not to be similar, because such animals will die in a cold in which vegetables do live; I therefore supposed that there was some other principle.

I did not confine these experiments to the walnut-tree, but made similar ones on several trees of different kinds, as pines, yews, poplars, &c., to see what was the difference in different kinds of trees. The difference proved not to be great, not above a degree or two: however, this difference, although small, shows a principle in life, all other things being equal; for as the same experiments were made on a dead tree, which stood with its roots in the ground, similar to the living ones, they became more conclusive.

In October I began the experiments upon the walnut-tree when its powers of action were on the decline, and when it was going into its passive life.

Exp. VI.   October 18th, at half-past six in the morning, the atmosphere at $51\frac{1}{4}°$, the thermometer in the tree was at $55\frac{1}{2}°$; but, on withdrawing and exposing it for a few minutes in the common atmosphere, it fell to $50\frac{1}{2}°$.

Exp. VII.   October 21st, seven o'clock in the morning, the atmosphere at 41°, the tree at 47°.

Exp. VIII.   October 21st, in the evening at five o'clock, the atmosphere at $51\frac{1}{2}°$, the tree at 57°.

Exp. IX.   October 22nd, at seven in the morning, the atmosphere at 42°, the tree at 48°.

Exp. X.   October 22nd, one o'clock afternoon, the atmosphere at 51°, the tree at 53°.

Exp. XI.   October 23rd, in the evening of a wet day, the atmosphere at 46°, the tree at 48°.

Exp. XII.   October 28th, a dry day, the atmosphere at 45°, the tree at 46°

Exp. XIII.   October 29th, a fine day, the atmosphere at 45°, the tree at 49°.

Exp. XIV.   November 2nd, wind east, the atmosphere at 43°, the tree at 43°.

Exp. XV.   November 5th, wet day, the atmosphere at 43°, the tree at 45°.

Exp. XVI.   November 10th.   Atmosphere at 49°, the tree at 55°.

Exp. XVII.   November 18th.   Atmosphere at 42°, the tree at 44°.

Exp. XVIII.   November 20th, fine day, the atmosphere at 40°, the tree at 42°.

Exp. XIX.   December 2nd.   The atmosphere at 54°, the tree at 54°.

In all these experiments, which were made at various times in the day, viz. in the morning, at noon, and in the evening, the tree was in some degree warmer than the atmosphere, excepting in one, when their temperatures were equal.   For the sake of brevity, I have drawn up my other experiments (which were made on different trees) into four tables, as they were made at four different degrees of heat of the atmosphere, including those made in the time of the very hard frost in the winter of 1775-6.   They were as follows:

TABLE I.

Atmosphere.	Names.	Height.		Dia-meter.		Heat.
		ft.	in.	ft.	in.	°
	Carolina poplar ...	2	0	0	2	29½
	English poplar....	4	0	0	2¼	29½
	Oriental plane	3	0	0	1¼	30
	Occidental plane ..	3	6	0	2	30
	Carolina plane....	1	0	0	1¾	30
	Birch	3	6	0	2¼	29½
29 deg.	Scotch fir........	3	6	0	4	28½
	Cedar of Lebanon..	2	2	0	4½	28½
	Arbutus	2	6	0	3½	30
	Arbor vitæ	2	8	0	3½	29
	Deciduous cypress.	3	0	0	2½	30
	Lacker varnish....	3	6	0	2	30
	Walnut-tree.......	5	0	2	4	31

The old hole in the walnut-tree, being full of sap, was frozen up; but a new one was made.

TABLE II.

Atmosphere.	Names.	Height.		Dia-meter.	Heat.
		ft.	in.	in.	°
	Spruce fir	4	0	2½	32
	Scotch fir........	1	5½	1½	28
	Silver fir	3	11	2½	30
	Weymouth fir....	4	6	2½	30
27 deg.	Yew.............	3	7	3	30
	Holly...........	2	6	2	30
	Plum-tree........	4	6	3	31½
	Dead cedar	3	11	3	-29
	Ground under snow	0	3 deep.	......	34

TABLE III.

Atmosphere.	Names.	Heat.
		°
	Spruce fir	23
	Scotch fir........	23
	Silver fir	23
24 deg.	Weymouth fir....	23
	Yew.............	22
	Holly...........	23
	Dead cedar	24

The same trees we mentioned when the thermometer was at 29°, in new holes made at the same height, and left some time pegged up till the heat produced by the gimlet was gone off; but in which, as they were moist from the sap, the heat could be very little, especially as the gimlet was not in the least heated by the operation.

TABLE IV.

Atmosphere.	Names.	Heat.
		°
	Carolina poplar ...	17
	English poplar....	17
	Oriental plane....	17
16 deg.	Occidental plane..	17
	Carolina plane....	17
	Birch	17
	Scotch fir........	16¼

It will be necessary to observe, that the sap of the walnut-tree, which flowed out in great quantity, froze at 32°. I did not try to freeze the sap of the others.

Now since the sap of a tree when taken out freezes at 32°; also, since the sap of a tree, when taken out of its proper canals, freezes when the heat of the tree is at 31°; and since the heat of the tree can be so low as 17° without freezing; by what power are the juices of the tree, when in their proper canals, kept fluid in such a cold? Is it the principle of vegetation? Or is the sap inclosed in such a way as that the process of freezing cannot take place, which we find to be the case when water is confined in globular vessels? If so, its confinement must be very different from the confinement of moisture in dead vegetables; but the circumstance of vegetables dying with the cold and then freezing appears to answer the last question. These, however, are questions which at present I shall not endeavour to solve.

I have made several experiments upon the seeds of vegetables similar to those on the eggs of animals; but as inserting them would draw out this paper to too great a length, I will reserve them for another.

PROPOSALS FOR THE RECOVERY OF PERSONS APPA-RENTLY DROWNED[a].

HAVING been requested by a principal member of the society esta-blished for the recovery of persons apparently drowned to commit my thoughts on that subject to paper, I readily complied, hoping, that al-though I have had no opportunities of making actual experiments upon drowned persons, it might be in my power to throw some lights on a subject so closely connected with the inquiries which for many years have been my business and favourite amusement: I therefore collected together my observations and experiments relative to the loss and re-covery of the actions of life, which I now offer to the public. The en-deavour to recover persons apparently drowned is a new practice, and has furnished, as yet, few important and clear facts: our knowledge of the animal œconomy is so imperfect, that I am afraid our reasoning from that alone must not be relied on in a question so interesting to the cause of humanity. But let us reason as well as we can from the few data we have, and let every man bring forward, freely, the observations he has made, that the subject thus fairly before the public may in time, by its united efforts, be more perfectly understood.

I shall consider an animal apparently drowned as not dead, but that only a suspension of the actions of life has taken place. The difference between a suspension of the actions of life and absolute death is well illustrated by the common snail when drowning. If a snail is immersed in water and kept there, certain voluntary and instinctive actions take place; but after remaining a certain time covered by the water, all these actions cease. Hence the animal, being relaxed, naturally comes out of the shell in that state; its stomach is filled with water, and the body appears larger than natural, but without motion. These actions con-tinue thus suspended till either the cause of suspension be removed or some other stimulus shall bring the parts into action: but under such circumstances life cannot be preserved for any considerable length of time; and when the stimulus which precedes death takes place, the whole animal is thrown into action, and in that contracted state, possibly, ab-solute death is produced. A state of relaxation should therefore (where

[a] [From the Philosophical Transactions, vol. lxvi.; read March 21, 1776.]

an universal violence has not been committed,) be considered as the criterion of life; and even in such cases should be for some time admitted as a probable reason for supposing life still to exist.

If an animal appears so far dead as to have lost all the actions characteristic of life, yet a certain degree of action in all the parts will be produced when absolute death is taking place; and that animal, being still susceptible of stimulus, is recoverable if the proper stimulus could be applied.

It is asserted that men have recovered the actions of life even after the contraction, in consequence of the stimulus which precedes death, has taken place. If this be true, which I very much doubt, the stimulus must first produce relaxation, which is an action dependent on life.

This is probably the case in the first appearances of death from all violent accidents, except those caused by lightning, electricity, an universal shock, a blow on the stomach, a violent affection of the mind, or some other modes by which absolute death may be instantaneously produced, which all appear to act in the same way, producing absolute and instant death. For in cases which have fallen under my observation, the concomitant circumstances have resembled those which attend death caused by lightning or electricity, such as a total and instantaneous privation of sense and motion without convulsions; consequently, no rigor of muscles having been produced, and the blood remaining uncoagulated, differing entirely in these respects from what appears in persons deprived of sense and life by any injury done the brain. It seems only possible to account for this effect of a blow on the stomach, from the connexion subsisting between that viscus and every part of the body, at least with vital parts; the blow most probably causing instant death in that organ, of which the death of the whole animal is the consequence*. When death takes place from violent affections of the mind, it must be referred to the universal influence which the mind has over the body.

To ascertain when a body is deprived of life it is first necessary to know in what manner apparent death took place; whether in the common way, or from the vital actions being too long suspended. In either case stiffness of the muscles is probably the most certain and most evi-

---

* I should consider the situation of a person drowned to be similar to that of a person in a trance. In both the action of life is suspended without the power being destroyed; but I am inclined to believe that a greater proportion of persons recover from trances than from drowning, because a trance is the natural effect of a disposition in the person to have the action of life suspended for a time; but drowning being produced by violence, the suspension will more frequently last for ever, unless the power of life is roused to action by some applications of art.

dent proof of absolute death, since that arises from the stimulus immediately preceding death having taken place. But if the privation of life
is produced by any of the modes above mentioned, which kill instantaneously and universally, the stimulus which produces stiffness is not
allowed time to act, and the muscles are all left in a relaxed state. Yet
this state of relaxation must not, on that account, be always considered
as a proof of life still remaining.

A degree of flaccidity in the eyeballs, which produces glassiness, is a
certain mark of death; but is, however, only a secondary mode of ascertaining it in those instances where the body becomes stiff; but may be
the first mode where absolute death takes place instantaneously; and
putrefaction will be the second; while in the other cases putrefaction
will be the third.

That I may more fully explain my ideas upon this subject, it will be
necessary to state some propositions.

First: that so long as the animal retains the susceptibility of impression, though deprived of the action of life, it will, most probably, retain
the power of action when impressed; therefore the action may frequently
be suspended, and yet recoverable: but when the susceptibility of impression is destroyed, the action ceases to be recoverable. Secondly:
it is necessary to mention, that I consider part of the living principle as
inherent in the blood*. Thirdly: that the stomach sympathizes with
every part of an animal, and that every part sympathizes with the stomach; therefore, whatever acts upon the stomach as a cordial, or rouses
its natural and healthy actions, and whatever affects it so as to produce
debility, has an immediate effect upon every part of the body. The last
proposition I have to make is, that every part of the body sympathizes
with the mind; for whatever affects the mind, the body is affected in
proportion. These sympathies are strongest with the vital parts; but
besides these universal sympathies between the stomach, the mind, and
all parts of the body, there are peculiar sympathies, of which the heart,
sympathizing immediately with the lungs, is an instance. If anything
is received into the lungs which is a poison to animal life, such as inflammable air, volatile vitriolic acid, and many other well-known substances, the motion of the heart immediately ceases, even much sooner
than if the trachea had been tied; and, from experiments, it appears that

---

* That the living principle is inherent in the blood is a doctrine which the nature of
this account will not allow me to discuss; thus much, however, it may be proper to say,
that it is founded on the result of many observations and experiments. But it may be
thought necessary I should here give a definition of what I call the living principle: so
far, then, as I have used the term, I mean to express that principle which preserves the
body from dissolution with or without action, and is the cause of all its actions.

anything salutary to life, applied to the lungs, will restore the heart's action after it has been at rest some time.

I shall divide violent deaths into three kinds: first, where a stop is put only to the action of life in the animal, but without any irreparable injury to a vital part, which action, if not restored in a certain time, will be irrecoverably lost. The length of that time is subject to considerable variation, depending on circumstances with which we are at present unacquainted. The second is, where an injury is done to a vital part, as by taking away blood till the powers of action are lost; or by a wound or pressure being made on the brain or spinal marrow while life remains in the solids sufficient for the preservation of the animal, if action could be restored to the vital parts. The third is, where absolute death instantly takes place in every part, as is often the case in strokes of lightning; in the common method of killing eels, by throwing them on some hard substance, in such manner as that the whole length of the animal shall receive the shock at the same instant; by a blow on the stomach; by violent affections of the mind; and by many diseases, in all which cases the muscles remain flexible*

How far that may be strictly considered as a violent death which is caused by affections of the mind, I will not pretend to say; but if it is to have a place in that class, it must be ranked with those which happen from lightning, and a blow on the stomach; and in most cases of persons drowned, I can easily conceive the mind to be so much affected prior to the immersion, and in the moment immediately succeeding it, as to make a material difference in the power of recovery. In many sudden deaths arising from violence, and even from disease, death shall take place so immediately that the muscles neither contract, nor does the blood coagulate.

The present consideration is, under which of the kinds of violent death drowning can be classed or arranged? I am of opinion it will most commonly come under the first, and upon that ground I shall principally consider the subject, always supposing the body to remain flaccid.

The loss of motion in drowning seems to arise from the loss of respiration, and the immediate effects which that has upon the other vital motions of the animal; except what may have arisen from the affections of the mind. The privation of breathing appears, however, to be the

---

* On the other hand, when an eel is killed by chopping it into a number of pieces, the powers of life are by those means roused into action; and as every part dies in that active state, every part is found stiff after death. This explains the custom of cutting fish into pieces while yet alive, in order to make them hard, usually known by the name of crimping.

first cause, and the heart's motion ceasing, to be the second or consequent; therefore most probably the restoration of breathing is all that
is necessary to restore the heart's motion; for if sufficient life still exists to produce that effect, we may suppose every part equally ready to
move the very instant in which the action of the heart takes place, their
actions depending so much upon it. What makes it very probable, that
in recovering persons drowned, the principal effect depends upon air
being thrown into the lungs, is what happens at the birth of children,
when too much time has intervened between the interruption of that
life which is peculiar to the fœtus and that which depends on breathing;
they then lose altogether the disposition for this new life; and in such
cases, there being a total suspension of the actions of life, the child remains to all appearance dead, and would certainly die if air were not
thrown into its lungs, and by such means the first principle of action
restored. To put this in a still clearer light, I will give the result of
some experiments which I made in the year 1755 upon a dog.

A pair of double bellows were provided, constructed in such a manner
as by one action to throw fresh air into the lungs, and by another to
suck out again the air which had been thrown in by the former, without mixing them together. The muzzle of these bellows was fixed into
the trachea of a dog, and by working them he was kept perfectly alive.
While this artificial breathing was going on I took off the sternum of
the dog, and exposed the lungs and heart; the heart continued to act
as before, only the frequency of its action was considerably increased.
When I stopped the motion of the bellows the heart became gradually
weaker, and less frequent in its contractions, till it entirely ceased to
move. By renewing the action of the bellows the heart again began to
move, at first very faintly, and with long intermissions; but by continuing the artificial breathing, its motion became as frequent and as
strong as at first. This process I repeated upon the same dog ten times,
sometimes stopping for five, eight, or ten minutes, and observed that
every time I left off working the bellows the heart became extremely
turgid with blood, the blood in the left side becoming as dark as that
in the right, which was not the case when the bellows were working.
These situations of the animal appeared to me exactly similar to
drowning.

Death in persons drowned has been accounted for by supposing that
the blood, rendered unfit for the purposes of life by being deprived of
the action of the air in respiration, is sent in a vitiated state to the brain
and other vital parts, by which means the nerves lose their effect upon
the heart, and the heart in consequence its motion. This, however, I
am fully convinced is false; first, from the experiments on the dog, in

which a large column of blood so vitiated (consisting of what had been propelled from the heart after respiration stopped, and might be supposed the cause of the heart ceasing to act, together with all that remained in the heart and pulmonary veins,) was again pushed forward without any ill effect having been produced; and next, from the return to life of persons drowned and children still-born, which, were such a supposition true, could never happen, unless we imagine a change of the blood to take place in the brain, prior to the restoration of the heart's motion. This restoration must therefore depend immediately on the application of air to the lungs, and not on the effects which air has upon the blood, or that blood upon the vital parts.

If the affections of the mind have had any share in the cessation of action in the heart, its motion will not be so easily restored as in other cases. In our attempts to recover those who have been drowned, it might therefore be proper to inquire if there had been time sufficient for the person to form any idea of his situation previous to his being plunged into the water, as it is not unlikely that the agitated state of mind might assist in killing him; and in such case I should very much doubt the probability of restoring him to life. In the history of those who have and who have not been recovered, could the difference be ascribed to any such cause, it might lead to something useful; as in those who have had an intention to destroy themselves, a great difference in the chance of recovery may arise, from the mind having been previously very much affected.

It frequently happens, in the case of drowning, that assistance cannot be procured till a considerable time after the accident; every moment of this delay renders recovery more precarious, the chances of which are not only diminished in the parts where the first powers of action principally reside, but also in every other part of the body.

In offering my sentiments on the method of treating persons who are apparently drowned, I shall say, first, what I would recommend to have done; secondly, what I would wish might be avoided.

When assistance is called in soon after the immersion, perhaps blowing air into the lungs may be sufficient to effect a recovery*; but if a considerable time, as an hour, has been lost, it will seldom be sufficient, the heart in all probability having by that time lost its intimate connexion with the lungs. It will in these cases, therefore, be proper to apply, mixed with the air, such stimulating medicines as the vapour of volatile alkali, which may easily be done, by holding spirits of hartshorn

* Perhaps the dephlogisticated air described by Dr. Priestley (oxygen gas) may prove more efficacious than common air. It is easily procured, and may be preserved in bottles or bladders for that purpose.

in a cup under the receiver of the bellows. I would advise the air and volatile alkali to be thrown in by the nose rather than the mouth, as the last mode of administering, by producing sickness, is more likely to depress than rouse the living principle. It will be still better if it can be done by both nostrils, as applications of this kind to the olfactory nerves certainly rouse the living principle and put the muscles of respiration into action, and therefore are the more likely to excite the action of the heart: besides, that affections of these nerves are known to act more immediately on the living principle; since while a strong smell of very sweet flowers, as orange flowers, will in many cause fainting, the application of vinegar will as immediately restore the powers to action again. All perfumes in which there is some acid rather rouse than depress, as the sweet-brier, essence of lemon, &c. If, during the operation of the bellows, the larynx be gently pressed against the œsophagus and spine, it will prevent the stomach and intestines being too much distended by the air, and leave room for the application of more effectual stimuli to those parts. This pressure, however, must be conducted with judgment and caution, so that the trachea and the aperture into the larynx may both be left perfectly free. While this business is going on an assistant should prepare bedclothes, carefully brought to the proper degree of heat. I consider heat as congenial with the living principle; increasing the necessity of action, it increases action; cold, on the other hand, lessens the necessity, and of course the action is diminished: to a due proportion of heat, therefore, the living principle owes its vigour; and, from observations and experiments, it appears to be a law of Nature in animal bodies, that the degree of external heat should bear a proportion to the quantity of life; when it is weakened, this proportion requires great accuracy in the adjustment, while greater powers of life allow a greater latitude*.

I was led to make these observations by attending to persons who are frost-bitten, the effect of cold in such cases being that of lessening the living principle. The powers of action remain as perfect as ever, but weakened, and heat is the only thing wanting to put these powers into action: yet that heat must at first be gradually applied, and proportioned to the quantity of the living principle, which increasing, the degree of heat may likewise be increased. If this method is not observed, and too great a degree of heat is at first applied, the person or part loses entirely the living principle, and mortification ensues. Such

* It is upon these principles that cold air is found of so much service to people who are reduced by disease, as the confluent smallpox and fevers, by diminishing heat in proportion to the diminution of life, or lessening the necessity of the body's producing its own cold.

a process invariably takes place with regard to men, and the same thing, I am convinced, happens to other animals. For if an eel is exposed to a degree of cold sufficiently intense to benumb it till the remains of life are scarcely perceptible, and still retained in a cold of about 40°, this small proportion of living principle will continue for a considerable time without diminution or increase; but if the animal is afterwards placed in a heat about 60°, after showing strong signs of returning life, it will die in a few minutes. Nor is this circumstance peculiar to the diminution of life by cold. The same phenomena take place in animals which have been very much reduced by hunger.

If a lizard or snake, when it goes to its autumnal hiding-place, is not sufficiently fat, the living powers are, before the season permits it to come out, very considerably weakened; perhaps so much as not to admit of the animal being again restored. If animals in a torpid state are exposed to the sun's rays, or placed in any situation which by its warmth would give vigour to those of the same kind possessed of a larger share of life, they will immediately show signs of increased life, but quickly sink under the experiment and die; while others, reduced to the same degree of weakness, as far as appearances can discover, will live for many weeks, if kept in a degree of cold proportioned to the quantity of life they possess.

I observed, many years ago, in some of the colder parts of this island, that when intense cold had forced blackbirds or thrushes to take shelter in outhouses, such of them as had been caught, and were, from an ill-judged compassion, exposed to a considerable degree of warmth, died very soon. The reason of this I did not then understand; but I am now satisfied that it was owing, as in other instances, to the degree of heat being increased too suddenly for the proportion of life remaining in the animal.

From these facts it appears that warmth causes a greater exertion of the living powers than cold; and that an animal in a weakly state may be obliged by it to exert a quantity of the action of life sufficient to destroy the very powers themselves*. The same effects probably take place even in perfect health; it appearing, from experiments made in a heated room, that a person in health, exposed to a great degree of heat, found the actions of life accelerated so much as to produce at last faintness and debility†.

If bedclothes are put over the drowned person, so as scarcely to touch him, steam of volatile alkali, or of warm balsams and essential

---

* It is upon this principle that parts mortify in consequence of inflammation.
† Vide Phil. Trans. for the year 1775, vol. lxv. p. 111.

oils, may be so conveyed as to come in contact with many parts of his body; and it will certainly prove advantageous if the same kind of steams can be conveyed into the stomach, as that seat of universal sympathy will be roused by such means. This may be done by a hollow bougie and a syringe; but the operation should be performed with all possible expedition, because the instrument, by continuing in the mouth, may produce sickness, an effect I should choose to avoid, unless it is intended to produce the action of vomiting. Some of the stimulating substances, which are of a warm nature and have an immediate effect, as spirits of hartshorn, peppermint-water, juice of horse-radish, and many others which produce a more lasting stimulus in a fluid state, and are found to quicken the pulse of a man in health, as balsams and turpentines, may be thrown into the stomach; but the quantity must be small, as they have a tendency to produce sickness: for it may be imagined that what would produce debility, or lessen action when in health, would in opposite circumstances prevent actions from taking place. The application of steams and other substances should also be thrown up by the anus; and the process recommended under the first head of treatment should still be continued while that recommended under the second is putting in practice, the last being only an auxiliary to the first. The first, in many cases, may succeed alone; but the second without the first must, I think, always fail where the powers of life are considerably weakened. Motion may possibly be of service, it may at least be tried; but, as it has less effect than any other of the usually prescribed stimuli, it should be the last applied*. I would recommend to the operator the same care in regulating the application of every one of these methods as I did before in that of heat, as each may have the same property of entirely destroying the feeble action which they have excited, if administered in too great a proportion. Instead, therefore, of increasing and hastening the operations on the first signs of returning life being observed, as is usually done, I should wish them to be applied more gently and gradually, that their increase afterwards may be directed, as nearly as possible, in a degree proportioned to the powers as they arise. As the heart is commonly the last part that ceases to act, it is probably the first part that takes on the action of recovery. When

---

* Electricity has been known to be of service, and should be tried when other methods have failed. It is probably the only method we have of immediately stimulating the heart; all other methods being more by sympathy. I have not mentioned injecting stimulating substances directly into the veins, though it might be supposed a proper expedient, because, in looking over my experiments on that subject, I found none where animal life received increase by that method.

it begins to move, I would advise lessening the application of air to the lungs, and enjoin those employed to observe with great attention when the muscles of respiration begin to act, that our endeavours may not interfere with their natural exertions, yet that we may be still ready to assist. I would by all means discourage bloodletting, which I think weakens the animal principle and life itself, consequently lessens both the powers and dispositions to action; and I would advise being careful not to call forth any disposition that might depress, by introducing things into the stomach which ordinarily create nausea; as that also will have a similar effect, except it can be carried so far as to excite the action of vomiting, by which the stomach could relieve itself. It will be prudent likewise to avoid administering by the anus anything that may be likely to produce an evacuation that way, every such evacuation tending to lessen the animal powers. I have purposely avoided speaking of the fumes of tobacco, which always produce sickness or purging, according as they are applied.

Whoever is appointed for the purpose of recovering drowned persons should have an assistant well acquainted with the methods intended to be made use of; that while the one is going on with the first and most simple methods, the other may be preparing what else may be proper, so that no time may be lost between the operations; and this is the more necessary, as the first means recommended will, in all cases, assist the second; and both together may often be attended with success, though each separately might have failed.

A proper apparatus is also essentially necessary to the institution : a description of which I here annex. First, a pair of bellows, so contrived, with two separate cavities, that by expanding them, when applied to the nostrils or mouth of a patient, one cavity may be filled with the common air, and the other with air sucked out from the lungs; and by shutting them again, the common air may be thrown into the lungs, and that which is sucked out of the lungs be discharged into the room. The pipe of these should be flexible, in length a foot or a foot and a half, and at least three eighths of an inch in width : as the artificial breathing may be continued by such means, while the other operations, except the application of the stimuli to the stomach, are going on; which cannot conveniently be done if the nozzle of the bellows be introduced into the nose. The end next the nose should be double, and applied to both nostrils. Secondly, a syringe, with a hollow bougie, or flexible catheter, of sufficient length to go into the stomach, and convey any stimulating matter into it, without affecting the lungs. Thirdly, a small pair of bellows, such as are commonly used in throwing fumes of tobacco up the anus, by which stimulating fluids or even fumes may be thrown in.

I shall conclude this account by proposing that all who are employed in this practice be particularly required to keep an accurate journal of the means used, and the degree of success attending them ; whence we may be furnished with facts sufficient to enable us to draw conclusions, on which a certain practice may hereafter be established.

AN ACCOUNT OF CERTAIN RECEPTACLES OF AIR IN
BIRDS, WHICH COMMUNICATE WITH THE LUNGS AND
EUSTACHIAN TUBE.

Since the account of these receptacles was read before the Royal
Society, in the year 1774, I have, by the dissection of a number of birds,
been able to make some additional observations relative to the extent of
the air-cells which communicate with the lungs in animals of this class.
These latter observations were not, however, made in consequence of
any regular design to investigate this subject further, as to have established the principle seemed all that was necessary; unless by general
observations we could hope to throw more light on the final intention
of this remarkable piece of mechanism.

Before the period I have mentioned, the communication subsisting in
birds, between the air-cells of the lungs and other cavities of the body,
had not been clearly explained, nor even much attended to by anatomists
or natural historians[a]. It is a singularity of structure peculiar to this

---

[a] [The continuation of the air-passages of the lungs into large membranous receptacles, situated in the abdominal cavity, was first discovered and described by Harvey
(On Generation, 8vo, 1653, p. 7; *Opera Omnia*, 4to, 1766, p. 185). The abdominal
air-cells of the ostrich are figured in Perault's Collection of Anatomical Memoirs of the
French Academicians. Borelli, in explaining the causes of the greater specific levity
of birds, observes, " Hoc patet, quia ossa avium fistulosa, valde excavata et subtilia sunt,
ad instar radicum pennarum scapulæ, costæ et brachia parum carnosa sunt; pectus et
abdomen amplas cavitates aëre plenas habent; pennæ tamen et plumæ levissimæ sunt."
(*De Motu Animalium*, 4to, 1685, p. 231, prop. 194.) Borelli appears, however, to
have believed both the quills of the feathers and the hollow bones to have contained
only a light marrow. The discovery that the bones of birds contained air was first
published in the year 1774,—in England in the Philosophical Transactions of that
year, which contained Mr. Hunter's 'Account,' &c. read before the Royal Society
February 27, 1774; and in Holland in the *Verhandeling van Bataafsche Genootschte*,
Rotterdam, 1774, in which Camper's discovery of the same structure was first published.
Camper transmitted, in the year 1773, an account of his researches on the air-bones of
birds to the French Academy, which was published in the *Mémoires de Mathématiques
et Physique*, 4to, in 1776. Whilst, therefore, we may be willing to admit that Camper's
Memoir was founded on an independent discovery, we must also conclude that the mass
of valuable observations on the air-receptacles of birds, communicated to the Royal Society some months before the first publication of Camper's discovery in the Dutch language,
was equally original. The French translator of Carus's Comparative Anatomy, in a
prefatory sketch of the History of the Science, introduces John Hunter to the reader's
notice as follows: " Le premier, il (Camper) a fait remarquer que les os longs du sque-

tribe of animals; and an account of it cannot, I imagine, be unacceptable to the public.

It is not my present intention to enter into minute descriptions of all the particular communications of this sort discoverable in birds by dissection, but only to mention such general facts as may serve to introduce the subject into natural history, and lead to an inquiry into the purposes which this structure was intended to answer. With this view I shall endeavour to give some idea of the construction of the lungs, and of the air-receptacles in birds, occasionally remarking the circumstances in which these principally differ from what is seen in other animals.

The mechanism of the lungs in birds, which renders them fit for conveying air to different parts of the body, consists principally in certain communications.

It has been asserted that birds have no diaphragm; but this opinion must have arisen either from a want of observation, or from too confined an idea of a diaphragm; for there is a moderately strong, but thin and transparent membrane, covering the lower surface of the lungs, and adhering to them, that affords insertion to several thin muscles which arise from the inner surfaces of the ribs. The use of this part seems to be that of lessening the concavity of the lungs towards the abdomen at the time of inspiration, and thereby assisting to dilate the air-cells, for which reason it is to be considered as answering one main purpose of a diaphragm. Besides this attachment of the lungs to the diaphragm, they are also connected to the ribs, and to the sides of the vertebræ[a].

Such adhesions are peculiar to this tribe of animals, and are of singular use, nay, in fact are absolutely necessary in lungs like those of birds, out of which it is intended the air should find a passage into other cavities. For if the lungs were loose in the cavity of the thorax, as is the case in many other animals, the cells of the lungs could not be expanded, either by the depression of the diaphragm, or the elevation of the ribs; since the air rushing in to fill up the vacuum produced in the cavity of the chest by these actions would take the straight road from the trachea through the passages, and of consequence would expand no part of the lungs which lay out of that line, whereby respiration would be totally prevented, and an effect produced exactly similar to what happens in other animals when the lungs are so much wounded as to allow a free exit to the air at that part[b].

---

lette des Oiseaux sont creusés de cavités dans lesquelles l'air a la facilité de s'introduire, parce qu'elles communiquent avec l'organe pulmonaire, découverte que Hunter eut l'impudeur de s'approprier quelques années après." (Jourdan's Carus, tom. i. p. xxxi.) Truly the ignorance of such an assertion can only be equalled by its impudence.]

[a] [See Harvey, On Generation, p. 6.]   [b] [Ibid., p. 7.]

The cells in the bodies of birds which receive air from the lungs are to be found both in the soft parts and in the bones, and have no communication with the cavity of the common cellular membrane. Some of these air-bags are placed in the larger cavities, as in the abdomen; and others are so lodged in the interstices of muscles, blood-vessels, and nerves, about the breast, axilla, &c., as at first to give the appearance of the common connecting membrane. Some communicate immediately with one another, and all may be said to have a communication by means of the lungs. They are of very different sizes, as may best suit the particular circumstances of the parts in which they are placed.

The bones which receive air are of two kinds; some, as the sternum, ribs, and vertebræ, having their internal substance divided into innumerable cells; whilst others, as the os humeri and os femoris, are hollowed out into one large canal, with sometimes a few bony columns running across at its extremities. Bones of this kind may be distinguished from those that do not receive air by several marks: first, by their less specific gravity; secondly, by being less vascular than the others, and therefore whiter; thirdly, by their containing little or no oil, and consequently being more easily cleaned, and when cleaned, appearing much whiter than common bones; fourthly, by having no marrow, or even any bloody pulpy substance in their cells; fifthly, by not being in general so hard and firm as other bones*; and sixthly, by the passage that allows the air to enter the bones, which can be easily perceived. In the recent bone we may readily discover holes or openings not filled with any soft substance, as blood-vessels or nerves; several of these holes are placed together, near that end of the bone which is next to the trunk of the bird, and are distinguishable by having their external edges rounded off, which is not the case with the holes through which either nerves or blood-vessels pass into the substance of the bone. When birds break any of the bones which contain air, the surrounding parts often become emphysematous.

There are openings in the lungs by which air is transmitted to the other parts; and the membrane or diaphragm above mentioned is perforated in several places with holes of a considerable size, which admit of a free communication between the cells of the lungs and the abdomen, a circumstance which has been frequently noticed. To each of these perforations is joined a distinct membranous bag, extremely thin and transparent, which bags being afterwards continued through the whole of the abdomen, and attached to the back and sides of that cavity, are

---

* The bones of some birds are so soft that they can be squeezed together with the finger and thumb; the bones of the extremities, however, have very solid sides.

kept firm in their proper situations, each receiving the air from their respective openings. There is no occasion to describe here all the bags, or their attachments, it being sufficient to have said that they extend over the whole abdomen.

The lungs at the anterior part, contiguous to the sternum, have openings into certain membranous cells which lie upon the sides of the pericardium, and communicate with the cells of the sternum. At the superior part the lungs have a communication with the large cells of a loose network, through which the trachea, œsophagus, and great vessels pass as they are going to and from the heart. When these cells are distended with air, the size of that part where they lie is very considerably increased, and this enlargement is in general a mark of either the passion of anger or love. It is plainly seen in the turkey-cock, the pouting-pigeon, &c., and is very visible in the breast of a goose when she cackles. These cells communicate with others in the axilla, under the large pectoral muscle, and in some birds are still further extended. In the pelican, for instance, the skin of the whole body, even to the tip of the wing, is united to the part underneath by means of these cells, which are equally formed; and when the skin is removed, the two separated surfaces appear as if honeycombed. When the cells are distended the skin is removed to a considerable distance, by which means the volume is proportionally increased[a]. In most birds, I believe in all that fly, these axillary cells communicate with the cavity of the os humeri, by means of small openings in the hollow surface near the head of that bone; in some they are continued down the wing, communicating with the ulna and radius; in others they reach even as far as the pinions. The ostrich, however, is an exception.

The posterior edge of the lungs (which lies on the sides of the spine, and projects backwards between the ribs,) communicates with the cells of the bodies of the vertebræ, with those of the ribs, the canal of the medulla spinalis, and the cells of the sacrum and other bones of the pelvis; from which parts the air finds a passage into the cavity of the thigh bone. This takes place in the greatest number of birds; but in some the air is even continued part of the way down the thighs. This account agrees with what we generally find, though some birds have

---

[a] [Whilst inflating the air-cells of a gigantic crane (*Ciconia Argala*), in which bird they are continued along the wing, beneath the skin, as in the pelican, the wings became extended as the air-cells were filled. This phenomenon suggested to me a secondary use of the air cells, which appears not to have been noticed, viz. to render mechanical assistance to the muscles of the wings, both by keeping the wing extended during the long hovering flight peculiar to this bird, and also by compressing and bracing the muscles, as is done by the fasciæ of the extremities in man.]

more, and some fewer of these communications; for, in the ostrich, no air gets into the os humeri, yet it enters into every other part, as before described, and in very large quantities. In the common fowl no air appears to enter any bone except the os humeri. The woodcock has no air-cells, either in the first bones of the wing or in the thigh-bones. On the other hand, in the pelican the air passes on to the ulna and radius, and into those bones which answer to the carpus and metacarpus of quadrupeds[a].

Thus the cells of the abdomen, those surrounding the pericardium, those situated at the lower and fore part of the neck and in the axilla, those in the cellular membrane under the pectoral muscles, as well as in that which unites the skin to the body, all communicate with the lungs, and are capable of being filled with air; and again, from them the cells of the sternum, ribs, vertebræ of the back and loins, bones of the pelvis, the humeri, the ulna and radius, with the pinions and thigh-bones, can in many birds be furnished with air.

It is not by the lungs alone that air is conveyed into the bones of birds, for the cells of the diploe between the two plates of the skull, in some birds, receive a considerable quantity of air by the Eustachian tube[*]. Of this the owl is a remarkable instance. The lower jaw of some kinds is likewise supplied with air, and often by the same canal[†].

---

[*] The only thing in other animals similar to this communication in birds, of the cells of bones with the external air, is that which takes place in the internal ear of quadrupeds, by means of the Eustachian tube[b].

[†] When I wrote this account to send it to the Royal Society, I did not then know by what means this was done; for in that I said, "but by what means I do not know"; that is, I did not know whether it was conveyed by the trachea, where it passes along the neck, or the Eustachian tube. Professor Camper, when he did me the honour to call upon me, was so obliging as to take some pains to show me, in the lower jaw of the hawk, the hole where the air entered, which makes me suspect he did not understand what I had written. For after having given the marks by which such openings were particularly distinguished, it will hardly be supposed I could say that I did not know the hole where the air entered[c].

---

[a] [In the hornbill the air is also extended into the phalanges of the toes, and in short into every bone in the skeleton; whilst in the penguin, on the other hand, the air-cells are confined, as in reptiles, to the thoracic abdominal cavity, and not a single bone of the skeleton is permeated by the atmospheric fluid. These birds present the two extremes of the condition of the respiratory apparatus described by Hunter in the present paper.]

[b] [Camper, besides citing the mastoid processes as an analogous structure in the mammalia, also adduces the extensive sinuses containing air in the cranium of the elephant. The air-cavities of the diploe of the cranial bones in the porcupine are also remarkable for their extent.]

[c] [In this note we have undesigned evidence that Hunter had never read the Memoir of Camper, or he would hardly have omitted to notice the error into which the Dutch anatomist falls with reference to the source whence the bones of the head derive

Some authors have considered the diploe in the cranium of a bird as a continuation of the mammillary process, and looked upon it as a circumstance peculiar to singing birds, which is not really true.

These facts, which had been formerly observed, led me in the year 1758 to make several experiments upon the breathing of birds, that might prove the free communication between the lungs and the before-mentioned parts.

First, I made an opening into the belly of a cock, and having introduced a silver cannula, tied up the trachea. I found that the animal breathed by this opening, and might have lived; but by an inflammation in the bowels coming on, adhesions were produced, and the communication was cut off.

I next cut the wing through the os humeri, in another fowl, and tying up the trachea, as in the cock, found that the air passed to and from the lungs by the canal in this bone. The same experiment was made with the os femoris of a young hawk, and was attended with a similar result. But the passage of air through the divided parts, in both these experiments, especially in the last, was attended with more difficulty than in the former one; it was indeed so great as to render it impossible for the animal to live longer than evidently to prove that it breathed through the cut bone.

I have made several preparations of these cells, by throwing into the trachea an injection, commonly called the corroding injection, which first filled the air-cells of the lungs, then all the others, such as the cells in the abdomen, anterior and superior part of the chest, axilla, os humeri, cells of the back-bone and thigh; and the whole being afterwards put into spirit of sea-salt, and corroded, the cast of injection came out entire.

The singularity of these communications in birds put me upon considering what might be their final intention. At first I supposed it might be intended to assist the act of flying, that being the circumstance which appears the most peculiar to birds; and it might be of service in that respect, I thought, by increasing the volume and strength with the same quantity of matter, without adding to the weight of the whole, which indeed would rather be diminished by the difference of specific gravity between the external and internal air. This opinion was strengthened

their internal supply of air. Camper states that it is received by the *meatus auditorii*, believing that birds had no Eustachian tubes: "l'air entre dans le diploë du crane entiér par les trous auditifs; car les oiseaux n'ont point de trompes d'Eustache comme les quadrupèdes et les amphibiés." (*Mém. de Mathém. et de Physique*, tom. vii. 1776, p. 334.)]

by discovering that the feathers of birds contained also a considerable quantity of air, in the very part which requires the greatest strength, and by the analogy which is observed between this mechanism in birds and what is discoverable in most kinds of fishes; for these last have air contained within their bodies, which I believe is commonly supposed to lessen their specific gravity, although this does not appear so necessary in fishes, which move in a much heavier element than birds*. But when I found that the ostrich (which is not intended to fly) was amply provided with these cells; and that the common fowl, and many others of that class, which are endowed with the faculty of flying, were less liberally supplied; when I saw that even the woodcock, which flies and is supposed to be a bird of passage, was inferior in this respect to the

---

* When we consider that the elevating and suspending apparatus is much smaller in fishes than in birds, we may reasonably conceive the air in them was intended as a kind of equilibrium between the fish and water; and that progressive motion was the only thing wanted in the actions of fishes. Were we to reason upon general principles alone, we should suppose that those fishes who have the largest air-bags should have their muscles of a greater specific gravity, and those fishes that have none should have the lightest flesh; therefore that the flesh of the salmon and cod, which have an air-bag, should be heavier than that of the shark, which has none. But to know how far this, which appeared to be reasonable, was a fact, I made the following experiments:

Experiment I. I took a portion of muscle of the shark, cod, and salmon, of the same weight in air; and first examined how far they occupied the same space, by immersing them in water, and observing the rise or fall of the water upon each of them being separately immersed in it.

The shark occupied the smallest space, the salmon a little more, and the cod the largest.

Experiment II. I then suspended the same three portions, upon a level, in a glass vessel filled with water about two feet high, and let them all go at the same instant, to see which would fall through the water in the shortest space of time. The shark got to the bottom first, the salmon next, and the cod last.

It is necessary to observe that, in both these experiments, the difference in bulk and in the times of their falling was very little, but, however, sufficient to ascertain the fact for which the experiments were instituted.

To see how far the muscular flesh of birds was specifically lighter than that of a quadruped, I repeated the above experiments upon a portion of a hind, of a pigeon, and of a sheep; but could discover no visible difference in their weight.

It may be observed there are in common two situations of oil in fishes: in one it is diffused through the fish, as if the body had been steeped in it, as in the salmon, herring, &c. In the other it is found in the liver, as in all of the ray kind, cod, &c., and in general those that have it in one part have none in the other; however, there are some, although I believe but few, who have their oil in form of what may be called fat, viz. in flakes in the interstice of parts, as the sturgeon. The liver, in those of the ray kind, is large, and extended through the belly; therefore it might be supposed to lighten the body, from oil being lighter than water or the flesh; but we have oil in the liver of the cod, and in the salmon and herring the oil is diffused through the whole; therefore I am afraid we are not yet acquainted with the full effect of the air-bladder in fishes.

ostrich, and that the bat differed not in structure from animals that do not fly[a]; I was compelled, by so many contradictions to theory, to suppose that this singular mechanism might be intended for some other purpose.

The next conjecture that offered was that these cells were to be considered as an appendage to the lungs; and to this I was led by the analogy observable between birds and amphibious animals. For although both in the bird and amphibious tribe, as the snake, viper, and many others, the lungs are continued down through the whole belly, in form of two bags[b], and therefore appear to be larger than the lungs in any other animal, yet in all of them the quantity of surface exposed to the air is much less than in the quadruped; for the cells of the lungs in the bird are larger, and in the snake, &c. the upper part only can perform the office of respiration with any degree of effect, the lower having comparatively but few air-vessels. The air must pass through this upper part before it gets to the lower in inspiration, and must also repass in expiration, so that the respiratory surface has more air applied to it than what the lungs of themselves could contain. It is not however to be supposed that the air can be made to pass to and fro in bones as in parts which admit of contraction and dilatation; the purpose answered by these bony cells must therefore be different, and perhaps they should be considered as reservoirs of air*. There is in fact a great

---

* It is not to be supposed that the air in the cells in birds will be changed while flying; only accumulated and retained; not in the least influenced by either inspiration or expiration. It might be asked, Where is the stricture upon the air when flying, so as

---

[a] [This is not absolutely true; for it is a remarkable fact,—and one which gives additional probability to the hypothesis of Borelli as to the final intention of the air-cells of birds in diminishing the specific gravity for the facilitation of flight,—that in one genus of bats (*Nycteris* of modern naturalists) remarkable for their lofty and continued flight, air-cells are continued beneath the integument, which are inflated from the cheek-pouches. "The skin adheres to the body," says Bell, in his excellent article *Cheiroptera* (Cyclop. of Anatomy, p. 599.), "only at certain points, where it is connected by means of a loose cellular membrane: it is therefore susceptible of being raised from the surface, on the back as well as on the under parts. These large spaces are filled with air at the will of the animal, by means of large cheek-pouches, which are pierced at the bottom, and thus communicate with the subcutaneous spaces just mentioned. When the animal, therefore, wishes to inflate its skin, it inspires, closes the nostrils, and then, contracting the cavity of the chest, the air is forced through the openings in the cheek-pouches under the skin, whence it is prevented from returning by means of a true sphincter, with which those openings are furnished, and by large valves on the neck and back. By this curious mechanism the bat has the power of so completely blowing up the spaces under the skin as to give the idea of a little balloon, furnished with wings, a head, and feet."]

[b] [In most snakes the abdominal air-bag is single, but a rudiment of the second lung exists.]

similarity between birds and that class of animals called amphibia;
and although a bird and a snake are not the same in the construction
of the respiratory organs, yet the circumstance of the air passing in
both beyond the lungs, into the cavity of the abdomen, naturally leads
us to suppose that a structure so similar is designed in each to answer
a similar purpose. This analogy is still further supported by the lungs
in both consisting of large cells[n]. Now in amphibious animals the use
of such a conformation of the lungs is evident, as it is in consequence
of this structure that they require to breathe less frequently than others;
and in this respect it may in birds have some connexion with flying,
as that motion might easily be imagined to render frequency of respiration inconvenient, and a reservoir of air would therefore become sin-
gularly useful. Although we are not to consider this structure in birds
to be an extension of lungs, yet I can easily conceive this accumulation
of air to be of great use in respiration. For it was observed before respecting the amphibia, that the air in its passage to and from these cells
must certainly have a considerable effect upon the blood in the lungs,
by allowing a much greater quantity of air to pass in a given time than
if there was no such construction of parts*; and this opinion will not
appear to be ill founded, if we consider that both in the bird and the
viper the surface of the lungs is small in comparison to what it is in

to keep the parts distended? Is it upon the outlets from the lungs, or is it at the glottis,
as in the quadruped? For we may observe that when an animal is using considerable
exercise, it never either expands the lungs, nor makes a full expiration, giving the ribs
and diaphragm as little extent of motion as possible, so that the body may be kept firm,
which obliges it to breathe oftener; and as this quantity of air is not sufficient for the
accelerated motion of the blood, the animal gets what is called out of breath, which is
no more than the two not being proportioned; and when it rests, it breathes as quick
and takes as long strokes as possible, to make up the loss. So that in exercise we probably breathe less air.

* It may, perhaps, occur to some, that the whole of these communicating cells are
to be considered as extended lungs; but I can hardly think that any air which gets
beyond the vesiculated lungs themselves is capable of affecting the blood of the animal,
as the other cavities into which it enters, whether of the soft parts or of the bones,
appear to be very little vascular.

---

* [The air-cells are smaller, and much more numerous in the lungs of birds than in
the corresponding anterior or true respiratory portion of the lungs of reptiles. The
analogy which Hunter here mentions, as also that between the abdominal air-receptacles of birds and the air-bladders of fishes, to which he previously alludes, had not
escaped the observation of Hervey, who says, "Quin etiam (quod tamen a nemine
hactenus observatum memini) avium bronchia, sive asperæ arteriæ fines, in abdomen
perforantur, aeremque inspiratum intra cavitates illarum membranarum recondunt.
Quemadmodum pisces, et serpentes intra amplas vesicas in abdomine positas eundem
attrahunt et reservant; eoque facilius natare existimantur."—De Generatione Animalium, Ex. III.]

many other animals which have not this extension of cavity. It is also
a corroborating circumstance, that in the fowl the air might have passed
by a much readier way than through the lungs into all the cells about
the breast, neck, axilla, wings, &c., as these could have been filled from
the lower end of the trachea, upon which many of them lie. But the
air must now take a roundabout passage both in its way in and its way
out, those openings being upon the exterior surface of the lungs. We
must not, however, give up the idea of such structure being of use in
flying; for I believe we may set it down as a general rule, that in the
birds of longest and highest flight, as eagles, this diffusion of air is extended further than in the others. This opinion is strengthened by
comparing the structure above described with the respiratory organs in
the flying insects, which are composed of cells diffused through the
whole body; these are extended even into the head and down the extremities; while there is no such appearance in the insects that do not
fly, as the spider : but why the pelican should be so amply provided I
cannot say, not knowing the natural history of that bird sufficiently to
be able to judge of this point. Do they carry weights in the large fauces
so great as to require such an increase of substance without increase of
weight?

How far this construction of the respiratory organs may assist birds
in singing deserves investigation, as the vast continuance of song, between the breathings, in a canary-bird would appear to arise from it.
This is a subject, however, which I shall not at present enter upon[a].

---

[a] [The objection offered by Hunter in the preceding note to the use of the air-cells
as accessory organs of respiration, is weakened, if not removed, by the anatomical fact
that the bronchiæ open into them by such direct and wide apertures as to render it most
probable that much of the air passes at once into the air-receptacles without having
previously been decomposed in the vesicles of the lungs. It may be concluded, therefore, that the respiratory function is heightened, in harmony with the increased energies
of the circulating and locomotive powers in birds, by means of the extensive system of
continuous air-receptacles above described, which operate both by effecting a change
in the blood of the pulmonary circulation in the return of the air of the cells through
the bronchial tubes, and also by the change which the blood undergoes in the capillaries of the systemic circulation, which are in contact with the air-receptacles.

A second use of the air-receptacles in reference to the respiratory function arises out
of the mechanical aid which they afford in the action of breathing. During inspiration
the sternum of the bird is depressed or recedes from the spine, the angle between the
vertebral and sternal ribs is made less acute, and the thoracic cavity proportionally enlarged; the air then rushes into the lungs and into the thoracic air-receptacles, while
those of the abdomen become flaccid: when the sternum is raised, or approximated towards the spine, part of the air is expelled from the lungs and thoracic cells by the trachea, and part driven into the thoracic receptacles, which are thus alternately enlarged
and diminished with those of the thorax. Hence the lungs, notwithstanding their fixed
condition, are subject to due compression through the medium of the contiguous air-

receptacles, and are affected equally and regularly by every motion of the sternum and ribs.

A third use, and one which Hunter inclines to admit, is that of rendering the whole body specifically lighter, in relation to the peculiar actions of flight. A diminution of specific gravity must necessarily follow the desiccation of the marrow and other fluids in those spaces which are occupied with the air-cells, and by the rarefaction of the contained air by the heat of the body. In harmony with this view are the facts, not only that the quantity of air admitted into the system is in proportion to the general powers of flight, but also that in birds where the skeleton is only partially permeated by air, this is especially distributed to those members which are most employed in locomotion: thus, it is admitted into the wing-bones of the owl, but not into the femur; while in the ostrich the air penetrates to the femur, but not the humerus or other bones of the wing.

I have already alluded to the secondary use which the air-cells may afford to some large and long-winged birds, which, like the Argala, or the Frigate Bird, hover with a sailing motion for a long-continued period in the upper regions of the air, by diminishing the necessity for muscular exertion by the tendency of the distended air-cells to maintain the wings outstretched. Of the same adventitious character is the use finally suggested by Hunter to the air-receptacles, of contributing to sustain the song of birds, and to impart to it tone and strength. It is no just objection to this function that the air-cells exist in birds which are not endowed with the mechanism and power of song, since it is not pretended that this is the primary or exclusive office of the air-cells. The latest writer on the pneumaticity of birds, M. Jacquemin, has indeed reproduced this suggestion of Hunter's as a novel idea.]

A DESCRIPTION OF THE NERVES WHICH SUPPLY THE ORGAN OF SMELLING.

THE nerves being in themselves perhaps the most difficult parts of an animal body to dissect, becomes a reason why we are still unacquainted with many of their minuter ramifications; yet if a knowledge of these, together with that of their origin, union, and reunion, is at all connected with their physiology, the more accurately they are investigated the more perfectly will the functions of the nerves be understood.

I have no doubt, if their physiology was sufficiently known, that we should find the distribution and complication of nerves so immediately connected with their particular uses, as readily to explain many of those peculiarities for which it is now so difficult to account. What naturally leads to this opinion is, the origins and number of nerves being constantly the same, and particular nerves being invariably destined for particular parts, of which the fourth and sixth pair of nerves are remarkable instances. We may therefore reasonably conclude, that to every part is allotted its particular branch, and that however complicated the distribution may be, the complication is always regular.

There are some nerves which have a peculiarity in their course, as the recurrent and chorda tympani; and others which are appropriated to particular sensations, as those which go to four of the organs of sense, seeing, hearing, smelling, and tasting; and some parts of the body having peculiar sensations (as the stomach and penis), we may, without impropriety, include the fifth, or sense of feeling. This general uniformity in course, connexion, and distribution, will lead us to suppose that there may be some other purpose to be answered than mere mechanical convenience; and many of the variations which have been described in the dissections of nerves, I believe to have arisen from the blunders of the anatomist, rather than from any irregularity in their number, mode of ramifying, course, distribution, or connexion* with each other.

We observe no such uniformity in vessels carrying fluids, but find particular purposes answered by varying their origin and distribution: the pulmonary artery answers a very different purpose in the circulation of

* Here it is to be understood I do not mean lateral connexion, such as two branches uniting into one chord and then dividing; or a branch going to a part, either single or double, for still it is the same nerve; or whether a branch unites with another a little

the blood from that of the aorta; yet both arise from the same source, the heart. The course of the arteries is such as will convey the blood most conveniently, and therefore not necessarily uniform, it not being very material by what channel, provided the blood is conveyed to the part; though in particular instances certain purposes may be answered by a peculiarity in origin and distribution, as happens in the testicle of quadrupeds. This observation respecting arteries is likewise applicable to veins, and still more to the absorbent vessels; in which last, regularity is even less essential than in the veins.

Whoever, therefore, discovers a new artery, vein, or lymphatic, adds little to the stock of physiological knowledge; but he who discovers a new nerve, or furnishes a more accurate description of the distribution of those already known, affords us information in those points which are most likely to lead to an accurate knowledge of the nervous system; for if we consider how various are the origins of the nerves, although all arise from the brain, and how different the circumstances attending them, we must suppose a variety of uses to arise out of every peculiarity of structure[b].

Indeed, if we reflect on the actions arising immediately from the will and affections of the mind, we must see that the origin, connexion, and distribution of the nerves ought to be exact, as there are parts whose

sooner or a little later, for still it is the same branch. Such effects may arise more from a variety in the shape of the bodies they belong to, than any variety in the nerves themselves[a].

---

[a] [See the observations of Swan on the exceptions which occur in the uniformity of the anatomical conditions of the nervous system, in his excellent 'Demonstration of the Nerves of the Human Body,' pp. 29, 30, 31.]

[b] [With reference to anatomical researches on the nervous system, Sir Charles Bell has observed: "Whilst the nerves are supposed to proceed from one great centre, to have the same structure and functions, and to be all sensible, and all of them to carry what has been vaguely called nervous power, these discoveries of new nerves and ganglia are worse than useless; they increase the difficulty, and repel inquiry."—*Exposition of the Natural System of the Nerves of the Human Body*, 1824, p. 70.

The different views entertained by Hunter on this subject doubtless arose from his belief that a variety of uses arose out of the various origins and other peculiarities of structure of the nerves. Hence he was led to trace the different nerves which are distributed to a single organ to their different origins, and to infer that the organ thereby received different sensitive endowments. It is this principle, in a more extended application from the nerves to their component filaments, so far as they have different origins, which forms the basis of the present improved doctrine of the nervous system. "The key to the natural system of the nerves," says Bell, "will be found in the simple proposition, that each filament or track of nervous matter has its peculiar endowment, independently of the others which are bound up along with it, and that it continues to have the same endowment throughout its whole length."—*Ibid.*]

actions immediately depend upon such circumstances. The brain may be considered as having an intelligence with the body; but no such intercourse subsists between the different parts of the body and the heart.

In the summer of 1754, being much employed in dissecting the nerves passing out of the skull, I was, of course, led to trace many of their connexions with those from the medulla spinalis; and was assisted by Dr. Smith, then pursuing his studies in London*. The better to trace these nerves through the foramina of the skull, I steeped the head in a weakened acid of sea-salt till the bones were rendered soft, and that the parts might be as firm as possible, and at the same time free from any tendency to putrefaction (it being summer), the acid was not diluted with water, but with spirit. When the bones were rendered soft, pursuing my intention, I dissected the first pair of nerves, and discovered their distribution; and having made a preparation of the parts in which they were found, I immediately had drawings made from them, with a view to have presented the account to the Royal Society; but other pursuits prevented it†. Engravings were afterwards made from these drawings, and the preparation was repeatedly shown by Dr. Hunter, in his courses of anatomy, who, at the same time, pointed out that alteration in the mode of reasoning upon those nerves which would naturally arise from this discovery. In this dissection I found several nerves, principally from the fifth pair, going to and lost upon the membrane of the nose; but suppose that those have nothing to do with the sense of smelling, it being more than probable that what may be called organs of sense have particular nerves, whose mode of action is different from that of nerves producing common sensation, and also different from one

* Dr. Smith was afterwards teacher in chemistry and anatomy in the university of Oxford; is now Savilian professor of geometry, and lecturer in physiology. This account of the first pair of nerves, as also of the branches of the fifth, is taken from the original description written by him, and taken from my dissection when I was tracing them.

† Dr. Scarpa, professor of anatomy at Pavia, while in London in 1782, acquainted me that he had dissected the ramifications of the olfactory nerves, and that on his return to Italy he meant to publish an account of them. At this time I showed him my drawings and engravings. I have lately been informed that he has published his account, but have not met with it: I have, however, seen one of his engravings, which was executed in London, and is very elegant. It only shows those on the septum narium, whose minuteness is rather carried further than the power of dissection, and the ramifications are more regular than we find them in Nature[a].

[a] [See Scarpa, *Anatomicæ Disquisitiones de Auditu et Olfactu*, fol. 1789, and *Anatomicarum Annotationum, Liber secundus De Organo olfactus præcipuo, deque Nervis nasalibus interioribus e Pari quinto Nervorum cerebri*, 4to, 1792.]

another, and that the nerves on which the peculiar functions of each of the organs of sense depend, are not supplied from different parts of the brain. The organ of sight has its peculiar nerve; so has that of hearing; and probably that of smelling likewise; and, on the same principle, we may suppose the organ of taste to have a peculiar nerve. Although these organs of sense may likewise have nerves from different parts of the brain, yet it is most probable such nerves are only for the common sensations of the part, and other purposes answered by nerves. Thus we find nerves from different origins going to the parts composing the organ of sight, which are not at all concerned in the immediate act of vision; it is also probable, although not so demonstrable, that the parts composing the ear have nerves belonging to them simply as a part of the body, and not as the organ of a particular sense: and if we carry this analogy to the nose, we shall find a nerve, which we may call the peculiar nerve of that sense; and the other nerves of this part, derived from other origins, only conveying common sensation, and we may suppose only intended for the common actions of the part. This mode of reasoning is equally applicable to the organ of taste; and if the opinion of peculiar nerves going to particular organs of sense be well founded, then the reason is evident why the nose, as a part of our body, should have nerves in common with other parts, besides its peculiar nerves; and, as the membrane of the nose is of considerable extent, and has a great deal of common sensation, we may suppose the nerves sent to this part for that purpose will not be few in number. It is upon this principle the fifth pair of nerves may be supposed to supply the eye and nose in common with other parts[a]; and upon the same principle, it is more than probable, that every nerve so affected as to communicate

---

[a] [Since the period when Hunter wrote this remarkable paper, in which the principle of different nerves having particular functions in relation to differences of origin and other anatomical conditions is so distinctly enunciated, the attention of physiologists has been more especially called to the fact of the organs of sense being supplied by nerves from different sources, for the purpose of different endowments, by the experiments of Majendie. He divided the fifth pair of nerves within the cranium, and thus contributed to define more exactly than had before been done the importance of common sensation to the safety of some of the organs of sense, as the eye, and also the share which touch bears in the impressions received by the organs of special sense, as in that of smell.

Physiological science does not perhaps afford a more striking example of the inferiority of mere experimental inquiry to that which is based on extensive anatomical induction, than the singular conclusions at which Majendie arrived after performing the experiment above alluded to. There are few physiologists, however, who do not adopt the conclusions of Hunter, that the organs of sense receive their endowments of ordinary sensation from the fifth pair, which is common to each, in preference to the well-known view originally adopted by Majendie. (See *Journal de Physiologie Expér.*, vol. iv. p. 169. "Le nerf olfactif est-il l'organe de l'odorat?")]

sensation, in whatever part of the nerve the impression is made, always gives the same sensation as if affected at the common seat of the sensation of that particular nerve*.

The first pair of nerves arriving at the part of its destination as soon as it escapes from the skull, and immediately ramifying, has rendered its distribution more obscure than that of the others, whose course to the part to which they are allotted is visible and to be traced. As the body of the nerve, while within the skull, is pulpy and composed of the brain itself, it easily breaks off at the very division and exit of the small branches; it therefore becomes impossible to trace them, as we usually do other nerves; and they have by most physiologists been considered as never forming chords, but going on in their pulpy form to be distributed on the membrane of the nose, in a mode somewhat similar to that of the optic nerve, and to what is commonly supposed to take place with respect to the portio mollis of the seventh pair. Winslow has suggested an idea that the first pair forms chords ; but it is only as an assertion, and not having described them, that alone was not sufficient to alter the former mode of reasoning.

Haller, who is to be considered as the latest anatomist and physiologist, who has published on the subject, on whom we can depend, says, that " The first pair of nerves makes its way into the nose covered by the pia mater only, very little altered from what it was when within the cavity of the skull*." This shows that Haller retained the old idea concerning these nerves ; but we shall find that they become firm chords immediately upon piercing the dura mater and cribriform plate of the ethmoid bone.

The first pair, while within the skull, differs in some respects from all other nerves : firstly, it seems to be made up of a cortical and medullary substance, while the others appear to consist of medullary alone ; and secondly, it is different, in that it does not seem to be composed of fasciculi, and has but one covering from the pia mater investing the whole nerve, whereas other nerves appear to have a covering round each

---

* I knew a gentleman who had the nerves which go to the glans penis completely destroyed by mortification, almost as high as the union of the penis with the pubes; and at the edge of the old skin, at the root of the penis, where the nerves terminated, was the peculiar sensation of the glans penis ; and the sensation of the glans itself was now only common sensation ; therefore the glans has, probably, different nerves, and those for common sensation may come through the body of the penis to the glans.

A serjeant of marines, who had lost the glans and the greater part of the body of the penis, upon being asked if he ever felt those sensations which are peculiar to the glans, declared, that upon rubbing the end of the stump, it gave him exactly the sensation which friction upon the glans produced, and was followed by an emission of the semen.

† Elementa Physiologiæ, vol. v. p. 151.

fasciculus; and this is probably the reason why the first pair is weaker while within the skull than the others. Its form is somewhat triangular, having three edges, from lying in a groove made by two convolutions of the brain. The course is forwards, a little upwards and inwards, and where it lies upon the cribriform plate of the ethmoid bone becomes somewhat larger, and divides into a great many branches, like so many roots, answering to the number of holes in that plate, except one left for a branch of the fifth pair; but these divisions we cannot see, they being covered by the body of the nerve, which cannot be raised without breaking off the small branches at their origin. As the branches of the nerve pass through this bone, they seem to take processes from the dura mater along with them, then becoming firm chords, similar to other nerves. These branches, after they have got through the bone, form themselves into two planes or divisions, one passing on the septum, the other on the turbinated bones. Those of the septum narium, in their passage to the nose, are first continued a little way down, in bony canals of the perpendicular lamella of the ethmoid bone, which holes become small grooves in that bone; and those on the opposite side, being more numerous and smaller, pass down through small holes that are on the inside plate of the ethmoid bone, which holes are likewise continued into grooves, for a little way, upon that plate. When the branches get upon the membrane of the nose, they subdivide into a great many smaller ones, which are somewhat flattened, and are only to be seen on that side of the membrane that adheres to the bones, not being visible at all on the other; so that the dissection of these nerves is no more than separating the membrane and bone from each other. They can hardly be dissected all round; and the further they are traced upon the membrane the fainter they become, and growing smaller they sink deeper and deeper into the membrane to get on its outer surface, where we must suppose they terminate. Those upon the septum pass down a little radiated, and the branches, especially at the upper part, or at their first setting out, unite with one another. Those on the side next the antrum, when they have reached the membrane of the nose, in their course to the superior turbinated bone, form a very considerable network or plexus; and when they reach that bone, do not all go round its convex curvated pendulous edge to the concave side, but some passing through its substance get immediately upon it, which is the reason why we find so many holes in that bone. It is difficult to trace them further; but we have reason to suppose that they go through the inferior turbinated bone in the same manner, since we find similar holes.

A DESCRIPTION OF SOME BRANCHES OF THE FIFTH PAIR OF NERVES.

In tracing the course of the olfactory nerves, I also discovered several branches of the fifth pair not commonly known, particularly two that were supposed to go to the membrane of the nose for the sense of smelling, but which only pass through that organ to their place of destination. The first is a small nerve from the first branch of the fifth pair; or, according to Winslow, the nervus ophthalmicuṣ Willisii, which small nerve is called by Winslow the nasal. This branch, after having passed out of the skull into the orbit, re-enters the cranium through the foramen orbitarium anterius, and gets on the cribriform plate of the ethmoid bone; from thence it passes down through one of the anterior holes of the cribriform plate, and after having continued its course in a groove on the nasal process of the frontal bone, runs forward and downward in a similar groove on the inside of the os nasi; from thence getting on the outside of the cavity of the nose, it runs along the cartilaginous part of the ala, and near the extremity of the nose mounts up upon the tip of the ala, and then dipping down between the two alæ, is lost on the anterior extremity of the cartilaginous septum. In its course it sends several small filaments into the alæ.

The second is a branch of the superior maxillary nerve; for that nerve, having passed through the foramen rotundum, divides and sends off several branches, one of which passing backwards and inwards, through the foramen commune, between the orbitar process of the palate, and the root of the ala of the sphenoid bone, gives a branch which gets into a fissure that seems to separate the root of the ala from the body of the sphenoid bone, where that bone makes the roof of the nose. This branch then passes along the under surface of the body of the sphenoid bone, in its way to the septum narium, and getting upon that part, passes along between its membranes and the bone: its course is downwards, and forwards towards the foramen incisivum, through which it passes and is lost in the gum behind the first dentes incisores, and on the membrane of the roof of the mouth at that part.

There is another branch of the superior maxillary nerve, which comes off from a large branch that is going down to the mouth, uvula, &c., and this branch, with its division into two, has been described by Professor Meckel, of Berlin; but after tracing one of these into the portio dura, he pursued the search no further. This branch of the superior maxillary nerve passes back through the foramen pterygoideum, accompanies the carotid artery as it passes across the posterior edge of the foramen, and there divides into two branches; one of which passes down along with the carotid artery, through the basis of the skull, and proceeding in a direction contrary to the course of the artery, in contact with that branch of the cervical ganglion that passes up with the carotid artery to join the sixth pair, then joins the first cervical ganglion. The other branch decussates that artery on its upper surface, and getting upon the anterior side of the petrous portion of the temporal bone, enters a small hole near the bottom of that large one which affords a passage to the seventh pair of nerves, joining the portio dura just where that nerve, making its first turn, passes along with it through what is called the aqueduct. This nerve, composed of portio dura, and the branch of the fifth pair, sends off, in the adult, the chorda tympani before its exit from the skull; and in the fœtus immediately after. The termination of the branch, called chorda tympani, I shall not describe; yet I am almost certain it is not a branch of the seventh pair of nerves, but the last-described branch from the fifth pair; for I think I have been able to separate this branch from the portio dura, and have found it lead to the chorda tympani; perhaps it is continued into it; but this is a point very difficult to determine, as the portio dura is a compact nerve, and not so fasciculated as some others are. However this may be, it is very reasonable to suppose that the chorda tympani is a branch of the fifth pair, as it goes to join another branch arising from the same trunk[a].

---

[a] [This is a point which it is undoubtedly very difficult to decide by dissection of the parts in the human body. Cloquet, Hirzel, and Majendie describe the chorda tympani according to the supposition of Hunter. In the horse and calf, however, where the portio dura is less dense in its structure, the Vidian branch of the fifth may be distinctly seen crossing that nerve after penetrating its sheath, and separating into many filaments, with which filaments of the seventh nerve are blended, and a ganglion formed by the superaddition of gray matter; the chorda tympani is here continued partly from this ganglion, partly from the seventh or portio dura.]

CROONIAN LECTURE ON MUSCULAR MOTION, No. I.

For the year 1776.

[Read before the Royal Society, by Mr. John Hunter, F.R.S.[a]]

A SELF-MOVING power is such a phenomenon as must call up the attention of the thinking mind (while ignorant of the cause); and when that very mind is connected with this power it becomes still more interested.

This power of motion was first discovered to be inherent in parts of an animal body of a certain construction, called muscles[b]. This construction appeared to be a composition of fibres, which were called muscular; and motion was supposed to be produced by these contracting in length, and all the varieties of motion in an animal the most complicated, to be the result of the manner in which these fibres were disposed.

It is no wonder, then, that the mode in which a muscular fibre produces motion has been esteemed an inquiry not unworthy the attention of the greatest philosophers, and has almost universally been one of the principal researches of the physiologist; especially when we consider that the substance, called muscular, alone constitutes the largest part of most animals; and indeed many are wholly composed of it.

The inquiries into the nature of self-motion have been principally

---

[a] [In Home's Account of the Life of John Hunter, prefixed to the treatise 'On the Blood, Inflammation, and Gun-shot Wounds,' 1794, p. xxviii. is the following passage:

"Besides the papers which he presented to that learned body (the Royal Society), he (Mr. Hunter) read six Croonian Lectures upon the subject of muscular action, for the years 1776, 1777, 1779, 1780, 1781, 1782. In these Lectures he collected all his observations upon Muscles respecting their powers and effects, and the stimuli by which they are affected; and to these he added comparative observations upon the moving powers of Plants. These Lectures were not published in the Philosophical Transactions; for they were withdrawn as soon as read, not being considered by the author as complete dissertations, but rather as materials for some future publication."]

[b] [Both Aristotle and Hippocrates were ignorant of the function of the muscular fibre: the important discovery that the animal motions were performed by the muscles is attributed to Lycus of Macedon, who wrote a voluminous work on Myology. It is certain that the use of the muscles was known to Herophilus, since he is quoted by Galen as having spoken of the happy disposition of the muscles for the movement of the limbs. To Herophilus belongs the honour of having first discovered in the nerves the organs of sensation and of voluntary motion.]

confined to animals; most probably from the power in them being more conspicuous, which almost prevented its being taken notice of in any other substance whatever. Inquiries into nature have, however, become less confined, and experiments and observations have induced men to leave the beaten track of others, and take their observations from nature herself; by which means a self-moving power has been observed and universally allowed in vegetables. And this principle, upon investigation, appears now to be as much a property in vegetables as in animals; and in such cases where the functions and uses are the same in both, it is perhaps as considerable in vegetables as animals. But where they are dissimilar in their actions, and the uses arising out of these actions are also different, it is reasonable to suppose the quantity of action will vary; and such difference must frequently occur in both animals and vegetables. In animals a considerable part of this motion is called muscular; in vegetables it has not yet got a name.

The immediate cause of motion in all vegetables is most probably the same, and it is probably the same in all animals; but how far they are the same in both classes has not yet been determined. But I think it will appear, in the investigation of this subject, that vegetables and animals have actions evidently common to both, and that the causes of these actions are apparently the same in both; and most probably there is not an action in the vegetable which does not correspond or belong to the animal, although the mode of action in the parts may not be the same, or muscular, in both,

There appear, however, to be actions in animals which are peculiar to them; these make them more complicated, and in them another stimulus to action is superadded, evidently for that purpose[a].

All actions may be considered of two kinds,—immediate and secondary.

The first is an action of the part itself, having no relation to anything else; as action in a muscle, or elasticity in a spring.

---

[a] [The actions here alluded to are the voluntary, which are consequent upon an act of sensation, and are the result of a determination or stimulus derived from the brain. The action in the muscle produced by this stimulus is, however, essentially the same as is produced by mechanical or chemical stimuli applied to the muscle out of the body, or as takes place in the muscle involuntarily as in sleep, or when an animal is stimulated while in a state of hybernation, or immediately after decapitation.

Instead therefore of saying that animals have *actions* of the moving powers peculiar to themselves, it is more correct to express, with reference to the voluntary actions, that they have parts superadded, for the purpose of exciting the actions of the moving powers, which the vegetable has not, viz. the nerves. It is true that the actions of the moving powers of an animal, whether automatic or voluntary, are different from those which produce the motions of parts in vegetables, as explained in the notes pp. 200, 206; but the observations in the text refer only to the voluntary actions.]

The second may be divided into two kinds,—first, where this action has an effect upon some other part, or moves it, which is the ultimate effect, as the heart moving the blood by contracting,—secondly, where the action is applied to some other body adapted for a particular motion, which is to produce the ultimate effect, such as the muscles of a joint.

We may in general observe, from what we know of motion or action in matter, that it is always preceded by something which we call the cause; and that the immediate cause is an irresistible impulse to action, which action becomes the effect. A body endowed with the power of self-motion is under the same influence of impulse as matter in general: it cannot move without an immediate cause for its motion.

Self-motion may be of three kinds in the more perfect animals. The first is where the motion is excited by a cause from within the animal itself, and is employed in the œconomical operations and functions of the machine, and with the materials the machine is already in possession of, which are only made use of in the growth of parts, secretion of fluids, &c. The second is where motion is excited from an internal cause, and is employed in particular functions and operations, but where such materials used are out of the body; as in those excited in consequence of hunger and thirst, the passion between the sexes, &c. The third is where motion is excited by external stimuli, and where whole parts are put in motion: as where the sight or voice of a person excites one to approach him; the application of a medicine which excites vomiting, &c. We can have no other idea of these motions in animals but that they are muscular: and as the two first of these actions exist in vegetables, it is natural to suppose that there is a similarity in the cause which produces the same final intention, although the same mode of action or a similar power is not made use of to produce it.

These immediate causes of action in an animal are called stimuli, and the capability in parts for action is termed irritability; but such a definition is too confined for the numerous actions excited in an animal body.

The word stimulus is pretty well determined in its signification; it is an incitement to an action of a proper or salutary nature: but the calling a part capable of being stimulated an irritable part, weakens the idea of the stimulus being the cause of the action; and indeed the expression of a part being irritated conveys a different meaning from what would be annexed to the effect produced by a stimulus. I would therefore define a ' stimulus' to be the cause of an increased natural action; and an ' irritation' to be the cause of an unnatural, disagreeable, or diseased action.

Vegetables as well as animals have their motions produced by these causes, and are subject to the very same laws. A stimulus or excitement to actions of a salutary or proper kind is simple, and depends on the original mode of action, or the original laws of the vital œconomy, and the action only changes in some degree as the properties of the matter which stimulates changes. An irritation or excitement to morbid action is according to the susceptibility of the body or part which is to be excited to action, and alters according to the power of the irritating matter, combined with the various susceptibilities of different animals and parts for irritation; for different animals and parts have different modes and powers of receiving the same power of irritation.

In the more perfect animals we have the senses, or parts so constructed as to be impressed by the various properties of matter, and, as it were, adapted to these properties alone. These are connected together by the brain, or common sensorium, which is common to the whole of the sensitive powers : to and from the brain pass the nerves, or conductors of sensation and voluntary stimulus. But as animals become more and more imperfect, the senses, or parts constructed so as to be impressed by the properties of matter, become fewer, and the common sensorium less perfect. There appear to be animals entirely deprived of these parts or senses, and consequently having neither brain nor nerves[a].

These senses give us intelligence of the various properties of matter, from whence we derive our acquired actions, and have been naturally led to suppose that there were no other causes of action in an animal body.

The eye gives us at once the shape or limits, and the various effects of the reflection of light from bodies at a distance ; the first of which could not be sufficiently effected by the sense of touch, and the second we could not have had the least idea of, the common powers of touch not being sufficiently acute.

The ear is adapted to receive the vibrations of air, giving us intelligence of bodies at a distance.

The nose is adapted for smelling, giving us the odorous properties of the matter of which bodies at a distance are composed.

The tongue is adapted to tasting, giving us a property in matter different from any discovered by the sense of touch.

The sense of touch gives us a vast variety of information respecting the form, construction, density, &c. of bodies. In giving us form and

---

[a] [Mr. Hunter nevertheless appears subsequently to have believed that the animals here alluded to, the *Acrita* of modern naturalists, had something similar to the materials of the brain diffused through the body; and that every other principle or elementary tissue, as the muscular fibre, was diffused through the whole, making every part alike contractile and stimulable, as in the fresh-water polype, *Hydra viridis.* See Vol. III. p. 116.]

construction it is somewhat similar to the eye; but it is obliged to run over the whole for this intelligence, whereas the eye takes in a larger scope of this intelligence at once. However, even the eye is obliged to do the same thing where the object is too large, or where it is examining minutely.

None of these senses are affected by a stimulus or an irritant, although either the one or the other may be carried so far as to produce sensation. This, however, is not a necessary effect, unless the stimulus or irritant is the immediate object of sensation; as the stimulus of light to the eye, or the irritation of too much light to the eye.

These organs of sense are parts constructed for sensation, and those animals that are endowed with all of them must be the most sensible; and those that are entirely deprived of them must be wholly insensible to every impression arising from the different modifications or external influence of matter.

The animals which receive no intelligence from external objects have their actions arising out of immediate stimuli and irritants[a], and their consequent sympathies, which last extend to the action beyond the part of impression. The perfect animals in some instances seem also to be under some general power of external influence, not referrible to any one sense or all of them taken together: it is a general observation that many animals go into shelter before a storm comes on, and before any of the particular senses can be affected. Many people are weather-wise, as it is vulgarly called, and, like the brutes, are sometimes previously apprised of the ensuing change. Many sleep soundest in a storm, especially when attended with thunder.

The natural salutary actions, arising from stimuli, take place both in animals and vegetables, and may be divided into three kinds.

The *first* kind of action, or self-motion, is employed simply in the œconomical operations, by which means the immediate functions are carried on, and the necessary operations performed, with the materials the animal or vegetable is in possession of, such as growth, support, secretion, &c. The blood is disposed of by the actions of the vessels, according to their specific stimulus, producing all the above effects. The juices of a plant are disposed of according to the different actions of the sap-vessels, arising also from their specific stimulus, which is different from that of blood-vessels, but equally produces growth: but a vine will grow twenty feet in one summer, while a whale probably does not grow so much in as many years[b].

---

[a] [i. e. Of stimuli which do not produce action through the medium of the brain.]
[b] [The insensible organic contractility of Bichat corresponds with the kind of action which Hunter here defines.]

The *second* kind of action is in pursuit of external influence, and arises from a compound of internal and external stimulus; it is excited by the state of the animal or vegetable, which gives the stimulus of want, and, being completed by external stimulus, procures the proper supplies of nourishment. It produces motions of whole parts : thus we see the *Hedysarum gyrans* moving its lesser foliola. This is an action apparently similar to breathing in animals, though perhaps it does not answer the same purpose; yet there is an alternate motion in both. The cirriferous plants, or those bearing tendrils or claspers, requiring to be supported by other bodies, as the passion-flower, briony, vine, &c., stretch out their tendrils as it were at random, moving them slowly in various directions. They are to lay hold of any substance that may be within their reach that can support them, and when they come in contact with a body on that side where their power of motion is greatest they begin to bend in that direction, grasp it, and continue turning round it. We see motions of the same kind in the stems of the *Plantæ volubiles*; some of these turn to the left, as the *Lonicera, Humulus,* &c.; some to the right, as the *Clitoria, Convolvulus,* &c. They are directed in this course by a lateral inclination, which takes place only on one side, they having little or no power of action on the other. Those which have one mode of action pursue that principally; but if prevented from doing it, their action then varies. In the vine and other plants the action of the tendrils is in different directions; and they may be seen at one time stretched out on one side of the stem, and in twenty-four hours' time on the opposite side; and some time after in the direction of the stem itself, or in the very contrary direction. These actions arise equally from stimulus; it requires, however, different powers of action, arising from such stimulus, to produce these effects in different plants[a]. The random action of the polypus is of the same kind as those of plants. It elongates itself and throws out its tentacula, moving them in various directions to catch food; the use of this action to the animal, however, is immediate, and therefore quicker than those above described[b].

---

[a] [In the plants of the genus *Cuscuta* the tendrils will only twine around other living plants, which shows that the phenomena of climbing plants are not explicable simply by supposing that the inclination of the extremities of the tendrils or stems towards one side is a necessarily inherent law of their growth, but that it is, as Hunter regards it, an action dependent on stimulus, which, in the case of the *Cuscuta*, would seem to be a species of organic affinity.]

[b] [In comparing the motions of a polype with those of a plant, the following difference must be borne in mind : the motions of a plant, like those of the parts of an animal after their communication with the brain has been cut off, are invariably the result of external stimulus : they follow, as it were mechanically, some appreciable change in the surrounding external circumstances or influences,—it may be alteration of tempe-

The *third* kind of motion is from external stimulus, and consists principally of the motion of whole parts, which is not inconsiderable in vegetables, as in the *Dionæa muscipula* and *Mimosa pudica* is very evident; for the first, upon being touched, closes up, and as it were confines tne stimulating cause; the second bends its leaves, from external stimulus. This kind of motion is very strongly illustrated in the *Tragopogon, Calendula pluvialis*, and many other plants, which shut up their flowers either towards night or when rain comes on; and in others of different genera which open in the evening, and shut up on the approach of the sun, as different species of the *Convolvulus, Mirabilis,* &c.; and in almost the whole class *Diadelphia,* which chiefly consists of the winged-leaved plants, which shut up their foliola towards night, not expanding them till morning, which is called by Linnæus the sleep of plants; and in the motion of the footstalk of the leaf of an inverted plant, which twists so as to bring the surface of the leaf naturally uppermost to its natural position, which is remarkable in the vine, where there is evidently an apparatus for motion, although not a joint.

These actions are similar to what arise in many animals from external stimulus, more especially those not endowed with sensation, and also to the actions of many parts of animals which do not appear to be directed or stimulated by the brain and nerves; as the actions of a polypus, which has no brain, and the peristaltic motion of the intestines in the more perfect animals, which does not arise from the stimulus of the brain and nerves[a].

---

rature, difference of light, the application of a chemical or mechanical stimulus; or, in an animal, loss of blood, &c. But whoever observes the actions of a living polype will see that although, for the most part, they may be traced to an external cause or stimulus, yet that one or more of the tentacula are occasionally extended or retracted without the slightest appreciable change in any of the external circumstances under which the animal exists. These motions evidently result from an internal impulse, and I would refer them to the presence, in the polype, of an organic element,—the nervous matter,—which is wanting in the vegetable; even in that plant, which, from the energy of its excitability, has been erroneously called sensitive. There is also an essential difference in the nature of the motion itself of the *Mimosa* and *Hydra*. If we touch one of the feelers of the polype it recedes from the irritant by a true contraction of the part within itself; which contraction appears to result from the injury experienced by that part of the nervous system which is disseminated through the feeler touched. In the case of the Sensitive plant there is nothing like that contraction of the part touched, but only an articular plication of the neighbouring part without any of the dimensions of the irritated leaf being altered.]

[a] [The more just comparison of the motions of plants adduced in the text would be with those automatic actions of whole parts which take place in animals, but which result from the power possessed by the central axis of the nervous system, or any part of it, to transmit the action of an excitable nervous fibril to the exciting one with which that central axis or part brings it into communication: I apply the terms *excitable* and

The apparent difference in these actions would in many cases induce us at first to believe they were produced by different principles; as in many species of the same genus of plants some open their flowers in the day, others at night (as in the *Mesembryanthemum*, or fig-marigold), similar to that which is the œconomy of some animals, as in many species of the same genus of moths (*Phalæna*, Linn.), some fly, seek their

---

exciting to the nervous fibres with reference to their intermediate relation, as to the muscular fibre and the external stimulus to its contraction. The excitable fibres are those usually termed sensitive; the exciting fibres those usually termed motive. When the communication between the excitable nervous fibre and the brain is entire or uninterrupted, the latter may take cognizance of the excitement and sensation be produced. When the exciting nervous fibres of muscular motion are in connection with the brain, the will, through the brain, may excite them to action, and this act of the brain may be felt. The essential character, therefore, of the actions of the brain, whether as a recipient or transmitter of impressions, is consciousness of the action. But this property of consciousness is not possessed by the spinal chord, probably not by the medulla oblongata. Whenever, therefore, an impression received by an excitable nervous fibre is transmitted through the unconscious part of the central axis to the exciting fibre of muscular motion, the latter phenomenon is unaccompanied with consciousness or sensation. That the spinal chord, or any segment of it, possessed the power of transmitting an impression from an excitable to an exciting nervous fibre, has been known and admitted as a fundamental fact in physiology since the experiments of Whytt, Blane, and Mayo. To the latter physiologist we are more especially indebted for the most decisive experiments in proof, and the clearest enunciation, of this property of the central nervous axis. Recently the automatic animal motions resulting from this property have been grouped together more extensively than had before been done, and the morbid phenomena resulting from them ably traced out by Dr. M. Hall. But I cannot perceive the necessity of a distinct class of excitable nervous fibres for transmitting an impression to the motive fibre through the medium of the spinal chord and brain, and of another class of nervous fibres for transmitting an impression to the motive fibre through the medium of the spinal chord alone; still less can I perceive the necessity for one class of exciting or motive fibres for transmiting the stimulus to the muscular fibre from the brain and spinal chord, and of another and distinct class for transmitting a stimulus received from the spinal chord independently of the brain. It remains to be seen whether anatomy will establish the existence of these four classes of nervous fibres, which, so far as I understand Dr. Hall's hypothesis of the reflex function, are called in to account for the voluntary and automatic muscular motions. There is not, however, a single phenomenon of automatic motion in parts supplied by spinal nerves which may not be accounted for on the demonstrated property of the central axis to transmit impressions from the excitable to the exciting nerves at any part where they are connected to it, independently of the rest; and I am at a loss to understand why impressions so received by the spinal chord should not also be transmitted to the brain (its continuity with that organ being uninterrupted,) without the necessity of supposing a class of nervous fibres for conveying, in this case, the impressions to the spinal chord, distinct from a second class which are supposed to transmit to the motive fibres those impressions which are not afterwards propagated to the brain. It would appear from the text that Hunter supposed that the animal motions which are unaccompanied by consciousness were altogether independent of the nerves; but they can truly be stated to be only independent of the brain.]

food, and procreate in the day; while others are inactive and fixed to one spot, without apparent motion, all day, but on the approach of night become all at once animated, fly abroad, seek their food, and procreate. These actions are, nevertheless, produced by one and the same cause.

The owl and hawk are similar in their food, yet dissimilar in their times of catching it: hunger is the first stimulus, animal food is the second; light stimulates the one to motion, darkness the other*. The action, however, in both arises from the same principle.

These three kinds of motion in plants are influenced by various circumstances, and sometimes are all totally suspended†. This is generally produced by cold, and shows them to be influenced by the seasons; often this cessation takes place when much weakened by transplanting, &c. I have kept a fir alive for three years without the least growth.

The second and third kind of actions commonly take place only when the first kind of action is in full vigour, because the first must produce the only parts which are capable of the second and third; and these two last can only be of service to the first when it is in full force, nourishing the vegetable and performing the action of propagation.

These actions are almost entirely suspended in some animals from cold, they being in this respect subject to seasons as well as plants. This is most remarkable in the simplest in their construction, and becomes less and less so in the more complicated, they being better adapted to the various seasons.

The first of these kinds of action is small and insensible, although its effects are great. The second is considerable in both vegetables and animals, but most so in animals. The third is almost peculiar to animals, as there are very few vegetables visibly affected by external stimulus, while all animals seem to be so.

The variety of motions is greater in animals, and more purposes are answered by them, which constitutes the great difference between the actions of a vegetable and an animal; for those powers in an animal not only move themselves, but also other parts of the same body, which in many instances are so mechanically constructed as to move common matter. A remarkable instance of this is the human hand; and it is by this means all our various operations on the matter of this globe are performed.

The first kind of action appears to be stronger in its power, although

---

* It may be supposed that there is a physical cause for the one seeing only in the day, the other only at night; but it is having a much more enlarged idea of an animal to suppose that the senses are adapted to the first principle than the first principle to the senses.

† Similar to drowned people.

less in quantity*, in vegetables than in animals; for a small vine was capable of sustaining and even of raising a column of sap 43 feet high†, while a horse's heart was only capable of supporting a column of blood 8 feet 9 inches high: both of which columns must have been supported by the action of the internal parts, for we must suppose the heart equal, or nearly so, to the strength or action of the other parts of the vascular system; and when we consider that the sap of the tallest tree must be supported and even raised from the root to the most distant branches, it must appear that the power of such vegetables far exceeds the power of any animal, and indeed it is such as the texture of a vegetable only can support. The power of supporting a leaf erect for a whole day is as great an effort of action as that of the elevator palpebrarum muscle of the eye of an animal.

If we consider the differences in the œconomy and the mode of life of vegetables and animals, we shall find the increased quantity of motion of the three kinds above mentioned, and the increased power of the third kind in animals are only adapting them to those differences.

Locomotion, for the purposes of procuring nourishment, concourse of different individuals for the propagation of the species, and destruction of each other, are the chief differences in animals. This power, however, is not given to all animals, and those which are deprived of it have their motion confined to the procuring food and the propagation of their species[a]. Many of these, although with great impropriety, have been considered as vegetables.

To see if the actions of plants were affected by a continuation of stimulus similar to those of animals, I made the following experiments.

As I took for granted that the analogy could go no further than as it related to the actions produced by external stimuli, my experiments were only on such plants as exhibited actions of this kind.

As those parts of plants which are capable of the second and third kinds of motion are in general small, as leaves, tendrils, flowers, &c., it is difficult to discover the mechanism upon which the motion depends: the sensitive plant is probably the best of this kind that we are as yet acquainted with.

As the motion of the petioli is confined principally to one part, and that differing from the others in external appearance, which difference

---

* I make a material difference between the power and the quantity of action. Some motions may be very small, yet act with great force; while others are of considerable extent, although very weak.

† Vide Hale's Veg. Statics, vol. i. p. 112, Exp. 36.

---

[a] [The two sexes are also necessarily united in the same individual, as in all attached and pedicellate animals, from the Coralline to the Barnacle, and in many others of slow motions. See note, p. 35.]

is its increased thickness and uniformity of surface, upon cutting the footstalk longitudinally, as also the stem on which it stands through its whole length, the following appearances may be observed[a] :—

For the purpose of making my experiments I took three sensitive plants, having several others for any comparative experiments which might be thought necessary. I first pitched upon one leaf in each plant which was capable of the greatest motion of collapsing and erection; and behind each of these leaves a board was placed, on which was marked the greatest extent of the two motions, so that the leaf was like the index or radius of an arc.

To have the greatest part of the day before me, I began my experiments at eight in the morning, while the leaves were in full expansion, and I continued them till four in the afternoon, as longer than this would not have been just, for they begin to collapse of themselves between five and six o'clock.

Comparative Trials of the Action and Relaxation of Three Sensitive Plants.

Exps.	The time.	The point they fell to.	The times they took to rise in.			The point to which they rose.
			No. 1. *Min.*	*No. 2.* *Min.*	*No. 3.* *Min.*	
1.	8 o'clock A. M.	To the lowest point, and became stationary.	51	24	32	The 1st and 3rd rose to the highest point, the 2nd not so high, and then became stationary.
2.	9½ A. M.	To the lowest point, but the second lower down.	77	18	38	The 3rd rose to the highest point, the 2nd and 1st not so high, and then became stationary.
3.	11 A. M.	The second & third lower than lowest point.	40	30	60	All three rose to within a little of the highest point, and there became stationary.
4.	12 Noon.	Below lowest point.	30	30	35	All three within a little of the highest point.
5.	40 min. P. M.	Below lowest point.	60	65	30	The 2nd and 3rd to highest point, the 1st not so high.
	2 P. M.	1st only below lowest point.	45	45	45	Ditto.
	3 P. M.	Ditto.	45	45	45	3rd to highest point, the 1st and 2nd not so high.
	3½ P. M.	Below lowest point.	15	15	15	1st and 2nd to highest point, 3rd not so high.

[a] [A blank in the manuscript here occurs, which leaves us ignorant as to the result of Hunter's examination of the structure of the irritable intumescence at the base of the leaf-stalks and stalklets of the Mimosa. With his usual sagacity, however, he rightly refers the motive power to this part, and it has been the subject of much diligent and minute investigation since these Croonian Lectures were read.]

From these experiments we may draw the following conclusions :

That there is no fixed time for the leaves of any of the plants to move through its course.

That they are less affected as they become accustomed to the stimulus, but the power of collapsing is increased (although not in the same degree), so that they do not move through the same arc.

That they require a stronger or quicker stimulus to produce motion after being some time accustomed to it, which was evidently seen in comparing these with others which had not been stimulated.

It may also be observed that when these plants collapse in the evening they have nearly the same quantity of flexion as when roughly touched at noon ; but if touched after they have collapsed from the effect of the evening, they become much more bent than by the same touch at noon. This would seem to arise from a disposition to collapse in the evening, and a power of increasing that disposition and action when stimulated.

Their collapsing more in the day, and erecting themselves less after a repetition of such actions, may assist in explaining the principle on which this depends.

Relaxation in Vegetables.

There is an action in plants which appears to be the contrary of expansion ; it may be considered as a relaxation, or an action of those parts antagonizing the others which acted through the day, or at other periods, and takes place at the time these other parts cease to act.

This action has hitherto been considered as analogous to sleep in animals, whereas sleep is a total loss of the sensitive principle and all the actions dependent on volition for the time, and therefore can only take place in animals endowed with sensation*. It is rather a defect in the animal than an action or the exertion of a principle.

This action of relaxation is seen in the sensitive plant when the folioli close upwards and are kept bent by the power of action in the flexors, till light and some other of its attendants affect it, when the extensors begin to act, and this action of the flexors ceases. The footstalk dropping down favours the idea of simple relaxation ; but this only arises from the position of the plant, for if turned upside down it still bends against its own gravity[a].

* The polypus does not sleep.

---

[a] [The powers which produce the depression and elevation of the leaf-stalk operate in a manner precisely the reverse of the flexor and extensor muscles in animals, pushing the moving part from, instead of pulling it towards, the fixed point. See Mayo's Physiology, p. 9 et seq.]

The one action is produced by the stimulus of light, the other by that of darkness; for if the sensitive plant is kept in a dark room it will keep bent, and perhaps as long as it lives; and if one part of the plant is kept in the dark and the other in the light, that in the dark will be bent, and continue so, while that in the light will expand itself.

Light and darkness become stimuli to the same plant, and have much more influence over vegetables than could at first be imagined. Many plants only grow through the day, others only grow after it is dark.

Sympathy in Vegetables.

Sympathy is the action of one part in consequence of an application being made to another part, or action in another part.

This power of action is extended to few plants, and even in these appears to have little variation. It is evident in the sensitive plant; for if one of the little leaves be wounded at its termination it will collapse immediately, as also its fellow on the other side. This action runs through the whole of the rachis of the compound leaves, the leaves bending regularly in pairs.

If it is a middle foliole that is wounded the same thing takes place; they all collapse towards the footstalk, but seldom towards the extreme end of the leaf, and in a little time the rachis is inflected and the whole leaf drops at the trunk. It may be remarked that a small flexion takes place towards the tip; but this principally arises from a disposition in the folioles, for a middle one cannot collapse without pressing or folding a little on the one next to it towards the end of the leaf which stimulates it and makes it collapse.

It is evident in the tendril of the vine, for these tendrils generally divide into two, near their ends : these two going out from the principal trunk in different directions, if one lays hold of any body and twines round it, the other immediately alters its direction and gradually approaches the same body till it comes in contact with it, and then bends round it and encircles it. This motion, however, is very slowly performed.

Sympathy in plants is very slow in producing its actions; the succession of stimuli in them being slow, the consequent actions must also move slowly along.

Plants have but one mode of sympathy, which arises from stimulus. Animals with no brain or nerves have but one also. Those, however, endowed with sensation have three : they have one mode from stimulus, one from sensation, and one compounded of both.

Sympathy in animals, arising from stimulus only, is slow, as in plants; but sympathy from sensation is often very quick.

MOTION IN ANIMALS.

Muscles would seem to act by vibration, although in a strong healthy man they are so short as not to be observed; yet if the muscles are made to act beyond their powers they plainly vibrate, but still more plainly in weak constitutions.

The weaker a muscle is, the longer would seem to be the vibrations, for if a weak person holds anything out in his hand it shakes.

In paralytic cases, whenever they are put to the smallest action, the vibration becomes very long, and the less the action the shorter the vibration.

Fear also increases the vibration in proportion as it weakens the muscle[a].

The Causes of Action in Muscles.

The actions of muscles have been hitherto attributed to the nerves as a cause; the mode of action of the nerves, however, not being known, most physiologists have thought themselves obliged either to make a new hypothesis, or support an old one; in all which they make it mechanical, depending either upon the motion of a fluid, or the vibration of a solid, or vapour; but there is not a single known fact attending the nervous system which could either give rise to, or support, these hypotheses, except the distance between the seat of the will and a voluntary muscle; and they have consequently been such as few thinking men could adopt.

As the brain and voluntary muscles are, with respect to our senses, in two different places, and are connected together by the nerves, it might be supposed there was some fluid in motion that would convey the impression to the mind, or the will of the mind to the voluntary muscles; but these informations are very probably the effects of sympathy.

---

[a] [The first part of Dr. Wollaston's Croonian Lecture for 1809 is devoted to the illustration of an opinion on the nature of muscular motion, corresponding with that which Hunter has above enunciated. Dr. Wollaston, as is well known, was led to infer that each act of contraction, apparently single, consisted in reality of a great number of contractions, repeated at short intervals, by reflecting on the sound perceived upon inserting the extremity of the finger into the ear. This sound, which resembles that of carriages at some distance passing rapidly over a pavement, is not perceived when the force applied to stop the ear is not muscular, unless the action of some distant muscle be communicated through some medium capable of conveying its vibrations. From experiment, associated with the above observation, Dr. Wollaston concluded that the vibratory alternations recur between twenty and thirty times in a second, varying in proportion to the degree of force exerted by the muscle; the greatest number being estimated at thirty-five vibrations in a second, and the lowest at fifteen. The more obvious illustrations of this mode of muscular action, presented by the aged and infirm, are also adduced by Dr. Wollaston, who, without doubt, was quite unconscious of the conclusion previously drawn by Hunter from the same phenomena.]

I am afraid we can go no further in the investigation of the cause of the action of muscles than by observing the phenomena which happen, and these all lead us to one cause of action.

The visible external cause of the action of a muscle is called ' stimulus,' and it is reasonable to suppose that all causes of such action are similar. This, however, may admit of dispute, the heart certainly having no visible stimulus for its motion, except the being called upon, by the sympathy which subsists between the combined powers of the animal œconomy, to exert itself in their favour, which will not account for the heart's motion when removed from that connexion.

The great question has hitherto been, whether a muscle is susceptible of impression without the medium of a nerve, or whether a nerve is in all cases necessary to its being called into action; for a stimulus must either affect the nerve which affects the muscle, or the muscular fibre itself must be susceptible of immediate impression from the stimulus.

A muscle would appear to be capable of being affected in both ways, for many animals certainly exist without nerves, and plants are susceptible of stimulus where it must be immediate, they never having been supposed to have nerves[a]. It is also evident in animals with nerves that by stimulating a nerve the muscle to which it goes will be immediately thrown into action, the nerve becoming the immediate stimulant, so that a muscular fibre may be stimulated by a nerve as well as by any other impression.

---

[a] [Those who admit that a muscle is susceptible of stimulus only through the medium of the nervous matter blended with its substance, do not scruple to ascribe nervous or sensitive globules to vegetables. But they here create the necessity which an undemonstrable organ is called in to supply. Now the more simple and philosophical mode of considering this question seems to be to examine whether the moving organs are stimulated in any new, distinct, and additional manner in those organized beings in which nerves have been detected; and if it be found that they all manifest spontaneous actions,—motions of parts independent of any external stimulus,—a phenomenon which has never been witnessed in any plant, then the next step would be to determine by experiment the relations subsisting between the new function and the superadded organ. The irritable fibre does not contract in a different manner when stimulated by the will than when stimulated mechanically out of the body; nerves, it is true, convey impressions which excite action, and are essential to the application of the voluntary stimulus, but not, therefore, to the muscular contraction. Hence, when we come to account for the cause of the spontaneous actions in animals in which no nerves have been detected, we are justified, by analogy, in attributing the spontaneous stimulus to the presence of undemonstrable nervous matter. But in the case of plants, if we attribute the contractions to anything but the irritability of the moving parts themselves, we must first hypothetically assume that nerves are necessary for the action, and then gratuitously infer their existence. This, however, only leads to a greater difficulty, to account, viz. for the non-existence of spontaneous motions in those organized beings to which nerves are, in the above theory, attributed.]

The modes of stimulating a muscle will be different according to the nature of the animal or of the muscle. In the more simple animals they will be few, increasing as the animal is more complicated.

The first kind of stimulus is that common to all animals and vegetables, which regulates the internal machine, producing growth, preparing the parts of generation, &c. &c.

The second is the internal stimulus, which respects external matter for the support and continuance of the first, as that producing breathing, hunger, the desire of propagating the species; all which are common to vegetables as well as animals, and require the assistance of a third kind to complete the action.

Vegetables are supposed with great reason to have an action analo-gous to breathing, for the same kind of air which kills animals which do breathe, certainly kills vegetables also[a]. Vegetables imbibe nourish-ment, which action arises from the same stimulus as in animals. They also require the stimulus of certain operations to be performed upon them by external matter to enable them to propagate. This external matter is either some other part of the same plant, as in the *Marchan-tia polymorphia calyce decemfido*, which has the filaments almost con-stantly in motion striking the antheræ[b]. The filaments of the flosculæ of the thistle produce the same effect, or it is done by some foreign stimulus, as the wind, driving the pollen of the male plants against the germina of females*. Most animals perform these actions them-selves, yet in both animals and vegetables a similar stimulus is necessary.

The third kind of stimulus is from external or extraneous matter immediately applied to the part, which is also common to animals and vegetables.

The fourth kind of stimulus arises from the nerves, which we may reckon twofold; one in consequence of the nerves being impressed by external matter, the other from their being impressed by the brain, or sensorium.

This is peculiar to animals, many of them receiving intelligence from without, which becomes the regulator of their actions towards that

* The antheræ of vegetables require some motion to make them burst; some have not the power of producing this motion, but if the power is given they burst immedi-ately. A blast of wind is often necessary, and in such plants propagation does not go on well in a calm place.

---

[a] [As azote, hydrogen, or any gas deprived of carbon and oxygen; for though vege-tables in health and sunshine give out oxygen, they absorb that gas, and emit carbon, but in less proportion, during the night.]

[b] [In the barberry the filaments supporting the mature anthers, when touched, bend towards the germen. In the tiger-lily the female part of the flower is endowed with irritability, and the style bends first to one stamen, then to another.]

matter which gives the intelligence. This leads us immediately to voluntary actions.

The actions of muscles have hitherto only been considered by physiologists in the more perfect animals where this (the voluntary or nervous stimulus,) is given, which becomes a different cause of action from those found in other animals and vegetables.

Those actions where the mind, being made sensible of them, may be considered as a cause, are called voluntary actions; and those actions over which the mind has no influence, and about which it is not in the least consulted, are called involuntary actions. The actions of the muscles which go on without the influence of the mind, but can be restrained, increased, or stopped by the mind, are called mixed. There are also actions which may be allowed to arise from a peculiarity in the state of mind, but not dependent on the will: these are common to both the voluntary and involuntary muscles. Thus an involuntary muscle, as the heart, increases its strokes, and the voluntary muscles of the hands, legs, tongue, &c. tremble when the mind is agitated by anger, fear, &c. These four kinds of action not only appear to arise from different causes, but produce different phenomena.

The first kind, or voluntary motions, last only for stated times, beyond which they cannot go, the muscles either losing the power altogether, or the mind becoming incapable of stimulating them; by which means a cessation of action takes place, which indeed is necessary for the preservation of the animal. For these actions, too long continued, weaken, hurt, or destroy the body; and therefore the mind which is under no restriction is thus prevented from continuing the action. We have this beautifully illustrated in some of the mixed motions: for where their involuntary motions are employed for the preservation of the animal, as in breathing, they are constant; and where the stimulus of necessity does not constantly take place they rest, as in the stomach, levator palpebrarum, &c.; but if we voluntarily increase the actions of these they soon tire.

The natural involuntary actions of muscles are such as never tire, while the voluntary always do; and we may observe that the muscles which are under the influence of both are never tired of their involuntary actions, while they are of their voluntary. This we might suppose was owing to this property being stamped upon them at first, and for very wise purposes; but it rather appears to be a property arising from the mode of impression, viz. not being impressed by the will, but probably acting from a general impression in the machine, viz. from general principles; whereas the voluntary actions are caused by a peculiar impression of the will, and the muscles are so constituted as to tire of that impression, or rather become incapable of acting, which gives the sensation called *tired*. But this is carried further, for in muscles that are entirely at the command of the will, if they take on involuntary actions they never tire. For instance, Lord L——'s hands are almost perpetually in motion, and he never feels the sensation in them of being tired. When he is asleep his hands, &c. are perfectly at rest; but when he wakes, in a little time they begin to move.

We tire of voluntary actions whether of voluntary parts or of parts that commonly act involuntarily, as the muscles of respiration. Tiring of action feels to the mind to be in the muscles themselves, but I imagine it must be in the mind, although it is referred to the muscles; for we cannot suppose that the mode of action of a muscle directed by the will is different from the mode of action when not directed by the will. This is not a tiring of the will itself, but probably a tiring of the action of the nerves of the will; and as the actions of these nerves is always referred to the part of their destination, the tiring is also referred there.

The second kind are the involuntary actions, which are lasting, as the parts themselves: these are always fit for action: and if they are inactive, it does not arise from the want of power in the part to act, but from a cessation of the stimulus, which cessation takes place whenever the action, from peculiar circumstances, is become unnecessary. Such actions are naturally so circumstanced as to be constantly wanted, being for the preservation of the animal, as the motion of the heart.

The nerves are only to be considered as conductors carrying impressions from every part of the body to the brain, or carrying the command of the will to those muscles whose actions can only be employed about such external objects as can affect the mind; but those parts whose actions are unknown to the mind appear not to be affected at all by the will.

That the nerves are the principal agents between the mind and the parts would appear from circumstances respecting their comparative size; for all those parts which convey a strong sensation, or are intended to perform extraordinary voluntary actions, have large nerves; while those parts of animals which neither give intelligence to the mind of their actions, nor are under the influence of the mind, have very small nerves. A stronger instance of this cannot be given than the electric organ of the torpedo, where the power of giving or restraining the shock depends upon the will: the actions are strong and violent, for he can soon exhaust himself by them; and the nerves which convey the power of the mind exceed, compared with the size of the animal, in bulk the nerves in any organ of any other known animal. It is a part whose actions, its growth excepted, depend entirely upon the will, having no power of action of its own; the communication between the will and the organ is large in the same manner as the communication between the senses in general and the brain is large.

The voluntary muscles have large nerves to command the action of the muscle, which is independent of the will, although in some degree subservient to it; but they are not so large as those of the senses or electric organs, where they give the part its whole action.

A nerve being cut going to a voluntary muscle, the muscle cannot obey the will, and thereby loses its voluntary actions; but it may be stimulated into action by immediate impression from other causes, as electricity.

The voluntary and involuntary muscles having their quantity of motion in an inverted proportion to their quantity of nerves, is a strong argument against the nerves being the cause of muscular motion.

If it is asked why the involuntary parts have nerves at all, the answer may be given that it is not for their common actions, but to keep up the connexion between the whole, for without them an animal would become two distinct machines, and one might be acting very contradictorily to the other; but by the intercourse between the will and voluntary parts, between the voluntary and involuntary, and also between these last and the mind, an universal and uniform agreement or regulation is kept up, which communication produces one kind of sympathy. This connexion between the living principle and the sensitive produces a compound action, which becomes the cause of the instinctive principle in animals.

Muscles are either employed upon the internal operations of the animal, as the heart, muscles of respiration, stomach, intestines, &c., or upon external matter for the support of both, as those of the extremities.

The first of these are nearly of the same strength in the robust strong man and the small woman or man, if equally healthy; and it is right it should be so, for the small man has nearly the same resistance to cope with; but it is the others which constitute the strong or weak man.

The power of muscles which are influenced by the will, although they have a common power of action with those independent of the will, sooner lose their powers than those which are wholly involuntary, as the heart, stomach, bladder, blood-vessels, &c., which would seem to show that the power of simple life lasts after the will is no more.

We might naturally suppose that the voluntary muscles have nearly the same quantity of power of action as the involuntary; but upon considering several circumstances, we should rather conceive the contrary; for when we consider the power by which the colon of a horse propels such a load of solid contents, we can hardly conceive the power of any voluntary muscle of the same thickness equal to it. For, as voluntary motion arises from two causes, or has two causes of action, the moment one of these ceases, the power which remains is either not so strong originally as the whole power of the involuntary muscle which has only this principle of action, or not so strong, from want of habit, not having been always employed as a principle of action in them.

It is not clear to me but that every muscle has a sphinctorial power of contraction so as to bring them to the middle state. This we may see in the temporal muscles; for by opening the jaws the muscle sinks, and by leaving the jaw to itself, not acting with it in the least, the jaw rises and the muscle in part fills up, so that the jaw is suspended by the half action of the muscle; however, this power may be much more in some muscles than others.

The great variety of causes of muscular motion make it almost inexplicable: they may be said to be three,—the will, passions of the mind, and external stimuli. Those actions arising from the will and the mind appear to be most simple, because they are totally unintelligible; but those arising from external stimuli are either voluntary or involuntary, for a muscle that acts by the command of the will at one time is also capable of being thrown into action by a particular state of mind or external stimulus.

Those actions which arise from the will have reason and habit for their continuance: they are such as arise out of imitation, reasoning, and all the powers collected by the senses.

Those actions which arise from the mind belong mostly to the passions, which affect more muscles of the body than the will; perhaps there is not a muscular fibre in the whole animal machine but is at different times affected according to the different affections of the mind, every different state of mind having its particular muscles to stimulate.

Upon many of these occasions reason is introduced, which is provided by this state of mind to call in the assistance of other muscles, to act according to that state, either to bring about an increased action which will destroy itself, or to prevent the increase and continuance of those actions.

From extraneous stimuli arise all our internal insensible actions, and these depend upon the principle of simple life, upon which depends also the action of medicines; and health is only the right action of such parts.

Some muscles must be put upon the stretch, and they will continue their action far beyond the easy point, or that which was so before this action, as the stomach, intestines, and bladder. Others wait to be stretched, as the uterus; this, however, is not the cause of its contracting again, it is only putting it in a state to act when another cause takes place, as a miscarriage or fœtus at the full time. This is nearly opposite to the other, for what endeavours to empty or relax the uterus becomes the cause of its contraction, not what stretches it.

Voluntary actions, when very violent, produce involuntary, as the cramp, from dancing, swimming, &c.

We feel every involuntary action of a voluntary muscle, while we do not feel the voluntary actions; nor do we feel the actions of an involuntary muscle. When such actions are slight we only feel them as little convulsions, contractions in different parts of the body, called creeping in the flesh, or quivering in the eyelids; but when these become violent, as in cramps or spasms, then the sensation is pain.

Voluntary muscles, the stronger they are, the more they are at the command of the will; and the weaker they are the more they seem independent of the power of the will, and seem to be either at their own command, or at that of the nerve. Strong people are less subject to spasms than weak, which may perhaps arise from custom; the strong muscles being more healthy, are oftener in use, and therefore become more at the command of the will.

Women, children, and sick men are subject to fits, for the reason just mentioned; perhaps also diseases of the uterus, for the same reason, are the cause of spasmodic complaints, it being very little at the command of the will, but of other circumstances; and from this disposition draws in other parts by consent, and so brings on general spasm.

Voluntary muscles always become tired when long continued in the same action, which accounts for animals tiring sooner by being kept in one position than if allowed to move; and we find a man can hardly stand five minutes in one position; he never stands equally upon both legs, but upon one as a base, the other as a prop, so as to be able to shift his legs as they tire.

Animals, also, by moving or producing alternate motions by their muscles, can go on for a considerable time, but their alternate motion must not be quick, as it always requires a certain time for muscles to regain the power which they lost in action, and if the alternate motion becomes quick and violent, it may tire sooner than constant motion.

The voluntary actions of young animals are not so strong, and are much less lasting than those of middle age; that strength they have they are not capable of employing for any great continuance without tiring, especially in actions where a considerable force is required.

Thus we have young horses soon fatigued with labour, which the same horses will easily perform some years after. This ability in the older horse does not arise entirely from a naturally greater degree of strength, joined with a natural capability of continuance, but in some degree from an acquired strength from employment, and a capacity of endurance from the habit of action. This might be thought sufficient to account for the whole difference, but dealers in horses affirm that one of seven and one of four years old, having equally done no work, shall not be equal in their continuance of it. In riding they also give weight according to age, and the aged horse always carries the greatest weight, if other parts are equal*.

When an animal is at its full strength is not easily ascertained, but it cannot be while growing; it must have arrived at its full extent, and perhaps it is even necessary to have been some time in that state.

The involuntary actions are stronger before this period than after; this is perhaps necessary for the animal's growth.

Besides the decrease in the size of a muscle from an atrophy, &c., and the restoration of them again to their natural size, which is disease and health, there is an increase which accompanies the whole body, till it arrives at its full size, when the whole seems to rest, except the muscles.

How long the muscles continue in this full size is not easily ascertained, but when old age begins to come on, the muscles begin to decay; but not becoming pale and flabby, like a diseased muscle, but retaining their redness and sound appearance.

A person grows thinner after a certain age, but not in proportion to the decrease of size of the muscles, for the interstices between the bundles of fibres, and also between the muscles themselves, are loaded with fat, and this takes place so constantly that an old man may be distinguished from a young one from only seeing the muscles, and the fat mixed with them.

Muscles in old people lose their quantity of contraction, and the joints are therefore never moved to their full extent. This is the loss of only the extreme motion, which is weak, and therefore may be supposed to arise from weakness alone; but I do not think this effect is produced in young people from weakness.

An old man stands with his knees, thighs, and all his joints bent, not being able to bring himself to the upright position.

The actions of the body that are both involuntary and voluntary are some of the most beautiful circumstances in the machine. I believe the muscles of respiration are the only perfect instances of it. The sphincters also have both; but in them it would seem to be an involuntary continuation of an action which is voluntary.

Fresh air was necessary for our existence, and it was therefore necessary that it should be regulated by some other principle than that of the will; for it is necessary when we sleep, and also when we *will* the contrary. Therefore our will has its limits of power over the involun-

---

* How accurate these gentlemen are I don't know.

tary actions, and the involuntary also have their limits over the actions of the will; each therefore can only go a certain length in opposition to the other.

As all animals which breathe air are probably endowed with the power of forming sounds, and as air is in common necessary for such an effect, Nature has made this air answer the purpose of sound as well as of life. For the purposes of life it was necessary the action should be kept pretty regularly constant, and therefore involuntary, because it required too much attention of the will to keep up the necessary action, and the will is not always in a state to attend to it; but for the purposes of sound it was necessary it should be at the command of the will, for sound is in some degree arbitrary; for although often attended or caused by a natural propensity at the time, yet it can be avoided, as in crying. Vocal sounds, however, do not entirely interfere with inspiration and expiration; it is performed by the last, which must have been preceded by the first, although not with the same ease.

Many other actions of the body interfere with involuntary respiration; all violent exertions of the body are a check upon it; but then in proportion to the intended exertion, the voluntary supersedes the involuntary, and they take in a proportionate quantity of air; but, both in sounds and exercise, if continued, the stimulus of necessity for a repetition of respiration takes place, and the person is obliged to take in a fresh supply of air, which again answers the former purpose.

The Colour of Muscles.

Most parts of an animal body are white, and when they have any other colour it generally arises from some adventitious though necessary matter, as the pigment of the eye, which in many persons is black, in some green, in others white, &c.; also the pigment of the skin, which in many people is dusky in its colour.

A muscle in all animals is in itself white, and its red colour found in living animals, and also immediately after death, arises from the blood; for if a red muscle be steeped in water it will become white; or if the arteries of a part which has red muscles be injected with water till it returns by the veins, the muscles soon become white. A red muscle exposed to the air loses the Modena red, becoming florid.

As the colour of muscles arises from the blood in their vessels, the muscles of every animal must have the same colour with the blood: if the blood is red, the muscle will be more or less so, according to its quantity; for in sick or unhealthy people they are pale.

If the blood is of any other colour the muscle will be tinged with that colour, and also in proportion to the quantity of the blood.

All muscles, however, have not the colour of the blood, for many animals having red blood have their muscles almost white; and even in the human body many muscles are much redder than others. The muscles of an arm or leg are much redder than those of the stomach or intestines; those of the face are much paler than the temporal or masseter, although nearly in the same situation.

The muscles of quadrupeds are not equally red, there being a great difference between those of a hare and rabbit.

The difference in the colour of muscles in the same animal, and in different animals of the same order, is very remarkable, but is equally to be observed in another order of animals, viz. fowls.

The blood in fowls is red; there are few, however, in which some muscles are not much redder than others, and in some birds they shall be almost wholly red, as in the black cock, while in others they shall be nearly all pale, as in the turkey. The muscles of birds are more generally pale than those of quadrupeds, from their having a smaller proportion of red blood, and that blood being more partially distributed.

The muscles in frogs, snakes, tortoises, &c. are generally pale, from their having a still smaller quantity of red blood, and that quantity more confined to the vital parts than in birds.

The muscular parts in fish are generally white, although I believe they have all red blood, but in smaller quantity than even frogs and snakes, so that the motion of red blood in them is much confined in its extent, appearing to go no further than those parts which are essential to life.

The muscles of many animals of a still inferior order are generally pale; the blood in them being not apparently of any colour, and in some almost transparent, as in the lobster, oyster, snail, &c.; and in this order of animals, if the blood is of any determined colour, it is generally so confined in its motion, not running minutely into parts, that they are hardly tinged with it, as in the slug, which is black, although the blood is of a milk white. The earth-worm, however, is an exception to these general observations on the more imperfect animals, for it has a great deal of red blood, which is seen through the whole body of the animal, from the external covering being pretty transparent.

The red blood in a muscle is in proportion as the red blood in the animal is to the quantity of muscle; and also in proportion to the quantity of action in the muscle and the quantity of red blood taken together.

The blood in the more perfect class of animals, as man and quadrupeds, and in which class whales are also included, is in greater quantity, and more loaded with red particles, than in other inferior orders[a]; therefore the muscles are in general redder, and the quantity of blood in this order of animals, and perhaps every other order in which they have red blood, is rendered greater by increasing the action of the muscles, the blood being driven or extended further into those parts by their increased action. This happens commonly in voluntary muscles only ; the involuntary, being employed in uses at all times equally necessary, are even and constant in their actions.

Muscles much at rest are pale, as in animals just come into the world, before the muscles have had much action, except the heart, which has been acting from the beginning; and all the muscles of a young animal, except the diaphragm, may be kept pale by keeping the animal in a state of rest*, for in that state the blood does not pass far into the muscle ; but as the animal grows up, the muscles become redder and redder, especially if they are allowed action by the animal taking exercise, and nearly in proportion to that exercise.

This, however, is not universally the case ; for the natural actions of a hare and rabbit are not very different, yet the muscles of a hare are very red, and those of a rabbit pale ; whereas I do not believe it possible by rest alone to make a hare's pale, although by rest they will become proportionably paler†.

This difference in animals so nearly allied would seem to arise from an original law in their nature; for although a hare may not have a greater quantity of motion in common, yet it is formed to be always in such a state as if it really had, that it may be constantly prepared to undergo such motion. The rabbit has no occasion for such a state of muscle, its sphere of action being much confined, and it is even not intended to run fast.

In an inferior order of animals, where the quantity of red blood is not so great, and the destruction of voluntary action not nearly equal through the whole muscular mass, we find a great difference in the colour of muscles.

A bird has two kinds of progressive motion, flying and walking. Some principally fly, others walk‡, and many perform both equally.

* This becomes a distinguishing mark between the hares of a barren mountainous country and a rich flat one.

† Such is the method of preserving veal white, for the proportional quantity of red blood is not allowed to increase or go far from the heart.

‡ Swimming in fowls I consider as walking, both being actions of the legs.

[a] [From the numerous experiments of MM. Prevost and Dumas (*Examen du Sang*, Bibl. Univ. de Genev., t. xvii.), it would appear that the red globules and fibrine are most abundant in the blood of birds, in which respiration is most active and animal temperature highest.]

In the walking bird the muscles of the leg are the reddest, as in the pheasant, partridge, and common fowl. In the flying bird the muscles of the wing are the reddest, as in the swallow and woodcock*.

In the frog, snake, turtle, alligator, &c. there is but little action, and the muscles are nearly equally employed through the whole animal except the heart; so that there is not that difference in colour in the muscles of the same animal, or of any two of this order, although in many it may be observable.

In fish we find a good deal of difference in the colour of muscles, and the heart, which is in constant action, is in them as red as any other animal[a]. The natural history of fish is very little known, but what variety there is we may attribute to the cause above mentioned[b].

The actions of the more inferior orders of animals we shall not at present enter into.

From the above observations we may conclude that red blood, in those animals that have it, is of essential use to muscular contraction.

That the quantity of red blood brought to a muscle is of service in its action is plain; for a muscle become paralytic from an injury to the nerve, or an anchylosis in the joint preventing its having contracted for many years, is found white, small, and somewhat ligamentous, retaining however a degree of transparency and gelatinous consistence, so that a muscle may become paralytic from too much rest alone.

The wasting of a limb which is seen externally takes place principally in the muscles, more especially where they are paralytic from an anchylosed joint; in that case the muscles alone can be supposed to be affected, they alone being concerned in the motion; but where it arises from a defect in the nervous system, that defect may be in all the nerves of the limb, and therefore all the parts may suffer alike.

---

* Epicures are sensible of this; therefore white veal, the leg of woodcocks, are delicious bits, and the feeders of domestic fowls indulge them. They rob the appetite, however, to please the eye, the flavour generally being in the muscles of action.

---

[a] [Most of the above facts, with their physiological inferences, were known to Grew, who alludes to them in the following digression while describing the digestive organs of the bird: "And as the strong and continual motion of all these muscles is taught, us from their structure, so likewise from their red colour, which, especially in the grinders" (the lateral muscles of the gizzard,) "is intense. Hence in a fish the muscles which move the fins are usually red, although the rest of the flesh is very white; and so the leg of a domestic fowl. Whereas the wings also of a wild fowl are of the same colour. So likewise the flesh of a driven calf, or of a hare, though that of a coney be white. And that which comes nearer, the heart in all creatures having the like continual motion is of a red colour."—Anatomy of Stomachs and Guts, fol., p. 41; 1681.]

[b] [See note [b], p. 147.]

Swelling of Muscles.

We may suppose that the blood is of great use in muscular contraction; for in violent and frequent actions of the muscles they swell and become considerably larger, not when in action only, but when relaxed immediately after the action, and will continue swelled for some time.

This swelling does not come on till the muscle is tired of acting: this must be from a greater influx of blood at that time, or that the action does not let the blood pass so freely through the veins. It must be owing to something of this kind which happens to animals which use much violent exercise, and are killed during the action, that they are redder, fuller, and eat much tenderer, but do not keep so long. There is a material difference between a hare or deer that is shot and one run down by dogs.

Muscles not only become really larger by acting, but also become larger in the time of acting, and for that time only, subsiding gradually after the action is over: this increase is in proportion to the violence of the action at the time, and appears to go on till they are tired, and is probably one cause of their being so.

In order to ascertain this fact as much as possible, I made the following experiments. Immediately after getting up in the morning, having used my arm as little as possible, I measured the circumference of my right arm across the belly of the biceps flexor, while in the relaxed state of all the muscles of this part, and found it measured ten inches and a half. I then bent the fore arm, in which action the biceps being contracted, I measured it again at the same place, and found it twelve inches one eighth, so that this part of the arm had gained one inch and five eighths.

After having thus ascertained the size of the arm, both when all the muscles were relaxed and also when contracted, I next worked an air-pump for about ten minutes with considerable violence, when my arm became quite tired. On repeating the above mensurations I found my arm in the relaxed state eleven inches and five eighths, and in the bent state twelve inches and five eighths; so that the arm, by acting ten minutes, had acquired an increase of six eighths of an inch in circumference even in the relaxed state of the muscles, and four eighths in the contracted state.

That the calf of the leg swells towards night is a common observation; and I suppose it is principally owing to its having acted so much through the day.

That the swelling in such cases is in the muscles themselves is evident from the stiffness felt in acting with tired muscles.

What produces this temporary increase in the muscle? It is probable that an extravasation of fluids has taken place, and the weakness induced in the muscles in consequence of their having acted more than usual, and with greater force, is the cause of extravasation.

Effects of Habit on Muscles.

Muscles are capable of being improved and increased in different ways by exercise, or employing the muscle much in its natural functions.

This improvement in action is most observable in the muscles of volition, as it is in consequence of the will that they become more familiar with the actions; and also they are more subjected to a variety of action, sometimes acting strongly, at others not at all.

The stimulus of the will never loses its influence by habit or by becoming familiar, but these stimuli may be called arbitrary or accidental, foreign, &c. Muscles not only improve in one particular, but in every respect whatever.

One improvement voluntary muscles acquire from habit is the readiness with which they take up their own actions, the will frequently only having to set them a going; there are instances of people playing tunes without attending to the notes or even thinking of the tunes.

From this facility of obeying the will in beginning actions, and of repeating actions they have been accustomed to, with the greatest variety of motions, in the voluntary muscles, particularly in man, and also from the frequent employment in any actions, muscles acquire a facility in obeying the mind in the performance of actions they had never tried before, going hand in hand with the mind; for as the mind, when it sets the body to perform actions, acquires a facility in immediately employing the proper muscles, they obey directly, and this even in actions they never performed before.

A man will learn one trade much more readily if he knows another, than if he knew no trade at all.

The habit of acting in a muscle, especially when employed in considerable exertions, increases the necessity of becoming stronger, which necessity, acting as a stimulus upon the muscles, becomes a real cause of increase of size, which augments their strength.

This effect is so evident, that painters and sculptors, as well as physiologists, have observed it. We have Charon and Vulcan always represented with large shoulders, brawny arms, and their lower extremities small, and apparently disproportioned.

This effect is still more nicely marked by the difference between the right arm and the left; the right being generally employed in preference, and more particularly in great exertions, is therefore the largest and strongest. People who play much at tennis, where the ball is always struck with the right hand, have that arm much thicker and stronger than the left; therefore a man originally well-proportioned shall lose that proportion by being employed in any action that does not require the whole body. From these facts it must appear, that if every animal was perfectly made, with respect to any standard proportion of its parts, that few would be allowed to grow to that standard, because few animals exert all their muscles equally, there being in most some circumstances in life which oblige them to exert one set of muscles more than another. This is probably more the case in man than in any other animal, and also in him less determined to any one set of muscles more than another; it, however, also takes place in animals, as there will be a considerable difference in the muscles of two birds' breasts of the same species, one being allowed to fly, and the other kept in a cage.

The increase in the voluntary muscles appears not to be without limitation, and indeed if it was we might see them increase beyond conception. What principle sets bounds to this increase from action is not known; the circumstance of these muscles tiring may become a cause.

This increase is not confined to the voluntary muscles, for the involuntary, when obliged from any circumstance to act with uncommon force, also enlarge, and become stronger, and in a much greater degree; than the voluntary.

The bladder has been found exceedingly thickened in its muscular coat where there are either strictures in the urethra or stones in the bladder, for in this last complaint, although it discharges the urine, yet it continues to act with more violence than usual, being irritated by the stone, which it cannot expel. I have seen it increased to three times its natural thickness[a].

Increase of thickness in the auricles and ventricles of the heart, in consequence of an aneurism in the arch of the aorta, is not uncommon.

The cremaster muscles I have seen very much enlarged in cases of hydrocele of long standing.

In the increase of involuntary muscles there appear to be no limits; the power of increasing seems to be in proportion to the necessity, and as they do not tire there is no end to their power of acting.

Whether this increase of the body of a muscle is a new addition of muscular fibres, or an increase in size of those already formed, is not easily determined, but I should be inclined to suppose the last.

---

[a] [Hunter has preserved many preparations in his Pathological Series illustrative of this fact, as Nos. 746, 752, 755, 758, 759, and 961, &c.]

CROONIAN LECTURE ON MUSCULAR MOTION, No. II.

[Read before the Royal Society in the year 1797, by John Hunter, F.R.S.]

THE CONSTRUCTION OF THE ANIMAL MACHINE, WITH THE ME-
CHANICAL EFFECTS PRODUCED BY THE MUSCLES AS MECHANI-
CAL POWERS.

Mechanical arrangement of the Fibres of Muscles.

THE most simple mode of investigating an animal body is first to consider the matter of which it is composed. In this inquiry we shall find
it more than probable that there is but one species of matter which is
peculiar to animals, and therefore I shall call it animal matter.

The blood appears to be the most simple modification of this matter:
it is the material from which all the solids are composed.

The next modification, or what may be called the simplest organization, is a certain arrangement of this matter so as to produce some action. This may be of two kinds: first, such an arrangement as may
take place in any kind of matter, so as to produce elasticity. The second is such as is capable of producing a motion in itself, without the
cause being mechanical as in elasticity : this is the composing of a muscular fibre.

A muscular fibre is one of the simplest constructions of an active
solid, and it is these fibres which compose almost the whole of many
animals.

The muscles are the powers in an animal body, and are perhaps the
most regular parts of the whole. They are apparently constructed of
fibres laid nearly parallel to one another ; in some they are extended
longitudinally from one end to the other of the muscle which they compose ; in others their direction is oblique to the body of the muscle ; this
obliquity in some is regular from one end of the muscle to the other,
while in other muscles the fibres lie in contrary directions. In some a
number of these oblique portions compose the muscle ; the parallelism,
however, in each portion is preserved. This parallelism is only found
in some of those muscles whose fibres all tend to one point of action, and
they are nearly of equal lengths in every part of such muscles ; but where
parts of a muscle produce different effects the fibres vary in length, suited
to the quantity of motion admitted by the directions of the joints.

The most simple muscle in an animal body is a bundle of fibres, distinct from end to end from all other portions, and having one determined use. The muscles which move the globe of the eye come the nearest to the idea of a distinct muscle; however, there are very few muscles in an animal body so unconnected with other muscles, which makes it difficult in many cases to say with certainty what may be called a distinct muscle.

If we take a view of what we call muscles in an animal body, the human for instance, we shall find that no definition can be given which will answer to them all.

A muscle is said to be distinct if it is so at its insertion only, although it may be connected with others at its origin, as the extensor indicis proprius. A muscle is distinct, although connected with another at its insertion, if there is a difference in the use; or although connected at its origin with one muscle, and at its insertion with another; but where two portions of flesh are united at their insertion, both having the same use, they are considered as one muscle. So that it is the particular effect which is produced by a portion or portions of flesh which in general has made anatomists either unite or divide them into separate muscles.

This, however, has not been universally followed; for in some particular muscles, in which the origin is of considerable extent, and the insertion but small, each part of the muscle having the power of acting separately, and producing different effects according to the parts which act, (the joint admitting of a variety of motions,) these have generally been considered as one muscle; and in such muscles, when the whole acts, it produces one general effect, as in the pectoralis major muscle. Also those muscles in which the origin and insertion are of considerable extent, and produce different motions of the same part, yet produce one general effect when the whole acts, are considered as distinct muscles, as the trapezius, the broad muscles of the abdomen, &c. When a muscle has a number of insertions, and each portion moves a distinct joint, while the whole mass, in the same action, moves all these joints, it is then considered as only one muscle. Of this kind is the longissimus dorsi, the use of which is to erect the whole spine; but its particular action (if it had any) could only be to move one or more joints, according to the number of portions in action.

External Figure of Muscles.

Muscles have various shapes and sizes; they are long, short, thick, round, flat. They have the fibres either in straight lines or in curved ones; they may be broad and thin, or hollowed and circular, making rings; all which varieties of size and shape are connected with their action and use, and have induced anatomists to give them different names, as *teres major, latissimus dorsi, longus colli, palmaris brevis, sphincter oris*, &c., *rhomboides, deltoides, pyramidalis*, &c. &c.

The form and size of muscles are adapted to the uses in which they are employed; and these in general arise from the nature of the parts or joints to be moved.

In some muscles the position of the whole leads to the general direction of all its fibres; but this does not always happen, being the case only in muscles of a more simple construction. A muscle, for example, lies between the os hyoides and the upper end of the sternum, which two points lying nearly in the same plane would lead one to presuppose the fibres of such a muscle to be rectilineal, which is really the case.

The figure of the muscle often shows the motion of the joint which it moves, particularly if it is a simple motion. This is the case in the rectilineal muscles and those which are nearly so, or those which are radiated, as the pectoralis, diaphragm, &c.

The different kinds of Muscles.

Muscles are more or less complex, arising generally from the different dispositions of their fibres, which difference is owing to the manner of their arising and being inserted, more particularly the former; and hence we say, muscles are straight, broad, radiated, half-penniform, complete-penniform, and complex.

The most simple muscle would be one whose fibres are in the direction of its body, or in a straight line between the two resisting points, and should be called rectilineal; but there is not in the human body a muscle truly rectilineal, and from what has been observed of the disposition of the muscles and their tendons, also of their origins, it is hardly possible to have one.

The straight muscles have fewer fibres in proportion to their size than the oblique, therefore their powers are less; some are round, or nearly so; others are flat and broad: some of these last are radiated.

The half-penniform muscle, although nearly as simple as any in the body, appears to be the first stage towards combination. It is composed of a series of fibres, arising from a bone, tendon, or fascia, but more commonly a tendon, of which the insertion runs nearly parallel to the origin, representing a quill with one side of the feathers taken off. This disposition of fibres, from the mode of origin or general disposition of the bones and fascia above described, is almost as common as any in the body.

The complete-penniform muscle is two half-penniform muscles joined together.

The complex-muscle is several complete-penniform muscles united into one.

There are many half-penniform and complex muscles in the human body, but hardly one instance of a distinct complete-penniform muscle.

In proportion to their combination their fibres are shorter, and a greater number in a given size, which must make them proportionally stronger.

Situation of Muscles.

Muscles which move bones, cartilages, &c. which are inflexible in themselves, generally lie upon them; for instance, the biceps flexor cubiti lies on the os humeri, the latissimus dorsi upon the back. Now the humerus and spine have little motion in themselves when these muscles have occasion to act. Muscles, however, lie sometimes upon the axis of motion, the body of the muscle going over the joint. This is most remarkable in parts near the centre of the body, as in the muscles of the spine, and in those of the first joints, or setting on of the extremities.

The necessity of this disposition will appear more evident when we consider the vast power which must often be brought into a small space. In the spine, for example, there is not surface sufficient in this chain of small bones for the origin and insertion of a sufficient quantity of muscle; therefore the fixed point of the most superficial muscles is removed to a distant and broader base, and they pass over several joints to their different insertions, as the longissimus dorsi, sacro-lumbalis, &c.

The same disposition is necessary in the first joints of the extremities; the extremities come out at once from the trunk, which is a broad or extended base for muscular attachment, so that the muscles are obliged to pass over the joint some way to find a surface for their insertion.

Muscles in general lie in the direction of the parts they are to move, there are, however, exceptions to this where there is an irregularity in the motion of the joint, as in the motions of the head, shoulders, ribs, thighs, &c.

In those animals which have one great centre of motion, to which a series of smaller ones are subordinate, as in man, the bodies of the muscles are in general nearer to the fixed point than to the moving one; and the muscular fibres often arise from the fixed point itself, without the interposition of a tendon; these muscles, however, do not come near to the moveable point, but are attached to it by a tendon, and frequently a very long one. This brings the body of the muscle, which is the heavy part, nearer to the centre or basis of the whole body, which is most able to support it; it also makes the part to be moved freer, more fit for motion, and better adapted for other purposes which may be required.

Tendons and Fasciæ, and their Uses.

In most machines constructed for motion by art, there is the machine itself, or all the different parts which are formed for motion, so disposed as to make one part when moved become the cause of motion in another, communicating it to every part of the machine; and the moving power is superadded, and is not to be considered as being a part of any such machine. A horse, for instance, cannot be considered as a part of any machine which he moves, although he is essential to its motion.

This is also the case in many parts of the more perfect animals where great variety of motion was necessary, parts being constructed for the purpose of motion only, having no power within themselves, but this power is superadded or applied to them, as in the extremities of many animals; but there is no known animal so mechanically constructed in all its parts as to have the power distinct from the parts to be acted upon in every part of its structure. There are in all animals parts constructed for motion which have the power of moving within themselves; those in the more perfect animals are the heart, stomach, intestines, &c. In the more simple animals all the parts of the body are composed of materials with the power of motion, so that in them the machine and power are combined in one, as in the polypus, leech, worm, &c.

In the parts of the compound animal constructed for motion each part is independent of another, so that one part may move, or have its motion complete, while all the other parts are at rest; but although the mechanical parts are so constructed as to have their motions independent, yet the simple effect is not always produced, for the powers are in many places so applied as for one power to move two, three, or more parts, as in the fingers. The same power has often a retrograde effect, moving the part which was its fixed point of motion.

In an animal body the machine constructed for motion is composed of bones, cartilages, &c., and the unions of these form the places for motion, called joints.

The construction of the bones at those parts which constitute the joints is only such as adapts them for motion on each other, not making them become themselves powers so as to move each other, as in the machines constructed by art.

The bones and cartilages are confined or kept together by strong pliable substances called ligaments.

There are also parts called tendons, which are the medium of union between the different parts of the machine and the powers. They have hitherto been considered as belonging to the powers; but I shall rather make them a part of the machine itself.

A tendon is a peculiar substance, placed between some muscles or powers and the parts of the machine to be acted upon by such powers. It is composed of white fibres placed parallel to each other, forming a chord, which is extremely flexible, has no sensible elasticity, and is much smaller than the power to which it is attached.

Its figure is in general a little rounded; sometimes, however, rather flattened, and in many situations it is broad and thin; in all cases it is extended between the body to be moved and the power.

It is sometimes spread out in breadth, and is then called fascia: this form answers various purposes. Its fibres in some situations run pretty parallel, but in general they are interwoven. It has flexibility, strength, and convenience in size. The application of this substance is extremely extensive, complicated, and various.

The parts adapted to motion in animal bodies, as bones, tendons, &c., are formed with greater nicety, and fitted for more exact motions in the more perfect animals, of which we have a striking instance in the human subject.

The purposes which this substance, called tendinous, answers in the animal machine are the following:

First, it intervenes between the body to be moved and the power, to keep up the exact proportion necessary between them to produce any determined motion, so that the length of the bones, or the distance between the joints or points of motion, the quantity of motion in the joint, and the quantity of contraction in the muscle, are proportioned to one another. But if this substance had been wanting, and the muscular fibres had extended the whole distance between many of those joints, the power of contraction in such a muscle would have been much too great, especially in the extremities[a]. The tendon is used for this purpose princi-

---

[a] [A most beautiful and forcible example of the use of tendon in limiting the length of a muscle to the extent of motion required to be produced in the part to be moved occurs in the sterno-thyroidei of the giraffe. Had these muscles been continued fleshy as usual, from their origin, through the whole length of the neck, to their insertion, it is obvious that a great proportion of the muscular fibres would have been useless, because such a condition of the muscle would have been equal to have drawn down the larynx and os hyoides more than one third of the extent of the neck, which is neither required nor permitted by the mechanical attachments of the parts. The sterno thyroidei, therefore, proceed from the head of the sternum blended together in one fleshy fascicu-

pally where the fibres of the muscle run parallel to the direction of motion ; for we shall find the tendons to which many muscles are attached longer than we could suppose necessary, from this reason singly. This, however, arises in them from the oblique manner in which the muscular fibres are placed, and the mode of their being attached to the tendon, as may be seen in the complete-penniform.

Secondly, tendons and fascia are in many places substituted for bone, there not being a sufficient surface of bone for the attachment of all the muscles in an animal body ; and, by being much smaller and thinner, they exclude the necessity of bone.

Thirdly, tendons and fasciæ, from their flexibility, answer in many parts better than bone; for if a long process or thin lamella of bone had united the ends of the muscles to the principal bones to be moved, no motion could have been produced by the endeavour of such muscles. In many situations, where flexibility is not required, they answer better than bone, from their yielding to external or internal pressure, which bone could not have done without being liable to be broken ; as in those situations where they give attachment to two muscles, and where they cover many muscles, as in the forearm. The advantage arising from the flexibility of tendon and fascia is seen in its full extent by comparing the muscles of the more perfect animals with those of the oyster, lobster, or turtle, where many of them are attached to external shells, instead of fasciæ. Flexibility also allows them to vary their direction, by which means they vary the motion of the parts, as in the tendon of the biceps flexor of the forearm winding round the head of the radius : the first action of the muscle (in some positions of the bone) gives it rotation upon its axis, the second bends it upon the os humeri. Similar actions are produced by the latissimus dorsi and teres major.

Fourthly, fasciæ from their strength answer in many situations better than bone, for a lamella of bone of the same thickness would in many cases have been broken by the contraction of the muscle to which it was attached.

Fifthly, it was necessary that some substance should be introduced

---

lus for about nine inches, and end in a tendon which is continued for six inches; this then divides and the muscles proceed again fleshy for about sixteen inches, when a second tendon intervenes in each between the preceding and the next fleshy portion, which is finally inserted into the thyroid cartilage, and, by a continued fascia, into the os hyoides : thus the quantity of contractile fibre is proportioned to the required extent of motion by intervening tendons ; the sterno-hyoidei being wanting, or their place supplied by the sterno-thyroidei, as in some other ruminants.

The analogue of the omo-hyoideus is, in the same animal, adjusted to its office by a different and more simple modification ; its origin is removed from the shoulder-blade to the nearest point (the third cervical vertebra) from which it could act with the requisite force and extent upon the os hyoides.]

as a medium between bones and muscles, to admit of the nicety of action and freedom of motion we find in many parts of the body, particularly in the fingers; which could not have taken place if the muscles had been continued from bone to bone.

Where flexibility is not necessary we find then that there is a continuation of bone, as in many birds, as in the leg of the turkey, partridge, &c., and through the whole body of most fishes; so that tendon is to be considered as a substitute for bone where that substance would be improper. Physiologists, however, have given a very different idea of it, supposing it to be a continuation and condensation of the muscular fibres; for which supposition there is no proof, even the smallest shadow of reason, either from analogy or from the parts themselves: it is therefore too absurd to deserve refutation.

Besides the uses of fasciae above described, we find them in many parts of the body covering muscles, giving origin to them, binding down the belly of the muscle, and also binding down the tendon which is attached to it: this application of them is chiefly found in the extremities, particularly the forearm and leg.

Where the fascia binds down the tendon at or near the joint it is called ' annular ligament,' which is in general little more than the fascia made strong; but where greater nicety in the motion of the parts is required we find annular bindings independent of the general fascia, as in the fingers and toes. These are to keep the tendons from having lateral motions, and where the joint makes an angle, to prevent their coming into straight lines, which would happen if not prevented by this annular ligament, and which would destroy the intention of the joint, as is evident in the fingers.

Where the fascia covers two muscles it is fixed to the tendon which lies between them, and generally covers their tendons.

Where it covers a tendon it almost surrounds it, making a kind of theca, and is fixed to the bone along which the tendon passes.

These circumstances only take place where muscles are placed at a considerable distance from the parts to be moved, and their tendons pass over more joints than one, as in the muscles of the forearm and leg, where the tendons go to the fingers and toes.

Fascia is sometimes very thin, called membrana communis musculorum, covering superficial muscles, particularly the broad ones, as the obliqui externi, latissimus dorsi, pectoralis, &c., and on some of the deeper-seated broad muscles, but thinner and looser in its connexion with the muscles. It is never met with in this state on the round muscles.

It would seem to be intended to connect the skin by its cellular membrane more closely to the muscles, by which means the skin may be in some measure moved by them.

The fasciæ in some instances give insertion to muscles, as in the thigh, and to the broad abdominal muscles.

Attachment of Muscles to Tendons.

As the body of a muscle is much thicker than the tendon to which it is attached, the fibres of the one cannot be continued to the other in a straight line; therefore the end of the tendon is not joined to that of the muscle in one line, but by a tapering point or an irregular edge, to gain surface for the insertion of the muscular fibres, the oblique ending of a small body being capable of becoming equal to the less oblique ending of a thick one; but the direction of the tendon cannot be the same with the muscular fibres, but must be more or less oblique, so that an angle must be formed at their union, the muscular fibres being bent a little in towards the tendinous ones. This obliquity in the direction of most of the muscular fibres, and of their attachments at both ends when they have tendons at both origin and insertion, makes the muscle become gradually thicker from the body of the first tendon to the most distant point of that tendon; and if the middle part of the muscle is free from tendon, that part will be everywhere equal in size, or if the tendon at its insertion goes higher than at its origin, the part where these tendons are opposite and parallel to one another will also be equal in size, the body of the muscle from that part becoming gradually smaller upwards towards its origin, and downwards towards its insertion.

From such disposition of fibres the bodies of most muscles are much

longer than their component fibres, which produces in the same proportion a shorter complete tendon. This circumstance lessens the thickness of the bodies of such muscles, and also of their extremities, which gives to the muscle a curve in its outer line.

The obliquity in the direction of the muscular fibres admits of there being a greater number, and lengthens the swell in the time of contraction, by which means the motion of the muscles in the cellular membrane becomes more free, the swell is smaller, and the smoothness of the whole body is preserved. The tendon at its origin is generally on one side, or surrounding the muscle, and the inserting tendon is on the opposite side, or next the centre of motion.

Origin and Insertion of Muscles.

In describing the origin and insertion of muscles the tendons are always included, and this is very necessary to be understood of the insertion, as it is the point of insertion which in some degree gives the use of the muscle.

The origin of a muscle is in general the most fixed point, and the insertion the point where the greatest motion is produced; in different muscles, however, these points are subject to variations, and on different occasions in the same muscle, most of them being capable of acting from either end. Some of these variations may be considered as natural, and others as a force upon Nature.

I shall call the variations natural where the effect is necessary in the natural movements of any part of the body, such as the extensors of the thigh, the glutæi, particularly the glutæus major, are commonly understood to produce; for these muscles, in the action of walking, when the leg is brought forwards or bent by the flexors, extend the body upon the thigh, by which action the body is brought forwards before and over the foot; also, after stooping or bending the body forwards, the glutæus muscle raises it; and these are as much the actions of this muscle as bringing the leg and thigh back upon the body.

Some muscles are capable of performing similar inverted actions, although not commonly so employed as the recti abdominis, whose ordinary use is to bend the body upon the pelvis, but which sometimes, however, bend the pelvis upon the body. Those which I call a force upon the natural effect of the muscle, or an inversion of the fixed point, are where the moving point is by art, or something foreign to the body made the fixed one, as the hand; and the action of the muscles, instead of bringing the hand to the body, draws the body to the hand.

In many animals, however, the effects of certain muscles are reciprocal, and these therefore cannot be said to have an origin and insertion, both the parts to which they are attached being equally moveable in themselves, and there being no power capable of keeping either the one or the other firm, as is very evident in animals where the two points of attachment, or parts to be moved, are similar or in pairs, as in the bivalve shell, where the motion in the two valves is equal.

The origins of muscles are in general more simple than their insertions, nothing being wanted but a sufficient surface for attachment, which is generally required to be pretty extensive; and for this purpose there are various contrivances, which have given rise to particular names, for the various kinds of origins.

The origin of a muscle is generally from an immoveable part with respect to the action of that muscle, and commonly from the most firm or solid parts of the body, as bones, cartilages, periosteum, tendons, and fascia; some muscles, however, arise from soft parts, as the lingualis, orbicularis oris, &c.

The insertions of muscles are less simple, for as the insertion is to produce the various motions of the parts, and, as the construction for motion is hardly the same in any two joints, more nicely and art is required; the insertions of muscles are commonly more determined than the origins.

Few muscles are so situated as to arise from surfaces at right angles to the direction of their fibres, as they generally pass nearly in the same direction with the surface from which they arise, whether bone, tendon, or fascia. They therefore take their origin from a part as they pass along it, which renders it very oblique, and produces the form of muscle called half-penniform. Some muscles, however, both arise from, and are inserted into, surfaces at right angles to the direction of their fibres, as many of the spine, &c.

The insertions of muscles are more general than their origins, for they must be inserted into every part of the body to be moved, and therefore we find them inserted into bones, cartilages, periosteum, tendons, fascia, and many of them into soft parts, as the skin, cellular membrane, the tongue, &c.

In describing muscles, they are never said to be inserted into, or to arise from, periosteum, but from the bone the periosteum covers, as it is upon the bone the effect is produced.

Muscles never arise from, or are inserted into, capsular ligaments, for although in some few cases they seem to run into, or are attached to them, the effect is not immediately on the capsular ligament, but on the bone beyond it, and the ligament is strengthened at this part in proportion to the power of the muscle; so that in this case, as far as regards the mechanical effect, the ligament and tendon may be considered as one.

Many tendons, in their course over joints, adhere to the ligaments, and bring them along with them in the action of their muscles. This adhesion, however, is only to bring out a secondary use, to save the ligament from being bruised between the bones, which otherwise might have been the case.

Many muscles besides these insertions give off fibres to the fasciæ, which cover other muscles, as is evident from the lower edge of the pectoralis major, biceps flexor cubiti, semitendinosus, &c., but what is intended by it is difficult to determine.

The origins of muscles are generally further from the centre of motion of the part to be moved than the insertion; remarkable instances of this are seen in the biceps flexor and triceps extensor of the forearm, and all the movers of the hand and fingers. This gives neatness to the parts to be moved; but its principal use is to give velocity to the motion, with a small quantity of contraction; what it gains, however, in velocity, it loses in strength. That velocity is the intention is evident, for if the muscular fibres had been continued to the most distant end of the bone to be moved, the muscle must have been longer, and must have contracted more, to produce the same effect, which contraction must have taken a greater length of time[a].

Many muscles arise near to the centre of motion of the part to be moved, and are inserted at a considerable distance, as the *deltoides*. This also produces a great deal of motion in the part to be moved, with very little contraction of the muscle; for when the greatest quantity of motion is produced, the insertion has approached very little nearer the origin.

This kind of insertion gives an advantage to the power of the muscle, which the other has not, viz. a much longer lever, and allows the muscles to communicate their strength to the moving parts more fully, although with less velocity; and being employed upon parts of considerable extent, as the arm and leg, and generally upon the first joints of them, the effects upon the hand and foot are very considerable.

In the formation of many parts of the body neatness is a principal object, as is visible, not only in the external form of the limb, but in the parts constructed for motion; as in the formation of the bones, and their situation with respect to one another, and the mode of removing the inserted tendon (when too close to the centre of motion to produce a sufficient effect) a little further off, by means of little moveable bones called patellæ or sesamoid bones, as in the knee, first joints of the thumb and great toe: and where this construction would be clumsy and inconvenient, as in the fingers and lesser toes, the two tendons which are obliged to pass along these parts to their insertions at the second and third joints, are so disposed in their course, that the profundus, or one nearest to the bone, acts as a patella to the other, keeping it at a distance from the centre of motion equal to its own thickness; and the sublimis or upper one is obliged to split into two near its termination before it can be inserted into the second bone. The advantage gained by this construction is, that the tendon of the muscle employed in the greatest action is removed further from the centre of motion than it otherwise could be, and from which the other sustains no disadvantage.

Adaptation of Muscles to Joints.

It is to be understood that the joints of an animal are fitted for motion, and that their form, with the application of the muscle or power, are, in a natural state, so adapted to each other that the power acts with the greatest advantage, and that any variation from the natural form or

---

[a] [The extent of the space through which the bone is moved is also greatly increased by this arrangement, in comparison with the extent to which the muscle itself contracts.]

position of the joint weakens the effect of the power.   This may be demonstrated in those who turn out their toes, as in a dancing-master,
who, before he makes a leap, turns his toes forwards.

Few joints in an animal body are confined to one motion, therefore
either a number of single muscles must be employed, or the direction of
the muscular fibres, of the tendons, and of the insertions, must be so disposed that a few muscles may produce the different effects.

Joints admitting of motion in only one direction come nearest to a
simple joint ; the joint of the elbow is perhaps as near this as any in most
animals, as also the joint of the lower jaw in the carnivorous animals,
and the fingers in most animals[a] : the muscles of such joints are tolerably
simple in their structure, direction, and insertion.

In the joints which admit of various or compound motions, the construction of the muscle, the course of its different fibres, the disposition
of the tendon in its course and insertion, produce a great variety of effects.

This, indeed, was absolutely necessary in a number of animals, more
especially those which have extremities, and particularly the human
subject, in which there are more motions produced than separate muscles to perform them ; nor was it possible, in the present construction
of bones, &c., to have placed particular muscles so as to perform all the
motions, without interfering in the opposite actions.   In the human
subject the number of muscles exceeds that of any other animal ; the
motions in the joints, however, are still greater than can be accounted
for by the increase in number of muscles, the difference in the construction of the muscles, as well as of the joints, producing this difference,
which is so remarkable in the joint of the shoulder, the rotatory motion
in the forearm, and the joint of the thigh.

Instances of the different motions produced by the shape of muscles,
their mode of application, and the disposal of tendons, are seen in the
biceps flexor cubiti, latissimus dorsi, &c. passing some way round the
bones into which they are inserted, so as to produce two very different
motions in the parts ; at one time they may move the part through some
space, at another time upon its own axis.   The muscles in the lower
jaw in graminivorous animals give a remarkable instance of this, there
being hardly any of them which do not perform more than one motion.

The disposition of tendons will often give a different direction to the
body moved from that of the muscle, arising from the tendon bending
over some fixed point and taking another direction, which is beautifully
illustrated in the trochlearis muscle of the eye, the body of it passing in
the same direction as the straight muscle of the eyeball, while from the
course of its tendon it counteracts the oblique, which passes in a dif-

---

[a] [In insects and crustacea every joint of the extremities, save that which is between the limb and the body, is ginglymoid, and limited to motion in one plane.]

ferent direction. The obturator internus of the thigh and circumflexus palati are both of this kind.

The different positions of tendons shall make two muscles produce the same effect in different ways, being inserted in the opposite sides of the same joint. The gastrocnemius, which is inserted into the heel behind the joint of the foot, pulls the heel up, which depresses the toes. The tibialis posticus and peronei muscles, which pass in the same direction, and are inserted before the joint of the foot by means of their tendon passing round the joint, also pull the toes down, which raises the heel.

Muscles, by the course and mode of insertion of their tendons, shall perform very differently a series of regular motions, bending some joints and extending others. Such are the uses of the lumbricales and interossei interni upon the fingers and toes; for their course is before the centre of motion in the first joint, but by winding round the second bone they get upon the back of the fingers and extend the two last joints. These, by their situation and insertion, produce an effect which could not be performed by the other flexors or extensors of the same parts.

From the various formations of joints, and the different positions and insertions of the muscles or powers, the greatest force of the power is required at different periods of the motion.

In all those where the power is between the centre of motion and the resistance, the greatest action of the muscle is required at the beginning, as a smaller contraction of the muscle produces a greater effect at this time than afterwards, as in the deltoid.

Where the power and weight are at the two ends and the fulcrum in the middle, as in the biceps extensor of the arm, or where the power and the fulcrum are at the two ends and the weight in the middle, as in the muscles of the tendo Achillis, the greatest force is required in the last part of the motion.

Where there is no lever, but one body moving round a centre as a pulley, which is the case in the extensors of the knee-joint, the same force is required through the whole of the motion.

We may observe that the ligaments of the joints are necessarily so constructed and placed with respect to their motion as to produce an effect analogous to that of a centre-pin in a plain circular joint, in all the various situations of the centre of motion.

There are few levers of the first kind in the body, on account of the unevenness in the effects of muscular contraction upon them, arising from the variation taking place in the angle of insertion of the muscle; they are therefore introduced where that is compensated by some other circumstance in the action.

The motion of the body upon the thigh is a lever of this kind, and is generally used in raising the body; but as the body becomes more and more bent it requires less power to overcome the power of gravity in the body, therefore the angle of insertion is becoming more and more in the same plane with the moving part. The same thing takes place in moving the heel.

The angle of insertion can only have its effects vary when the insertion is some way from the centre of motion, and this only when in levers.

When in levers of the first kind (which extend joints) the effect is gradually becoming less; as, for instance, the extensors of the forearm, which are inserted into the olecranon, because the angle is becoming less and less; but perhaps the velocity which the parts may commonly acquire may make up this loss. When inserted into levers of the second kind they are gaining in their effect, the angle becoming greater, as in the flexors of the forearm.

In the lever of the first kind the quantity of effect, according to the quantity of contraction, is becoming more and more as the angle becomes less. In the second it is becoming less and less as the angle becomes greater.

Muscles going over more Joints than one.

Many muscles, or their tendons, go over two joints while they only move one, and the joint which they do not move is often moving in a contrary direction, from the action of another muscle; this happens in the biceps flexor and extensor of the forearm, the flexors of the leg, &c. This disposition saves a great deal of muscular contraction; for by the biceps going over two joints while it is employed in bending the forearm upon the arm, the arm is bending back upon the scapula, which last action would produce in some degree a flexion of the forearm, even if the biceps flexor did not contract at all, but only remained without relaxing. This arises from the motion of these joints going zigzag to one another.

Muscles whose tendons pass over two joints keep the joint not to be moved, firm; which is of great service, as when we bend the forearm by the biceps flexor, the two heads rising from the scapula, especially the long head which runs through the joint, keeps the joint of the shoulder firm. In this motion there are muscles acting on both sides of the joint. Had it not been for this purpose, the biceps flexor might as well have arisen from the head of the os humeri.

Muscles often go over two, three, or four joints, and only move the third and fourth, as the flexors of the last joints of the fingers; but to prevent the first and second joints being moved by this action, the extensors of the intermediate joints are obliged to interfere and keep them from bending.

Every joint has a certain quantity of motion, and the quantity of contraction of the muscles of that joint are adapted to that motion; we have therefore in joints of considerable motion long muscles, as those of the knee, and in joints with little motion we have short muscles, as those of the spine.

Of the Strength of the Body as compounded.

The strength of a part and the strength of the whole body is in proportion to the natural resistance, which arises either from some body to be propelled, as the blood, urine, &c., or from the position of our bodies to overcome gravitation; for every muscle in the body is just able to move the part to which it is fixed with tolerable ease in the most difficult position, and any additional weight in that position will fatigue it, it being unable to support it any time. From this it would appear that the different parts of our bodies are not much stronger than can support their own motions with ease; and whatever motion the body can perform with ease, by exerting itself it can give it a considerable velocity, or support a greater weight for a continuance.

If our muscles are capable of moving our bodies in every position, they must be able to move much more in some positions than others. If I can raise my body from the ground perpendicularly up when my feet are fixed upon the ground and my knees bent at right angles, I can support or raise a much greater weight when upright or nearly so.

If a horse raise himself from the ground when his legs are bent, he can support a greater weight when erect or standing; and if loaded with no more than he can stand under upon three feet, he can walk with it. A leg also that can raise the quarter of a horse from the ground can move the parts of which it is constructed only with great velocity.

If you load a man with no more than he can stand under upon one foot, he can walk with the load. A man can raise his whole body upon his hands, and therefore can move his hands with great velocity when they are put into motion without the body.

The Effects arising from the different Constructions of Muscles.

The straight narrow muscle, whose fibres run parallel, generally employs all its fibres, so that when it acts, the whole muscle is in action at the same time.

The broad and radiated muscles do not always employ the whole of

their fibres at the same time, each part often acting separately, like separate muscles; they are capable of taking on an action at any one part,
and of continuing from that part a succession of actions to any other
part, or through the whole muscle; and they are capable, by an action
of the whole muscle, of producing one general effect. The action of
the lateral portions of such muscles affects the tendon somewhat similar
to the complete-penniform; therefore the middle fibres must either be
longer than the lateral, or have a greater power of contraction, which
will be better understood after the explanation of the action of the complete-penniform.

The temporal muscle is an exception to the rule of muscles being
made radiated to produce a succession of actions; for whatever part of
this muscle acts, nearly the same effect is produced; such muscles, *cæteris
paribus*, produce effects proportioned to their length of fibres.

These muscles have one advantage, which is, that their fibres are
much longer than those of any other muscle whose body is of an equal
length; they can therefore contract much more, and are always used
in the more extensive motions.

The half-penniform muscle is, I believe, similar in its action to the
foregoing; for although the fibres are more oblique, the tendon is moveable laterally, so as to move nearly in the same line with the fibres.
This kind of muscle is never used in extensive motions, except where
there is considerable distance between the origin and insertion, to admit
of sufficient length of fibres.

Although there is hardly an instance of a
complete-penniform muscle in the body, yet
as all the complex penniform act upon the
same principle, I shall explain the effects in
a supposed complete-penniform, and show
that this disposition of fibres produces a
greater effect than any of the foregoing.

In the action of these muscles we suppose
that the inserted tendon is always moved in
the middle line, between the two origins of
the muscle, and therefore the muscular fibres
in this action do not lose their obliquity, as
in the half-penniform, but have it increased,
which produces a greater effect.

Let A C and B C represent two fibres of
a penniform muscle in their extended state,
A and B being their origin, and C the point
of insertion into the tendon C D.

Suppose these fibres contracted to the points E and F, it is evident that such contraction will bring the point of insertion from C to G, and that the motion of the tendon will be to the contraction of the muscle as C G is to C F or C E; for A G is equal to A E, and B G equal to B F, or A and B are the centres of the circles A G E and B G F.

The advantage arising from this construction of muscle is great, as it allows of a great number of fibres in small bulk, and is therefore used where strength is required. It is also used where the quantity of motion required is greater than the distance between the origin and insertion would admit of in any other construction of muscle.

CROONIAN LECTURE ON MUSCULAR MOTION, No. III.

[Read before the Royal Society in the year 1779, by John Hunter, F.R.S.]

Of the Effects of Muscles.

IN the spring of 1776 I had the honour of delivering to this Society the Croonian Lecture upon the self-moving power in animals seated in the muscles, in which I also made some observations on the analogy between this power in animals and a similar power in vegetables.

I was then desired to prosecute this subject, and accordingly, in the winter following I presented a paper, in which I considered the most remarkable circumstances relative to this power in animals, through which they are enabled to perform all their various motions,—such as the arrangement of the fibres in the construction of all the muscles; the distinct muscles, their figure, kinds, and situation; the tendons, and fasciæ, with their uses; the applications of muscles to tendons, their origin and insertion, and the fitness of them to the joints.   It was here noticed that their effect in some cases is equal to their quantity of contraction; in others not.   The different quantity of contraction in the same length of fibres in different muscles was observed, and the effect arising from the different construction of muscles.

As the muscles are, by their contraction, the cause, either immediate or remote, of every action in the animal, and as animals are so constructed as to produce evident mechanical effects, arising from an application or combination of the mechanical powers (the contraction of the muscles being the power or original cause), I shall now consider this mechanical application and its effects, with which I shall slightly compare the applications and effects of the mechanical powers as applied in machines which are the productions of art.

Muscles are the first simple powers in an animal by which all the mechanical effects are ultimately produced; but an animal body is very differently constructed from that of a machine.

A machine is composed of a series of parts, having a regular dependence on each other; and the power which produces motion is applied only at one end of these parts, although two, three, or more effects may ultimately be produced, which effects, notwithstanding, must therefore arise from the multiplication of the parts of the machine, and not from the increased number of powers.

But an animal is composed of parts, each part, and each motion of each part, having its own moving power, capable of producing its immediate and remote effects independent of each other: so that in animals many effects may be going on at one and the same time, and each actuated by its own peculiar power, by which means an innumerable variety of effects are carried on at the same time, and without the least confusion or interference with each other.

A muscle, as to itself, may be considered in two lights, one respecting its quantity of contraction, and the other its power, both of which produce considerable effects in the body, and each is employed according to circumstances.

Every muscle in an animal body may be considered as a simple independent power; and if we attend to the effects that many animals are capable of producing, particularly the motion of fishes and the flight of birds, we shall see great reason to admire the immense velocity and great force with which their muscles are contracted; and if we compare the effects produced by the contraction of their muscles with the weight of each muscle and the part which is to move, it may lead us to conclude that there probably is not in nature a more active simple power than the contraction of the animal muscles. An animal is perhaps the only machine that has the power of overcoming its own gravity.

In considering animal bodies in general in a mechanical light, we should first attend to the most simple mode of action in the animal, or the mode of action of the muscles in the most simple animal, and proceed from the most simple to the most compound or complicated, in which latter may be discovered applications and combinations of the several mechanical powers (which for beauty, simplicity, regularity, and aptness far excel all human applications), in order to produce the manifold effects of animal motion, and to accommodate the ultimate velocity or force at the same time to the particular effects to be produced, as well as to the simple power of contraction in the several muscles which act as first movers in producing that effect.

In many animals the parts endowed with the first principles of motion, viz., the muscular fibres, are themselves formed in various shapes, so as to constitute complete animals of the most simple fibres; and even in the most complicated animal many distinct parts are composed of those moving powers, forming regular bodies, called organs, commonly producing of themselves a vast variety of effects, by which means many of the numberless internal actions respecting the animal œconomy are carried on; so that even in those more complicated animals we have the first organization formed of muscular fibres alone, in the same manner as in the more simple animals[a].

This would lead us to consider the effects of muscular contraction in very different views, viz. according to the various effects they are capable of producing in animals of all the various constructions and complications.

In many of the more simple animals there is little else besides those formations or organizations composed of muscles.   A polypus is little more than a muscular bag, and by the contraction of its fibres in different parts, and in different directions at different times, the bag is changed into various forms and sizes.

A worm seems a little more complicated ; however it is in reality little more than a body formed of different parts, each of which is composed of muscle.   A slug, a maggot, as also numberless tribes of sea-animals, come under the same description.

But as animals emerge from this simplicity of construction, becoming more and more complicated, having particular parts added, and those parts being composed of something besides muscle, and it also being necessary that these should move, and be so constructed as to direct, circumscribe, increase, or limit the motion, we find the muscular fibres of such animals collected into various portions and forms, in order to give all the different motions to these superadded parts which were taken notice of in the former lecture.   Those additional parts are composed of more rigid matter than muscle, viz. bones, cartilages, &c., on which the muscles can have no other influence than by giving them motion.   There are a number of those bones, cartilages, &c. in many animals, some having more, some fewer; and they are connected in such a way as to form between them intervals fit for motion, called joints : in most parts of the body there is a series of those bones and joints, as the spine, the extremities, &c.

Many of these bones are so formed, and so placed and connected with one another, as to form levers (and those of all the various kinds), which direct and limit the motions, so as to produce a regularity in the whole.

As the relative inclinations and positions of those several bones which are immediately connected and joined together are very various, it fol-

---

[a] [Hunter here compares the first-formed parts of the vertebrate embryo, derived from the mutually receding layers of the germinal membrane and the folding of those layers, with the simple homogeneous tissue of the hydra or other acrite animal. And, as he applies the term *muscular* to the contractile tissue of these animals, so he would also regard the homogeneous gelatinous parietes of the newly formed digestive sac of the embryo of the higher organized species as being in like manner endowed with contractility, and therefore 'formed of muscular fibres' or contractile substance 'alone.']

lows that there must be a variety in the angle of insertion of the several muscles, to accommodate them to the particular circumstance of each joint. And as those inclinations vary in the motions of the joint, so must the angle of insertion of the muscles, which will produce a difference in the effects, both in the power and quantity of contraction.

To this great variety of these levers and joints we have the muscles adapted.

We may observe, that the more perfect the animal is, the more curiously these levers and joints are formed, the joints commonly consisting of compound curves (which is the most remarkable in the more perfect animals), by which means their own motions admit of greater variety.

The human subject is a striking instance of this, having the joints more compounded, and the motions less limited, than in any other animal that I know, which circumstances require a greater variety of muscle, and the greater nicety in the adapting of each muscle to produce its peculiar motion.

In the most perfect animals there are very few joints whose motion is simple, or which are confined on all occasions to move in one direction; for whatever may be their chief or ordinary motion, in many there is some other motion compounded with it; nor are there many joints which move upon one centre in all their motions, but they shift their centre as the curve varies*.

These firm inflexible substances are kept together by soft, yielding, yet sufficiently strong parts, called ligaments, which are necessarily so constructed and placed, with respect to the motion of the joint, as to produce an effect analogous to that of a centre pin in a plain circular joint, and in all the various situations of the centres of motion.

I may be allowed to observe, previous to entering upon the mechanical motions produced by the muscles in an animal body, that, without external resistance, there would be no such thing as progressive motion in an animal; for although a muscle has the power of contraction in itself, and is capable of moving all its different parts upon itself, yet it cannot move any other part without having some fixed point to act from, which is the greatest point of resistance. There is in every animal, therefore, a fixed point from which the parts of the body take their principal motions. In the human body this fixed point seems to be in the joints of the thigh-bones; which point, being in the middle of the body, must be common to the extremities. We see, therefore, that the body either moves on the legs, or that the legs move on the body or trunk. Besides this, there are many fixed points, so that the body is to

---

* A remarkable instance of this we have in the joint of the lower jaw in graminivorous animals.

be looked upon as a chain of joints whose general centre of motion is in the joints of the thighs; but each has its fulcrum, or centre of motion, which is always on that side next to the first, or the general centre of motion of the whole, by which means the smaller moves upon the greater, the toe upon the foot, the foot upon the leg, the leg upon the thigh, and the thigh upon the body. The same in the arms, the wings of birds, the tails of fishes, the oars of a boat, &c. But those motions can be, and often are, inverted, so that the greater can be made to move upon the smaller; as, for instance, the body upon the thigh, the thigh upon the leg; or, in birds, the body upon the wing, &c.; but then the smaller must be so circumstanced as to be the fixed point, which cannot be without external resistance. It is the inverted motions, then, which produce the progressive; but it is necessary, for the production of a succession of them, to bring in also the motion of smaller parts upon greater; the two kinds of motion are, therefore, acting alternately whenever the progressive motion is continued beyond the first action.

The animals which move upon the earth have it for their point of resistance. Birds are supported and propelled in their flight by the resistance of the air; and fishes, like boats, by the resistance of the water.

The effects of muscular contraction may be divided into three kinds.

The first is, where the effects are in those parts of the body which are principally composed of muscle: these simply vary their configuration without extending their power beyond themselves, as in the actions of many of the more imperfect tribes of animals, as the leech, polypus, &c., and in many parts of the more perfect animals, as the heart, stomach, intestines, bladder, and all the vascular system[a].

The second is where the effect is more extended and reaches beyond the muscles themselves to such adjoining parts as are either formed simply for motion, as bones, cartilages, &c., or whole parts of the body, such as an eye, a lip, the skin, &c.

The third is where the effects are mixed, viz. partake of both the preceding, as in those produced by the muscles of the tongue, of respiration, of the abdomen, &c., where they both move parts and alter their configuration.

The first and third kind of effects of muscles, when considered in the more perfect animals, are more connected with the internal œconomy of the animal than with the mechanical application of the power of mus-

---

[a] [This is not exactly true of these viscera, for their contents ejected by the contraction of the surrounding fibres act upon the parts into which they are propelled, as the bone moved by the muscle inserted into it also carries the parts connected with it along with it in its motions.]

cular contraction; therefore in them it is the second which comes properly under consideration, as mechanical, since it produces visible mechanical effects upon parts formed for motion, and evidently calculated to vary the velocity from that of the first.

The application of muscles in an animal body is either to produce a quantity of motion equal to the quantity of contraction of the muscle; or, by the application of levers, to give a greater motion than could be produced by the simple contraction of the muscle. This in general is not the case in machines composed by art; for in art the principal reason for the introduction of mechanics is to acquire power in the effect, which obliges us to increase the velocity in the moving cause, as in levers and pulleys. However, this is not universal in machines; for some have it reversed, as the catapulta, the lock of a gun, and also in many machines where strength is not the object but velocity in some particular movements, as in watches, jacks, &c.

Whether the effect of a given quantity of contraction in a muscle be or be not equal to that quantity depends upon the construction and disposition of the parts to be moved, or the form which the whole muscle is thrown into. Thus the effects of some muscles upon the parts are just equal to the contraction of the muscular fibres; such are those which simply draw parts to them, not varying the position of the part moved from the right line, as many of the muscles of the larynx, the trapezius, rhomboideus, and all of the panniculus carnosus kind, as the muscles of the face, platysma myoides, and the muscles of the skin of animals.

Another class, whose effects are always known, or are the same in all cases, are those muscles which produce their effects from the shape which the muscle is thrown into, for instance, a curve. Curved muscles are of two kinds, viz. those which are fixed at their ends, as the abdominal muscles, pharynx, &c., and those which are circular, as the sphincters, heart, and the whole vascular system. These muscles always reduce the circumference and, of course, the diameter of the circle, which they themselves compose, in proportion to their quantity of contraction; but the ultimate effect here is not in proportion to the quantity of contraction, but decreases as the squares of the diameters of such vessels. But most parts of the body are so mechanically formed, acting as levers, and the muscles so advantageously inserted, as to produce a much greater degree of velocity in the motion of the part than is equal to the contraction of the muscle. But those mechanical applications are so various that there are no two muscles which act with the same advantages, excepting those that are in pairs. On this application of muscles to levers depends the distinction between the absolute and apparent force of muscles, neither of which can possibly be ascertained with any degree of certainty.

Every muscular fibre is capable of contracting with a given power, which power simply must be always its absolute force; but from the construction of parts to be moved, and the application of muscles to those parts, either an increased or decreased effect is produced.

It is impossible to ascertain the absolute force of a muscle because there is no one known muscle in the body that we can throw into action separately, and independently of the collateral effects of others. And, if we could, there are many whose power could not be measured by any given quantity of resistance to be overcome, so as to ascertain the power of contraction of that muscle, as, e. g. all those which simply pull bodies in a straight line: but, in those muscles which act upon the bones in the form of levers, if any could be made to act singly its power could easily be known. But whatever this power is it must be always the same; nothing can alter it excepting real weakness in the muscular fibres themselves.

As we cannot separate and ascertain the absolute force of a single muscle, so it is impossible to find out the apparent force; and exactly for the same reasons that we cannot find out the absolute. The apparent force of circular muscles will be in a ratio proportionably to their diameters, and in those which are inserted into levers it will always be as the distance of the insertion of the muscle from the centre of motion, the angle of insertion, &c. But the relative force is not always the same, or it loes not always act alone in the motion of the parts, for it is often joined with velocity, and then it may become vastly greater. But if not joined with velocity it will always be less than the absolute, as the length of lever in the resisting power is longer than in the acting one.

The absolute force of a muscle will always be employed in the most simple action of the parts. The most simple action will be where a muscle passes in a straight line from some fixed point to a moveable one and by its contraction simply pulls the moveable one towards the immoveable one, such as many of the muscles of the os hyoides, and in many other parts of the body.

As the circular muscles are commonly employed in propelling bodies, and principally fluids, they will keep up an equal power upon the body to be expelled; for, the power increasing as the fluid decreases, it is capable of throwing out the same quantity in the same time*.

* It may be asked, at what point of the contraction of a muscle has it the greatest power? Or, does it contract with the same force through the whole contraction?

I observed that the muscles, as moving powers in an animal, differ from the moving powers in a machine, the production of art, inasmuch as every part had its power adapted to the motion it is capable of, and therefore the motion of any one part did not depend entirely upon its own configuration and connexion with some other. Although this is in a great measure the truth, yet the motion in most parts is assisted by actions or the contrary in other parts, so that there is a kind of dependence and mutual assistance through the whole. This does not, however, arise from any mechanical construction, but from a connexion of the living principle in the powers of one part with those of another, which may be termed a species of intelligence.

The motion of parts generally is the motion of a smaller upon a greater, and the greater becomes the fixed point upon which the smaller may be said to move; but we find that there are few motions, however trifling, but what affect the greater part; therefore that this motion in the smaller part may be more effectual and answer the intended purpose, the greater part is either thrown into a counter-motion by its own muscles, or it is supported in its place by them, or it is thrown into the same action with the small part, so as to increase it. Hence the actions of these powers may be said to be of two kinds, immediate and secondary.

The first is that which produces the immediate action of the part; the second produces the assistant, supporting, regulating actions, &c. For instance, when a man walks, it at first might appear that the only thing necessary to produce the ultimate effect was the motion of the two legs, the body being first thrown sufficiently forwards, so as always to require that motion of the legs to support the centre of gravity. But this is not sufficient; it is necessary that the muscles of the trunk should act, and regulate the body so as to support the centre of gravity on all sides. If the right leg moves, the muscles of the left side of the trunk act to support the whole on the left leg, and *vice versâ*; so that the body plays upon the motion of the legs, by which means the legs have much less to do, and therefore can support it longer.

In many of the actions of parts of the body other parts are kept immoveable, although they would appear to have nothing to do with any such actions. A man never performs any considerable action, even with any of the extremities, without the trunk being more or less affected, so as to favour the motion of the extremity. We find that we first make a full inspiration and that all the muscles of respiration act, also the muscles of the glottis, and of the soft palate, so as to confine the air which makes the trunk as rigid and firm as possible to support or sustain the actions and motion of the extremity.

If an action takes place in an extremity, where a considerable effect is to be produced, which can only be produced by a considerable velocity, then the whole body gives it assistance so far as it is possible for it to do.

If a man throws a stone, or a blacksmith swings his sledge-hammer, the whole body humours the action, and the fixed point is thrown to a greater distance than the setting-on of the arm : the whole moves from the loins, or perhaps lower.

Those secondary actions are brought in as auxiliaries, and answer two very important purposes : they increase the quantity of action when necessary, and they assist in easing the immediate action, so as to allow of a continuance of it, by which means animals are capable of performing greater actions, with more ease, and a longer continuance.

Muscles regulate the actions of others not only by their contraction but by their relaxation, which last is a kind of negative action. When a man walks I have already observed that there are many muscles acting as secondary agents in the body, so as to assist the immediate motions of the part to be moved; but, besides this, there are many of the same muscles that are gradually relaxing, so as to allow the alternate motions by imperceptible degrees to creep regularly into one another.

Perhaps I cannot give a more striking idea of those primary and secondary actions, with the relaxations, which I have called negative actions, than to present to the minds of those who have some knowledge of the subject what must be going on with the muscles of a man balancing himself on a slack or tight rope, when the first or immediate order of muscles are acting with their utmost force; where the secondary are assisting in the secondary actions of the body, and as it were playing into the hands of the first; where others again are relaxing in proportion as the first and second are acting; and where the entirely relaxed are waiting the opportunity to act, when called upon by any change that shall take place in the position of the body, which in such circumstances is in a continued agitation.

CROONIAN LECTURE ON MUSCULAR MOTION, No. IV.

[The manuscript of this Lecture appears not to have been among those which were accessible to Mr. Clift, and from his copies of which the Lectures in the present volume have, with his permission, been printed. Its absence may, however, be accounted for, from the fact that the substance of the Fourth Croonian Lecture was incorporated by Hunter in his work ' On the Blood,' (see the Chapter on the Vascular System,) as is evident from the Abstract of the Lecture in the Archives of the Royal Society, the subjoined copy of which Abstract Mr. Palmer, with the permission of the President and Council, has obtained for the use of the present edition of Hunter's Works.]

[The Croonian Lecture on Muscular Motion, by Mr. John Hunter, was read on the 25th of May and 1st of June, 1780.]

" THE construction and general application of muscles in the animal body having been discussed by our author in three former lectures, he now proceeds to treat of the action of muscles on the blood-vessels, an inquiry which, however essentially it may contribute to our better acquaintance with the animal œconomy, has yet, it seems, till now been but little attended to, the existence of muscular fibres in the system of blood-vessels being by no means obvious.

" Mr. H. finds it necessary previously to lay down some general principles concerning muscles, which he derives from their operations in those parts of the animal where their uses are well understood.

" A muscle he defines such an arrangement of animal matter as, whilst it is endowed with life, is fitted for self-motion. This motion, he says, consists in the contraction of the muscular fibres, in which light he considers it as totally distinct from elasticity. And he ventures to assert that no part of an animal except the muscles is endowed with this power of self-motion. He acknowledges soon after that this power cannot be the sole effect of contraction, but that there must also be a power of relaxation, acting alternately, without which no effect could be produced. But even this relaxation, he says, is not sufficient to produce any effect without a previous elongation ; and as no muscle is, as such, possessed of this power of elongation, he considers it as the effect of antagonists of some kind or other, or of what may be called the elongators of the muscles, and says, that it is not in all cases muscular, but sometimes the effect of elasticity, and sometimes even of matter foreign to the body. This leads him to distinguish it into three kinds; the first, where it is immediately muscular, or when antagonist muscles act immediately upon each other; the second, when a muscle acts upon some other matter, and gives it the power of an antagonist, as is the case in all those muscles that enter into the formation of canals or cavities, whose elongation is produced by other muscles, which have no immediate connexion with them, but which force them to an extension by propelling the contents of the canal, instances of which we find in the œsophagus, the intestines, and the bladder; and thirdly, when the elongation is owing to elastic substances, which sometimes cooperate with, and sometimes resist the action of muscles; and of other powers, such as gravitation, velocity, &c.

" The second section treats of the application of the muscular and elastic powers, where both indisputably act. The joint application of these two powers we are told is very common, though hitherto it has been but little noticed. Elasticity operates where constant or stationary action is wanted. Muscles are applied where occasional action is required; and where both effects are wanted both powers cooperate. This is illustrated by various examples, among the rest that of a bivalve, which has a muscle between the two shells, for the purpose of closing them, and an elastic ligament in the joint, which constantly tends to diverge them.

" Another instance, much more to the present purpose, is that of the elastic cartilages and membranes of the trachea and its branches, which maintain an equilibrium by counteracting the tendency the muscles of respiration have to contract that channel.

" In most parts of the body the muscles are so well defined that their existence is evinced by merely viewing their structure and colour. But this is not always the case, and we especially find that in the bloodvessels no traces of muscles are distinguishable by mere inspection.

" Here then other modes of information are requisite, and our author proposes two. The one is their effect when we see actions that are in every respect muscular, although no muscle be distinguishable by the eye; and the other the change that takes place after death, when, as Mr. H. has observed, in many cases the power of contraction preponderates so as to stiffen all the muscular parts; and when, if the muscles thus contracted be afterwards stretched or put into what in the living body may be called its relaxed state, they remain thus relaxed without showing the least tendency to any further contraction. These circumstances mark the difference between muscular and elastic parts, since this latter power continues to act after death much in the same manner as it did during the life of an animal.

" These two modes of information are next applied in the examination of blood-vessels, which, our author previously observes, seldom bear any visible marks of muscular construction, and scarce ever admit of examination from their effects in the living body, on which account the second mode of information must be adopted as the likeliest to furnish some lights in this inquiry. He made a set of experiments on the blood-vessels of a dead horse, which were taken out so carefully as not to affect in the least either their texture or degree of contraction. They were examined both in their natural state and after they had been opened, and stretched different ways, by which means the different actions of the muscular and of the elastic powers become easily discernible. The following are the principal facts that resulted from this examination:

" Every part of the vascular system is not equally endowed with muscles; the larger vessels, especially the arteries, being chiefly composed of elastic substances, whilst many parts of the smaller, or what are called the capillary vessels, appear to be almost entirely muscular.

" In the middle-sized arteries two substances are visible to the eye, that towards the inner coat being evidently darker in colour, and of a structure somewhat different from the outward. The relative thickness of these coats differs as we recede from the heart, the interior becoming considerably thicker in proportion to the exterior; whence it evidently follows that the external diameter of the duct is not to be inferred from its external thickness, this being always proportionably greater as the vessel diminishes in size. Both these coats are in some measure elastic, but the external is more so than the internal; whence it may be judged that it is the internal that is endowed with muscular properties. This indeed is confirmed by a variety of experiments, in which it was found that the inner surface after death was considerably more contracted than the outward, the latter being thrown into longitudinal corrugations, which could only be the effect of the greater transverse or circular contraction of the latter.

" It has further been observed that this muscular contraction is chiefly in the transverse direction, and seldom if ever longitudinal.

" The physiological application of these facts, especially to arteries, is briefly this. The muscular contraction being chiefly circular, and tending to lessen the diameter of the vessel, the animal œconomy would suffer greatly if in the larger arteries, where this contraction is greater in proportion as its diameter increases, some power did not counteract this tendency so as to maintain a middle state or equilibrium. Thus also when muscular parts are too much distended, which in large arteries will often happen on account of their vicinity to the heart, a similar power is requisite to contract it to its natural size or tone. In both cases the elastic power produces this necessary effect, and it seems to follow hence that this power must always be proportionally greater in the larger vessels than in the smaller ones.

" A Table, exhibiting at one view the results of the above-mentioned experiments concludes this lecture[a]."

---

[a] [The irritability, or muscularity, of part of the coats of the artery contended for in the preceding lecture by Hunter, has since been demonstrated experimentally, first, by Dr. John Thompson of Edinburgh, and subsequently by many other physiologists; in whose experiments distinct contraction of the small arteries was produced, not only by mechanical (Wilson Philip, Hastings, Kaltenbrunner) but by galvanical irritation. (See *Wiedemeyer, Experimenta circa Statum Sanguinis et Vasorum in Inflammatione*, Monachii, 4to, 1826, and the Bibliography of the Vascular System, vol. iii. p. 233.) The muscular action is easily seen by dropping water colder than the atmosphere upon the capillaries in the mesentery of a frog, which thereupon contract both longitudinally and transversely, and after a little while resume their ordinary dimensions. Nevertheless the best chemists agree in classing the fibrous coat of arteries with the non-albuminous textures, as cellular tissue, cartilage, &c. (See *note*, vol. iii. p. 161.) The ultimate fibres of the middle coat, viewed microscopically, are smooth, branched, and anastomose reticularly, like the fibres of involuntary muscle: they present a remarkably clear dark outline.]

CROONIAN LECTURE ON MUSCULAR MOTION, No. V.

FOR THE YEAR 1781.

[Read before the Royal Society, June 14, by Mr. John Hunter, F.R.S.]

Of the Contraction and Relaxation of Muscular Fibres.

MUSCULAR motion differs from every other motion in matter; it is a motion taking place in the component parts of a muscle, and not a change of their relative situation. It is an uniform approximation, and receding in all the parts; the size, construction, and connexion of these are as yet not known: it is similar, as far as we can discover by our senses, to elasticity; in both cases the motion is produced in the component parts, which we are as yet unacquainted with, and only see the ultimate effect.

For the better investigating this motion in muscles, we may divide the general motions in matter into four kinds.

The first is the motion of whole bodies by means of an external impulse, the *vis inertia* of the body being overcome.

The second is the motion from attraction of one species of matter to itself or to another species, as wholes. Of this kind is gravitation, perhaps magnetism and electricity, probably also cohesion.

The third kind of motion is from chemical attraction, where, besides the attraction of whole parts, there is an elective attraction between the particles of one kind of matter and those of another, as it were drawing them out from the general mass. This can only happen when suspended in a fluid or in the form of vapour, no other form admitting of the motion of particles among themselves. Repulsion produces a similar motion among the parts.

The fourth kind of motion is muscular, arising most probably from construction, and a principle in action very different from the attractions in common matter.

This action and the others are equally unintelligible, the general effect alone being evident to our senses.

From the effect in muscular motion, we should be inclined to suppose that there is an approximation of the parts in one direction, which in the whole produces a visible contraction.

It is natural to suppose that all muscular fibres act alike; that every fibre in every muscle when in action is under exactly the same circumstances : therefore whatever variety may appear in muscular action, or difference between the action of different muscles, must depend upon the various causes and intentions of these actions.

A muscle in action as it contracts becomes more dense or hard, and therefore *a priori* we should suppose it becomes less, as we can form no adequate idea of the same substance becoming firmer or harder without either an approximation of its parts, or an addition of new matter introduced into all its parts, or a particular position of the constituent parts of a muscular fibre, so as to become immoveable while in that position.

One circumstance, however, which makes muscular fibres firmer when contracted in the living body is, their always overcoming some resistance in such contraction, which puts them more or less in the situation of a stretched cord.

Take the unattached hairs which compose the strings of the bow of a fiddle, and they will feel pliant or soft; but when put upon the stretch they will feel much firmer. An elastic body also, as India-rubber, feels much firmer while stretched than when contracted and at ease, by its natural elasticity. A muscular fibre, however, in the state of tension between the two points is little indebted to this cause for its firmness, although it will increase the effect produced by the position of its component parts; for a muscular fibre unattached is very much increased in hardness while contracted, as in crimped fish[a], and in the flesh of all animals allowed to die so gradually that the muscles, from the stimulus of death taking place, contract : but a muscle is as firm and as strong in all its degrees of contraction as it is in its full contraction, if not firmer and stronger than in its ultimate ; therefore cannot be called contraction. It is its proximity of its parts arising from that attraction, not from the proximity of such parts mechanically, but attractively.

Many authors of authority, as well physiologists as others, have attempted to explain the contraction of a muscular fibre ; but, however ingenious their opinions may be, none of them completely account for any one particular, relative to muscular contraction : I shall, however, mention them, with the objections to which they are liable.

In the investigation of this subject the following apparent alteration in the figure of a muscular fibre has been principally attended to :

---

[a] [Sir Anthony Carlisle found that the contracted muscles in crimped fish had not only acquired a sensible rigidity, but also an increase of specific gravity. See his 'Croonian Lecture for the year 1804,' Philos. Trans., 1805, p. 1.]

When a muscle acts, it increases in thickness, and becomes visibly firmer in texture, therefore each component fibre of the muscle must be supposed to undergo the same change; and many experiments have been made to ascertain whether this increase of thickness in a muscular fibre is in proportion to its decrease in length, but hitherto without effect: probably the only method of ascertaining this fact is, to determine whether a muscle in the state of contraction is really increased or diminished in its bulk.

Haller, in his Elements of Physiology, asks the following questions: "Does a muscle really increase in bulk in its action? As a muscle, when it acts, becomes shorter, and swells, we may next ask, Do these two changes, contraction and dilatation, compensate each other? that is, Is there the same quantity of matter in it at both these periods? Or does a muscle in action really lose in its size? or does it gain in bulk what it loses in length? Both sides of the question have had their advocates."

Borelli, to find out whether a muscle really had an addition of new matter in its contracted state, and thereby became heavier, made the following experiment:

He placed a naked man upon a table suspended upon a point, which supported it directly under his buttocks, in which situation he was perfectly balanced. He was then desired to act with the muscles of the lower extremities, but he still kept his balance, no change taking place in the equilibrium. (Borelli, vol. ii. p. 39.)

This experiment was made most probably upon the supposition that some additional matter was to flow from the brain along the nerves, or from the heart along the vessels to the muscles of the extremities, so as to render the upper part lighter, and the lower part heavier. If it was to come from the brain, it was conceiving the supposed animal spirits to be heavier than air, of all of which we are wholly ignorant.

The celebrated experiments of Goddard, Glisson, and Swammerdam are quoted, to prove that muscles lose in their bulk while in action. They put a muscle or a whole limb into a glass vessel, and filled it up with water; they then made all the muscles act at once; or if a single muscle, they irritated the nerve, and made it contract, during which time they attended to the motion in the water, and its rising or falling was to determine whether the size of the muscle was increased or diminished.

Swammerdam, in trying this experiment with a single muscle (the heart of a frog), saw the water sink in the contraction of that muscle, and rise in its relaxation.

The result of this experiment has been very differently explained.

Swammerdam himself doubted its being conclusive, believing the air might be compressed during the heart's action; but we have no proof of the presence of air in a muscle in the simple state of air.

Boerhaave and Sauvages accounted for the water descending by the blood being pressed out by the contraction of the muscle, which blood was returned into it by the relaxation, and raised the water. This certainly would be the case in the experiment made upon a whole limb; for we know, from every day's experience, that in bleedings from the arm the blood is thrown out more forcibly while the muscles are in action; therefore there is less blood in the vessels of the limb when the muscles are contracted than in a state of relaxation, and of course the limb is less in bulk at that time than in the other; but when a single muscle or a whole animal is immersed in water, whatever loss the muscle has in its substance must be gained by the water, so that the whole can neither be diminished nor increased.

Hambergerus tied a string round a man's arm, and found that during the action of the muscles it cut him; he therefore thought that muscles in action were increased; but the experiment only proved that it became thicker, which is generally allowed.

It has been objected to such experiments, that if a person acts only with one set of muscles, their opponents become stretched or relaxed in proportion, keeping up an equilibrium in the part: as antagonizing muscles, however, never bear a just proportion to one another in strength, it follows, that if we act with the strongest set of mucles the limb will of course become thicker in the proportion that the strength of the acting muscles bears to the strength of the relaxing ones, and *vice versâ*.

To ascertain with as much precision as possible whether a muscle really alters in size or not when contracted, I repeated the experiments of Goddard, Glisson, and Swammerdam, but in such a way as to have little or no doubt what was the effect. I got a glass blown which contained almost a gallon; its mouth was about three inches over, to admit its receiving a pretty large muscle, and was fitted with a ground-glass stopper, which was water-tight, and a glass tube was fitted into this stopper, so as to communicate with the cavity of the glass, being at the same time water-tight. This apparatus could be filled with water, and have the water stand at any height in the tube which might be required, so as to give with great nicety the comparative size (should there be any difference,) of a muscle when contracted and when relaxed, while immersed in it.

The muscles best adapted for experiments of this kind are those which have no antagonists, for in that case the contraction of one muscle produces the elongation of the other. The muscle should be wholly detached, having neither origin nor insertion, as a muscle cut out of the body, or cut from its attachment, as in crimped fish; those muscles however are best which have no natural attachment, as the heart.

In repeating such experiments it will be hardly possible to have the result of two exactly the same, for no two muscles will be equally relaxed at the beginning of the experiment, nor will any two muscles contract equally; but if there is one universal general effect taking place in all of them, that general effect becomes the result of the experiment intended, and is what is to be attended to.

Experiment 1. I killed a dog instantaneously, and took out the heart as expeditiously as possible, and put it into the glass filled with water, and immediately after putting in the stopper with the glass tube fixed in it. I now observed the height at which the water stood in the tube.

The heart had so far lost its action as not to contract and relax alternately, having only the power of contraction from the stimulus of death, and when put into the water was perfectly relaxed. It was allowed to remain in the water some hours; and it was observed, that by its apparent loss of bulk it had contracted considerably; and we also found that the water in the tube had fallen*. The next thing to be done was to ascertain how much the heart had lost in size, which was known by the quantity necessary to fill up the glass to the first height, which was sixteen grains.

The size of the heart was equal to two ounces six drachms, and thirty-eight grains of water, that is, 1328 grains, so that the contracted state was to the relaxed as 82 to 83, or $\frac{1}{83}$rd part of the whole.

Experiment 2. I took the heart of a sheep, whose size was equal to 13 ounces or 104 drachms of water; it lost in contraction 1 drachm; so that the contracted state was to the relaxed as $\frac{1}{104}$th part of the whole.

Experiment 3. I took a live eel, which was gutted, to remove as much as possible everything not muscular, and then crimped, to destroy the attachment of most of the muscles. The eel was equal to 14 ounces and 133 grains, or 6853 grains of water, and it lost in contraction 39 grains, or $\frac{1}{177}$th part of the whole[a].

* It is to be observed that the water was kept in the same degree of heat through the whole of the experiment.

---

[a] [In the experiments above detailed Hunter drew his conclusions, as to the change of bulk in a muscle during contraction, from the effects observed in the level of the surrounding fluid, after the last contraction of the part or ' rigor mortis.' In Mr. Mayo's well-known experiment, which is similar to the first of Hunter's, the ordinary contractions of the ventricles of a dog's heart, alternating with relaxations of the same parts, produced no perceptible change in the level of the water in the tube[1]. In comparing the above

---

[1] [Anatomical and Physiological Commentaries, vol. i. p. 12.]

As this animal was composed of muscles, bones, &c., some allowance is to be made for these parts, which will account in some measure for the difference in the result between this and the hearts, although in the experiments on the hearts there is a considerable difference between the two, arising from the reasons above mentioned.

It appears, however, upon the whole, that a muscle loses more of its length than it gains in thickness, unless the apparent difference arises from an universal approximation of all its parts.

As a muscle loses in its general size by the contraction of the length of its fibres, we cannot suppose that contraction to arise from the introduction of additional matter into those fibres; therefore the opinions that a muscular fibre is a hollow tube from end to end, or a chain of cells of various shapes, either rhomboidal or circular, according to the ideas of the authors of such opinions, and these cells being filled with foreign matter, must fall to the ground[a]; indeed, this idea of a muscular

experiments, one cannot fail to be struck with the difference in the period during which the muscular contractions of the dog's heart continued. But as Hunter killed his dog *instantaneously*, it was probably by some sudden concussion or injury to the brain, when the action of the heart would be arrested, and the last contraction only would be witnessed, notwithstanding the expedition with which it was taken out. In Mr. Mayo's experiment the dog was killed by hanging, and the ventricles of the heart continued alternately to contract and dilate for a considerable time. Barzolotti, Prevost and Dumas, who performed similar experiments on smaller portions of flesh, also found no change of level to take place in the surrounding fluid during the contraction of the muscle. Gruithuisen and Ermann[1], on the contrary, observed, like Hunter, a slight change in the bulk of the muscle during contraction. Ermann introduced into a glass vessel the posterior half of an eel, the intestines being removed. A metal wire was inserted into the spinal marrow, and a second into the flesh, and these were directed so as to be brought into communication with the pole of a galvanic battery. The vessel was then filled with water, so that a narrow tube, in which the apparatus ended above, was filled. In completing the chain, and during the contraction of the muscles, the water fell in the tube four or five lines, and again rose to the opening, when the muscle relaxed.

If, however, the muscular fibre, which is generally admitted to have increased in density, and, according to the experiments of Sir Anthony Carlisle, in specific gravity, during contraction, has really diminished in bulk, the difference is so trifling that we can hardly avail ourselves of it in elucidating the nature of muscular contraction.]

[a] [It is now generally admitted by microscopical observers that the ultimate muscular fibre is solid. The voluntary muscular fibres ('secondary fibres' of Prevost and Dumas, 'ultimate fasciculi' of Müller,) in the vertebrate classes, and those of insects, arachnidans, crustaceans, and cirripeds, present a microscopical character which distinguishes them from every other animal tissue: it consists of close-set, parallel, transverse, or slightly oblique and sometimes slightly curved striæ. The fibres which present these striæ are divisible into component fibrillæ, which have a knotted or beaded structure; this I have myself observed in the human voluntary fibre, and in that of the

fibre being a chain of cells does not account for any one phenomenon attending muscular motion, and is directly contradicted by two circum-stances attending muscular contraction : the first of these is the muscle becoming rather less than larger in its contraction, which is just contrary to what must have happened if the contraction had been owing to that cause; the second is, that a muscle is capable of contracting much more than one third of its length, and indeed, as far as we yet know, having no limitation, which could not possibly happen if they were tubes capable of receiving foreign matter into their cavities; for according to that idea, a muscular fibre should become thicker in its contraction in proportion as the diameter of a sphere is greater than that of a cylinder of the same area, which would be an immense increase.

Although a muscle becomes on the whole somewhat less in its con-traction, and has its ends brought considerably nearer together, yet it cannot be called attraction, for there is nearly the same reason for sup-posing a lateral repulsion, as the muscle swells out laterally almost as much as it contracts in the other direction.

I do suppose that a muscular fibre is not one uniform body from end to end, but is made up of parts, which may be called the component parts of a muscular fibre; and I am apt to suppose that a change takes place in the position of those parts, during contraction, and this alteration diminishes the extent of those parts in one direction while it is increas-ing them in the other, although from the experiments it appears not to be in the same proportion; but what that alteration is I shall not pretend to determine[a].

---

mole-cricket. Some physiologists suppose that the transverse striæ result from the la-teral apposition of the knots on the parallel fibrillæ. The muscular fibres of the mol-lusca and radiata, and the involuntary muscular fibres of the vertebrata, with the excep-tion of those developed in the vascular layer of the germ disc, as the fibres of the heart, do not present the striated character.]

[a] [According to the observations of Hales (*Hæmastatics*, p. 59.), and of Prevost and Dumas (Magendie, *Journal de Physiologie*, iii. p. 301.), the change in the muscular fibre, at the moment of contraction, is from a straight to a zigzag line: the observation has been generally made on the rectilinear parallel fibres of one of the thin abdominal mus-cles (the *rectus*) of a young frog, stimulated to contract while under the microscope ; and the conclusion is admitted as an established fact in the most recent works on physiology. I have been led to doubt this fact, from observing the contraction of the muscular fibres in small *Filariæ* (such as commonly infest the abdominal cavity of the cod), and more especially from observing the contraction of the retractor muscles of the tentacles of a species of *Vesicularia* of Vaughan Thompson, a compound polype-like animal, which, under the guise of a *Sertularia* manifests a much higher type of organization. Here each separate fibre of the retractor muscles is seen with great distinctness, and is cha-racterized by a single knot or swelling in the middle. In the act of retracting the ten-tacles the fibres become shorter and thicker, especially at the central knot, but do not fall out of the straight line. After the retraction has been effected, the fibres fall into

Muscles have a disposition to throw themselves into wrinkles or corrugations when not in action, and when the position of the part moved by these muscles is such as allows the muscle to be in its shortest state, as in the biceps-flexor-cubiti after having bent the arm. If it is kept in that position by any other power, the biceps will leave acting and fall into wrinkles, adapting itself to the short distance between its origin and insertion; so that these wrinkles are a kind of substitute for the contraction that was in the muscle.

The greatest strength in a muscle while in action is probably when it is half contracted, as we find that in all great exertions of muscular strength, where ultimate actions are to take place, the muscles employed are never allowed to relax their full relaxation, or contract to their full contraction.

When a man walks with a heavy load his knees are a little bent, even of the leg he stands upon, which supports the whole while he is moving the other. The same thing takes place if he is weary; but if strong and in full activity his perpendicular joints may be kept pretty straight.

The same thing also takes place in old people from the same cause; for as they become naturally weak, they become, like the strong, loaded with a heavy burden, therefore take on the same modes of action: the knees are never straightened, the back bent forwards, and all the parts that are constantly in the action of support are all getting out of the perpendicular, in which perpendicular state, although they might be mechanically stronger, yet they are muscularly weaker, therefore get into that position in which the muscles can act with the greatest advantage.

The relaxers, which become the sustainers of the muscles in action, never allow themselves to relax to their full extent while the contractors are carrying on the motion of a part, as it would produce weakness.

The relaxation of muscles when contracted involuntarily, but from obnoxious stimuli, will not relax by the *will*; nothing but a counter-

---

a wavy or zigzag position: but this is characteristic of their state of relaxation under the circumstances which bring their two attached extremities nearer each other. In like manner, in the parallel longitudinal fibres of the *Filaria*, it is most evident that, at the moment of contraction, they become shorter and thicker, but do not alter their rectilinear position until the action has ceased, when they fall, like the parallel nervous chord, into zigzag folds, which continue until effaced by the restoration of the part to its usual length through the action of the exterior transverse fibres.

On relating these observations to my friend Dr. Allen Thompson, he informed me that, on repeating the experiment of Hales and Prevost on the frog, he had observed single fibres continuing in contraction, and being simply shortened, and not falling into the zigzag plicæ; and he was led to suspect, from this and other appearances, that the zigzag arrangement was not produced till after the act of contraction had ceased.]

stimulus of necessity can, and even that with difficulty.   For instance, if we attempt to breathe obnoxious air, or if anything touches the glottis, it immediately shuts, and it is out of the power of the will to relax it; but the stimulus of the necessity of breathing brings it to again. A muscle that has but one determined use, or rather a muscle that has but one point of origin and one point of insertion, always acts wholly when put into action, so as to bring about its effect on the part of insertion; I believe never one part of the muscle only, or only a few of its fibres, but the whole. This is not the case with muscles whose origin is broad and its insertion narrow, whose insertion is broad and its origin broad, or whose origin is narrow and insertion broad.

But in spasm in a muscle a very few fibres may be seen to act; in short, any number may act, as it is not motion of the part that is the intent of the action.

Relaxation.

Muscular fibres have a greater power of contraction than what is barely sufficient for the extent of the motion of the parts upon which they are designed to act.   This is illustrated in the shell-fish called bivalve, for the muscle in that fish brings the two shells together; but if one of the shells be broken, so as to allow of a nearer approximation of the two insertions of the muscle, we find that they are brought nearer. It is also evident where the tendo Achillis or patella is broken, for when that happens the fibres are allowed to contract to the full extent of their original contraction, and the parts heal in that position: in such cases the muscle is become shorter the whole length of its natural contraction, and the tendon is become so much longer; and in this case, if the muscle was not possessed of a greater power of contraction than was before made use of, or did not acquire a greater power, no motion could now take place, whereas we find the ultimate quantity of motion produced.

If the power of contraction was limited to the quantity produced in a straight muscle, the same kind of fibres, when forming sphincter muscles, could not answer the intended purposes, as a greater power of contraction is required.

That the same length of fibre is not absolutely necessary to produce in all cases the same effect, is strongly evinced, by the fibres of the gastrocnemius muscle in the African negro, being shorter than in the European, yet producing exactly the same quantity of motion in the joints which they move.   This takes place universally in the Africans, and now and then is met with in men of other nations.

This difference in the length of muscular fibres is a principal reason of the difference in the outline of most men from one another; it is at least a secondary cause, and should be particularly attended to by painters and sculptors, as it is a distinguishing mark between original nations.

The contraction of a muscular fibre is produced by the following causes: simple mechanical pressure, as touch, the pricking of a pin, &c.; simple impression on another part which acts upon this by sympathy.

It is also produced by properties of matter which are not mechanical, as the essential oils, salts, acids, &c.; by affections of the mind and intentions of the will by means of the nerves; by the circumstances of the body itself at the time, as want, repletion, &c.; and even by death itself.

An animal that dies so slowly as to allow the stimulus of death to be felt by its muscles, has those muscles so contracted as to become stiff; whether this contraction is equal to the greatest power of contraction of the same muscle, in such a position of the parts in the living body, I do not know.

In order, however, to ascertain how much a common muscle contracts from the stimulus of death, I cut out a muscle from a horse just after it was killed, and found that in the action of death it had contracted one third, and that the muscle so contracted had become one fourth thicker in its diameter, a proportion I believe it would have kept in the living body; also the same muscle, when stretched, or when put into what in the living may body be called the relaxed state, did not again contract.

The contraction of mucles from the stimulus of death is a stronger contraction than the attraction of cohesion of the muscles themselves; therefore when a muscle so contracted is attempted to be elongated it generally tears asunder: but this is not always the case, it only takes place under certain circumstances; it is with respect to the muscle itself in proportion to the power of contraction of the muscle, for we find it takes place much oftener in those that die of violent deaths, especially when they die of strong convulsions; it seldom or ever takes place in those which die of a disease of some standing, for in them the muscles have lost in some degree their absolute power of contraction; as also the disease may be such as has in some degree destroyed the stimulus of death upon the muscles, so that their contraction will be less, although their power may be pretty strong.

It would appear from the above that muscular contraction is not simply an approximation of the parts of which a muscular fibre is composed.

What the difference is in a muscular fibre between its relaxed state and the contracted, perhaps may never be known.

Relaxation would appear to be a natural consequence of the contraction having answered its end or fulfilled its purpose; or it may be supposed to have got rid of its stimulus by this action, the stimulus ceasing to have power when the action has taken place; therefore relaxation naturally occurs till excited to action by another stimulus, of which it is susceptible.

Relaxation might be supposed to be a simple cessation of action, but I think it is not; it appears to me to be a power as much depending on life as contraction; for if it was simply a cessation of action, muscles would become relaxed that had contracted by the stimulus of death whenever absolute death took place, which is not the case; on the contrary, it takes probably as much force to overcome this contraction as the same muscles would have done when acting with all the power of the will in the living body.

From the violence necessary for the elongation of a muscular fibre after death, it would appear that the position of the component parts of a fibre in any degree of contraction is such as requires force to alter or remove it, and, whatever that position is, it can be in part drawn out as if only in part contracted, or wholly drawn out; and in this operation of drawing out or relaxing a muscular fibre after death, we may observe there is a recoil or reaction in a certain degree when the elongating force is removed, becoming in this respect similar to elasticity. This recoil, however, is not extensive, although it takes place in every degree of relaxation, from the most contracted state to the almost totally relaxed state.

I first observed this recoil in a man who died in convulsions in St. George's Hospital, from a fever, attended with delirium, which was brought on by a hurt on his arm, which inflamed considerably. A few hours after death his muscles were stiffer than usual, and extremely well marked through the skin, which induced me to make the following experiment on the relaxation of muscles. I laid bare the rectus muscle of the thigh, and separated it from the other muscles without stretching it; I then passed a thread behind it and inclosed the muscle, and cut the thread off where the ends met. Upon bending the knee the muscle was stretched, and I found that the ends of the thread were lapped over each other. Upon measuring the difference it was one eighth of an inch diminished from what it was in the contracted state.

I was much surprised by a considerable degree of contraction in the muscles, similar to elasticity, for they evidently contracted a good deal after being stretched. I suspected that this had arisen from some remains of life, and therefore waited till the next day, when the same thing happened.

If, in stretching a contracted muscle after death, the fibres are not drawn out beyond this power of recoil, the whole contraction of the muscle (whatever quantity it is,) continues the same; but if the muscle is drawn out further than this power of recoil, then the muscle becomes so far relaxed, but no further; for instance, if the recoil is the one twelfth of an inch, and the muscle is only stretched so far, then the muscle will contract again one twelfth of an inch; but if it is stretched one sixth of an inch, then it will still only recoil one twelfth, the other one twelfth being the absolute relaxation of the muscle.

From all that is mentioned above, I think it will appear that relaxation of a muscular fibre depends upon life as much as the contraction, neither the one nor the other being produced after death by any property in the muscle.

The causes of relaxation are few; the will is perhaps the principal one, although not in all muscles. Emotion of the mind would appear to have a power of stopping the action of the heart, but is perhaps only hindering a new contraction.

The contraction and relaxation of a muscle are always adapting themselves to the motions of the parts on which they are to act, so that if a joint continues bent for some time the muscle will retain it in that situation, and any extension of that joint will put the muscular fibres on the stretch. This is not, as has been supposed, a contraction of the tendon, but a contraction in the muscle, to adapt it to the remaining motion in the joint, this half contracted state becoming now the state of relaxation from which the muscle is in future to produce its action. The point of relaxation of a muscle, therefore, is always the extent of motion in the joint, and the quantity of contraction of a muscle is always equal to the full motion of the joint on which it acts, and if the joint loses part of its motion the muscle also loses a proportionable degree of contraction, so as still to be adapted to it.

Muscles, however, so contracted, may be gradually stretched to their original length, and recover their original action, as the biceps flexor cubiti after inflammations, and abscesses in the arm.

Muscles may be also stretched beyond their original length, and still retain their use, as those of the belly in dropsies.

These circumstances prove that accidents to the body are provided against in its construction; for if the muscles remained in the half-bent state in the cases above mentioned, the length of muscle would be too great for the quantity of motion, and the first part of its action would produce no effect upon the joint.

CROONIAN LECTURE ON MUSCULAR MOTION, No. VI.

For the Year 1782.

[Read before the Royal Society June 13th, by Mr. John Hunter, F.R.S.]

An inquiry how far, and in what instances, the density or firm-
ness of a Muscle contributes to its strength.

IN comparative experiments respecting animals, where the actions of
life are attempted to be imitated in the dead body, we should attend to
every circumstance and see whether there is really any kind of similarity in the experiment. But, where life is absolutely necessary for the
action, on one side, and the action is imitated only so far as regards the
mechanical mode of performing it, the resemblance between the vital
action and the experiment is in reality very remote.

To suppose that the action of a muscle should be equal, more or less,
with its mechanical strength when dead is absurd, because they bear no
analogy. The action of a muscle is as unlike its mechanical resistance
as the effects of the irritability of a living body upon impression is like
the mechanical effects of the same impression; the mechanical effects
being the same in the living as the dead.

The action of a muscle is stronger than its mechanical resistance in
the dead body; that is, its power of contraction is greater than the attraction of the cohesion of its fibres.

These facts can only be ascertained by experiments on the power in
the living body, opposing them with the resistance in the dead; but as
a muscle is in very different states in contraction and relaxation, even
in the living body, and as the experiment is opposing contraction to the
state of relaxation, the experiment is not conclusive: it does not prove
what it is meant to prove.

The subject can and should be viewed in several lights. A muscle is
first to be considered in two points of view; the relaxed state, where it
is only united by the common attraction of cohesion of that muscle, and
is probably as mechanically strong in the dead as the living; but they
may be considered in the contracted state both in the dead and the living, for although a muscle does not contract after death, yet it often
contracts in the act of dying; and death does not produce a relaxation,
therefore it is to be presumed that the position of the parts of the muscle

so contracted remains in the same state, and therefore such muscle affords an opportunity of making comparative experiments between it and one in the living body so contracted.

How far the same muscles in the dead body, when fully contracted, could be relaxed by the same force as when in the living state, I do not know. It is certain that a muscle in health, and which feels the stimulus of death strongly, contracts with considerable force, and requires a considerable power to overcome it ; therefore the relaxation of a muscle, voluntarily contracted, must always be an act of the mind, or a cessation of action of the mind upon that muscle. But when a muscle takes on an action without the mind, either in diseases, as the involuntary actions of voluntary muscles, or by the stimulus of death (the immediate cause of action being, I conceive, the same in both), then a relaxation from the mind cannot take place in either, because the mind had nothing to do with the first, and it did not exist in the second. So that those involuntary actions of voluntary muscles arise from a stimulus independent of the will, and in those where it goes off it is because that stimulus can cease, and the part being alive a relaxation can ensue ; whereas in death a relaxation cannot ensue, because a cessation of the stimulus cannot ensue, that cessation being an act of the living body.

To oppose an experiment on muscles in the dead body with one in the living, the muscles should be always in similar states, for a muscle contracted is thicker than natural, and therefore stronger in its transverse direction ; and if when in a contracted state the particles of which it is composed are really brought nearer to each other, then it should be doubly strong, viz. in proportion to its increased size and closer approximation of its particles. But as the state of a muscle in contraction is totally different from its natural state, or that state which constitutes the natural structure of a muscle, no comparative experiments can be made which can explain anything.

It is evident from observation, that in the construction of a muscular fibre it was not necessary that they should be all of equal density, for we find some fibres denser than others. We find this difference in the different tribes of animals ; in some the fibres are extremely soft, while in others they are very firm.

The firm fibre is found in the more perfect animals, called quadrupeds, especially when full-grown ; and this difference of density of muscular fibres would appear to be in a pretty regular gradation from the most imperfect to the most perfect, from the muscles of the Medusa to those of the full-grown quadruped.

We may also observe that the first rudiments of every animal are extremely soft, and even the rudiments of the more perfect are similar to the full grown imperfect, and as they advance in growth they become firmer and firmer in texture.

It may likewise be observed that there is a very considerable difference in the densities of the muscles in some of those animals that are of distinct sexes, the male (probably in most) having by much the densest muscles; and the muscles of the same animal, whether perfect or imperfect, are not of equal densities, some being denser than others.

This arises from two causes,—one natural, growing up with the animal, the other acquired by frequent action.

This difference in density of the muscular fibres in different animals, and in the same animal at different ages, in different sexes of the same species, and even in the same sex, also the increased density arising from action, must answer some material purpose, and, from every observation, it would appear to produce strength or power in the contraction of the muscular fibre.

From every circumstance attending muscular contraction, it is obvious that those muscles employed in, or intended for the strongest actions, are the firmest in texture of any animal body, at least from many circumstances it is natural to suppose so; that they are the strongest would appear from the situation in which the firmest muscles are placed, for where the strongest actions are found in the living body, there we find the firmest muscles after death.

There are two causes for this situation of the firm or strong muscles; the first is an original or natural one, a principle in the animal œconomy, depending upon the natural growth of the animal as much as the formation of a leg or any other part. The second is action.

If we take a general view of the first or natural cause, we shall see from these general observations where we are to expect the strongest, and of course the hardest, muscles in any given animal whose mode of action is known.

In animals which have progressive motion it will generally, if not always, be found that this action will be one of their greatest, because the parts intended for progressive motion bear a small proportion to the whole animal, which they are obliged to move; whereas, every other part has its peculiar muscle, and the muscle is only obliged to move that one part, which is small in proportion to the others.

Another action which many animals are endowed with, and which requires very considerable strength, is fighting; this is an action which always requires great powers in the muscles, because it is an action in a part which is to overcome the whole strength and weight of its antagonist, which is more than the natural weight of the same muscle, or the resistance of the same muscle, or the resistance of any muscle in the same body.

Another partial cause of strength in some animals is for catching their prey, which is to overcome a resistance considerably beyond the motion of the part itself which is to perform the action.

If such parts of animals as are adapted for progressive motion, for fighting, or for catching prey, require the greatest strength in the muscle adapted for such purposes, and if we find that such parts as are endowed with the firmest muscles are the strongest, where all those purposes are united in the same part in any one animal, we must find there the greatest strength, and of course the firmest of all the muscles in the body, especially if every one of these actions is considerable or violent.

Thus, then, we find the muscles in the arm of a lion where all these three purposes are performed, are extremely firm in texture, and we must suppose are also exceedingly strong. The muscles of the thigh of a fighting-cock are employed in fighting and progressive motion, and are extremely firm.

The muscle which has the greatest resistance in an animal body to overcome is the heart, especially in quadrupeds, and this is perhaps the firmest in the body, being even firmer than those which have the above-mentioned resistances to overcome; but the firmness of this muscle may in some measure arise from its action, which I called the second cause of firmness.

Some muscles in the more imperfect animals are much firmer than others in the same animal; such is the muscle which draws the snail into its shell, and retains it there against almost any power that can be applied: also the muscle which shuts the two shells of the bivalve is very firm in its texture, and we know that it is exceedingly strong.

A difference is sometimes found in firmness between the muscles of the male and female; this, however, is not universal, not taking place in fish: but in all animals where the males have a disposition to fight and the females not, or at least in a less degree, I believe the muscles of the male are much firmer than those of the female, and this in proportion as their disposition for fighting is greater; therefore in beasts of prey, where the disposition to fight is nearly equal in the male and female, the difference in strength is not so remarkable as in many other animals, there being very little difference between a male and female cat, a dog and bitch, a male and female hawk, &c.; but the muscles appropriated for catching prey, and also for fighting, are much firmer than the other muscles in the same body allotted for common purposes, and according to our reasoning they must be much stronger.

We find, however, in animals which do not catch prey, and where the male has a strong tendency to fight with the males of its own species, while the female has this disposition very little, if at all, that there is a very considerable difference in the strength of the same parts in the male and female while alive, and a similar difference in the firmness of their muscles after death.

There is a considerable difference between the muscles of a bull and cow, and also between those of a cock and hen.

Besides the general strength of the muscles of those males who fight, as they have parts which are intended for this purpose, we find that the muscles of those parts far exceed all their other muscles in firmness; as the muscles in the neck of the bull, and the legs of the cock, far exceed in firmness all the other muscles in the body, and exceed, therefore, in a much greater degree the muscles of the female

We may also observe, that all those muscles in the male immediately employed in fighting, although not intended for this action alone, having other actions which are common to the female, besides being firmer than those of the female, are very considerably increased in size; thus the muscles of the neck of the bull, and of the stone horse, those of the legs of the cock, &c., are much thicker and larger than in the female.

The second cause of firmness in a muscle, and which contributes to its strength, is action, or what is commonly called exercise, and which has in general been considered as the principal cause of strength, size, and firmness.

This may be called accidental, as it is not confined to any order of animals, or any one set of muscles; it may, however, be observed, that the muscles employed in progressive motion and the purposes above mentioned, are more subject to this accidental cause of firmness than any other in the body, both from the natural actions of the body, and also, being naturally firm and strong, from more readily being employed in violent actions.

Thus we find the muscles employed in progressive motion are much firmer than any other muscles in the same animal, both from nature and action, except in those in the fighting males (who do not catch their food by violence,) which are employed for that purpose, as in the neck of the bull.

The heart of all animals partakes strongly of the two causes of firmness, and is perhaps the firmest muscle in the body. This firmness in the heart is very early in life, for in the small embryo the heart is a pretty firm manageable part, while every other muscular part of the animal is as tender as jelly.

Constant action not only gives firmness to muscles, but increase of size.

The epicure is no less sensible of the effects of these causes of firmness than the physiologist, and therefore prefers the inactive parts; and the leg of the woodcock, the breast of a partridge, pheasant, turkey, &c. are held in high estimation.   He even takes pains to diminish the effects which arise from exercise, &c., by feeding animals in such a way as to prevent them taking place.   Upon this principle house lamb, veal, &c. are made tender.   How delicious to the sensualist must the flesh of the sloth be, if the account of its motion being far exceeded by a snail is true!

From the above account it must appear that muscles, in proportion as they are firm in texture, will be strong in action; it is at least demonstrable in the muscles of the same animal whose texture is different, and in similar muscles in the male and female of the same species, and we may reasonably suppose that it will hold good in different species; and therefore, when we find the muscles very firm in any one species, we may conclude that this species is stronger than any other species in which the muscles are tender and soft.

This firmness in a muscular fibre we may suppose to arise from the density of its component parts, or those parts being closer together, the uniting medium being less in quantity; this, however, it is perhaps impossible to determine exactly.

That this idea may be better understood, I shall suppose that a part composed of dense parts (aggregated) at a given distance, will be firmer than a part composed of less firm parts at the same distance; and it is plain that a part composed of any given substance will be dense in proportion as the parts of that substance are near to each other.

It may probably be similar to iron and steel; in the iron the parts or crystals which compose the mass are large, and perhaps not regular. In the steel they are small, and probably more regular in their figure, by which means they can adapt themselves better to each other, and still more so if tempered, according to the degree of temper, so that their crystals shall become still smaller, and of course the whole becomes harder.

To ascertain whether the firm muscles really contained more matter, and were therefore specifically heavier than the soft, I made several experiments upon muscles of different densities.   The experiments were made upon the same muscle of two animals of the same species, whose muscles are of different densities, viz. the muscles of the neck of the ox and bull*.

* My reason for choosing those muscles in preference to others was, that they admit a greater degree of difference in firmness, and that they have no tendons intermixed, so as to give density from that cause.

Nine ounces and a half of muscle from a bull's neck, and the same quantity from that of an ox, were weighed in water, when the bull's was thirty-one grains heavier, which is about $\frac{1}{130}$th[a].

From this experiment it appears that there is some difference in weight between a firm muscle and one that is naturally soft or lax, although not great, not even so much as one might at first imagine, at least not so much as the apparent difference in density.

As it appears, from the above observations, that with the same given size the firmer muscles are the strongest, it becomes a question why every muscle in the bodies of the more perfect animals, and in the young of such animals, as also the muscles of the more simple animals in general, should not all have been of this texture, which constitutes the greatest power of contraction? This is perhaps not yet to be fully answered. It certainly would have rendered many parts of the more perfect animals much smaller than what they now are, and would have had the same effect upon the whole body of the young of the more perfect animals, as also of the more simple animals universally; we must, however, suppose that it would have been attended with some inconveniences, although at present what these inconveniences would have been may not be perfectly understood.

[See note a, p. 256.]

THE USE OF THE OBLIQUE MUSCLES.

MUSCLES are the active parts in an animal body, producing different effects, according to the circumstances in which they are placed; and the greater number of parts requiring a variety of motions, it became necessary to have a variety of muscles suited to such motions.

The function of a muscle depends on the contraction of its fibres; and the most general effect produced by this contraction is to move some one part of the body upon another. But we may observe, that when motion in a part is performed by one set of muscles, there are other muscles employed in regulating that motion, as in most joints; and in a whole part, destined to a variety of motions, and composed of smaller parts, intended likewise to have their distinct motions, we find muscles appropriated for the purpose of keeping some of those parts fixed in a particular position, while the whole part is to be moved by other muscles, according to the nature of the action to be performed. This will, perhaps, be best illustrated by attending to what takes place in the eye, considering it as part of the head.

The eye being an organ of sense, which is to receive impressions from without, it was necessary it should be able to give its motions that kind of direction as would permit its being impressed by objects whether at rest or in motion, or moving from object to object; and it was also necessary that there should be a power capable of keeping the eye fixed upon an object when our body or head was in motion.

For the better understanding this action of pointing the eye towards objects under the various circumstances of vision, it will be necessary to mention that the eye is furnished with muscles, some of which, in the quadruped, bird, amphibia, and fishes, are called straight, from their being placed in the direction of or parallel to the axis of the eye; and two, I believe, have always been named oblique. Of the straight, some animals have more than others. There are four straight muscles common to most animals; and those which have more have the additional muscles inserted immediately in the eye-ball on its posterior surface, and surrounding the optic nerve. The four straight muscles, which are common to all quadrupeds, pass further forwards, and are rather inserted towards the anterior surface of the eye.

For vision at large it was not only necessary that the eye should be capable of moving from object to object, or of following any object in motion, but also necessary that there should be a power to keep it fixed on any one object to which the mind might be attentive; therefore the muscles are formed so as not only to be able to move the eye from object to object, but likewise to keep its point of vision fixed upon any particular one, while the eye is moving progressively with the head or body. This is the use of these muscles, when the parts from whence they arise are kept fixed respecting the objects the eye is pointed to; but it is often necessary, while the eye is fixed upon a particular object, that the eyeball and the head in which it is fixed should shift their situation respecting that object; and this would alter the direction of the eye, if the muscles had not the power of taking up an action that produces a contrary effect, that is, keeping the point of insertion of the muscles as the fixed point, by causing their fibres to contract according as the origins of the muscles vary their position respecting the object. From this mechanism we find these three modes of action produced: first, the eye moving from one fixed object to another; then the eye moving along with an object in motion; and, last, the eye keeping its axis to an object, although the whole eye, and the head, of which it makes a part, are in motion. From either of these motions taking place singly, or being combined, the eye is always kept towards its object. In the two first modes of action the origins of the muscles are fixed points respecting the object; and, in the last, the object becomes as it were the centre of motion, or fixed point, commanding the direction of the actions of the eye, as the north commands the direction of the needle, let the box in which it is placed be moved in what direction it may. These two first modes of action are performed by the straight muscles; for the head being a fixed point, they are capable of moving the eye up and down, from right to left, with all the intermediate motions, which, taken together, constitute a circular movement; or, when the eye is to become the fixed point, then the head itself performs the circular movement. Thence appears the necessity why the object, the axis of the eye, and the point of sensation, should all three be in the same straight line. But this does not take place in all movements of that whole of which the eye makes a part; for besides those which we have already taken notice of, the head is capable of a motion from shoulder to shoulder, the axis of which is through the axis of the two eyes, from the fore to the back part. It should be here observed, that for distinct vision the object must be fixed as respecting the pupil of the eye, and not in the least allowed to move over its surface*. To prevent any progressive motion

* Optical writers seem to have been entirely ignorant of this; for they not only suppose distinct vision compatible with the object having a motion over the different parts

of the object over the retina of the eye, either from the motion of the object itself, or of the head in some of the motions of that part, the straight muscles are provided as has been explained; but the effects which would arise from some other motion of the head, as from shoulder to shoulder, cannot be corrected by the action of the straight muscles, therefore the oblique muscles are provided. Thus when we look at an object, and at the same time move our head to either shoulder, it is moving in the arch of a circle whose centre is the neck; and of course the eyes would have the same quantity of motion on this axis if the oblique muscles did not fix them upon the object. When the head is moved towards the right shoulder the superior oblique muscle of the right side acts and keeps the right eye fixed on the object; and a similar effect is produced upon the left eye by the action of its inferior oblique muscle: when the head moves in a contrary direction the other oblique muscles produce the same effect. This motion of the head may, however, be to a greater extent than can be counteracted by the action of the oblique muscles. Thus, for instance, while the head is on the left shoulder the eyes may be fixed upon an object, and continue looking at it while the head is moved to the right shoulder, which sweep of the head produces a greater effect upon the eyeballs than can be counteracted by the action of the oblique muscles; and in this case we find that the oblique muscles let go the eye, so that it immediately returns into its natural situation in the orbit. Whether this is performed by the natural elasticity of the parts, or whether the antagonist oblique muscles take up the action and reinstate the eye, I do not know. If the head still continues its motion in the same direction, then the same oblique muscles begin to act anew, and go on acting, so as to keep the eyes fixed on the object. As this motion of the head seldom takes place uncombined with its other motions, some of the straight and oblique muscles will be employed at the same time, according as the motions are more or less compounded.

---

of the retina, but even explain the effects which would be produced by it on the mind of the observer. Keill makes the following observation:

" Since optics teach us that every body which is visible has by means of the rays which proceed from that object its image painted on the bottom of the eye or retina, it follows that those objects will seem to be moved whose images are moved on the retina, that is, which pass over successively the different parts of the retina whilst the eye is supposed to be at rest; but those objects will be looked upon as being at rest whose images always occupy the same part of the retina, that is, when the motion of those images are not perceived in the bottom of the eye."—Keill's Introduction to Natural Philosophy, p. 79.

ON THE COLOUR OF THE PIGMENTUM OF THE EYE IN DIFFERENT ANIMALS.

IN the eyes of all animals which I have examined there is a substance approaching to the nature and appearance of a membrane, called the pigmentum, which lines the choroid coat, and is somewhat similar to the rete mucosum which lies under the cuticle of the human body; and there is also some of the same kind of substance diffused through the cellular membrane which unites the choroid with the sclerotic coat. My intention at present is only to communicate the observations I have made on this subject and its use, confining myself to the consideration of that kind of it which lines the tunica choroides of the class Mammalia, and of birds: in doing which I shall also take occasion to speak of the difference of colour occurring in animals of the same species. Although an accurate examination of the appearances of a similar substance in the eyes of some fishes might illustrate the subject, we cannot avail ourselves of that, as from not being sufficiently acquainted with the effects of light on the eyes of that class of animals.

The propagation or continuance of animals in their distinct classes is an established law of Nature, and in a general way is preserved with a tolerable degree of uniformity; but in the individuals of each species varieties are every day produced in colour, shape, size, and disposition. Some of these changes are permanent with respect to the propagation of the animal, becoming so far a part of its nature as to be continued in the offspring.

Animals living in a free and natural state are subject to few deviations from their specific character; but Nature is less uniform in its operations when influenced by culture*. Considerable varieties are produced under such circumstances, of which the most frequent are changes in the colour. These changes are always, I believe, from the dark to the lighter tints, and the alteration very gradual in certain species, requiring in the canary-bird several generations; while in the crow,

* From the variations produced by culture it would appear that the animal is so susceptible of impression as to vary Nature's actions; and this is even carried into propagation. Whether this takes place at the very first union of the principles of the two parents, so as to derive its existence from both; or whether it takes its formation from the mother, after the first formation of the embryo, are perhaps not easily determined.

mouse, &c. it is completed in one. But this change is not always to white, though still approaching nearer to it in the young than in the parent, being sometimes to dun, at others to spotted, of all the various shades between the two extremes. This alteration in colour being constantly from dark to lighter, may we not reasonably infer that in all animals subject to such variation the darkest of the species should be reckoned nearest to the original; and that where there are specimens of a particular kind, entirely black, the whole have been originally black? Without this supposition it will be impossible, on the principle I have stated, to account for individuals of any class being black. Every such variety may be considered as arising in the cultivated state of animals; but whether, if left to themselves, they would in time resume their original appearance, I do not know *.

The colour of the pigmentum of the eye always corresponds, I believe, with that of the hair and skin, especially if the animal be only of one colour, but is principally determined by the hair; and the most general colour is a very dark brown, approaching to black, from whence it had the name, nigrum pigmentum †. The colour differs in different classes of animals, often in the same class, and even in the same species. In the human it is most commonly dark, in the ferret kind always light, and its difference of colour in the same species is evident from the variety observable in the eyes of different people. There is even a difference of colour in the same eye in many classes of animals, in all of the cat and dog kind, and perhaps in most part of the granivorous. In some it is partly black, and partly of the appearance of polished silver; and in many classes the variation from dark is of two colours: for in the cow, in sheep, deer, horses, and I believe in all animals feeding on grass, there are in the same eye certain portions of it white, and others of a fine green colour. The difference in colour of this pigmentum in the eyes of different animals of the same species is very remarkable: in the human species it is of all the different shades between black and almost white, and the same variety is seen in rabbits, mice, crows, blackbirds, &c., but in these it is of one colour only in the same eye. Every species is, perhaps, subject to such variations; and some of these are so extraordinary as with propriety to be denominated monstrous ‡.

* In vegetables, I believe, it invariably holds good that, however improved by culture, if neglected, they soon degenerate into their first state.

† As the colour of this membrane corresponds with the colour of the skin and hair of the person, it is probable that the people among whom it first got the name were dark.

‡ Perhaps the word monstrous is too strong, or not exactly just. It certainly may be laid down as one of the principles or laws of Nature to deviate under certain circumstances. It may also be observed, that it is neither necessary, nor does it follow that

The variation in the colour of the pigmentum in different species of animals seems to depend on a fixed law of Nature; but the varieties which are met with in the same species are much less constant, being merely different shades approaching to black or white. But the extraordinary circumstance is its being sometimes unusually lighter or darker in individuals of the same species; and this difference not seldom starting up in the young without any hereditary principle to account for it.

The human species is a striking example of the colour of the pigmentum corresponding with that of the skin and hair; and though the skin and hair of one person differs very considerably from the skin and hair of another, yet it is not in so great a degree as in many animals. There are cattle perfectly white, white sheep, white dogs, white cats and rabbits; but there are few of the human species that we can say are perfectly white. They rather pass from the black into the brown, red, and even light yellow; and we find this pigmentum, although only of one colour, varying through all the different corresponding shades. In the African negro, the blackness of whose hair and skin are great distinguishing characteristics, this pigmentum is also very black. In the mulatto, who has not the skin so dark as the African, but the hair nearly as black, this pigmentum is of a shade not quite so deep; yet still it does not approach so near to the middle tint as the skin, rather following the colour of the hair. In people of a swarthy complexion, as Indians, Turks, Tartars, Moors, &c. we find the hair always of a jet black, and this substance of a much darker brown than in those that are fair. In those of very dark complexions, and having very black hair, although descended from fair parents, the same thing holds good. There are few species of animals, or even individuals of a species, whose bodies are only of one colour. Crows and some others, are exceptions; but the greatest number are of two or more, being variously spotted or streaked either with different colours, or with shades of the same. Many species are constantly lighter in some parts of the body than in others; and, with a few exceptions, animals are generally lighter, as to colour, on the lower, or what may be called the foreparts, than on the upper or backparts. The fair man or woman may strictly be considered as a spotted or variegated animal. In many persons the hair of the head, eyebrows, eyelashes, beard, and hair on the pubes, all vary in colour. The hair of the three first may be called fœtal, and are oftener all of the same than of a different colour; the two last are to be considered as adult hair, and are commonly alike in colour, which yet fre-

all deviations from the original must be a falling off; it appears just the contrary, therefore we may suppose that Nature is improving her works, or at least has established the principle of improvement in the body as well as in the mind.

quently varies from that of the fœtus, which last is more liable to change its colour than the other; and the change is generally that of growing darker, especially on the head and the eyelashes*. This difference in the colour of the hair on different parts of the body is not so observable in those nations who are dark or swarthy, as in people inhabiting many of the northern climates.

In animals which are variegated let us observe the colour of this pigmentum, and we shall find it regulated by some general principle, and corresponding with the colour of the eyelashes. The magpie, for instance, is nearly one third, or fourth part white; and the two colours, if blended, would make the compound grey; but the eyelashes being black the pigmentum is black also. We sometimes meet with people whose skin and hair are very white and yet the iris is dark, which is a sign of a dark pigmentum; but if we examine more carefully we shall also find that the eyelashes are dark, although the eyebrows may be the colour of the common hair.

As the colour of the iris in the human species is probably a presumptive, though not a certain sign of the colour of this pigmentum, we may be led to suppose that in those who have the iris in one eye different from that of the other, this substance will likewise differ; but this I cannot determine, never having examined the eyes of any person with such a peculiarity. It is not an uncommon circumstance in some species of animals, the Angola cat seldom having the colour of the iris the same in both eyes.

In people remarkably fair, whether they are of a race that is naturally so, or what may be called monstrous in respect to colour, as white Æthiopians, still we find this pigmentum following the colour of the skin and hair, being in some of a light brown, and in others almost white, according to the colour of the hair in such people.

All foals are of the same colour, and whatever that may be, as they grow older it generally becomes lighter, therefore the pigmentum in them is almost always of the same colour, and does not seem to change with the hair. This change, however, is only in the hair, and not in the skin, the skin of a white or grey horse being as dark as the skin of a black one: yet there is a cream-coloured breed which has the skin of the same colour, whose foals are also of a cream-colour; and by inspecting the parts not covered with hair, such as the mouth, anus, sheath, &c., these, and the pigmentum of the eyes of such horses, are found of a cream-colour likewise.

In the pigmentum of the rabbit kind there are all the degrees of

---

* The hair growing grey is not in the least to the present purpose.

dark and light, corresponding with the colour of the hair; yet there seem to be exceptions to this rule in some white rabbits with black eyes, and therefore with black pigmentum; but in all such there is either a circle of black hair surrounding the eye or the eyelashes, and the skin forming the edge of the lid is also black. In many white cattle this is also observable; and in that breed of dogs called Danes some have the hair surrounding one eye black, while the hair surrounding the other is white; and the iris of the one is often lighter than that of the other. This circumstance, of the iris of one eye being lighter in colour than that of the other, is a common thing in the human species; and sometimes only one half of the iris is light, without any difference in the colour of the eyelash or eyebrow. Whether this difference in the colour of the iris of the two eyes in the same animal is owing to the pigmentum being different in colour, I do not know, although I rather suspect it is something similar to the white iris in horses, which makes them what is called wall-eyed.

The variation of colour appears most remarkable when a white starts up, either where the whole species is black, as in the crow or blackbird, or where only a certain part of the species is black (but permanently so), as a white child born of black parents; and a perfectly white child, whose hair is white, and who has the pigmentum also white, though born of parents who are fair, should as much be considered as a play of Nature as the others. All these lusus naturæ, such as the white negro, the pure white child of fair parents, the white crow, the white blackbird, white mice, &c. have likewise a white pigmentum corresponding with the colour of the hair, feathers, and skin.

Besides the circumstance of animals of the same species differing from one another in colour, there are some distinct species which are, as far as we know, always of a light colour, and in them, too, this pigmentum is white: the animal I allude to is the ferret.

When the pigmentum is of more than one colour in the same eye, the lighter portion is always placed at the bottom of the eye, in the shape of a half-moon, with the circular arch upwards, the straight line or diameter passing almost horizontally across the lower edge of the optic nerve, so that the end of the nerve is within this lighter coloured part, which makes a kind of semicircular sweep above it. This shape is peculiar to the cat, lion, dog, and most of the carnivorous tribe; in the herbivorous the upper edge being irregular; in the seal, however, the light part of this pigmentum is equally disposed all round the optic nerve, and is, on the whole, broader than it is commonly found in quadrupeds. How far this increase of surface is an approach towards the fish kind, in which it is wholly of this metallic white, I will not pretend to say, but it is probable, as the animal is to see in the water as well as in the air, that it may be formed circular, the better to correspond with the form of the eyelids, which open equally all round, which seems to accord with what is observable in fishes, they being without eyelids.

The colour of the pigmentum, whether white or green, or both, has always a bright surface, appearing like polished metal, which appearance animal substance is very capable of taking on, as we see in hair, feathers, silk, &c.

After having taken notice of the various colours of this pigmentum in different animals, both where permanent and where it appears to be a play of Nature, let us next examine what effect it has upon vision in both cases, whether these effects are similar, or if one case illustrates the other.

It may be asserted as an undoubted fact, that the light which falls on the retina covering a white pigmentum has more effect than when it falls on the retina which covers a dark one; which is known by comparing the vision of those of the same species who have the pigmentum wholly dark with those who have it perfectly white; and something may be learned by a similar comparison of animals who have it only in different species, it being reasonable, from analogy, to suppose that some such effect is produced in the eye which is possessed of both.

I shall first consider the effect produced when the white or light colour makes only part of the pigmentum. This will lead me to observe, that all animals having the pigmentum diversified, though they are capable of bearing as much light as others, and can see as perfectly when light is in an equal degree; can likewise see very distinctly when the light is much less than will serve the purposes of animals having it wholly dark. May we not, therefore, ascribe this advantage to the pigmentum being partly white? One might be almost tempted to suppose that such animals have a power of presenting the different parts of the eye to the light, according to the quantity of light required; or of moving the crystalline humour higher or lower: but we are at present unacquainted with any power in the eye by which these actions can be performed.

We may observe, that when a cat or dog looks at us in the twilight the whole pupil is enlarged and illuminated, but in a full light there is no such appearance. It is plain there must be a reflexion of light from the bottom of the eye to produce the above effect, especially as the light reflected is always of the colour of the pigmentum in such animals, which in the cow is of a light green.

I shall secondly consider those animals which have the whole pigmentum of a white colour, whether it is accidental or natural, and that see much better in the dark, or with less light than those in which it is of a dark colour: of the first of these I shall take my instance from the human species; of the second the ferret will serve as an example.

Those of the human species who have the pigmentum of a light colour see much better with a less degree of light than those who have it dark; and this in proportion to their fairness; for when the hair is quite white they cannot see at all in open day without knitting their eyebrows and keeping the eyelids almost shut. In many of these instances there is an universal glare of light from the pupil, tinged with a shade of red, which colour, most probably, arises from the blood in the vessels of the choroid coat. I have likewise observed that the pigmentum is thinnest when it is light, so that some of the light which is reflected from the point of vision would seem to be thrown all over the inner surface of the eye, which being white, or rather a reddish white, the light appears to be again reflected from side to side*. This seemed to be the case in a boy at Shepperton, when about three years of age, of whom I have a portrait, to show that appearance. He is now about thirteen years of age†: the common light of the day is still too much for him; the twilight is less offensive. When in a room he turns his eyes from the window, and when made to expose his face to the light, or when out in the open air, he knits his eyebrows, half shuts his eyelids, and bends his head forwards, or a little down: yet the light appears to be less obnoxious to him now than formerly, probably from habit. Such persons appear to be nearer sighted than people in common, but I apprehend that appearance to arise from the position into which they throw the eyelids and eyebrows, which not only in a great degree excludes the light, making the object faint in proportion to the contraction of the pupil and shade made by the eyelids and eyebrows, but at the same time fits the eye to see near objects; for if we nearly close our eyelids and knit our eyebrows we can see a small object much nearer than if we did not perform such actions, and it will make above a foot difference in the focal distance of the eye.

In many rabbits who have white eyelashes, and in white mice, the pigmentum is entirely white, which is likewise observable in a certain distinct species of animals, the ferret, which we have adduced as an example of the pigmentum being naturally white; for these animals being intended to see in the dark, and their mode of life not exposing them

* How far this is really the case I do not absolutely say; for whatever light comes through the pupil must be reflected from the point of vision; but I imagined I saw the light passing through the substance of the iris.

† The period here alluded to is 1786, when the first edition of this work was published.

to the light, they are liable to be affected by strong light to a greater degree than many others.

If it is allowed as probable that in animals having the pigmentum diversified the object to be viewed is thrown upon the lighter coloured portion, how does it happen that such are able to bear the light better than those who have the pigmentum altogether of a light colour? Perhaps it is not the illuminated object itself that is offensive to the retina, but that diffusion of light in the one kind of eye which does not happen in the other.

Having stated the facts, and the general effect arising from the diversified pigmentum, let us next consider the manner in which it is brought about, that such animals see better with little light than those which have the pigmentum wholly black.

Let us then suppose the retina to be the organ of sight, and that by the rays which fall upon it being properly refracted it gives or conveys to the mind an idea of a distinct object, corresponding with the sensation of touch. This is the most common and simple manner in which vision is performed, and is that mode which takes place where the pigmentum is black, or nearly so, and where the greatest quantity of external light is required.

The retina, although somewhat opaque, is yet so transparent as to allow a considerable quantity of light to pass through it. For if this was not the case there could not be those differences in the appearance of the eye which I have been describing. The rays which pass through, we may suppose, do or do not give sensation in their passage; and we may also suppose that only those which strike against the retina are the cause of sensation: but this is not the present inquiry; the rays which pass through the retina are what I am alone to consider, which falling upon the pigmentum are there disposed of according to the reflecting powers of that substance. If the pigmentum is black the rays will then be absorbed, and entirely lost, therefore in such eyes vision can receive no assistance from it, and consequently a considerable quantity of light is required to produce distinct vision; but in those who have some part of this pigmentum white, we find that the rays of light which pass through the retina are reflected back again; and in this case it is not unnatural to suppose that the reflected rays, in their passage back, will strike against the retina, and increase the power of vision. It is evident that a considerable portion passes forwards through the retina, which, I suspect, is partly lost on the inner surface of the lateral and forepart of the eye, where the pigmentum is black, while the remainder passing through the pupil is again thrown on the object looked at. The next thing to be considered is, whether the shape of the eye is such as will throw the rays, which passed through the retina, back upon that membrane, in the same or nearly in the same place as that through which they originally came. The eye being a sphere, or approaching to that figure, makes it probable; but whether the curve is such as will reflect the rays exactly in the same direction is not so easily determined. If the curve be a true one, then the rays that are not obstructed in their return by the retina must pass forwards through the pupil, and, being refracted in their passage through the crystalline humour, will be sent out of the eye in the same lines in which they entered, and be thrown on the very object from whence they came; which seems to be in a great measure the case, if we may judge by the degree of illumination in the cat's eyes. If the rays reflected from the light part of the pigmentum should not, in their return, strike exactly on the same points in the retina, through which they first passed, yet if they are thrown nearly on the same place it will be sufficient, for we know that our sensations are not capable of conveying to the mind mathematical exactness. And the same circumstance will be a sufficient answer, should it be objected that the time lost in the passing and repassing of the rays may prevent distinct vision; for it is known that if an illumined body is made to move quickly in a circle, it will appear to the eye a circle of fire.

SOME FACTS RELATIVE TO THE LATE MR. JOHN HUNTER'S PREPARATION FOR THE CROONIAN LECTURE.

By Everard Home, Esq., F.R.S.

[Read November 14, 1793.]

MR. HUNTER having announced to the Royal Society that he would make the structure of the crystalline humour of the eye the subject of the Croonian lecture for the present year, and having, unfortunately for science, died before his observations on that subject were rendered complete, I feel it a duty I owe to his memory as well as to the Society, to state the facts respecting this humour with which he had acquainted me; and shall subjoin an unfinished letter from Mr. Hunter to Sir Joseph Banks on the same subject.

It is now many years that Mr. Hunter has had an idea that the crystalline humour was enabled by its own internal actions to adjust itself, so as to adapt the eye to different distances; and when the *Tænia hydatigena*[a] first came under his observation as a living animal, he was surprised to see the quantity of contraction that took place in a membrane devoid of muscular fibres, but made use of the fact in his investigation of the structure of the crystalline humour of the eye.

Some time after this, having occasion to dissect the eye of the cuttle-fish, which he had frequently done before, but not with exactly the same view, he discovered in the crystalline humour a structure which corresponded with the idea he had formed of its actions in the human eye. He found it composed of laminæ, whose appearance was evidently fibrous for some depth from the external surface; but becoming less and less distinct, till at last this fibrous appearance was entirely lost, and the middle, or central part of the humour, was compact and transparent, without any visible laminæ. From this structure it would appear that in the eye of the cuttle-fish the exterior parts of the humour are fibrous, the interior parts not; so that the central part is a nucleus round which the fibrous coverings are placed. The preparations which demonstrate these facts will be laid before the Society[b].

As the structure of the crystalline humour in the cuttle-fish differs in nothing from that of the same humour in other animals but in the

---

[a] [The hydatid commonly found in the abdominal cavity of the sheep,—*Cysticercus tenuicollis*, Rudolphi.]

[b] [The Hunterian preparations demonstrating the peculiarities of the eye of the cuttle-fish are not fewer than twenty. See Physiological Catalogue, vol. iii. p. 140.]

distinctness of the fibrous appearance, Mr. Hunter was led to consider that the exterior part in all of them was similar, although no appearance of fibres could be demonstrated.

What I have here explained I was acquainted with at the time I had the honour of giving the Croonian lecture, in which I examined the different structures endowed with muscular action, and was desirous that Mr. Hunter would, either of himself or through me, communicate these observations to the Society; but this he declined doing till he had ascertained by experiment whether any muscular effect was really produced; and the hope of being assisted by Mr. Ramsden made him, from time to time, put off making his experiments.

In the course of this season he began his experiments, which were founded upon the analogy that ought to exist between this humour, if muscular, and others of a similar structure, which led him to expect that they would be acted upon by the same stimuli : and having found that a certain degree of heat, applied through the medium of water, will excite muscular action after almost every other stimulus had failed, it was proposed to apply this to the crystalline humour, and ascertain its effects.

The crystalline humour taken from animals recently killed must be considered as being still alive.   Such humours were to be immersed in water of different temperatures, and placed in such a manner as to form the image of a lucid well-defined object, by a proper apparatus for that purpose, so that any change of the place of that image from the stimulating effects of the warm water upon the humour would be readily ascertained. These were the experiments which Mr. Hunter had instituted and begun; but in which he had not made sufficient progress to enable him to draw any conclusions.

To Sir Joseph Banks, from Mr. Hunter.
     " Sir,
     " When I did myself the honour of giving in my claim to the discovery of the crystalline humour being muscular, and proposed to make it the subject of the Croonian lecture, I did not foresee that anything could prevent me from fulfilling my promise; but since that time, what with my state of health, which does not allow me to be very active, the hurry of official business on account of the war, and my brother-in-law, Mr. Home, being employed on the medical staff, I have not had the power of repeating my experiments, and drawing out, to my satisfaction, the many conclusions which are the result of such a power in this humour.

"The laws of optics are so well understood, and the knowledge of the eye, when considered as an optical instrument, has been rendered so perfect, that I do not consider myself capable of making any addition to it: but still there is a power in the eye by which it can adapt itself to different distances far too extensive for the simple mechanism of the parts to effect. This power writers upon this subject have been at great pains to investigate and explain. The motion of the crystalline humour forwards and backwards was asserted by some to be the cause, while others supposed in the eye a power to alter its shape, so as to shorten or lengthen its axis, which altered the distance between the crystalline humour and the point of impression; but we should consider that a part of the eye is itself a refractor, and that if its shape be altered so as to remove the crystalline humour from the point of impression, in order to enable it to bring a distant object to its proper focus on the retina, this effect will be in some degree counteracted by the anterior part of the eye refracting more than before, by being rendered more convex. But we have, in fact, no power capable of producing this effect: for the straight muscles, so far from appearing to have this power, have been even supposed to flatten the eye, and shorten its axis: and it is very possible that the action of these muscles is such as tends to both effects; but, being in opposition to each other, the eye retains its shape, the insertion of these muscles being much more forwards than appears to be necessary for the simple motions of the eye. Further, when we consider that in many animals the shape of the eye is unalterable, as in all of the whale tribe, the sclerotic coat being above half an inch thick and composed of a strong tendinous substance;—that in many fish this coat is composed of cartilage; and in all birds the anterior part of it is (I believe) composed of bone;—from all these considerations, I saw no power that could adapt the eye to the various distances of which we find it capable in the human body, unless we suppose the crystalline humour to be varied in figure, which can only be effected by a muscular action within itself. With this idea strongly impressed upon my mind, and finding that in many animals, when the crystalline humour was coagulated, it had a fibrous structure like muscles, I confess it seemed to me to confirm it; but as this might to others appear only conjecture, requiring some proof, I set about such experiments as were best adapted for that purpose. Knowing that in all violent deaths the muscles contract, I supposed the crystalline humour, if muscular, would show signs of this effect; for which purpose I got the eyes of bullocks when removed from the sockets, the moment the animal was knocked down, and while the eyes were warm the humours were removed."

Mr. Hunter had proceeded thus far in the account of his experiments, when he was suddenly, and very unexpectedly, carried off; and as he has left no notes upon this subject, I am unable to make any addition to the account I have already given.

Mr. Hunter's laying claim to the discovery of a fibrous structure in the crystalline humour, which had been observed long before, and described by the accurate Leuwenhoek, may appear to require some explanation. The discovery of a fibrous appearance in that humour appertains to Leuwenhoek; but the discovery of an eye in which this structure of the crystalline humour was perfectly distinct, and in which all the circumstances of course and situation could be determined, is due to Mr. Hunter[a]: and if it should be found, by future observation and experiments, that this structure, which is different from any that has hitherto been described, is capable of producing consequent actions and effects, sufficient to explain the adjustment of the eye to different distances, it will not be considered as a small or unimportant discovery.

---

[a] [In this investigation by Hunter of the intimate structure of the crystalline lens we may perceive the continuation of the series of discoveries which, commenced by Leuwenhoek, have, in the hands of Sir David Brewster, produced such unexpected results, and opened so interesting a field for philosophical experiment and teleological speculation with regard to this part of the mechanism of the instrument of vision.

Notwithstanding the anatomical remarks of Hunter, the observations of Professor Blair (*Edinburgh Transactions*, vol. iii.), and the experiments of Young, Wollaston, Wells, and Frauenhofer, we still find, even in very recent physiological works, a mere repetition of the simple statement of Paley that the lens consists of concentric layers, which gradually increase in density from the circumference to the centre; and, under the influence of an apt comparison, the principle of the construction of the lens is asserted to be the same as that of the compound or achromatic object-glass, and the invention of Dollond to be a repetition, though an imperfect one, of this the natural type and perfection of a dioptric instrument which is supposed to converge the rays of light into a focus without any dispersion of the rays, and consequently without the production of false colours round the image. Now the fact is that the image given by the eye is not perfect with regard to colours in its ordinary exercise: there is not only dispersion of the rays of light, but the quantity of dispersion has been measured, and the different focal lengths of the eye for red and violet lights have been accurately determined by Young and Frauenhofer; the latter philosopher, indeed, has found it necessary to correct the dispersion of the eye in the construction of his achromatic object-glasses. But to return to the structure of the crystalline lens,—this complex and beautiful part consists, according to Sir David Brewster, of innumerable fibres of nearly the same length, each of which tapers from its middle part to its two extremities, like the gores or gussets of a globe. In the lenses of some animals the extremities of all the fibres terminate in two opposite poles; in others, in a line at each pole, the line at the posterior pole being at right angles to the line at the anterior pole, and all the fibres except a few being bent into the most beautiful curves of contrary flexure. In some lenses the fibres terminate in the lines of a rectangular cross at each pole, the

The melancholy event which has deprived this learned Society of so valuable a member, and which has taken from me so able an instructor,

---

line of the cross at one pole being inclined 45° to the lines at the other pole; in others, the terminations of the fibres form more complicated figures. In the.largest number of animals the arrangement of the fibres is the same at both poles; but in a few, such as the turtle, the fibres terminate in a different manner in the two surfaces of the lens. But the structure of each of the fibres is still more wonderful than their arrangement. The sides of each fibre are formed with teeth, like those of a watch-wheel, and the teeth of one fibre lock into those of the adjacent ones, apparently to strengthen them and give body to the frail morsel of transparent jelly into which they are so marvellously moulded.

In the lens of a cod-fish, four tenths of an inch in diameter, Sir D. Brewster calculates the number of fibres to be about five millions, and the number of teeth by which the fibres are bound together to be *sixty-two thousand five hundred millions*; and as every tooth has three surfaces, the number of touching surfaces will be *one hundred and eighty-seven thousand five hundred millions*; and yet this little sphere of tender jelly is as transparent as a drop of the purest water, and allows a beam of light to pass across these almost innumerable joints without obstructing or reflecting a single ray!

With respect to the muscular theory of the lens, and its supposed power of adjusting the eye to vision at different distances, by an alteration of its own form or dimensions, it is hardly necessary to state that these views have derived no support since the time of Hunter, and of Dr. Young, who also entertained the theory of the irritability of the crystalline fibres. It has, on the other hand, been shown, in the well-attested case of Henry Miles[1], that the eye may retain its power of adjustment after the removal of the lens.

The supposed function of the lens, as an achromatic instrument, has been deduced from the structure which it presents in the human body, where the density of the fibrous layers diminishes from the centre to the surface: a structure of which the purpose is undoubtedly to correct spherical aberration; but the lenses of quadrupeds display three different structures of varying density, separated by neutral lines, in which lines a density decreasing outwards passes into a density increasing outwards. This structure is well displayed in the lens of the horse; and when the animal has attained a great age the densities of the central and superficial structures have become uniform throughout, while the middle one exhibits a varying density more strongly marked than in the young lens, and exhibiting by polarized light a brilliant yellow colour, like the most perfect films of regularly crystallized bodies. That these structures are intended to correct spherical aberration or to improve vision cannot be doubted; but the principles are yet to be discovered on which that correction or improvement depends. Meanwhile it is the duty of the physiologist to set plainly before himself, and to offer fairly to his pupils these unexplained or residual phenomena of the theory of vision; not to hide them beneath an easily comprehended but insufficient illustration. An achromatic lens, though highly desirable, indeed essential to the construction of a good telescope or microscope, is not therefore necessary in the eye: it is well known to be less adapted for the purposes of a *camera obscura* than a common lens; but the organ of vision has a much closer analogy to a *camera obscura* than to a telescope. In a telescope, if there be colour, or dispersion of the object-glass, this must be greatly magnified by the eye-piece; and, what is still more essential, there is an eye behind the instrument which takes cogni-

---

[1] See the Croonian Lecture, Phil. Trans., 1802, vol. xcii. p. 8.

so rare an example, and so inestimable a friend, is too recent to make any apology necessary for the shortness or incorrectness of this account. I thought it due to the memory of my friend that no promise of his, however inadequate I feel myself to the performance, should be left unfulfilled; and the circumstances of distress under which it has been drawn up will procure for me every indulgence from this learned Society.

EVERARD HOME.

Leicester Square, Nov. 4, 1793.

---

zance of those imperfections, and for whose sake they are endeavoured to be remedied. But there is no eye behind the retina to view in the same manner the image which is thrown upon that membrane. It is well known that the retina is incapable of transmitting a distinct idea of any spectrum depicted upon it save of that which is situated in or near its axis: the colours of the lateral pencils cannot be seen, and hence it is of no importance whatever to render the image achromatic at a distance from the axis. When we wish to examine an object, or a part of an object, with minute attention, we direct to it the axis of the eye; and in order to obtain a sensibly colourless vision in or near the axis achromatic compensation is not necessary. It is no doubt true that even in this axis there is a non-coincidence of the foci of the differently-coloured rays; but owing to the shortness of the focal distance of the eye, and the low dispersive power of the humours, this non-coincidence of the different foci does no injury to our ordinary vision.]

AN ACCOUNT OF THE ORGAN OF HEARING IN FISHES[a].

NATURAL history, having ever been considered as worthy the attention of the curious philosopher, has in all ages kept pace with the other branches of knowledge; and as both arts and sciences have of late years been cultivated to a degree perhaps beyond what was ever known before, we find that natural history has not been neglected. All the nations of Europe appear solicitous to encourage the study; and in this island it has been pursued with more philosophic ardour than was ever known in any country. It has become an object of pursuit to men possessed of affluent fortune; which they have not only dedicated to the cultivation of this science, but have even risked their health and lives in exploring unknown regions to increase the sources of information, and in settling correspondences everywhere, so as to bring materials into this country that might render it the school of natural history. It is no wonder then that a spirit of inquiry is diffused through almost all ranks of men; and that those who cannot pursue it themselves, yet choosing at least to benefit by the industry of others, are eager to be informed of what is already known.

These reflections have induced me to publish this short account of the organ of hearing in fishes; for, though the existence of such an organ is now known to many, it is still a subject of dispute with others whether they possess the sense or not[b].

---

[a] [Originally communicated to the Royal Society, and printed in the Philosophical Transactions (vol. lxxii. p. 379) for the year 1782.]

[b] [Cuvier justly states that the structure of the organ of hearing was better known to some of the ancient anatomists in the class of fishes than even in the human subject. Casserius has given moderately good figures of the semicircular canals and the ossiculum auditus of the pike in his work entitled Pentestesion (p. 224), published in the year 1600. Steno, in the *Acta Medica* of Copenhagen for 1673, described the internal ear of the *Squalus Mustelus*, Linn., with tolerable exactness, although without figures.

Klein, in his *Missus Historiæ Piscium permovendæ*, printed in the year 1740, gives a detailed description and accurate figures of the ossicula of the ear of the pike, salmon, trout, umber, marene (*Salmo Marœna*, L.), herring, cod, dorsch (*Gadus callarius*, L.), ling, pike-perch, perch, gremille, stickleback, turbot, sole, barbue (*Pleuronectes Rhombus*, L.), carp, barbel, and many other species of Cyprinus.

In 1753, Etienne-Louis Geoffroy, a physician of Paris, presented to the Academy a memoir *ex professo* on the organ of hearing in fishes; but this was not printed till the

Some time before I quitted my anatomical pursuits, in the year 1760[a], and went with the army to Belleisle, I had discovered this organ in fishes, and had the parts exposed and preserved in spirits. In some the canals were filled with coloured injection, which showed them to great advantage, and in others were so prepared as to fit them to be kept as dried preparations*. My researches, in that and in every other part of the animal œconomy, have been continued ever since that time. I am still inclined to consider whatever is uncommon in the structure of this organ in fishes as only a link in the chain of varieties displayed in its formation in different animals, descending from the most perfect to the most imperfect, in a regular progression†.

* I have injected these parts in other animals, both with wax and metals; which, the bone being afterwards corroded in spirit of sea-salt, make elegant casts of these canals.

† The preparations to illustrate these facts[b] have been, ever since, shown in my collection, to both the curious of this country and foreigners. In showing whatever was new, or supposed to be new, the ears of fishes were always considered by me as one important article[c].

---

year 1778. He has described generally the ear of the eel, the cod, the pike, the carp, the gardon (*Cyprinus idus*, Blo.), the flounder, and the perch; but he errs in ascribing to certain holes in the cranium the office of a meatus auditorius externus, which they do not fulfil. The figures annexed to this memoir, Cuvier informs us, were mislaid and lost, and therefore they did not appear in the printed essay. The description of the ear of the ray was given by Geoffroy in a Memoir on the Ears of Reptiles, presented in 1752, and printed in 1755.]

[a] [Camper's researches on this subject were made in the year 1761: they appeared first in the Haerlem Memoirs for 1762. He afterwards sent a more detailed memoir on the same subject to the Academy of Sciences of Paris in 1767, which was printed in the 'Recueil des Savans Etrangèrs, t. vii.,' in 1774. He describes in detail the organ of hearing of the ray, the cod, the pike, and the lophius, with figures in his style, i. e. somewhat vague. He added but little to that which Geoffroy had advanced, except that he denied too generally the external canal, and that he speaks of an organ which he terms *tensor bursæ*, which seems only to be an appendage, or rather a ligament, more distinct in the pike than in most other fishes.

In the year 1773, in the 17th vol. of the *Novi Commentarii* of St. Petersburgh, Kolreuter gave some very precise and detailed descriptions and figures of the ear, in two species of sturgeon, the common one (*Acipenser Sturio*, Linn.), and the huso (*Acipenser Huso*, Linn.).

Monro described, better than any of his predecessors or successors, the external ear of the Chondropterygii, in his Anatomy of Fishes, published in 1785.

Scarpa denies the external communication in the ray, which Hunter correctly describes in the present memoir.]

[b] [He here alludes to the series of other organs in his collection analogous to those of the ear; and it is interesting to observe these incidental evidences of the philosophical tendency in Hunter to view the varieties of structure, which his numerous dissections displayed to him, as modifications of one type, or a graduated and connected chain of varieties.]

[c] [See the Preparations in the Gallery of the Hunterian Museum, numbered from 1560 to 1574 inclusive.]

As in this age of investigation a hint that such an organ existed would be sufficient to excite a spirit of conjecture or inquiry, I was aware that there would not be wanting some men who, whether they only imagined the fact might be true, or really found it to be so, would be very ready to assume all the merit of the discovery to themselves. My attention was more strongly called to this point by hearing, in conversation, that some anatomists in France, Germany, and Italy, had discovered the organ of hearing in fishes, and intended to publish on the subject. I therefore thought that it would be only justice to myself to deliver to the Royal Society a short account of that organ, a discovery of which I had made more than twenty years before. This account I shall reprint here, without adding anything to what I had before written, reserving a more complete examination of this subject for a larger work, on the structure of animals, which I one day hope to have it in my power to publish.

I do not intend to give a full account of this organ in any one fish, or of the varieties in different fishes, but only of the organ in general; those therefore who may wish to pursue this branch of the animal œconomy will think it deficient perhaps in the descriptive parts. If it was a difficult task to expose this organ in fishes I should perhaps be led to be more full in my description of it, but in fact there is nothing more easy.

It may be proper just to observe here, that the class called Sepia has the organ of hearing, though somewhat differently constructed from what it is in fishes[a].

The organ of hearing in fishes is placed at the sides of the cavity which contains the brain, but the skull makes no part of it, as it does in the quadruped and the bird, the organ being a distinct and detached part. In some fishes, as in those of the ray kind, the organ is wholly surrounded by the parts composing the cavity of the skull; in others it is in part within the skull, or cavity which contains the brain, as in the salmon, cod, &c., the skull projecting laterally, and forming a cavity.

---

[a] [This is the first announcement of the existence of an organ of hearing in the Cephalopoda. It differs from that of fishes in the absence of the semicircular canals, and exhibits a simpler stage of structure, consisting of a vestibule, with the nerve, fluid, sacculus, and ear-stone or otolithe. The low-organized Cyclostomous fishes manifest their character as transitional links between the invertebrate and vertebrate animals in several parts of their structure, but more especially in the organ of hearing. The myxine has a vestibule, with one canal extended from it. The lamprey shows a further stage of complication, in having two canals continued from the vestibule. All the osseous fishes have three semicircular canals, as described in the text; and the plagiostomous cartilaginous fishes, as the sharks and rays, exhibit a higher type of structure, in having the internal ear inclosed within the parietes of the cranial cavity, and in the external communication or meatus which some of the species present.]

The organ of hearing in fishes appears to increase in dimensions with the animal, and nearly in the same proportion, which is not the case with the quadruped, &c., the organs being in them nearly as large in the growing fœtus as in the adult.   Neither is its structure, by any degree, so complicated in fishes as in all those orders of animals which may be reckoned superior, such as quadrupeds, birds, and amphibious animals; but there is a regular gradation from the first of these to fishes.

It varies in different genera of fishes; but in all it consists of three curved tubes, which unite one with another; this union forms in some only one canal, as in the cod, salmon, ling, &c., and in others a tolerably large cavity, as in the ray kind.   In the jack[a] there is an oblong bag, or blind process, which is an addition to these canals, and communicates with them at their union.   In the cod, &c. this union of the three tubes stands upon an oval cavity; and in the jack there are two; the additional cavities in these fishes appearing to answer the same purpose with the cavity[b] observed in the ray or cartilaginous fishes, which is at the union of the three canals.

The whole organ is composed of a kind of cartilaginous substance, very hard or firm in some parts, and in some fishes crusted over with a thin bony lamella, to prevent it from collapsing; for as the skull does not form any part of these canals or cavities, they must be composed of a substance capable of keeping its form.

Each tube describes more than a semicircle, resembling, in some sort, what we find in most other animals, but differing in the parts being distinct from the skull*.

Two of the semicircular canals are similar to one another, may be called a pair, and are placed perpendicularly; the third is not so long, and in some is placed horizontally, uniting as it were the other two at their ends or terminations.   In the skate this is somewhat different, the horizontal canal being united only to one of the perpendicular canals.   The two semicircular canals, whose position is perpendicular, are united, forming one canal; at their other extremities they have no connexion with each other, but join the horizontal one, near its entrance into the common cavity.   Near the union of these canals they are swelled out into round bags '(ampullæ),' and become much larger.

In the ray kind all these canals terminate in one cavity, and in the cod in one canal, placed upon the additional cavity or cavities, in which there is a bone or bones.   In some there are two bones; and in the

* The turtle and the crocodile have a structure somewhat similar to this; and the intention is the same, for their skulls make no part of the organ.

---

[a] [*Esox Lucius*, L.]   [b] [*Sacculus vestibuli*.]

jack, which has two cavities, we find in one of them ' (the accessory sacculus of the vestibule,)' two bones, and in the other ' (the ordinary sacculus of the vestibule,)' one; in the ray there is only a chalky substance*.

In some fishes the external communication, or meatus, enters at the union of the two perpendicular canals, which is the case with all the ray kind, the external orifice being small, and placed on the upper flat surface of the head; but it is not every genus or species of fishes that have the external opening[b].

The nerves of the ear pass outwards from the brain, and appear to terminate at once on the external surface of the enlarged part of the semicircular tubes above described[c]. They do not appear to pass through these tubes so as to get on the inside, as is supposed to be the case in quadrupeds; I should therefore very much suspect that the lining of the tubes in the quadruped is not nerve, but a kind of internal periosteum.

As it is evident that fishes possess the organ of hearing, it becomes unnecessary to make or relate any experiment made with living fishes, which only tends to prove this fact; but I will mention one experiment, to show that sounds affect them much, and is one of their guards, as it is in other animals. In the year 1762, when I was in Portugal, I observed in a nobleman's garden, near Lisbon, a small fish-pond full of different kinds of fish. The bottom was level with the ground, the pond having been made by forming a bank all round, and had a shrubbery close to it. Whilst I lay on the bank observing the fish swimming about, I desired a gentleman who was with me to take a loaded gun and fire it from behind the shrubs. The reason for desiring him to go behind the shrubs was, that there might not be the least reflection of

---

* This chalky substance is also found in the ears of amphibious animals[a].

---

[a] [In these it is lodged in a small blind sac, communicating with the vestibule, and representing the cochlea in a rudimental state. In the ray also, the vestibule, after receiving the orifices of the semicircular canals, opens into a large oval sac, which gives off two appendages, one anterior, the other posterior; this sac is analogous to the rudimental cochlea in reptiles, as is also the sacculus vestibuli in the osseous fishes.]

[b] [Hunter had a drawing made of these orifices in the monk-fish (*Squatina Angelus*, Dum.), which has been engraved and published in the third volume of the Physiological Catalogue of the Hunterian Museum, pl. xxxiii. fig. 1, *a*.]

[c] [The acoustic nerve comes off from the brain, nearly opposite the junction of the sacculus with the vestibule; it sends off from its upper part a filament to each of the semicircular canals: this filament penetrates the ampulla of the canal to which it appertains, and is there lost. Another division of the nerve goes to the vestibule, but by far the greatest part of it spreads out into a number of filaments which form a very beautiful apparatus, under the parietes of the sac which contains the large stone.]

light.   The moment the report was made the fish seemed to be all of one mind, for they vanished instantaneously, raising a cloud of mud from the bottom.   In about five minutes afterwards they began to appear, and were seen swimming about as before.

Mons. Geoffroi, who has written on this organ, considers the ray as in the class of reptiles, and with that idea has examined their organ of hearing.   He is by no means clear in his description, so that it is almost impossible to follow him; yet it is but doing him justice to allow that he has discovered what is analogous to the three semicircular canals in other animals, together with their union into one cavity.   He mentions the chalky substance contained in that cavity, and also the nerves; but it is by no means clear that he was acquainted with the external opening which leads to these canals.   He says, "The entrance of the organ of hearing (by which one would suppose he means the meatus auditorius externus) is not easily discovered;" but that which he describes does not correspond with the real situation of the external communication; we may therefore reasonably conclude that he is describing something else.   He is not more clear in his mode of reasoning on the application of the parts to produce the sense of hearing.   He observes that the organ of hearing is very imperfect in this species of animals, but supposes this to be compensated by the medium in which they live, and by which sound is conveyed to them, being more dense than that of the air, by which sound is communicated to animals living on the land; and of this idea he is certainly the author.   Mons. Geoffroi cannot indeed be said to have given a perfect account of the organ of hearing in fishes, yet on the whole he should be considered as a discoverer; for though he only made his observations on the ray, as belonging to the class of reptiles, yet as it may be properly considered of the fish kind, he has a just claim to that credit.   Had I formerly been acquainted with this author's researches and pretensions, I should not have claimed that to which I had not a prior right; nor should I have held the discovery of the external communication alone, an object of consequence enough to induce me to dispute the honour with Mons. Geoffroi.

In looking over the works of the different authors who have treated of the organ of hearing in fishes, I find from a passage in Willoughby[*], who published prior to Mons. Geoffroi, and indeed is quoted by him, that my claim, even to the discovery of the external opening, is not so strong as I believed it to be, as he mentions an external orifice in the skate contiguous to what he supposes the organ of hearing in that fish. If what he alludes to is really the external opening of the ear, it gives

[*] Willughbeii Historia Piscium, Oxonii 1686, lib. iii. cap. viii.

him a prior claim to the discovery of that part of the organ, although from his account, he does not seem to have been acquainted with the organ itself; for, as in describing the external ear of the thornback, he has evidently mistaken the nose of it, of which he gives a tolerably full account, it is very obvious that he was ignorant of the opening into the ear*.

Although Professor Camper published an account of the organ of hearing in fishes so late as 1774, he did not seem at that time to have been acquainted with the external opening of the ear in the ray. After giving a description of the organ of hearing in the pike, he makes some general observations on the similarity of this organ in other fishes, but excepts the shark and ray†. This exception we might suppose alluded to the auditory canal, but further on he explains what is meant by this exception, and does not mention the external opening in the ray, from which we may fairly conclude that he was not acquainted with it‡.

* Lib. iii. cap. xiv.

† " Il est très-vraisemblable que toutes les autres espèces de poissons, tant *malacopterygii* qu' *acanthopterygii*, aussi-bien que les *branchiostegi* & les *chondropterygii* d'Artedi, à l'exception des squales & des raies, ont l'organe de l'ouïe construit à peu près de la même façon ; je n'excepte pas l'esturgeon, quoique M. Klein, *ibid.* ait donné la description du conduit auditif, *page* 19, *figure A, Tab.* 2. *b* ; ce poisson étant rare parmi nous, je n'ai eu occasion de l'examiner qu'une seule fois sans avoir trouvé ce conduit." Memoirs Etrangers de l'Academie des Sciences, 1774, tom. 6, page 190.

‡ " Au contraire, les chiens de mer, les *galeis* de Rondelet & les poissons qu'il a décrits, *lib.* XII. ; les *squalis* d'Artedi & les raies, ont bien l'organe à peu près de la même composition, mais il est enfermé dans une caisse tout osseuse ou cartilagineuse, ce qui ne fait pas une différence essentielle ; ils entendent donc comme les églefins, les morues, les baudroyes & les brochets, en un mot comme tous les autres poissons non amphibies : M. Geoffroi s'est trompé en comparant leurs organes avec celui de reptiles, tels que la vipère, les lézards, &c. qui entendent le son comme les quadrupèdes, les oiseaux & les amphibies aquatiques, savoir par le moyen de l'air & d'un tambour, comme j'ai dessein de le prouver dans une autre occasion." Memoires Etrangers de l'Academie des Sciences, 1774, tom. 6, page 190.

OF ABSORPTION BY VEINS[a].

[Dr. Hunter introduces the account of his brother's experiments on this subject as follows.]

IN both my courses of the winter 1759–60, I went so far as to say, I *believed* that the red veins did not absorb; and gave my reasons for thinking so; and in different parts of my lectures I used to treat of the transudation and absorption of fluids in animal bodies in the following manner:

" I have often considered with myself how the interstitial fluid gets into the smaller and greater cavities of our bodies; how the water of an anasarca, for instance, gets into the cellular membrane. The common opinion, I think, is, that there are everywhere exhalant arteries, which open and terminate on the superficies of such cavities, and throw out the watery fluid which they contain. But for my own part, I cannot help believing that it is entirely by transudation through the coats or sides of the vessels. My reasons for thinking so are these:

" First, so far as I can find, all the arguments of the latest and best anatomists, taken from injecting the arterial system in dead and living bodies, only prove that a thin fluid passes readily from the arteries into the interstices of parts. They do not prove the existence of exhaling branches more than they prove transudation.

" In the second place, the phenomena of injections, so far as I have been able to make observations, agree better with the notion of transudation than with that of exhaling arteries. I have had great experience of injections, and I have made experiments with all sorts of fluids injected into the arteries and veins of dead bodies. I have always observed that subtile and penetrating fluids pass with ease from the arteries into the cavity of the intestines, and into the cellular membrane in any part of the body: such fluids are water, gum-water, whites of eggs strained, glue, isinglass dissolved in water or spirits, any fluid oil, melted butter or axunge, &c. But when these fluids were coloured with vermilion I always observed that none of the vermilion passed out of the arterial system but when there were manifest appearances of extravasation and rupture of the vessels: I never observed vermilion pass into the cavity of an intestine from the mesenteric arteries, without seeing

---

[a] [Medical Commentaries, Part I., p. 39.]

a hundred ruptures and extravasations in the villi of the gut.   All this looks as if the fluid oozed through the coats rather than was poured out by the branches of arteries.

" In the third place, I have observed that the cellular membrane is not so immediately filled by injecting the arteries; it requires some time, and I have plainly seen, when I have let an injected part lie by a little while, that the cellular membrane became gradually more loaded as the arterial system became more empty : a strong argument, in my mind, that it got out of the arteries by transudation.

" In the fourth place, water and even red blood soaks through all our vessels and membranes in dead bodies; as you may see by steeping the apex of a heart well washed, or the convolution of a piece of fresh intestine in clear water; in both cases the water will become bloody.

" But still it is said that in all these cases the fluids pass by fine exhaling vessels, though these vessels cannot be seen.   To this I answer that if our interstitial fluid was of a strong marked colour, we should then by dissection be able to observe whether it was poured out by small arteries, or whether it soaked through the natural pores in the coats of vessels.   Now, very fortunately for us in this dispute, there is one such fluid in the body : it is the bile.   Its colour is pretty deep, and very different from anything that lies near the gall-bladder.   No man can have opened any number of bodies without allowing that the gall does pass through all the coats of the gall-bladder, and pervades the substance of the neighbouring parts, not by exhaling nor by inhaling vessels, but by manifest transudation or soaking.

" It might be asked, why the red blood does not transude through the vessels in living bodies; for I think it certainly does not.   In answer to this it may be said that our fibres and vessels have perhaps some degree of tension and firmness in life which they lose with life; and it must be observed too, that in proportion as the blood putrefies it becomes thinner : whence we see, in opening a putrid body, all the cavities more or less filled with a bloody water, and all distinction of colour in the muscles and cellular membrane quite lost.   But what I suppose to be the principal reason that red blood does not transude through the vessels in living bodies is its glutinous quality, its thickness while it is equally mixed up with its coagulating part.   That part coagulates as certainly as the blood stagnates even in living bodies; and when the universal stagnation happens in death, this part of the blood collects itself into irregular polypi and coagulations all over the body, and the rest of the blood is no longer the thick viscid fluid it was before, but rather a bloody serum, that will ooze through all the vessels and membranes."

Such were my notions of the source of our interstitial fluid. With regard to its absorption, I was of opinion that Nature had provided a system on purpose, viz. the lymphatics. I considered these vessels and the lacteals as an appendage to the venal system, by which the stores were brought in for supplying the circulation; and the glands and secretory vessels all over the body I considered as an appendage to the arterial system, by which the proper separations were made, and the redundancies thrown off.

My only doubt was whether the veins did or did not absorb a certain quantity, especially in the intestines. From my own observations on injections I should have concluded that they did not, and that there was no passage for liquors between an intestine and the mesenteric veins otherwise than by transudation. But authors of the best credit had given such arguments and experiments in favour of absorption by veins, that I dared not, even in my own mind, determine the question.

At this time my brother was deeply engaged in physiological inquiries, in making experiments on living animals, and in prosecuting comparative anatomy with great accuracy and application. It is well known that I speak of him with moderation when I say so. He took the subject of absorption into his consideration, and from all his observations was inclined to believe that in the human body there was one, and but one, system of vessels for absorption. He knew so well that many things had been asserted by one person after another which were not true, that so many mistakes had been made from inattention, so many errors introduced from other causes, that he could easily suppose the veins might not perhaps absorb, after all the demonstrations that had been given of the fact; and therefore was determined to see how far this point could be cleared up by plain experiments and observations. With that intention he made the following experiments, in my presence and in the presence of a number of gentlemen, who all of us assisted him, and made our own observations upon what passed before us. I shall quote the experiments from him, and can bear testimony to the fairness with which they were made and with which they are here related.

" *Animal First*.—Experiment I. On the 3rd of November, 1758*," says he, " I opened the belly of a living dog. The intestines rushed out immediately. I exposed them fully; and we observed the lacteals filled with a white liquor at the upper part of the gut and mesentery; but in those which came from the ileon and colon the liquor was transparent.

* In presence of Doctors Clayton, Fordyce, and Michaelson, and Messrs. Blount, Jones, Churchill, and Richardson.

" I tied up the mesenteric artery and vein that was going to about half a foot of intestine, and put a tight ligature upon the upper part of the intestine, including a little of the mesentery; then emptied that part of the gut by squeezing it downwards, and put a similar ligature upon the lower part of the gut. In the next place, I made a small hole in the upper end of this part of the gut, and by a funnel poured in some warm milk, and confined it by making a third ligature upon the gut close to this hole. These ligatures prevented the circulation of blood in this part of the bowel. Lastly, I punctured the vein beyond the ligature that had been made upon the mesenteric vessels, and by gently stroking with the end of the finger soon emptied it of its blood.

" Experiment II. I immediately after this made the same experiment, and in the same manner, on a part of the intestine lower down, where the lacteals were filled with a transparent liquor.

" In the first experiment the lacteals continued to be filled with a milky or white fluid : in the second, the lacteals, which before contained only a transparent lymph, were presently filled with white milk.

" In both these experiments we could not observe that the least white fluid had got into the veins. After attending to these appearances a little while, I put all the bowels into the abdomen for some time, that the natural absorption might be assisted by the natural warmth; then took out and examined attentively the two parts of the gut and mesentery upon which the experiments had been made : but the lacteals were still filled with milk, and there was not the least appearance of a white fluid in the veins; on the contrary, what little blood was in them was just as thick and as deep-coloured as in the other veins, and when squeezed out from them coagulated as the blood of other veins.

" Experiment III. I tied up and filled another piece of the intestine with milk in the same manner, but did not make a ligature upon the mesenteric vessels, leaving a free circulation in the part. We looked very attentively at the colour of the blood in the vein of that part, both with our naked eyes and with glasses : we compared it with that in the artery and in the neighbouring veins, but could not observe that it was lighter-coloured, nor that it was milky, nor that there was any difference whatever.

" Experiment IV. Lastly, we took that part of the gut which was filled with milk in the first or second experiment, and squeezed and pressed it very gradually, in order to see whether any milk would by these means pass into the empty mesenteric veins. This we did gradually, with more and more force, till the gut at last burst; but still there was not the least appearance of anything milky in the veins.

" *Animal Second.*—Experiment I. November 13, 1758*, I opened the abdomen of a living sheep, which had eat nothing for some days, and upon exposing the intestines and mesentery we observed the lacteals were visible, but contained only a transparent watery fluid. I made a hole in the intestine near the stomach, and by a funnel poured in some thin starch, coloured with indigo, so as to fill several convolutions; then tied up the hole in the gut, and put all the bowels into the abdomen for some time. Upon taking them out after this we observed all the lacteals of that part filled with a fluid of a fine blue colour[a]. We

* In presence of Doctors Wren, Fordyce, and Michaelson, and Messrs. Blount, Tickell, Churchill, Paterson, and Skeette.

---

[a] [Martin Lister, in 1682, injected twelve ounces of the tincture of indigo into the small intestines of a living and fasting dog. At the time of the experiment there "was not the least appearance of lacteal veins in the mesentery" : after full three hours the mesentery was examined, and many lacteals were found of an azure colour; and some of the biggest of them being cut, a thick bluish chyle was seen to issue forth. (Phil. Trans., vol. xiii. p. 9.) The conclusion which Lister drew from this experiment with reference to the power of the lacteals to absorb extraneous matters along with the chyle, was opposed in his time by some writers, and it was stated "that people may be deceived with blue tinctures, for this is the natural colour of these lacteals when they are almost or altogether empty." See Phil. Trans., No. 275, October 1701, p. 996.

In order to try the value of this objection, Dr. Wm. Musgrave instituted the following experiments:

"Feb. 1682-3. I injected into the jejunum of a dog, that had for a day before but little meat, about twelve ounces of a solution of indigo in fountain water, and after three hours, opening the dog a second time, I observed several of the lacteals of a bluish colour, which, upon stretching of the mesentery, did several times disappear, but was most easily discerned when the mesentery lay loose; an argument that the bluish colour was not properly of the vessel, but of the liquor contained in it.

"A few days after this, repeating the experiment in another company, with the solution of stone blue in fountain water, and on a dog that had been kept fasting thirty-six hours, I saw several of the lacteals become of a *perfect blue colour* within very few minutes after the injection: for they appeared so before I could sew up the gut. About the beginning of March following, having kept a spaniel fasting thirty-six hours, and then syringing a pint of a deep decoction of stone blue with common water into one of the small guts, and after three hours opening the dog again, I saw many of the lacteals of a *deep blue colour*. Several of them were cut, and afforded a blue liquor (some of the decoction), running forth on the mesentery.

"After this I examined the ductus thoracicus (on which, together with other vessels near it, I had upon my return made a ligature), and saw the receptaculum chyli and that ductus of a bluish colour, not so blue indeed as the lacteals, from the solution mixing in and near the receptaculum with lympha, but much bluer than the ductus uses to be, or than the lymphatics under the liver (with which I compared it) were. I trusted not my own eyes in any one of these experiments, but in each of them had the company and assistance of several physicians, who all agreed with me as to the colouring of the lacteals." (Phil. Trans., No. 275, October 1701.)

The same objection, the force of which was invalidated by the experiments of Mus-

thought at first that the blood in the veins of this part was of a darker colour, but on comparing it carefully with that in the other veins it was manifestly the same.

"Experiment II. I opened a vein upon this part of the mesentery, and catched a table spoon full of its blood. I set it by to congeal and separate into its coagulum and serum. On the next day and the day after that I examined the colour of the serum, but it had not the least bluish cast.

"Experiment III. I fixed an injecting pipe in an artery of the mesentery, where the intestine was filled with the blue starch, and tied up all communications both in the mesentery and intestine (as in Animal First, Exper. I.), but left the corresponding vein free; then I injected warm milk by the artery till it returned by the vein, and continued doing so till all the blood was washed away, and the vein returned a bright white milk. This was done with a view of seeing if the milk in the vein acquired any bluish cast, but there was no perceptible difference between the arterial and venal milk.

"Experiment IV. After this I opened the vein with a lancet, and discharged most of the milk, then put a ligature upon both the artery and vein, and waited some time to see if they would fill, but they did not, nor did the remaining contents of the vein acquire the least bluish cast. Then I opened the gut at this part, but we could not observe any appearance of the milk having got into the cavity of the intestine.

"Experiment V I filled another part of the intestine with milk. All that we observed after doing this was, that the lacteals became fuller, though not of a white colour, and the veins remained of the same complexion.

"Experiment VI. I fixed a pipe into a vein of the mesentery, and injected milk towards the intestine, to see if any would pass into the cavity of the gut; but presently innumerable extravasations happened, so that the experiment was fruitless.

---

grave, has been in recent times urged against the experiments of Hunter, related in the text; but it is obvious that it cannot apply where care is taken to observe the colour or appearance of the empty or transparent lacteals before throwing the coloured fluid into the intestine, and to contrast that appearance of the lacteals with the colour which they present after the experiment has been performed. Now this precaution Hunter invariably adopted.

With reference to the experiments on the lacteals recorded in the early numbers of the Philosophical Transactions, it may be observed that they differ from those of Hunter in the absence of observations and modifications which the latter physiologist combined with them, in order to test the share which the veins might take in the absorbing processes;—a question which does not appear to have occupied the attention of either Lister or Musgrave.]

" Experiment VII. I fixed a pipe into an artery, and tied up the vein and all the communications; then injected milk for some time into the artery till the vein became quite turgid and tight; this was continued for some little time, and with as much force as we thought the vessels would bear without bursting; then we opened the intestine at that part, and there was no appearance of milk in its cavity.

" Experiment VIII. I took a piece of the intestine that was quite empty and clean, and filled it with warm water. The returning blood in the vein of this part appeared not at all diluted or thinner than in the other veins. Then I tied up the artery and all the communications, and attended to the state of the vein for some time; it did not grow more turgid, nor did its blood become more watery, nor was there any appearance whatever of the water's having got into the veins.

" The animal was quite alive all the time of our making these experiments and observations, which lasted from one o'clock till half an hour after three. I chose a sheep rather than a dog, both because the animal was much larger, and therefore its mesenteric vessels were fitter for being easily injected, and besides, because it is much more patient and quiet. These advantages we were all sensible of when we made the experiments.

" *Animal Third.*—June 22nd, 1759. We repeated most of these experiments on another sheep, to see if the effect would be the same, but in this animal the viscera were diseased, inflamed, and thickened in most parts, so that the experiments were much less successful, less satisfactory, and conclusive. After injecting milk into the mesenteric artery for some time, and allowing it to return by the vein, we opened that part of the intestine which had been previously emptied, and found in it a watery fluid of a whitish cast, as if a few drops of milk had been mixed with it.

" *Animal Fourth.*—In July, 1759*, I repeated most of the experiments related in article *Animal Second*, upon another sheep. The effect of all of them was so nearly the same that I need not be particular.

" I shall only observe, that when the intestine was filled with starch-water and indigo, and milk injected by the artery till the vein was washed clean of blood, and a ligature put upon the artery and vein, so as to leave them about half full of pure white milk, after waiting more than half an hour we could not observe that the vein was in the least more filled or turgid, nor had the milk in the veins acquired the least of a bluish cast, not even in the small veins upon the gut itself, where

* In presence of Doctors Macaulay, Ramsey, and Michaelson, and Messrs. Edwards and Tomlinson.

we should suppose the absorbed liquor must have been apparent if any had been taken up by the veins from the cavity of the intestine.

" After the animal was dead I blowed into a mesenteric vein, and the air found a passage into the cavity of the gut; though in making the experiment when the animal was alive, I could not force the milk by injection from the vein into the gut.

" *Animal Fifth.*—If any animal could be supposed a fitter subject for such experiments than a sheep, it would be an ass. He is not so large nor so strong but that he may be managed; he is patient in the greatest degree; his mesentery and vessels being larger, it is so much more easy to fix injecting pipes, make ligatures, &c.; and, what is a very great advantage in making such experiments, his mesentery is very thin, without fat, so that the vessels are conspicuous and distinct. Hence it is easy to separate the artery from the vein, to fix pipes, to tie up anastomosing vessels by a needle, &c.

" Therefore I got an ass, and on the 24th of August, 1759*, put him upon his back in an open garden, and tied him fast to four stakes drove into the ground, then opened his abdomen, &c.

" Experiment I. I poured a solution of musk in warm water into a piece of the intestine, and confined it there by two ligatures. In doing this the animal struggled, and a little of the liquor was spilt upon the outside of the intestine and mesentery.

" After waiting a little while, I opened with a lancet some lacteals of this part, which were full of a watery fluid, and catched a little of their contents in a small spoon. It smelled strongly of the musk, and though it could hardly be doubted that the musk had been taken up from the intestine by absorption, yet as some of the musk-solution had been spilt upon the external surface of the parts, and as it was impossible to collect the lymph from the lacteals without resting the edge of the spoon upon the mesentery, the smell of the spoon might be owing to that circumstance.

" After this I wiped a vein upon the mesentery very clean, and opened it with a lancet: a gentleman who had kept out of the way of the musk came immediately with a clean spoon, and filled it from the stream of blood without touching any part of the animal, and carried it directly off, but it had not the least smell of musk.

" Experiment II. We poured some starch-water, made very blue with indigo, into a part of the gut in the same manner as in some of the former experiments, tied the vein and artery of this part, then punctured the vein close to the ligature, and pressed out almost all the blood; then

---

* In presence of Doctors Macaulay and Michaelson, and of Messrs. Edwards, White, and Gee.

tied up the empty vein, and put all into the cavity of the belly for a quarter of an hour. After that we examined the part, found the lymphatics very turgid, as the fluid could not pass through them towards the thoracic duct on account of the ligatures made upon the mesenteric vessels; but we found the veins of this part empty, except indeed that a little blood had got into them from the neighbouring vessels, which, from the appearance, had evidently passed the ligatures tied round the ends of the gut, a circumstance which it is very difficult to obviate.

"Experiment III. I next repeated the Third Experiment of Animal Second exactly in the same manner, and precisely with the same effect.

"Experiment IV. Then I repeated the Fourth Experiment of Animal Second, and the effect was still the same.

"N.B. It may not be amiss to observe that the lacteals continued to absorb the bluish liquor all this time, even at the part upon which this Fourth Experiment was made, where the nerves must necessarily have been tied up with the artery.

"Experiment V. I squeezed a piece of the intestine so as to empty it as entirely as well might be, then tied up all the lateral communications of the vessels, and injected warm milk into the mesenteric vein till it returned by the artery, and continued this operation for some time after all the blood was washed out. Then I opened that part of the intestine through its whole length, and found it quite empty.

"I made this experiment again upon another part of the intestine, in the same manner, and exactly with the same success."

Here is a new doctrine proposed in physiology, viz. that the red veins do not absorb in the human body. The fair inquirer after truth will be convinced, by the observations which occurred to me, that the common opinion, that they do absorb, is supported by some proofs that are at least doubtful or equivocal, and that the other opinion is not without plausibility; and he must allow that my brother's experiments render it highly probable[a].

---

[a] [In attempting to form a correct estimate of the merits of Mr. Hunter as a discoverer in reference to the absorbent system, it becomes necessary, in the first place, to distinguish between the discovery of the vessels themselves, whether lacteals or lymphatics, and that of their functions and anatomical relations to the other parts of the vascular system.

With respect to the *Mammalia*, it is scarcely necessary to observe that the existence of both lacteals and lymphatics had been determined in that class long before the time of Dr. William Hunter.

The discovery of the lacteals by Asellius was first made publicly known in 1628; and that of the thoracic duct by Pecquet in 1651.

In 1652 our countryman Joliff, having placed a ligature round the spermatic cord, saw, upon squeezing the testicle, that certain vessels, which he termed 'vasa lympha-

tica, became turgid; he did not, however, himself publish this observation, and it might
never have seen the light, had not, in the meanwhile, the attention of the anatomical
world been drawn to the lymphatic vessels by Bartholinus, an illustrious philosopher
of Denmark, in 1651, and by Rudbeck, a Swede, and professor at Upsal, in 1652.

In 1668, M. Louis de Bills appears to have traced lymphatic vessels from the 'jugu-
lar glanduls' of a dog to the thoracic duct.   See Phil. Trans., iii. (1668.) p. 791.

But the lymphatic absorbents had never been distinguished as a system, either anatomically or physiologically, from the capillary vessels.

Noquez, who of all anatomists before the Hunters, had dwelt more particularly on
the lymphatics, and who was cited by some of the contemporaries of the Hunters as
having anticipated them in this department of their anatomical labours, divided the
lymphatics into four classes: one of these corresponded with the capillary blood-
vessels of modern physiologists; a second, with the serous exhalent arteries; a third,
to the veins corresponding with these arteries, and to which Noquez gave the name of
'conduits absorbents,' until they became large enough to be sensible to the naked
eye, and began to receive red blood.   His fourth class of lymphatics includes the absorbent vessels of the Hunters, and were described by Noquez as ending in the receptaculum chyli, the thoracic duct, the vena cava, and the vena portarum.

It is therefore obvious that the Hunterian doctrine of the absorbent system was in
no way anticipated by Noquez, who appears to have been a mere compiler, undistin-
guished by any original research, and whose anatomical treatise was professedly an
improvement upon Keill's.

With respect to the extension of our knowledge of the condition of the lymphatic
system in the human subject, it appears that Mr. Hunter greatly contributed to this
important branch of anatomy.   Dr. Hunter describes one of his preparations, which
showed the lymphatic vessels extending from the ham upwards to the thoracic duct,
as well as the inguinal and lumbar glands, and the larger lacteals at the root of the
mesentery, the receptaculum chyli, or what is so called, all finely filled with mercury.
He acknowledges his brother's discovery in 1753 or 1754, that the lymphatic glands,
and the lymphatic vessels going from them, could be filled uniformly by pushing a pipe
into their substance; and states it to have been Mr. Hunter's intention to have traced
the lymphatic vessels all over the body, and to have given a complete description and
figure of the whole absorbing system.   This work was unfortunately arrested by a
very indifferent state of health, the effect of too much application to anatomy, which
obliged Mr. Hunter to be much in the country.   It was afterwards, as is well known,
ably accomplished by another ornament of the Hunterian school, the celebrated Cruikshank.

When the question of the office of the lymphatics first began to be agitated, one of
the arguments against their being the exclusive agents of the absorbing processes was
founded on their supposed absence in the oviparous vertebrata[1].   The discovery of
this system of vessels in birds formed, therefore, no unimportant support to the views
of Dr. William Hunter, and to this discovery Mr. Hunter is justly entitled.   Mr. Hewson, who first published on the lymphatics of birds, and who discovered their lacteal
absorbents, acknowledges that " it is but doing justice to the ingenious Mr. John Hunter
to mention here that these lymphatics in the necks of fowls were first discovered by
him many years ago."   (Phil. Trans., 1768, p. 220.)   And it appears from Dr. Monro's

[1] ["Lacteal vessels have not as yet been certainly observed in birds, or in the more
common fishes, nor in general in the animals called oviparous; and, from a considerable number of experiments I have made, I am convinced they want the lymphatics
as well as the lacteal vessels."—Monro, Observations Anatomical and Physiological,
8vo. Edinb., p. 57. 1758.]

reply to Mr. Hewson, that this discovery of Mr. Hunter's had been communicated to Dr. Cullen by Dr. George Fordyce, and had materially influenced Dr. Monro's opinions respecting the absorbent system.

Mr. Hewson also informs us, that prior to his own publication on the Absorbent System of Amphibia, Mr. Hunter had discovered and demonstrated to him the chyle, and we must suppose the lacteal vessels, of a crocodile.

With respect to the absorbent system in fish, the discovery of this must be awarded to Mr. Hewson.

As early as 1701 experiments had been instituted with a view to discover the function of the lacteal vessels, indicated of old by Erasistratus, and rediscovered by Asellius. Martin Lister and Musgrave satisfied themselves that coloured matter was taken up by these vessels, which they termed lacteal veins, from the intestine[1]. Nevertheless, until the observations and experiments of the Hunters, the lymphatics generally were believed by Haller and other physiologists to be simply continuations of capillary or lymphatic arteries, and they were supposed to have no other function than to carry back into the circulation the serum or lymph of the blood. Dr. William Hunter having observed that he could not inject the lymphatics from the arteries excepting the injection were extravasated in the cellular substance, but that he could readily inject the lymphatics both from the common cellular substance and that which assists in forming the parenchyma of the glands, as the testis, spleen, &c.; observing also that the course of the venereal poison, when introduced into the system, indicated that it was carried along by the lymphatics, affecting the inguinal glands when applied to the glans penis or prepuce, and in like manner affecting the glands of the armpits when applied to the hands, and the cervical glands when communicated by the lips; perceiving also the close analogy of the lymphatics to the lacteal absorbents, in their valvular structure and mode of termination; he concluded from all these circumstances that they had an analogous function; that they were not reflected capillary arteries, but originated from all the interstices and cavities of the body, forming the absorbing vessels of the general system, as the lacteals were allowed to be of the alimentary canal.

This doctrine was supported by the experiments of John Hunter given in the text, which were first published in 1762, while he was abroad with the army at Belleisle, by his brother, Dr. William Hunter, in the Medical Commentaries. It would seem, however, that Mr. Hunter did not consider these alone as sufficiently conclusive to be submitted to the public, since he left them in manuscript with his brother, who made use of them, four years afterwards, in the controversial essay with the Monros, while John was abroad with the army at Belleisle. They were unaccompanied by any additional proof or observation, but were considered by Dr. William Hunter as being decisive in depriving the veins of the power of absorbing altogether. Mr. Hunter, however, continued these experiments in other classes, as is shown in the following manuscript note in the possession of Mr. Clift. "The experiments upon the bird, to ascertain whether the mesenteric veins absorbed or not, were nearly the same with those made upon the ass, in 1758, with musk, as also with spirits of wine; and although in those researches I did not discover the lacteals in the bird, yet I discovered that the red veins in the mesentery in them most probably did not absorb, because I never could find any of the liquors which had been thrown into the gut mixed with the blood of the veins of the mesentery; and which I look upon as one of the first steps towards proving another system." Subsequent experiments, especially those of Tiedemann and Gmelin, Meyer

---

[1] [See Experiments for transmitting blue-coloured Liquor into the Lacteals. Musgrave, Phil. Trans., vol. xii. p. 996. Experiments for altering the Colour of the Chyle in the Lacteal Veins, by M. Lister, Phil. Trans., vol. xiii. p. 6. Powdered Blues pass into Lacteal Veins, ibid, vol. xxii. p. 819.]

and Segalas, have shown that a power of absorption cannot be denied to the veins; yet the admission of this power, (which must be granted on anatomical grounds to the veins of all invertebrate animals, and to some parts, probably of the vertebrata, as the eye and the brain,) does not invalidate or diminish the credit due to those experiments and enlarged conceptions of the uses and anatomical relations of the lymphatics, by which the true function of these vessels was ascertained. I say the true function: for though it be admitted that the veins absorb, yet every physiologist [1],—with the exception of one who has held the sympathetic nerve to be no nerve, and who, in the nineteenth century, denied that reptiles and fishes had lymphatic vessels,—allows that absorption, and the effecting a certain change in the nature of the absorbed liquors are the only functions which the lymphatic vessels perform.

I would here for the present willingly leave the subject, but that I feel it incumbent upon me, in regard to the character of an author whose works have exercised so great and salutary an influence over the surgical profession, to show that the charge of imperfection and negligence [1] which has been cast upon the Hunterian experiments,—whose want of exactness, according to M. Majendie, can only be excused by the rude state in which the art of physiological experiment was at the period when they were made,—rests entirely on the culpable oversight of the accuser.

In relating one of his experiments, Mr. Hunter states: "Nov. 13, 1758. I opened the abdomen of a living sheep, which had eaten nothing for some days; and upon exposing the intestines and mesentery we observed the lacteals were visible, but contained only a transparent watery fluid."

Is it conceivable that any succeeding physiologist would have ventured, in his commentary on Mr. Hunter's experiments, to object to them, "because the experimenter had neglected to notice whether the animal experimented on was full or fasting; or whether the lacteals were or were not distended with chyle?"

To give a colour to this objection, all reference to the experiment above quoted is avoided in the 'Précis Elémentaire'; but even in the very experiment of which M. Majendie gives a mutilated version, Mr. Hunter expressly premises that, "having exposed the intestines fully, he observed the lacteals filled with a white liquor at the upper part of the gut and mesentery; but in those that came from the ileon and colon the liquor was transparent."

In the herbivorous quadruped, the sheep, in which Mr. Hunter employed starch as the menstruum of the indigo, the transparent watery nature of the contents of the lacteals was especially noted before the colouring material was thrown into the intestine: they were afterwards observed to be filled with a fluid of a fine blue colour. And yet M. Majendie (ibid, p. 210.) would have us believe that no alteration had been observed; that the lacteals were of the same blue colour before the injection of the indigo and starch had been performed as after.

Whether, however, the coloured matter had passed into the lacteals or not, it could

---

[1] [" L'état d'imperfection où était l'art des expériences physiologiques à l'époque où J. Hunter a fait celle-ci peut seul excuser ce célèbre anatomiste de n'avoir pas senti combien il y manque de circonstances importantes pour que l'on puisse, en la supposant exacte, en tirer quelques conséquences. En effet, pour que cette expérience pût être de quelque utilité il faudrait savoir si l'animal était à jeûn lorsqu'on l'a ouvert, ou s'il était dans le travail de la digestion; il aurait fallut examiner l'état des lymphatiques au commencement de l'expérience; étaient-ils ou n'étaient-ils pas pleins de chyle." &c. And again, "Hunter fait une fausse théorie sur l'une de fonctions les plus importantes de la vie, il l'étaie à peine de quelques expériences inexactes, et dans tous les cas insuffisantes."—Précis Elémentaire de Physiologie, (3me ed.) tom. ii. pp. 199, 201.]

not, by the most careful and varied experiments, be detected in the veins. Great precaution was taken to ascertain that fact. Since the natural colour of the blood rendered it difficult to perceive a change of hue, the contents of the veins were collected and suffered to coagulate, in the expectation of the serum manifesting the presence of the indigo; but it had not the least bluish tint.

Warm milk was then made to circulate from the artery into the vein; and it might surely have been expected, especially if the doctrine of non-vital imbibition advocated by M. Majendie were true, to have then had a trace of the coloured contents of the intestine in the venal milk; but no such result took place.

The experiment upon the ass, in which the odour of musk was present in the chyle, but not in the venous blood, is not referred to by M. Majendie.

In making these comments it is by no means intended to uphold the infallibility of Mr. Hunter; but it may be safely averred that a candid and careful perusal of his experiments on absorption, recorded in the text, will not only exonerate him from any charge of haste or negligence, but must impress the unprejudiced reader with the conviction that those experiments have rarely been equalled and never excelled, either in the ingenuity and foresight manifested in their contrivance, in the skill and precaution against error displayed during their performance, in the fairness of the conclusions deduced from them, or in the minute accuracy and candour which pervade their narration.

To prove the absorbent power of the lymphatics, however, is one thing; that the veins are thereby deprived of the power of absorbing altogether is another; and it is in reference to this latter question that the experiments of M. Flandrin, recorded by M. Majendie, become interesting to the physiologist. But we may observe, *en passant*, that if M. Majendie and his collaborateur failed to obtain the same results as Hunter from similar experiments, other and as able experimenters in recent times have been more successful. Schroeder von der Kolk, for example, filled a loop of intestine in a living dog with a solution of the ferro-prusiate of potass, and included the distended loop between two ligatures. He then placed the loop and its contents in a solution of sulphate of iron. The blue compound, which could be formed by no other means except by the union of the two chemical fluids, was manifested in the lacteals alone, and not in the veins. (*Müller's Physiologie*, p. 229.) Viridet and Mattei also found that the chyle derived from yolk of egg was yellow, while that from food mixed with madder was red.

It is allowed indeed by all physiologists, and even by M. Majendie, that the lacteals absorb the chyle. But various experiments seem to show that other fluids, and especially those of a poisonous nature, are taken up from the intestines by the veins. Such was the general result of the numerous experiments of Tiedemann and Gmelin[1]. Those related by Majendie are not, however, free from objection. He opened the abdomen of a dog; a loop of intestine was included between two ligatures and separated from the rest of the canal, all other connection between the intestine and the rest of the body was destroyed except a single mesenteric artery and vein. Two ounces of the decoction of nux vomica were then injected into the detached portion of gut. In six minutes the effects of the poison manifested themselves with the ordinary intensity. Great precaution was taken to obviate the doubt which any lacteals remaining attached to the coats of the vessels might have occasioned; but as this objection might still be urged, the following more conclusive experiment was performed: a limb of a dog was amputated with the exception of a single artery and vein, which alone kept up the communication between the limb and the trunk; upas poison was then inserted

---

[Versuche über die Wege auf welchem Substanzen aus dem Magen und Darm Kanal ins Blut gelangen.]

into the foot (*enfoncés dans la patte*). Its effects became evident in less than four minutes; in less than ten the animal was dead. To avoid the objection of invisible lymphatics in the tissue of the vessels, a segment of both artery and vein was removed, after having substituted a portion of quill, so that there remained no other communication between the limb and the animal excepting by the blood which circulated from one to the other. The poison introduced into the foot (*introduit dans la patte*) produced its effects in about four minutes. What makes it so evident, adds M. Majendie, that the crural vein was the sole medium of introduction to the poison is this; that simple compression of this vessel arrested the deadly effects of the upas, which again immediately manifested themselves on a remission of the pressure [1].

Now, although the objection of lymphatics in the coats of the vessels is obviated in this experiment, yet its conclusiveness may be questioned on this ground, that the poison is applied to a wound where it can enter the circulating fluids by *open and divided veins*; but this is by no means the condition which is understood in the theory of venous absorption, which relates only to an action attributed to the veins in their natural state, and through the medium of their organic pores. If this objection be invalidated by the experiment in which the decoction of nux vomica was applied to an entire mucous surface, as when injected into the intestine, yet this may be accounted for by the paralyzing effects of the narcotic upon the animal tissues with which it comes in contact: it may be objected that their vitality is destroyed, that inorganic imbibition then takes place, and that the poison thus passes into the cavity of the vessels, and is carried along the returning currents to the heart.

But objections from the permeability of the tissue of a paralyzed vein are endeavoured to be overcome by the assertion that all absorption is the effect of non-vital imbibition, that it is a property which the living animal tissues possess in common with inorganic substances.

Thus M. Fodéra having repeated the experiment of MM. Majendie and Segalas, in which the solution of nux vomica was injected into the intestine, afterwards incloses the same poisonous solution in a dead portion of intestine, inserts this into a loop of the intestines of a living animal, and from the effect produced by the transudation of the poison through the parietes of the dead intestine, and through the paralyzed surface of that of the animal experimented upon, draws a sweeping conclusion as to the nature of absorption in general.

M. Majendie also rejects the theory of the vital action of the absorbents, and strongly condemns the supposition of a selecting power in absorbent pores as gratuitous and unphilosophical. He threw into the thorax of a dog a solution of nux vomica, and he found that in proportion as the obstacles to a free circulation were increased, by distending the blood-vessels with warm water, the effects of the poison on the system were retarded. This experiment is of the same species as that by M. Segalas, who limited the field of observation by confining the poison within a loop of intestine, and interrupted the venous current altogether by a ligature; it is consequently less conclusive, though liable to the same objections. When M. Majendie removed the obstacles which he had imposed on the circulation by opening a vein and relieving the distended vessels, the imbibed solution of nux vomica rapidly produced its effects. Thus the ordinary laws of the living tissue being suspended by the application of a narcotic or other poison to them, and mechanical imbibition being thereby permitted,—or when similar poisons are directly applied to divided vessels;—it may be concluded, from the experiments above quoted, that whatever arrests the return of the empoisoned blood to the heart, whether atmospheric pressure, produced by the action

---

[1] [*Loc. cit.*, p. 255, 256.]

of an exhausted cupping-glass, or by the direct pressure or ligature of the vein, or a general impediment to the circulation by a plethoric or artificial distension of vessels, will proportionately retard the deadly operations of the poison. M. Majendie has also shown that the rapidity of its action is increased by artificially diminishing the quantity of circulating fluids, and this observation is of great value in a practical point of view; but much is still wanting to sustain his conclusion that the ordinary and natural absorbent processes are arrested by a plethoric or distended state of the vessels, and *vice versâ*.

The experiments by which M. Majendie endeavours to support the theory of non-vital imbibition or capillary attraction as the immediate cause of absorption are these:—A saturated solution of nux vomica applied to the denuded vein of a living animal passes through the coats of that vein into the circulation and kills. The poison takes a longer time to soak through the coats of an artery; but having done so produces the same deadly effect. (*loc. cit.*, pp. 279, 280.) The nux vomica had certainly affected the system by transuding through the coats of the vessels, for its bitter taste could be detected in the blood which adhered to the inside of the coat of the paralyzed vessels. Dead vessels and animal membranes exhibited the same permeability as those which M. Majendie imagines to have retained their vital properties unchanged after four or ten minutes' contact with the narcotic extract. Ink injected into the serous cavities of the body of a living animal stains the lining membrane and contiguous parts. (p. 282.)

From these experiments the author concludes, " Il me parait donc hors de doute que tous les vaisseaux sanguins, artériels et veineux, morts ou vivans, gros ou petits, présentent, dans leurs parois, une proprieté physique propre à rendre parfaitement raison des principaux phénomènes de l'absorption."—*Ibid.*

To be consistent in this application of the theory of physical imbibition to the actions of organized bodies, we ought to conclude from observing the serum transuded after death into the pericardium, that such was the condition in the living state of the parts; and a physiologist could no longer infer from the different appearance of the parts in the immediate proximity of the gall-bladder, when examined in a living and dead animal, that the condition of the coats of that receptacle as to permeability must be influenced by the two states; and that the living tissue resists the percolation which the dead membrane readily allows. M. Majendie is, in fact, compelled by his theory to deny such difference; " the bile," says he, " does transude through the coats of the living gall-bladder, but the sanguineous current which exists in the small vessels which form in great measure those parietes, carries it off in proportion as it transudes." Yet the same currents in the serous membranes, which at p. 258 he admits are more abundant in vessels than the mucous, have no such effect in preventing the passage of the ink, &c.

But it is evident that he is himself not satisfied with his explanation, for in an account of one of the Hunterian experiments, in which means were adopted to ascertain whether water injected into the intestine of a living animal would be absorbed by the vein, M. Majendie observes that the vital action of the vein might be interrupted by the ligature of its corresponding artery. Now this objection ought to have no weight if, as he supposes, the veins absorb by a property of simple inorganic imbibition with which their coats are endowed. But laying aside for a moment the consideration of experiments, in all of which the vital operations are more or less interrupted, and the parts in question forced into unnatural conditions, let us attentively consider those phænomena of absorption which Nature plainly puts before our eyes. The chyle is known to contain globules of a definite size and form. It is admitted by M. Majendie that this fluid is exclusively taken up by the lacteal absorbents. The escape of the lacteal globules from the intestine could not be accounted for on the theory of imbibition or permeability of tissue; organic pores must be supposed to exist of a size adequate to their transmission. These pores have been described by Cruikshank as they were seen by himself and Dr. Wm. Hunter in the human subject; they have been witnessed by Majendie in a dog. But, says Majendie, it is unphilosophical, a mere physiological romance, to suppose that they can act in any way different from dead animal tissues; physical imbibition, inorganic capillary attraction is the only cause of the transmission of fluids through animal membranes that we are acquainted with, &c. Yet these organized pores of the lacteal absorbents permit nothing to pass them, according to his own admission, except the chyle.

Still it is contended this must be a mechanical action, because lacteal absorption has been observed to go on in a dog for two hours after death; but what does this prove but that the automatic or involuntary actions continue for a certain time after the sensorial power is lost,—after apparent death has ensued?

Thus the only natural absorbent process in the living body that we can reason upon from the evidence afforded by the nature of the substance absorbed, and the ascertained structure of the mechanism employed in its absorption, is totally at variance with the theory of non-vital imbibition as the cause of absorption, and can only be explained by a vital or organic endowment of the parts concerned, whether it be regarded as a power of selection or mutual attraction, or an action whose peculiar stimulus is the contact of chyle.

The various phenomena of excretory absorption, as it may be termed, render the theory of the capillary attraction of the tissue, whether of veins or lymphatics, as their cause, equally unsatisfactory. A property of dead matter cannot account for the rapid absorption of fat in disease; or of the parts of muscles, &c., which, from some accident to a joint, have become useless; or of alveoli of shed teeth; or of the parts which in the progress of growth become inconveniently situated, as the first deposit of osseous matter in long bones; or of parts which, at the conclusion of growth, are equally inconveniently situated in regard to some tumour or collection of matter, the discharge of which is salutary to the constitution, &c. A mere physical endowment of animal tissues ought always to be acting, and acting in but one way; and we therefore conclude, with Hunter, that these various and partial operations of the lymphatics are effected by the vital actions of organic pores, in a manner analogous to that which determines in the lacteals the exclusive absorption of chyle.]

EXPERIMENTS AND OBSERVATIONS ON THE GROWTH OF BONES, FROM THE PAPERS OF THE LATE MR. HUNTER.

[*Published by Mr. (afterwards Sir Everard) Home, in the Second Volume of the Trans-actions of a Society for the Improvement of Medical and Chirurgical Knowledge.*]

Read October 4, 1798.

MR. HUNTER'S Observations on the Growth of Bones have been mentioned in his lectures ever since the year 1772, the first year in which he gave lectures, and have been since adopted by the principal teachers of anatomy in London; it was therefore natural for me to suppose that they were generally known. In this, however, I find I have been mistaken, since the present Professor of Anatomy in Edinburgh, in a late publication, declares himself an advocate for the doctrine of Du Hamel; and from what he advances, it appears that he was not at all acquainted with Mr. Hunter's experiments upon this subject.

Under these circumstances I lay before the Society Mr. Hunter's experiments and observations, that they may be made known to the public[a].

It was some time anterior to the year 1772 that Mr. Hunter began to investigate this subject, and an account of the experiments and observations was given to me to copy in that year, as a part of his future lectures.

Du Hamel had published a very ingenious theory upon the growth of bones, which he endeavoured to support by experiments tending to prove that bones grow by the extension of their parts. With this doctrine Mr. Hunter was not satisfied, and instituted experiments to determine the truth of Du Hamel's opinion.

Mr. Hunter began his experiments by feeding animals with madder, which has a property of tinging with a red colour that part only of the bone which is added while the animal is confined to this particular food[b].

---

[a] [This record contains little more than a brief notice of the general results of Mr. Hunter's Observations and Experiments on the Growth of Bone.]

[b] [This effect of madder upon bone (first described in England by Belchier, Phil. Trans., vol. xxxix., 1736, p. 287.) depends on the following chemical properties. The colouring principle of the *Rubia Tinctorum* has a strong affinity to phosphate of lime, which earth, if artificially precipitated from a solution of madder, carries down with it the colouring matter in a state of combination, which water does not disturb.

The colouring principle of madder is hardly soluble in water, but is readily and abundantly soluble in albuminous fluids, and, consequently, when taken into the sy-

He fed two pigs with madder for a fortnight, and at the end of that period one of them was killed; the bones, upon examination externally, had a red appearance; when sections were made of them, the exterior part was found to be principally coloured, and the interior was much less tinged.

The other pig was allowed to live a fortnight longer, but had now no madder in its food; it was then killed, and the exterior part of the bones was found of the natural colour, but the interior was red.

He made many other experiments of the same kind upon the increase of the thickness of the neck and head of the thigh bone. From thence it appeared that the addition of new matter was made to the upper surface, and a proportional quantity of the old removed from the lower, so as to keep the neck of the same form, and relatively in its place[a].

---

stem as food, it is carried along, dissolved in the serum of the circulating blood, and is deposited, combined with the phosphate of lime, wherever that salt is separated from the blood to contribute to the increase or reparation of bone.

There are still, however, some points connected with this subject to be determined before the reasoning from experiments with madder on the growth of bone can have all the desirable exactness. Whether, e. g. the colouring principle of madder, after having been precipitated from the blood in combination with the phosphate of lime, remains in the bone until the particles of the earth are themselves removed,—or whether the colouring matter may again be redissolved in the serum of the blood circulating through the substance of the bone,—are questions not yet definitively settled; but there is much reason for believing that the colouring matter may be removed without the earth with which it had been combined. Accordingly, although an inference may be safely drawn with respect to the part of a growing bone which receives the accessions of osseous substance, by observing the part which is coloured with madder, yet we cannot so certainly conclude that a superficial colourless layer, in an animal killed after remission of the madder, is a new deposit, since it may be the old, from which the madder has been removed, after having been redissolved in the serum.

That the madder " tinges with a red colour that part only of the bone which is added," as is stated in the text, is an assertion, not only unsupported by any physiological reasoning, but directly in contradiction to Hunter's own statement; "that any part of a bone which is already formed is capable of being dyed with madder, though not so fast as the part that is forming." See Vol. ii. p. 17.

I may observe, incidentally, that the phænomena under consideration throw light upon the chemical condition under which phosphate of lime is contained in the living body. Since the colouring principle of madder has no affinity for lime or calcium alone, it is clear that the phosphate of lime is not contained in the blood or the bones as phosphorus, oxygen, and calcium, but that it exists as a binary compound, and is mixed as phosphate of lime with the cartilage or animal basis of the bones.]

[a] [Amongst the original drawings of the bones coloured by madder in the Hunterian experiments, besides those of the thigh-bone referred to in the text, there are three which illustrate the mode and direction of increase of the lower jaw, showing that the new bone is deposited in greatest proportion on the upper and posterior part of the ascending ramus, by which the rest of the jaw is pushed forwards, while the bone is absorbed from the anterior part of the ramus, and thus the sockets of the posterior grinders are gradually brought into line, with a free space above for the teeth to come

To ascertain that the cylindrical bones are not elongated, by new matter being interposed in the interstices of the old, he made the following experiment: he bored two holes in the tibia of a pig, one near the upper end, and the other near the lower; the space between the holes was exactly two inches: a small leaden shot was inserted into each hole. When the bone had been increased in its length by the growth of the animal, the pig was killed, and the space within the two shot was also exactly two inches.

This experiment was repeated several times on different pigs, but the space between the two shot was never increased during the growth of the bone[a].

Besides these experiments on the growth of bones, he made others, to determine the process of their exfoliation. He cauterized portions

---

forth. This mode of growth, with absorption at the symphysis of the jaw, continues throughout life in the elephant, in which new grinders are thus brought forwards into use in uninterrupted succession.

The preparations of bones coloured with madder in the Hunterian Collection are as follows. Nos. 190 to 201 inclusive, Physiological Series; Nos. 742 to 751, Osteological Series.]

[a] [Meckel has rightly observed (supposing the above to be a correct statement of Hunter's experiments on this point,) that they are invalidated by the careful and numerous experiments of Duhamel, which prove that the middle portion of the long bones does increase in length, though in a less degree than the extremities.

It is not easy to understand how the unqualified assertion came to be published, since the preparation and record of an experiment confirmatory of those made by Duhamel are still preserved in the Hunterian Museum.

The preparation (No. 188, Physiological Series,) is the left tarso-metatarsal bone of a common fowl, exhibiting two perforations at equal distances, two thirds of an inch from the extremities of the bone. The original record of the experiment is preserved with the specimen.

| | | .. | | .. | | |

" The two extreme lines are the present length of the bone from the head to the joint of the inner toe. The two inner lines are the length when cauterized. The outer dots are the present distance of the holes cauterized. The two inner dots are the distance of these holes when cauterized; so that the bone between the two holes has grown about two eighths of an inch, while the other parts have grown half an inch."— Physiological Catalogue, vol. i. p. 40.

In another experiment, in which shots were inserted into the holes, the result was spoiled by the shots passing into the medullary cavity of the bone, while the perforations became obliterated, as in Duhamel's experiment with the ring of wire, by the deposition of new bone from the periosteum. The shots being liberated from the osseous texture, could no longer serve to indicate its growth. The subject of the experiment, the tarso-metatarsal bone of a fowl, is No. 189, Physiological Series. It is remarkable that there is not a single preparation of the long bone of a pig, exhibiting the experiments with shot alluded to in the text. The notes of the experiments on the bones of fowls above mentioned are in the hand-writing of Mr. Wm. Bell, Mr. Hunter's talented artist and assistant, and must therefore have been written in or before the year 1789, when Mr. Bell left England for the East Indies.]

of bone in the same way in several different animals, so as to be able to examine the bones in the different stages of this process, and found that the earthy part of the living bone in contact with the dead portion was first absorbed; afterwards the animal mucilage itself, so as to form a groove between the two, which became deeper and deeper, till the dead bone was entirely detached, the dead portion itself having undergone no change[a].

From these experiments he ascertained the changes which take place in bones during their growth, and the readiness with which the materials of bone are absorbed; and from these facts, laid it down as an established principle, that the absorbents are the agents by means of which the bones, during their growth, are modelled as it were, and kept of the same shape.

Bones, according to Mr. Hunter's doctrine, grow by two processes going on at the same time, and assisting each other; the arteries bring the supplies to the bone for its increase; the absorbents at the same time are employed in removing portions of the old bone, so as to give to the new the proper form. By these means the bone becomes larger, without having any material change produced in its external shape[b].

[a] [See Preparations Nos. 197 to 204 inclusive, Pathological Series.]

[b] [The difference between the Hunterian theory of the growth of bone and that of Duhamel will be readily appreciated by attending to the explanation given by Duhamel of the phænomena which he observed during his investigations on this subject. Let us, for example, select from the number of his ingenious and instructive experiments, that in which he placed a ring of silver wire round the middle of the shaft of the thigh-bone of a young pigeon; and found at a subsequent period the ring in the medullary cavity of the bone, instead of embracing the exterior of the shaft, where he had placed it. It need scarcely be observed that the Hunterian physiologist would explain these facts by stating that the arteries of the periosteum had deposited new bone on the external surface of the ring, while the absorbents had removed the old bone in contact with the internal surface of the ring, by which its relations to the osseous parietes of the femur became reversed. But this physiological view of the phænomena, arising out of a knowledge of the powers and actions of great and important vascular systems in the frame, was wholly unsuspected by and unknown to the predecessors of Hunter. Duhamel explains the facts on mechanical principles; assuming that the bony layers of the shaft of the thigh-bone were expanded by the interposition of additional osseous matter, and that the layers were cut through in this process of expansion by the unyielding wire which he had placed around them. All his explanations bear the same mechanical character, in which processes of growth are assumed which are negatived by observation; and they are frequently vitiated by overstrained analogies, as where, in explaining the process of union in a fractured bone, he compares the periosteum to the bark of trees. But the numerous experiments of Duhamel[1], which are characterized by much precision and ingenuity, well merit the attention of the student of physiology.]

[1] [Sur le développement et la crue des os. Mémoires de l'Acad. des Sciences. Paris, 1742, p. 497; and 1743, p. 187.]

OBSERVATIONS TENDING TO SHOW THAT THE WOLF, JACKAL, AND DOG, ARE ALL OF THE SAME SPECIES.

THE true distinction between different species of animals must ultimately, as appears to me, be gathered from their incapacity of propagating with each other an offspring capable again of continuing itself by subsequent propagations: thus the horse and ass beget a mule capable of copulation, but incapable of begetting or producing offspring. If it be true that the mule has been known to breed, which must be allowed to be an extraordinary fact, it will by no means be sufficient to determine the horse and ass to be of the same species; indeed, from the copulation of mules being very frequent, and the circumstance of their breeding very rare, I should rather attribute it to a degree of monstrosity in the organs of the mule which conceived, as not being a mixture of two different species, but merely those of either the mare or female ass.   This is not so far-fetched an idea, when we consider that some true species produce monsters, which are a mixture of both sexes, and that many animals of distinct sex are incapable of breeding at all.   If then we find Nature in its most perfect state deviating from general principles, why may it not happen likewise in the production of mules; so that sometimes a mule shall breed from the circumstance of its being a monster respecting mules?

The time of uterine gestation being the same in all the varieties of every species of animals, it becomes a necessary circumstance towards determining a species.

The affinity between the fox, wolf, jackal, and several varieties of the dog, in their external form and several of their properties, is so striking, that they appear to be only varieties of the same species.   The fox would seem to be further removed from the dog than either the jackal or wolf, at least in disposition, being naturally a solitary animal, and neither so sociable respecting its own species or man; from which I should infer that it is only allied to the dog by being of the same genus.   It is confidently asserted by many that the fox breeds with the dog; but this has not been accurately ascertained; if it had, the inquiry would probably have been carried further; and once breeding, according to what we have said, does not constitute a species; this, however, is a part I mean to investigate.   I do not know if, in a wild state, there ever is in the same country a variety in any species of animal, but am

inclined to think there never is; if so, as both wolves and foxes inhabited this country, they cannot then be of the same species.

Wolves, as also jackals, are found in herds; and the jackal is so little
afraid of the human species, that, like a dog, it comes into houses in
search of food, more like a variety of the dog, the consequence of cultivation rather than of chance. It would appear to be much the most
familiar of the two; for we shall find that in its readiness to copulate
with the dog, and its familiarity with the dog afterwards, it is somewhat
different from the wolf; however, this may depend on accident. The
wolf being an animal well known in Europe, the part of the world where
natural history is particularly cultivated, some pains have been taken to
ascertain whether or not it was of the same species with the dog; but
I believe it has been hitherto considered as only belonging to the same
genus.

Accident often does as much for natural history as premeditated plans,
especially when Nature is left to herself. The first instance of the dog
and wolf breeding in this country seems to have been about the year
1766. A Pomeranian bitch of Mr. Brookes's, in the New Road, was
lined only once by a wolf, and brought forth a litter of nine healthy
puppies. The veracity of Mr. Brookes is not to be doubted, respecting
the bitch having been lined by a wolf; yet as it was possible she might
have been lined by some common dog without his knowledge, the fact
was not, in that, clearly made out; but it has since been ascertained
that the dog and wolf will breed. One of the above-mentioned litter
was presented to me by Mr. Brookes, who likewise informed me that
others had been purchased by different noblemen and gentlemen, and
named Lord Clanbrassil as having bought a bitch puppy. I reserved
mine for the purpose of experiment; and from observation it appeared
that its actions were not truly those of a dog, having more quickness
of attention to what passed, being more easily startled, as if particularly
apprehensive of danger, quicker in transitions from one action to another,
being not so ready to the call, and less docile. From these peculiarities
it lost its life, having been stoned to death in the streets for a mad dog.

Hearing that Lord Clanbrassil's bitch had bred, Sir Joseph Banks was
so obliging as, at my request, to write to his Lordship, who sent the
following account:

" Sir,

" About seventeen or eighteen years ago, the late Lord Monthermer
and I happened to see a dog-wolf at Mr. Brookes's, who deals in animals,
and lives in the New Road. The animal was remarkably tame, and it
struck us, for that reason, that a breed might be procured between him
and a bitch.

" We promised Mr. Brookes a good price for puppies if he succeeded. In about a year a bitch produced nine, and Lord Monthermer bought one; and I had another, which was a bitch. Lord Monthermer's died of fits in about two years : mine lived longer, and had puppies only once. One I gave to Lord Pembroke, but what became of it I do not remember. It was grand-daughter of the wolf by the dam, and got by a large pointer of mine.

" It might be considered that Mr. Brookes's word was not sufficient proof that the puppies were really got by the wolf, but the appearance of the animals, so totally different from all others of the canine species, did not leave a doubt upon our minds ; and I remember Hans Stanley, who had adopted Buffon's opinion, was thoroughly convinced upon seeing mine. The animals had the shape of the wolf refined; the fur long, but almost as fine as that of the black fox.

" I am afraid I have trespassed too much upon your time, and will only beg you will be assured nothing can give me more pleasure than any opportunity of assuring you how truly

" I am, Sir, &c.

" Jan. 7, 1787.   " CLANBRASSIL."

Upon the supposition that Mr. Brookes's bitch was not lined by a dog, but by the wolf, which I think we have no reason to doubt, the species of the wolf is ascertained; but choosing to trace this matter still further, and hearing that Lord Pembroke's bitch had likewise bred, I was desirous to know the truth of it ; and as his lordship was in France I took the liberty of writing to Lord Herbert, and received the following answer :

" Sir,   Wilton House, Dec. 20, 1786.

" The half-bred wolf-bitch you allude to was given, as I always understood, to Lord Pembroke by Lord Clanbrassil. She might, perhaps, have been bought at Brookes's by him. She had four litters, one of ten puppies, by a dog between a mastiff and a bull-dog. One of these was given to Dr. Eyre, at Wells in Somersetshire, and one to Mr. Buckett at Stockbridge. The second litter was of nine puppies, some of which were sent to Ireland, but to whom I know not. This litter was by a different dog, but of the same breed as the first. The third litter was of eight puppies, by a large mastiff. Two of these were, I believe, sent to the present Duke of Queensberry. The fourth litter consisted of seven puppies, two of which were sent to M. Cerjat, a gentleman who now resides at Lausanne in Switzerland, and is famous for breaking dogs remarkably well. These two puppies, were, however, naturally so wild and unruly, that he found it impossible to break them.

She died four years ago, and the following inscription was put over the place where she is buried in this garden, by Lord Pembroke's orders :

Here lies Lupa,
whose grandmother was a wolf,
whose father and grandfather were dogs, and whose
mother was half wolf and half dog.   She died
on the 16th of October, 1782,
aged 12 years.

"I am sorry it is not in my power to give you any better account; but if you think proper to write to Lord Pembroke, who is at Paris, I am convinced he will be very happy to give you any further information.
"I am, &c.
"HERBERT."

Buffon, whose remarks in natural history are well known, made experiments to ascertain how far the wolf and dog were of the same species, but without success.   He says, "A she-wolf, which I kept three years, although shut up very young, and along with a greyhound of the same age, in a spacious yard, could not be brought to agree with it, nor endure it, even when she was in heat.   She was the weakest, yet the most mischievous, provoking, attacking, and biting the dog, which at first only defended itself, but at last killed her."   And in another part of his work he makes the following observation : "The dog, the wolf, the fox, and the jackal, form a genus, of which the different species are really so nearly allied to each other, and of which the individuals resemble each other so much, particularly by the internal structure and parts of generation, that it is difficult to conceive why they do not breed together*."

This part of natural history lay dormant, till Mr. Gough, who sells

---

* In the Supplement to his Works he gives the following account which had been sent to him.   "A very young she-wolf, brought up at the Marquis of Spontin's, at Namur, had a dog, of nearly the same age, kept with it as a companion.   For two years they were at liberty, coming and going about the apartments, the kitchen, the stables, &c. lying under the table, and upon the feet of those who sat round it.   They lived in the greatest familiarity.

"The dog was a strong greyhound.   The wolf was fed on milk for six months; after that, raw meat was given her, which she preferred to that which was dressed. When she ate no one durst approach her, but at other times people might do as they pleased, provided they did not use her ill.   At first she made much of all the dogs which were brought to her, but afterwards she gave the preference to her old companion, and from that time she became very fierce if any strange dog approached her. She was lined for the first time on the 25th of March; this was frequently repeated while her heat continued, which was sixteen days; and she littered the 6th of June, at eight o'clock in the morning; the period of gestation was therefore seventy-three

birds and has a collection of animals on Holborn-hill, repeated the experiment on a wolf-bitch, which was very tame, and had all the actions of a dog under confinement. A dog is the most proper subject for comparison, as we have opportunities of being acquainted with its disposition and mode of expressing its sensations, which are most distinguishable in the motion of the ears and tail; such as pricking up the ears when anxious, wishing, or in expectation.; depressing them when supplicant or in fear; raising the tail in anger or love, depressing it in fear, and moving it laterally in friendship; and likewise in raising the hair on the back from many affections of the mind. This animal became in heat in the month of December 1785; and Mr. Gough having an idea of obtaining a breed from wild animals, as monkies, leopards, &c., he was desirous to have the wolf lined by some dog; but she would not allow any dog to come near her, probably from being always chained, and not accustomed to be with dogs. She was held, however, while a greyhound dog lined her, and they fastened together exactly like the dog and bitch. While in conjunction she remained pretty quiet, but when at liberty endeavoured to fly at the dog; yet in this way was twice lined. She conceived, and brought forth four young ones; and though the time she went with young was not exactly known, it was believed to be the same as in the bitch. Two of these puppies were like the dog in colour, who had large black spots on a white ground; another was of a black colour; the fourth of a kind of dun, and would probably have been like the mother[a]. She took great care of them, yet did not seem very anxious when one was taken from her by the keeper; nor did

days at the most[1]. She brought forth four young ones of a blackish colour, some of whose feet, and a part of the breast, were white; in this respect taking after the dog, which was black and white. From the time she littered she became surly, and set up her back at those who came near her; did not know her masters; and would even have killed the dog if it had been in her power."

---

[1] This is a longer period than in the bitch by at least ten days, but as the account was made from the first time of her being lined, and she was in heat for a fortnight, and lined in that time, it is very probable, if the time was known when she conceived, that it would prove to be the same period as in the dog.

---

[a] [Here it may be observed, that, from the known disposition of varieties to revert to the original, it might have been expected, on the supposition that the wolf is the original of the dog, that the produce of the wolf and dog ought rather to have resembled the supposed original than the variety. In a litter lately obtained, in the Royal Menagerie at Berlin, from a white pointer and a she-wolf, two of the cubs resembled the common wolf-dog, but the third was like a pointer with hanging ears[2].]

---

[2] [Lyell, Principles of Geology, vol. ii. p. 438, who cites Wiegmann for this fact.]

she seem afraid when strangers came into the room. Unfortunately these experiments were carried no further : one of the puppies being sold to a gentleman, who carried it to the East Indies; and the other three, one of which I was to have had, were killed by a leopard. The same wolf was in heat in December 1786, and was lined several times by a dog. She pupped on the 24th of February 1787, and had six puppies, one of which, a bitch, I had, and kept it till it was in heat; but missed the opportunity of having her lined. That loss, however, was made up by a wolf-bitch belonging to James Symmons, Esq., of Grosvenor-house, Milbank : the history of which is as follows :

This female wolf had been in his possession some time, had been lined by a dog, and brought forth several puppies, which I saw in company with Sir Joseph Banks, soon after Mr. Gough's wolf, the subject of my former paper, had produced her litter; so that these puppies were nearly of the same age with mine. Mr. Symmons reared them all; but one only was a female, which more resembled the mother or wolf kind than any of the others. I communicated to Mr. Symmons my wish that we should endeavour to prove the fact of the wolf and dog being of the same species, by having either his female or mine lined by a dog. This he very readily acceded to; and his bitch received the dog on the 16th, 17th, and 18th of December, 1788; and the 18th of February following she brought forth eight puppies, all of which she reared.

If we reckon from the 16th of December, she went sixty-four days; but if we reckon from the 17th, the mean time, then it is sixty-three days, the usual time for a bitch to go with pup. These puppies are the second remove from the wolf and dog, and similar to that given by my Lord Clanbrassil to the Earl of Pembroke, which likewise bred again. (See Philosophical Transactions, vol. lxxvii. p. 255.) It would have equally proved the same fact if she had been lined either by a wolf, a dog, or one of the males of her own litter[a].

---

[a] [This assertion, that the fertility of a hybrid with an individual of a pure breed proves the fact of identity of two supposed distinct species equally with the production of offspring from the connection of hybrid with hybrid, cannot be admitted. To prove the identity of two supposed distinct species, granting that the fertility of the hybrids from the two to be the proof required, it should be shown that such hybrids are fertile *inter se*, and capable of propagating indefinitely an intermediate variety. Now this is precisely the fact which is wanting in the evidence adduced in the text. All that Hunter proves is that two species very nearly allied to each other will produce a hybrid offspring, and that the hybrid is again productive with an individual of the pure breed; but this only illustrates a general law by which the reversion of the hybrid to the pure breed is provided for; while, on the other hand, the intermixture of the distinct species is guarded against by the aversion of the individuals composing them to sexual union: an aversion which we see in the case of Mr. Gough's female wolf to have been only overcome by force.]

It is remarkable that there seems to be only one time in the year in which impregnation is natural to the wolf, which is the month of December: for Mr. Gough's wolf has always been in heat in that month; so was that of Mr. Symmons. The time of heat in his of the half-breed (which is nearly of the same age with mine) corresponded likewise with that of the mother, and of those bred from Mr. Gough's wolf.

OF THE JACKAL.

This animal being so nearly allied to the dog, and only found wild like the wolf, I became desirous of ascertaining of what particular species it was; and while pursuing the subject, I was informed that Captain Mears, of the Royal Bishop, East Indiaman, had brought home a bitch-jackal with young, which brought forth soon after his arrival; and that he had given the bitch-jackal and one puppy to Mr. Bailey, bird-merchant, in Piccadilly. I went to see them, and purchased the puppy, the subject of the following experiment, which we found to have dispositions very similar to those of the half-bred wolf before-mentioned, which I had from Mr. Brookes.

To have a true history of this animal, I took the liberty of writing to Mr. Mears, who politely called upon me, and, at my request, sent me the particulars in a letter, of which the following is a copy:

" Sir,

" I had the honour of yours of the 15th instant; and with regard to the female-jackal, I can assure you that she took a small spaniel dog of mine on board my ship, the Royal Bishop. I had her, when a cub, at Bombay; and a very short time before I arrived in England she got to heat, and enticed this small dog into the long-boat, where I saw them repeatedly fast together. I brought her to my house in the country, where she pupped six puppies, one of which you have seen. Mr. Plaw, at No. 90, Tottenham-court Road, has a dog-puppy, which will be at your service at any time you chuse to send for him, to make further experiments: I called on Mr. Plaw, and got his promise to let you have the dog.

" I have the honour to be, Sir, &c.

" WM. MEARS.

" No. 107, Hatton-street, 16th Jan. 1786.

" P.S. I had the bitch on board fourteen months."

Having taken this puppy into the country, and chained it up near a mastiff-dog, they became very familiar, and seemingly fond of each other. When the bitch became first in heat I could not get a proper dog: but about the latter end of September, she being again in the same state, several dogs were procured and left with her. They appeared indifferent about her, probably from being in a strange place; nor did she seem inclined to be familiar with them. One was a large dog, which might not perhaps be able to line her; but she was twice tied by a terrier on the 3rd of October. In a few weeks she was evidently bigger; and on the 30th of November, in all fifty-nine days, brought forth five puppies. A few days before this period she dug a hole in the ground, by the side of her kennel, in which she littered; and it was some time before she would allow the puppies to stay in the kennel when put there. Some of these began to open their eyelids in about eight, others of them in nine days.

Here then being an absolute proof of the jackal being a dog, and the wolf being equally made out to be of the same species, it now therefore becomes a question whether the wolf is from the jackal, or the jackal from the wolf (supposing them but one origin)? From the supposition that varieties become more tame in their nature than the originals, we should be led to believe the wolf to be the original, and that the jackal was a step towards civilisation in that species of animal, and that therefore the jackal should be considered as a variety of the wolf. There are wolves of various kinds, each country having a kind peculiar to itself; but the jackals that I have seen have been more uniform in resemblance to each other, probably because only to be found in one country, the East Indies. I am informed, however, that they vary in size. Whether the wolves of different countries are of one species, or some of them only of the same genus, I do not know; but I should rather suppose them to be all of one species. An argument with me in favour of this supposition is, that if there were wolves of distinct species, we should have had by this time a great variety of every species of wolf, with the various dispositions arising from variation in other respects; and those varieties would now have been turned to very useful purposes, as in the case of the dog: for all the wolves we are yet acquainted with should have naturally the principle of cultivation in them (as much probably as any animal), as much at least as those wolves we now know by the name of dogs. The not having a civilised species with all the characteristics of the wolf is, indeed, with me a proof that they are all of the same species with the dog. If they are all of the same species with the dog, then the first variety that took place would be still in the character of a wolf, differing only in colour or some trivial circumstance, which could only arise from a difference in climate. The wolf is naturally, I believe, the inhabitant of cold climates, and little variety could take place while it remained in such a situation; but if the jackal was originally a wolf, which had strayed by accident more to the southward, a greater variation from the genuine character might be produced, the difference of

climate, and perhaps of food, becoming causes of variety. By continuing to inhabit a warm climate, this circumstance would in time lose
part of its influence on the animal, and the jackal would admit of little
more variety. This, however, is a point not now to be determined; it
being difficult (perhaps impossible) to say where the wolf became jackal,
or (what we call) dog; and, as dogs differ much from one another, what
particular dog may be considered as the first remove; or whether the
jackal is the intermediate link connecting the wolf and dog. In any
case we may reckon three great varieties in this species, wolf, jackal,
and dog; which again branch into their respective less obvious varieties.
If the dog proves to be the wolf tamed, the jackal may probably be the
dog returned to its wild state; which leads to another curious question :
Whether, as animals vary from climate, cultivation, or what may be
called differences in mode of living, they would return to their genuine
character if allowed to go wild again in the original country ?

To ascertain the original animal of a species, all the varieties of that
species should be examined, to see how far they have the character of
the genus, and what resemblance they bear to the other species of the
genus : for it is natural to suppose that the original animal, or that which
is nearest to it, will have more of the true character of the genus, and
a stronger resemblance to the species nearest allied to it, than any of
the other varieties of its own species.

If we apply this to the dog, and consider the fox as a distinct species,
which there is great reason to believe it is, that variety which has the
greatest resemblance to the fox is to be looked upon as the original of
all the others : which will prove to be the wolf.

Another mode of considering this subject, which is however secondary
to the above, is by supposing that all animals were at first wild; and
therefore that those animals which remain wild are the original stock;
and that when we find animals far removed from their originals in appearance the variation takes place in consequence of cultivation, yet so
that we can still trace the gradation. What gives some force to this
idea is, that where the dogs have been least cultivated there they still
retain most of their original character, or similarity to the wolf or the
jackal, both in shape and disposition. The shepherd's dog, all over the
world, has strongly the character of the wolf or jackal; so that but little
difference is to be observed, except in size and hair. That of size may
perhaps take place under a variety of circumstances; but difference in
hair is in general, although not always, influenced by climate. Thus
the wolf has longer and softer hair than the jackal, because a more
northern animal; while the jackal of the East, and shepherd's dog in
Portugal and Spain, have shorter and stronger hair than those of Ger-

many or Kamtschatka, from inhabiting warmer climates. But when
we consider their general shape, the character of countenance, the quick
manner, with the pricked and erect ears, we must suppose them varieties of the same species. The smelling at the tail has been mentioned
as characteristic of the dog ; but I believe it is common to most animals,
and only marks the male, for it is the most certain way the male has of
knowing the female, and by another scent discovering whether the female is disposed to receive the male, which is perhaps the final intention.

The Esquimaux dog, and that found among the Indians as far south as
the Cherokees, the shepherd's dog in Germany, called Pomeranian, the
shepherd's dog in Portugal and Spain, have all a strong similarity to
the wolf and jackal.

Buffon, on the origin of dogs, seems to have had nearly the same idea :
for he says the shepherd's dog is the original stock from which the different kinds of dog have sprung.

As the wolf turns out to be a dog, it seems astonishing that there
was no account of dogs being found in America. But this I consider
as a defect in the first history of that country, as there are wolves ; and
I must think, in spite of all that has been said to the contrary, that the
Esquimaux and Indian dog is only a variety from a wolf of that country
which had been tamed. Mr. Cameron, of Titchfield-street, who was
many years among the Cherokees, and considerably to the westward of
that country, observes that the dog found there much resembles the
wolf, and that the natives consider it to be a species of tame wolf; but
as we come more among the Europeans who have settled there, the dogs
are more of a mixed breed. Why the Cherokees should have had only
this kind of dog transported among them, while every other part of
America has the varieties of Europe, is not easily solved.

The voice of animals is commonly characteristic of the species ; but
I should suppose it to be only characteristic of the original species, and
not always of the variety, and the supposition holds good in the dog
species. Dogs may be said to have a natural voice, and a variation,
arising either from a variety having taken place in the species, or a kind
of imitation. It would appear that the voice of the wolf and the jackal
is very similar, being the natural voice, and is principally conveyed
through the nose, and exactly resembling that noise in dogs which is a
mark of longing or melancholy and also of fondness, but having no resemblance to the bark of the dog, which they do not perform. However,
in catching a jackal, when the animal found it could not escape, it yelped
like the dog, which is a kind of barking, and which is probably the natural sound. Barking is peculiar to certain varieties of the dog kind,
and even of those that bark some do it less than others : the dogs in

the South Sea Islands do not bark, our greyhound barks but little, while the mastiff and many of the smaller tribe, as spaniels, are particularly noisy in this way. There is reason to believe that the frequency of this noise may arise from imitation: for the dogs in the South Sea Islands learn to bark, the half-bred jackal barked, and so did the half-bred wolf, although but little; and others, as the hound, have a peculiar howl, by huntsmen called the tongue, which noise, and the barking also, are both made by opening the mouth. A variety in the voice or some parts of the voice, in varieties of the same species, is not peculiar to the dog.

It is a curious circumstance that variety not only takes place in colour and form, from the change of habits in the parents, but that the dispositions are also changed; and that the dispositions are most commonly changed in such a way as appears best adapted to the form of the animal. The change in the habits of the parent animal arise principally from its connection with the human kind, which has now succeeded in training dogs so as to fit them, both in body and mind, for almost every purpose of human œconomy, as if man himself had formed them expressly with such intention, while at the same time he can only be considered as an occasional cause, for we may observe that all the males of the wolf kind are nearly the same, and so are likewise those of the jackal, having little or no variety in their dispositions. Those of the half-breed, and even those that are three removes, although tame, yet have not the docility of dogs, nor are they so immediately at the command of the human will; neither are they perfectly satisfied with an artificial life, having when left to themselves a propensity to fall back into their original instinctive principles[a].

The following account from Mr. Jenner, of Berkeley, to whom I gave a second remove, viz., three parts dog, is very descriptive of this propensity:

" The little jackal-bitch you gave me is grown a fine handsome animal; but she certainly does not possess the understanding of common dogs. She is easily lost when I take her out, and is quite inattentive to a whistle. She is more shy than a dog, and starts frequently when

---

[a] [The range of deviation from the original type appears to be greater in the dog than in any other known species. Besides the well-known and considerable differences in the quantity, colour, and texture of the hair, and in the size, form, and proportions of the body, in some individuals an additional false grinder appears; and there is a race of dogs which have a supernumerary toe on the hind-foot, with the corresponding tarsal bones [1];—a variety analogous to the Dorking (or five-toed) fowl, and to the six-fingered families of the human race.]

---

[1] [Cuv. Disc. Prelim. Ossem. Fossiles, Ed. iv. tom. i. p. 205.]

a quick motion is made before her.   Of her inches she is uncommonly fleet, much more so than any dog I ever saw.   She can turn a rabbit in the field; she is fond of stealing away and lying about the adjacent meadows, where her favourite amusement is hunting the field-mouse, which she catches in a particular manner."

As animals are known to produce young which are different from themselves in colour, form, and dispositions, arising from what may be called the unnatural mode of life, it shows this curious power of accommodation in the animal œconomy, that although education can produce no change in the colour, form, or disposition of the animal, yet it is capable of producing a principle which becomes so natural to the animal that it shall beget young different in colour[a] and form, and so altered in disposition as to be more easily trained up to the offices in which they have been usually employed, and having these dispositions suitable to such change of form.

It also becomes a question, whether they would not go back again to their original state, if put into the situation of the original from whence they sprang; or acquire a form resembling the original of that country where they are placed.   I do not conceive that they must necessarily go back through the same changes; but I have some reason to suppose they would gradually return to a resemblance of that original[b].   And it would be difficult to prove whether, in many of the gradations, they are progressive or retrograde.   But this is a subject that requires particular attention and investigation, and upon which I hope, some time or other, to be able to throw more light.

---

[a] [This has recently been exemplified in the produce of a male and female Dingo, or wild dog of Australia, brought forth at the Zoological Gardens, and under circumstances which precluded the possibility of connection between the female and any other dog than the male with which she was kept confined.   Two, out of the litter of five puppies brought forth, had the uniform red-brown colour of the parents, the rest were more or less pied, brown and white.]

[b] [If the wolf were actually the original of the dog, it might have been expected that the Dingo of Australia, supposing it to have originated from some dog accidentally introduced into that continent, would have been found reverted to its original condition, or as a wolf.   But there appears to have been no further progress towards the acquisition of the characters of the wolf, in this instance, than may be supposed, on the theory of reversion, to have taken place in the time of Cook.   The existence of wild dogs which are not wolves, as the Dingo of Australia and the Dhole of India, which have either lost or have never acquired the common character of domestication, variety of colour, is itself a strong argument against the original of the domestic dog ever having been a wolf.]

OBSERVATIONS ON THE STRUCTURE AND ŒCONOMY OF WHALES. BY JOHN HUNTER, ESQ., F.R.S.[a]

THE animals which inhabit the sea are much less known to us than those found upon land; and the œconomy of those with which we are best acquainted is much less understood; we are, therefore, too often obliged to reason from analogy where information fails, which must probably ever continue to be the case, from our unfitness to pursue our researches in the unfathomable waters.

This unfitness does not arise from that part of our œconomy on which life and its functions depend, for the tribe of animals which is to be the subject of this Paper has, in that respect, the same œconomy as man, but from a difference in the mechanism by which our progressive motion is produced.

The anatomy of the larger marine animals, when they are procured in a proper state, can be as well ascertained as that of any others, dead structure being readily investigated.   But even such opportunities too seldom occur, because those animals are only to be found in distant seas, which no one explores in pursuit of natural history; neither can they be brought to us alive from thence, which prevents our receiving their bodies in a state fit for dissection.   As they cannot live in air, we are unable to procure them alive.

Some of these aquatic animals yielding substances which have become articles of traffic, and in quantity sufficient to render them valuable as objects of profit, are sought after for that purpose; but gain being the primary view, the researches of the Naturalist are only considered as secondary points, if considered at all.   At the best, our opportunities of examining such animals do not often occur till the parts are in such a state as to defeat the purposes of accurate inquiry, and even these occasions are so rare as to prevent our being able to supply, by a second dissection, what was deficient in a first.   The parts of such animals being formed on so large a scale, is another cause which prevents any great degree of accuracy in their examination, more especially when it is considered how very inconvenient for accurate dissections are barges,

---

[a] [Originally published in the Philosophical Transactions, vol. lxxvii. 1787.]

open fields, and such places as are fit to receive animals or parts of such vast bulk.

As the opportunities of ascertaining the anatomical structure of large marine animals are generally accidental, I have availed myself as much as possible of all that have occurred; and, anxious to get more extensive information, engaged a surgeon, at a considerable expense, to make a voyage to Greenland, in one of the ships employed in the whale fishery, and furnished him with such necessaries as I thought might be requisite for examining and preserving the more interesting parts, and with instructions for making general observations; but the only return I received for this expense was a piece of whale's skin, with some small animals sticking upon it. From the opportunities which I have had of examining different animals of this order, I have gained a tolerably accurate idea of the anatomical structure of some genera, and such a knowledge of the structure of particular parts of some others, as to enable me to ascertain the principles of their œconomy.

Those which I have had opportunities of examining were the following:

Of the *Delphinus Phocæna*, or Porpoise (Pl. XLV.), I have had several, both male and female.

Of the Grampus I have had two; one of them, (*Delphinus Orca*, Linn. Tab. XLIV.), twenty-four feet long, the belly of a white colour, which terminated at once, the sides and back being black; the other about eighteen feet long, the belly white, but less so than in the former, and shaded off into the dark colour of the back.

Of the *Delphinus Delphis*, or Bottle-nose whale (Tab. XLVI.), I had one sent to me by Mr. Jenner, surgeon, at Berkeley. It was about eleven feet long.

I have also had one twenty-one feet long, resembling this last in the shape of the head, but of a different genus, having only two teeth in the lower jaw (Tab. XLVII.); the belly was white, shaded off into the dark colour of the back. This species is described by Dale in his Antiquities of Harwich. The one which I examined must have been young, for I have a skull of the same kind nearly three times as large, which must have belonged to an animal thirty or forty feet long.

Of the *Balæna rostrata* of Fabricius I had one seventeen feet long (Tab. XLVIII.).

The *Balæna Mysticetus*, or large whalebone Whale, the *Physeter Macrocephalus*, or Spermaceti whale, and the *Monodon Monoceros*, or Narwhale, have also fallen under my inspection. Some of these I have had opportunities of examining with accuracy, while others I have only

examined in part, the animals having been too long kept before I procured them to admit of more than a very superficial inspection[a].

---

[a] [Cuvier, in his masterly Chapter on existing Cetaceans (Ossem. Foss., tom. v. pt. i.),
divides the *Balænæ* or true whales, (cetaceans having the roof of the mouth furnished
with baleen or whalebone,) into those which have, and those which have not a dorsal
fin. Of the latter he admits but one species, frequenting the northern latitudes, to be
accurately defined, viz. the *Balæna Mysticetus* of Linnæus, and which Hunter, from
the relative size of its baleen-plates terms the 'large whalebone whale.' The species
of *Balæna* found in the southern latitudes differs, according to Cuvier, from the *Bal.
Mysticetus*, in having all its cervical vertebræ anchylosed, while in *Bal. Mysticetus* the
five posterior cervical vertebræ remain detached; and in the number of ribs, which are
thirteen pairs in the *Bal. Mysticetus*, and fifteen in the *Bal. Australis*: there are also
well-marked differences in the form of the skull in the two species.

Of the fin-backed whales or *Balænopteræ*, Cuvier considers the existence of the species without ventral plicæ, called gibbar or finfish, as reposing on more than doubtful authority: in the original figure by Martens (*Voyage du Spitzberg*, 1671), Cuvier supposes
that the plicæ were accidentally omitted, rather than absent in nature, since he finds
that the skull of the so called gibbar, figured by Camper, and its skeleton figured by
Albers (*Icones ad Anat., Comp. illustr.*), are identical with those of the *Rorquals* or
Balænopteræ with the skin of the throat and fore part of the abdomen disposed in longitudinal folds. Mr. Hunter had evidently never met with a specimen of the supposed
gibbar, and, as he derived his observations from Nature alone, he did not contribute
towards perpetuating the error of Martens, as most nomenclative naturalists and com-
pilers had done up to his time, and continued to do until the publication of the works
of Scoresby and Cuvier.

The principal characters by which the Rorquals (*Balænoptera*) differ from the *Balænæ*
are the greater flatness of the head, the lower jaw projecting beyond the upper, the skin
under the throat, chest, and anterior part of the abdomen longitudinally plicated and
dilatable; the short and hard baleen-plates, terminating in stiff and brittle bristles,
a short and thick fin on the hinder region of the back.

Of the *Balænopteræ* which frequent the northern latitudes three species have been
admitted into the Zoologists' Catalogues, *Balænoptera Boops, Bal. musculus, Bal. rostrata*. Cuvier submits these species to a criticism, severe, as usual, but just: he finds
that no two of the species have ever been compared or seen by one naturalist, either
together or at different periods; that the only appreciable differences he can gather
from the best of their accounts resolve themselves into those of size or degrees of mutilation of the dorsal fin: and he asks, " Qui oseroit, d'après l'observation d'individus
vus isolément à de grandes distances de temps et de lieux, et par de personnes di-
verses, soutenir que ces différences ne venoient pas de l'âge?" Fabricius, however, assigns three rows of low ridges on the upper part of the head, extending forwards from
the blow-holes, as a character distinguishing his *Balæna Boops* from *Balæna rostrata*:
a more important distinction is afforded by the number of vertebræ. (See note, p. 340.)

The *Bal. musculus* attains, according to Scoresby, the length of seventy or eighty
feet; the *Bal. Boops* of the same author that of forty-six feet. The *Bal. rostrata* of
Fabricius is variously described as seventeen, twenty, and twenty-five feet in length.

The young Rorqual dissected by Hunter was but seventeen feet long, and he accordingly refers to it the *Bal. rostrata* of Fabricius. In speaking of it he generally uses
the term applied by Sibbald to the species of which this is supposed by Cuvier to be the
young, viz., 'piked whale;' and sometimes from the relative size of the baleen plates,
calls it ' smal lwhalebone whale,' in contradistinction to the ' large whalebone whale,'

From these circumstances it will be readily supposed that an accurate description of all the different species is not to be expected; but having acquired a general knowledge of the whole tribe from the different species which have come under my examination, I have been enabled to form a tolerable idea, even of parts which I have only had the opportunity of seeing in a very cursory way.

General observation would lead us to believe that the whole of this tribe constitutes one order of animals, which naturalists have subdivided into genera and species; but a deficiency in the knowledge of their œconomy has prevented them from making these divisions with sufficient accuracy; and this is not surprising, since the genera and species are still in some measure undetermined, even in animals with which we are better acquainted.

The animals of this order are in size the largest known, and probably, therefore, the fewest in number of all that live in water. Size, I believe, in those animals which feed upon others, is in an inverse proportion to the number of the smaller; but I believe this tribe varies more in that respect than any we know, viewing it from the whalebone

---

or *Balæna mysticetus*; not referring to the relative difference in the general bulk of the body, in which the ' small whalebone whale' (*Balænoptera Boops*, Cuv.) has the advantage, since it attains the length of from eighty to one hundred feet, while the ' large whalebone whale' was never seen by Scoresby to exceed the length of sixty feet, nor was ever reported to him to have been longer than sixty-seven feet.

The whale described by Dale, in Taylor's Antiquities of Harwich (p. 411, pl. xiv.), of which species Hunter dissected an individual, twenty-one feet in length, is generally called by him the ' great bottle-nose whale,' in contradistinction to the *Delphinus tursio*, which he calls also ' bottle-nose,' or ' small bottle-nose whale.' Dale's whale is distinguished chiefly by the presence of only two small teeth in the lower jaw, and a number of horny tooth-like projections from the roof of the mouth, which Cuvier conjectures may be the rudiments or analogues of the baleen of the true whales. This Cetacean is now considered the type of a new genus, called by Lacépede ' *Hyperoodon*,' and the only well-ascertained species is generally designated, after its original describer, Dale, ' *Hyperoodon Dalei*.' The individual described by Dale was fourteen feet in length. Another described by Chemnitz, which was captured at Spitzbergen, measured twenty-five feet. A female, which was taken with her young one, near Harfleur, in 1788, was twenty-three feet in length. Nevertheless, the skeleton of the Hunterian specimen manifests all the characters of immature age, in the separation of the epiphyses; although it is to be observed that these parts are anchylosed less early in the Cetacea than in the land mammalia.

The small bottle-nose whale of Hunter is not the common dolphin, *Delphinus delphis*, L., as he supposed, but the *Delphinus Tursio* of Fabricius, as is shown by the skull and other parts which are preserved in the Hunterian Collection, as well as by the size of the specimen which Hunter describes. The *Delphinus delphis* is from six to seven feet in length, and has from forty-two to forty-seven teeth on each side of each jaw. The *Delphinus Tursio* attains the length of ten and eleven feet, and has from twenty-one to twenty-three teeth on each side of each jaw; which teeth are conical, but proportionally larger and more obtuse than in *D. delphis*.]

whale, which is seventy or eighty feet long[a], to the porpoise, that is five or six: however, if they differ as much among themselves as the salmon does from the sprat, there is not that comparative difference in size that would at first appear. The whalebone whale is, I believe, the largest; the spermaceti whale the next in size (the one which I examined, although not full grown, was about sixty feet long); the grampus, which is an extensive genus, is probably from twenty to fifty feet long; under this denomination there is a number of species.

From my want of knowledge of the different genera of this tribe of animals, an incorrectness in the application of the anatomical account to the proper genus may be the consequence; for when they are of a certain size they are brought to us as porpoises; when larger they are called grampus or fin-fish. A tolerably correct anatomical description of each species, with an accurate drawing of the external form, would lead us to a knowledge of the different genera, and the species in each; and, in order to forward so useful a work, I propose, at some future period, to lay before the Society descriptions and drawings of those which have come under my own observation.

From some circumstances in their digestive organs we should be led to suppose that they were nearly allied to each other, and that there was not the same variety in this respect as in land animals.

In the description of this order of animals I shall always keep in view their analogy to land animals, and to such as occasionally inhabit the water, as white bears, seals, manatees[b], &c., with the differences that occur. This mode of referring them to other animals better known will assist the mind in understanding the present subject. It is not, however, intended in this paper to give a particular account of the structure of all the animals of this order which I have had an opportunity of examining: I propose at present chiefly to confine myself to general

---

[a] [This, as an average size, can only be attributed to the largest of the *Balænopteræ* or fin-backed whales. The usual length of the largest cachalots (*Physeter macrocephalus*, Shaw,) taken in the South Seas is about sixty feet; but this size refers only to the males, for there is a remarkable disproportion in the size of the two sexes in this species of Cetacean, the full-grown female of which rarely exceeds thirty-five feet. The difference is principally in the length of the jaws, which are twice as long in the male as in the female, reminding one of the sexual characters afforded by the mandibles in the Lucani or stag-beetles.]

[b] [The aquatic mammalia which Hunter includes under this name are associated by Cuvier, in consequence of the absence of hinder extremities with the true Cetacea. They include the manatee of South America (*Manatus*), the dugong of the Indian Ocean and Red Sea (*Halicore*), and the manatee of the Arctic Seas (*Rytina*). They are all herbivorous, and differ in many anatomical particulars from the true cetacea, which are the subjects of Hunter's observations; connecting these mammalia with the quadrupeds of the Pachydermatous order.]

principles, giving the great outlines as far as I am acquainted with them, minuteness being only necessary in the investigation of particular parts.

In my account I shall pay some attention to the relations of men who have given facts without knowing their causes, whenever I find that such facts can be explained upon true principles of the animal œconomy, but no further.

This order of animals has nothing peculiar to fish, except living in the same element, and being endowed with the same powers of progressive motion as those fish that are intended to move with a considerable velocity; for I believe that all that come to the surface of the water (which this order of animals must do) have considerable progressive motion ; and this reasoning we may apply to birds, for those which soar very high have the greatest progressive motion.

Although inhabitants of the waters they belong to the same class as quadrupeds, breathing air, being furnished with lungs and all the other parts peculiar to the œconomy of that class, and having warm blood ; for we may make this general remark, that in the different classes of animals there is never any mixture of those parts which are essential to life, nor in their different modes of sensation[a].

I shall divide what is called the œconomy of an animal :

First, into those parts and actions which respect its internal functions, and on which life immediately depends, as growth, waste, repair, shifting or changing of parts, &c., the organs of respiration and secretion, in which we may include the powers of propagating the species.

Secondly, into those parts and actions which respect external objects, and which are variously constructed, according to the kind of matter with which they are to be connected, whence they vary more than those of the first division. These are the parts for progressive motion, the organs of sense and the organs of digestion; all of which either act upon, or are acted upon, by external matter.

This variation from external causes in many instances influences the shape of the whole, or particular parts, even giving a peculiar form to some parts which belong to the first order of actions, as the heart, which in this tribe, in the seal, otter, &c., is flattened, because the chest is flattened for the purpose of swimming. The contents of the abdomen are not only adapted to the external form ; but their direction in the cavity is, in some instances, regulated by it. The anterior extremities,

---

[a] [That is, there is never any combination of the modifications of vital organs characteristic of two different classes of animals in the same species, as of a double heart of the mammal with the branchiæ of a fish ; nor is the structure of the organ of hearing, or of any other sense characteristic of a higher class of vertebrata, ever combined with a modification of the vital organs peculiar to a lower class.]

or fins, although formed of distinct parts, in some degree similar to the anterior extremities of some quadrupeds, being composed of similar bones placed nearly in the same manner, yet are so formed and arranged as to fit them for progressive motion in the water only.

The external form of this order of animals is such as fits them for dividing the water in progressive motion, and gives them power to produce that motion in the same manner as those fish which move with a considerable velocity. On account of their inhabiting the water, their external form is more uniform than in animals of the same class which live upon land; the surface of the earth on which the progressive motion of the quadruped is to be performed being various and irregular, while the water is always the same.

The form of the head or anterior part of this order of animals is commonly a cone, or an inclined plane, except in the spermaceti whale, in which it terminates in a blunt surface. This form of head increases the surface of contact to the same volume of water which it removes, lessens the pressure, and is better calculated to bear the resistance of the water through which the animal is to pass; probably on this account the head is larger than in quadrupeds, having more the proportion observed in fish, and swelling out laterally at the articulation of the lower jaw. This may probably be for the better catching their prey, as they have no motion of the head on the body; and this distance between the articulations of the jaw is somewhat similar to the swallow, goat-sucker, bat, &c., which may also be accounted for from their catching their food in the same manner as fish; and this is rendered still more probable, since the form of the mouth varies according as they have or have not teeth. There is, however, in the whale tribe more variety in the form of the head than of any other part, as in the whalebone, bottle-nose, and spermaceti whales; though in this last it appears to owe its shape in some sort to the vast quantity of spermaceti lodged there, and not to be formed merely for the catching of its prey. From the mode of their progressive motion they have not the connection between the head and body that is called the neck, as that would have produced an inequality inconvenient to progressive motion.

The body behind the fins or shoulders diminishes gradually to the spreading of the tail; but the part beyond the opening of the anus is to be considered as tail, although to appearance it is a continuation of the body. The body itself is flattened laterally, and I believe the back is much sharper than the belly.

The projecting part, or tail, contains the power that produces progressive motion and moves the broad termination, the motion of which is similar to that of an oar in sculling a boat; it supersedes the necessity of posterior extremities, and allows of the proper shape for swimming. That the form may be preserved as much as possible, we find that all the projecting parts found in land animals of the same class are either entirely wanting, as the external ear; are placed internally, as the testicles; or are spread along under the skin, as the udder.

The tail is flattened horizontally, which is contrary to that of fish[a], this position of tail giving the direction to the animal in the progressive motion of the body. I shall not pursue this circumstance further than to apply it to those purposes in the animal œconomy for which this particular direction is intended.

The two lateral fins, which are analogous to the anterior extremities in the quadruped, are commonly small, varying however in size, and seem to serve as a kind of oars.

To ascertain the use of the fin on the back is probably not so easy, as the large whalebone and spermaceti whales have it not; one should otherwise conceive it is intended to preserve the animal from turning.

I believe, like most animals, they are of a lighter colour on their belly than on their back; in some they are entirely white on the belly, and this white colour begins by a regular determined line, as in the grampus[b], piked whale, &c.; in others, the white on the belly is gradually shaded into the dark colour of the back, as in the porpoise[c]. I have been informed that some of them are pied upwards and downwards[d], or have the divisions of colour in a contrary direction.

The element in which they live renders certain parts which are of importance in other animals useless in them, gives to some parts a different action, and renders others of less account.

The puncta lachrymalia with the appendages, as the sac and duct, are in them unnecessary; and the secretion from the lachrymal gland is not water, but mucus, as it also is in the turtle; and we may suppose only in small quantity, the gland itself being small.

The urinary bladder is smaller than in quadrupeds, and indeed there is not any apparent reason why whales should have one at all.

The tongue is flat and but little projecting, as they neither have voice

---

[a] [This difference in the position of the tail-fin relates chiefly to the difference between the whale and fish in the mode and amount of respiration; the warm-blooded whale requiring a frequent ascent to the surface of the water to breathe the air, which the horizontal tail enables it to do. In the air-breathing Ichthyosaurus, the presence of a pair of horizontal flattened posterior paddles, for directing the snout to the surface of the water, enabled that extinct reptile to have lungs in combination with the vertical tail of the fish.]

[b] [See Plate XLIV.]   [See Plate XLV.]

[d] [This irregular distribution of the dark and light shades is remarkable in the *Phocœna Rissoana* of Fred. Cuvier.]

nor require much action of this part, in applying the food between the teeth for the purpose of mastication or deglutition, being nearly similar to fish in this respect as well as in their progressive motion.

In some particulars they differ as much from one another as any two genera of quadrupeds I am acquainted with.

The larynx, size of trachea, and number of ribs differ exceedingly. The cæcum is only found in some of them. The teeth in some are wanting. The blow-holes are two in number in many, in others only one. The whalebone and spermaceti are peculiar to particular genera; all which constitute great variations. In other respects we find an uniformity, which would appear to be independent of their living and moving only in the water, as in the stomach, liver, parts of generation of both sexes, and in the kidneys. In these last, however, I believe it depends in some degree upon their situation, although it is extended to other animals, the cause of which I do not understand.

All animals have, I believe, a smell peculiar to themselves; how far this is connected with the other distinctions I do not know, our organs not being able to distinguish with sufficient accuracy.

The smell of animals of this tribe is the same with that of the seal, but not so strong, a kind of sour smell, which the seal has while alive; the oil has the same smell with that of the salmon, herring, sprat, &c.

The observations respecting the weight of the flesh of animals that swim, which I published in my Observations on the Œconomy of certain parts of Animals[a], are applicable to these also; for the flesh in this tribe is rather heavier than beef: two portions of muscle of the same shape, one from the psoas muscle of the whale, the other of an ox, when weighed in air, were both exactly 502 grains; but weighed in water, the portion of the whale was four grains heavier than the other. It is probable, therefore, that the necessary equilibrium between the water and the animal is produced by the oil, in addition to which the principal action of the tail is such as tends either to raise them or to keep them suspended in the water, according to the degree of force with which it acts.

From the tail being horizontal, the motion of the animal, when impelled by it, is up and down: two advantages are gained by this, it gives the necessary opportunity of breathing, and elevates them in the water; for every motion of the tail tends, as I said before, to raise the animal; and that this may be effected, the greatest motion of the tail is downwards, those muscles being very large, making two ridges in the abdomen; this motion of the tail raises the anterior extremity, which always tends to keep the body suspended in the water.

---

[a] [Pages 182, 272.]

Of the Bones.

The bones alone, in many animals, when properly united into what is called the skeleton, give the general shape and character of the animal. Thus a quadruped is distinguished from a bird, and even one quadruped from another; it only requiring a skin to be thrown over the skeleton to make the species known. But this is not so decidedly the case with this order of animals, for the skeleton in them does not give us the true shape. An immense head, a small neck, few ribs, and in many a short sternum and no pelvis, with a long spine terminating in a point, require more than a skin being laid over them to give the regular and characteristic form of the animal.

The bones of the anterior extremity give no idea of the shape of a fin, the form of which depends wholly upon its covering. The different parts of the skeleton are so inclosed, and the spaces between the projecting parts are so filled up, as to be altogether concealed, giving the animal externally an uniform and elegant form, resembling an insect enveloped in its chrysalis coat.

The bones of the head are in general so large as to render the cavity which contains the brain but a small part of the whole; while in the human species and in birds this cavity constitutes the principal bulk of the head. This is, perhaps, most remarkable in the spermaceti whale; for, on a general view of the bones of the head, it is impossible to determine where the cavity of the skull lies till led to it by the foramen magnum occipitale. The same remark is applicable to the large whalebone and bottle-nose whale; but in the porpoise, where the brain is larger in proportion to the size of the animal, the skull makes the principal part of the head.

Some of the bones in one genus differ from those of another. The lower jaw is an instance of this. In the spermaceti and bottle-nose whales, the grampus, and the porpoise, the lower jaws, especially at the posterior ends, resemble each other; but in both the large and small whalebone whales the shape differs considerably. The number of some particular bones varies likewise very much.

The piked whale has seven vertebræ in the neck, twelve which may be reckoned to the back, and twenty-seven to the tail, making forty-six in the whole[a].

---

[a] [In the skeleton of the *Balæna rostrata* preserved in the Museum of the College of Surgeons, there are only eleven pairs of ribs, and two or three vertebræ are wanting at the extremity of the tail; but the total number of vertebræ could not have exceeded fifty. In the *Balænoptera Boops* the number of vertebræ exceeds sixty; there being seven cervical, fourteen dorsal, and from forty-one to forty-four caudal vertebræ. In the skeleton of this species, exhibited in the year 1827. in London, at Charing-cross, sixty-two vertebræ were distinguishable, and two or three more must have been concealed in the portion of the tail which had been preserved *in situ*. There were fourteen pairs

In the porpoise there are five cervical vertebræ, and one common to the neck and back, fourteen proper to the back, and thirty to the tail; making in the whole fifty-one [a].

The small bottle-nose whale, caught near Berkeley, in the number of cervical vertebræ resembled the porpoise: it had seventeen in the back, and thirty-seven in the tail; in all sixty [b].

In the porpoise four of the vertebræ of the neck are anchylosed; and in every animal of this order which I have examined the atlas is by much the thickest, and seems to be made up of two joined together, for the second cervical nerve passes through a foramen in this vertebra. There is no articulation for rotatory motion between the first and second vertebræ of the neck.

The small bottle-nose whale had eighteen ribs on each side, the porpoise sixteen [c]. The ends of the ribs that have two articulations, in the whole of this tribe, I believe, are articulated with the body of the vertebræ above (or before) and with the transverse processes below (or of the succeeding vertebra), by the angles; so that there is one vertebra common to the neck and back. In the large whalebone whale the first rib is bifurcated, and consequently articulated to two vertebræ.

The sternum is very flat in the piked whale, it is only one very short bone; and in the porpoise it is a good deal longer. In the small bottle-nose it is composed of three bones, and is of some length. In the piked whale the first rib, and in the porpoise the three first, are articulated with the sternum [d].

As a contraction, corresponding to the neck in quadrupeds, would have been improper in this order of animals, the vertebræ of the neck are thin, to make the distance between the head and shoulders as

---

of ribs. Cuvier, in the second edition of his 'Leçons d'Anatomie Comparee,' assigns sixty-five vertebræ to the *Balænoptera Boops*, of which fourteen are dorsal. In the *Balæna Mysticetus* there are forty-eight vertebræ, viz. seven cervical, thirteen dorsal, and twenty-eight caudal.]

[a] [In the skeletons which we have examined there are seven cervical vertebræ, the six first being anchylosed, thirteen costal or dorsal, and forty-six lumbar and caudal, making in all sixty-six.]

[b] [In the *Delphinus Tursio* there are seven cervical, the two first being anchylosed, thirteen dorsal or costal vertebræ, corresponding with the pairs of ribs, and forty-three to the tail, making in all sixty-three vertebræ.]

[c] [We have never found more than thirteen pairs of ribs in either the *Delphinus Tursio*, or *Phocæna communis*. In the Grampus there are seven cervical vertebræ, twelve costal, and forty-four lumbar and caudal; making in all sixty-three vertebræ. The Cachalot has sixty-one vertebræ, and fourteen pairs of ribs. The number of ribs in *Balænoptera rostrata* is eleven pairs.]

[d] [In our dissections we find five pairs of ribs articulated to the sternum in the porpoise. In the *Hyperoodon* there are also five pairs of sternal ribs. In the piked whale (*Bal. rostrata*) the floating extremities of the ten posterior pairs of ribs are attached to strong ligamentous decussating bands, which form a middle tendinous raphe, in the place of a sternum.]

short as possible; and in the small bottle-nose whale are only six in number[a].

The structure of the bones is similar to that of the bones of quadrupeds: they are composed of an animal substance, and an earth that is not animal; these seem only to be mechanically mixed, or rather the earth thrown into the interstices of the animal part. In the bones of fishes this does not seem to be the case, the earth in many fish being so united with the animal part as to render the whole transparent, which is not the case when the animal part is removed by steeping the bone in caustic alkali; nor is the animal part so transparent when deprived of the earth. The bones are less compact than those of quadrupeds that are similar to them.

Their form somewhat resembles what takes place in the quadruped, at least in those whose uses are similar, as the vertebræ, ribs, and bones of the anterior extremities have their articulations in part alike, although not in all of them. The articulation of the lower jaw, of the carpus, metacarpus, and fingers are exceptions. The articulation of the lower jaw is not by simple contact either single or double, joined by a capsular ligament, as in the quadruped, but by a very thick intermediate substance of the ligamentous kind, so interwoven that its parts move on each other, in the interstices of which is an oil. This thick matted substance may answer the same purpose as the double joint in the quadruped[b].

The two fins are analogous to the anterior extremities of the quadruped, and are also somewhat similar in construction. A fin is composed of a scapula, os humeri, ulna, radius, carpus, and metacarpus, in which last may be included the fingers, because the number of bones are those which might be called fingers, although they are not separated, but included in one general covering with the metacarpus. They have nothing analogous to the thumb[c], and the number of bones in each is different: in the fore finger there are five bones, in the middle and ring finger seven, and in the little finger four. The articulation of

---

[a] [The true number of cervical vertebræ is seven in all the carnivorous Cetacea, as the holes for the transmission of the cervical nerves distinctly demonstrate. In the manatee there are only six. The more or less anchylosed condition of these vertebræ gives fixity to the head. The corresponding region of the spine in fish is rendered inflexible; and in the burrowing armadillos some of the cervical vertebræ are anchylosed, which structure in all these cases is designed to afford the requisite power to the head for overcoming pressure.]

[b] [See the Preparation No. 240, Physiological Series, Hunterian Museum.]

[c] [i. e. No digit analogous in the opposable property which essentially characterizes a thumb; but he homologous digit, the fifth on the radial side, is present in most cetacea. It has two phalanges in the Porpoise, and four phalanges in the Black-fish (*Delphinus Globiceps*). It is wanting in the *Balænoptera Australis*.]

the carpus, metacarpus, and fingers is different from that of the quadruped, not being by capsular ligament, but by intermediate cartilages
connected to each bone. These cartilages between the different bones
of the fingers are of considerable length, being nearly equal to one half
of that of the bone : and this construction of the parts gives firmness,
with some degree of pliability to the whole.

As this order of animals cannot be said to have a pelvis, they of course
have no os sacrum, and therefore the vertebræ are continued on to the
end of the tail, but with no distinction between those of the loins and
tail. But as those vertebræ alone would not have had sufficient surface
to give rise to the muscles requisite to the motion of the tail, there are
bones added to the fore part of some of the first vertebræ of the tail[a],
similar to the spinal processes on the posterior surface.

From all these observations we may infer that the structure, formation, arrangement, and the union of the bones which compose the forms
of parts in this order of animals are much upon the same principle as in
quadrupeds.

The flesh or muscles of this order of animals is red, resembling that
of most quadrupeds, perhaps more like that of the bull or horse than
any other animal; some of it is very firm, and about the breast and
belly it is mixed with tendon.

Although the body and tail is composed of a series of bones connected together and moved as in fish, yet it has its movements produced by long muscles, with long tendons, which renders the body
thicker, while the tail at its stem is smaller than that of any other
swimmer, whose principal motion is the same. Why this mode of applying the moving powers should not have been used in fish is probably
not so easily answered ; but in fish the muscles of the body are of nearly
the same length as the vertebræ.

The depressor muscles of the tail, which are similar in situation to
the psoæ, make two very large ridges on the lower part of the cavity of
the belly, rising much higher than the spine, and the lower part of the
aorta passes between them.

These two large muscles, instead of being inserted into two extremities as in the quadruped, go to the tail, which may be consi-

---

[a] [These bones protect the great vascular trunk below, as the upper processes protect the spinal chord above, the bodies of the vertebræ. The former or inferior arches
are termed by Geoffroy paraaux, or paravertebral elements ; the latter the periaux, or
perivertebral elements. I have proposed to denominate those which protect the vascular
trunks 'aimapophyses'; those which protect the nervous trunk 'neurapophyses'.
The aimapophyses are articulated in the Cetacea at the interspaces of the bodies of
the vertebræ, and connected with the intervertebral substance. In the dorsal vertebræ of the tortoise, and in the sacrum of the ostrich, the neurapophyses, or superior
arches, are similarly placed with respect to the vertebral centres or bodies.]

dered in this order of animals as the two posterior extremities united into one.

Their muscles a very short time after death lose their fibrous structure, become as uniform in texture as clay or dough, and even softer. This change is not from putrefaction, as they continue to be free from any offensive smell, and is most remarkable in those of the psoæ muscles and those of the back.

Of the Construction of the Tail.

The mode in which the tail is constructed is perhaps as beautiful, as to the mechanism, as any part of the animal. It is wholly composed of three layers of tendinous fibres, covered by the common cutis and cuticle; two of these layers are external, the other internal. The direction of the fibres of the external layers is the same as in the tail, forming a stratum about one third of an inch thick[a]; but varying in this respect as the tail is thicker or thinner. The middle layer is composed entirely of tendinous fibres, passing directly across, between the two external ones above described, their length being in proportion to the thickness of the tail: a structure which gives amazing strength to this part.

The substance of the tail is so firm and compact that the vessels retain their dilated state even when cut across; and this section consists of a large vessel surrounded by as many small ones as can come in contact with its external surface: which of these are arteries and which veins I do not know.

The fins are merely covered with a strong condensed adipose membrane.

Of the Fat.

The fat of this order of animals, except the spermaceti, is what we generally term oil. It does not coagulate in our atmosphere, and is probably the most fluid of animal fats; but the fat of every different order of animals has not a peculiar degree of solidity, some having it in the same state, as the horse and bird. What I believe approaches nearest to spermaceti is the fat of ruminating animals, called tallow.

The fat is differently situated in different orders of animals, probably for particular purposes; at least in some we can assign a final intention. In the animals which are the subject of the present paper it is found principally on the outside of the muscles, immediately under the skin, and is in considerable quantity. It is rarely to be met with in the interstices of the muscles, or in any of the cavities, such as the abdomen or about the heart.

---

[a] [In the *Bal. rostrata.*]

In animals of the same class living on land the fat is more diffused; it is situated, more especially when old, in the interstices of muscles, even between the fasciculi of muscular fibres, and is attached to many of the viscera; but many parts are free from fat, unless when diseased, as the penis, scrotum, testicle, eyelid, liver, lungs, brain, spleen, &c.

In fish its situation is rather particular, and is most commonly in two modes: in the one diffused through the whole body of the fish, as in the salmon, herring, pilchard, sprat, &c.; in the other, it is found in the liver only, as in all of the ray kind, cod, and in all those called white-fish, there being none in any other part of the body*. The fat of fish appears to be diffused through the substance of the parts which contain it, but is probably in distinct cells. In some of these fish, where it is diffused over the whole body, it is more in some parts than others, as on the belly of the salmon, where it is in larger quantity.

The fat is differently inclosed in different orders of animals. In the quadruped, those of the seal kind excepted, in the bird, amphibia, and in some fish, it is contained in loose cellular membrane, as if in bags, composed of smaller ones, by which means the larger admit of motion on one another and on their connecting parts; which motion is in a greater or less degree, as is proper or useful. Where motion could answer no purpose, as in the bones, it is confined in still smaller cells. The fat is in a less degree in the soles of the feet, palms of the hands, and in the breasts of many animals. In this order of animals and the seal kind, as far as I yet know, it is disposed of in two ways: the small quantity found in the cavities of the body and interstices of parts is in general disposed in the same way as in quadrupeds; but the external, which includes the principal part, is inclosed in a reticular membrane, apparently composed of fibres passing in all directions, which seem to confine its extent, allowing it little or no motion on itself, the whole when distended forming almost a solid body. This, however, is not always the case in every part of animals of this order; for under the head, or what may be rather called neck, of the bottle-nose, the fat is confined in larger cells, admitting of motion. This reticular membrane is very fine in some, and very strong and coarse in others, and even varies in different parts of the same animal. It is fine in the porpoise, spermaceti, and large whalebone whale; coarse in the grampus and small whalebone whale†: in all of them it is finest on the body, becoming coarser towards the tail, which is composed of fibres without any fat, which is also the case in the covering of the fins. This reticular net-work in the seal is very coarse; and in those which are not fat, when

---

* The sturgeon is, however, an exception, having its fat in particular situations, and in the interstices of parts, as in other animals.]

† Where it is fine it yields the largest quantity of oil, and requires the least boiling.

it collapses, it looks almost like a fine net with small meshes. This structure confines the animal to a determined shape, whereas in quadrupeds fat when in great quantity destroys all shape.

The fat differs in consistence in different animals, and in different parts of the same animal, in which its situation is various. In quadrupeds some have the external fat softer than the internal, and that inclosed in bones is softest nearer to their extremities. Ruminating animals have that species of fat called tallow, and in their bones they have either hard fat, or marrow, or fluid fat, called neat's-foot oil. In this order of animals the internal fat is the least fluid, and is nearly of the consistence of hog's-lard; the external is the common train oil. But the spermaceti whale differs from every other animal I have examined, having the two kinds of fat just mentioned, and another, which is totally different, called spermaceti, of which I shall give a particular account.

What is called spermaceti is found everywhere in the body in small quantity, mixed with the common fat of the animal, bearing a very small proportion to the other fat. In the head it is the reverse, for there the quantity of spermaceti is large when compared to that of the oil, although they are mixed, as in the other parts of the body.

As the spermaceti is found in the largest quantity in the head, and in what would appear on a slight view to be the cavity of the skull, from a peculiarity in the shape of that bone, it has been imagined by some to be the brain.

These two kinds of fat in the head are contained in cells, or cellular membrane, in the same manner as the fat in other animals; but besides the common cells there are larger ones, or ligamentous partitions, going across, the better to support the vast load of oil of which the bulk of the head is principally made up.

There are two places in the head where this oil lies; these are situated along its upper and lower part, between them pass the nostrils, and a vast number of tendons going to the nose and different parts of the head.

The purest spermaceti is contained in the smallest and least ligamentous cells: it lies above the nostril, all along the upper part of the head, immediately under the skin and common adipose membrane. These cells resemble those which contain the common fat in the other parts of the body nearest the skin. That which lies above the roof of the mouth, or between it and the nostril, is more intermixed with a ligamentous cellular membrane, and lies in chambers whose partitions are perpendicular. These chambers are smaller the nearer to the nose, becoming larger and larger towards the back part of the head, where the spermaceti is more pure.

This spermaceti, when extracted cold, has a good deal the appearance of the internal structure of a water-melon, and is found in rather solid lumps.

About the nose, or anterior part of the nostril, I discovered a great many vessels, having the appearance of a plexus of veins, some as large as a finger. On examining them, I found they were loaded with the spermaceti and oil, and that some had corresponding arteries. They were most probably lymphatics[a]; therefore I should suppose that their contents had been absorbed from the cells of the head. We may the more readily suppose this from finding many of the cells or chambers almost empty; and as we may reasonably believe that this animal had been some time out of the seas in which it could procure proper food, it had perhaps lived on the superabundance of oil.

The solid masses are what are brought home in casks for spermaceti.

I found, by boiling this substance, that I could easily extract the spermaceti and oil which floated on the top from the cellular membrane. When I skimmed off the oily part, and let it stand to cool, I found that the spermaceti crystallized, and the whole became solid; and by laying this cake upon any spongy substance, as chalk, or on a hollow body, the oil drained all off, leaving the spermaceti pure and white. These crystals were only attached to each other by edges, forming a spongy mass; and by melting this pure spermaceti, and allowing it to crystallize, it was reduced in appearance to half its bulk, the crystals being smaller and more blended, consequently less distinct.

The spermaceti mixes readily with other oils, while it is in a fluid state, but separates or crystallizes whenever it is cooled to a certain degree, like two different salts being dissolved in water, one of which will crystallize with a less degree of evaporation than the other; or, if the water is warm and fully saturated, one of the salts will crystallize sooner than the other while the solution is cooling. I wanted to see whether spermaceti mixed equally well with the expressed oils of vegetables when warm, and likewise separated and crystallized when cold; and on trial there seemed to be no difference. When very much diluted with the oil, it is dissolved or melted by a much smaller degree of heat than when alone; and this is the reason, perhaps, that it is in a fluid state in the living body.

If the quantity of spermaceti is small in proportion to the other oil, it is perhaps nearly in that proportion longer in crystallizing; and when it does crystallize, the crystals are much smaller than those that are formed where the proportion of spermaceti is greater. From the slowness with which the spermaceti crystallizes when much diluted with its oil, from a considerable quantity being to be obtained in that way, and

---

[a] [See the Preparation No. 862, Physiological Series, Hunterian Museum.]

from its continuing for years to crystallize, one would be induced to think that perhaps the oil itself is converted into spermaceti.

It is most likely that if we could discover the exact form of the different crystals of oils, we should thence be able to ascertain both the different sorts of vegetable oils, expressed and essential, and the different sorts of animal oils, much better than by any other means; in the same manner as we know salts by the forms into which they shoot.

The spermaceti does not become rancid or putrid nearly so soon as the other animal oils, which is most probably owing to the spermaceti being for the most part in a solid state; and I should suppose that few oils would become so soon rancid as they do if they were always preserved in that degree of cold which rendered them solid; neither does this oil become so soon putrid as the flesh of the animal, and therefore, although the oil in the cells appeared to be putrid before boiling, it was sweet when deprived of the cellular substance. The spermaceti is rather heavier than the other oil.

In this animal then we find two sorts of oil, besides the deeper-seated fat, common to all of this class, one of which crystallizes with a much less degree of cold than the other, and of course requires a greater degree of heat to melt it, and forms, perhaps, the largest crystals of any expressed oil we know : yet the fluid oil of this animal will crystallize in an extreme hard frost much sooner than most essential oils, though not so soon as the expressed oils of vegetables. Camphire, however, is an exception, since it crystallizes in our warmest weather, and when melted with expressed oil of vegetables, if the oil is too much saturated for that particular degree of cold, crystallizes exactly like spermaceti.

In the ox the tallow, and what is called neat's-foot oil, crystallize in different degrees of cold. The tallow congeals with rather less cold than the spermaceti, but the other oil is similar to what is called the train oil in the whale.

I have endeavoured to discover the form of the crystals of different sorts of oil, but could never determine exactly what that was, because I could never find any of the crystals single, and by being always united the natural form was not distinct.

It is the adipose covering from all of the whale kind that is brought home in square pieces, called flitches, and which, by being boiled, yields the oil on expression, leaving the cellular membrane. When these flitches have become in some degree putrid, there issue two sorts of oil; the first is pure, the last seems incorporated with part of the animal substance, which has become easy of solution from its putridity, forming a kind of butter. It is unctuous to the touch, ropy, coagulates, or becomes harder by cold, swims upon water, not being soluble in it; and the pure oil, separating in the same manner from this, swims above all.

What remains after all the oil is extracted retains a good deal of its form, is almost wholly convertible into glue, and is sold for that purpose.

The cellular, or rather what should be called the uniting membrane, in this order of animals is similar to that in the quadruped; we find it uniting muscle to muscle, and muscle to bone, for their easy motion on one another.

The cellular membrane, which is the receptacle for the oil near the surface of the body, is in general very different from that in the quadruped, as has been already observed.

Of the Skin.

The covering of this order of animals consists of a cuticle and cutis.

The cuticle is somewhat similar to that on the sole of the foot in the human species, and appears to be made up of a number of layers, which separate by slight putrefaction; but this I suspect arises in some degree from there being a succession of cuticles formed. It has no degree of elasticity or toughness, but tears easily; nor do its fibres appear to have any particular direction. The internal stratum is tough and thick, and in the spermaceti whale its internal surface, when separated from the cutis, is just like coarse velvet, each pile standing firm in its place; but this is not so distinguishable in some of the others, although it appears rough from the innumerable perforations.

It is the cuticle that gives the colour to the animal; and in parts that are dark I think I have seen a dirty-coloured substance washed away in the separation of the cuticle from the cutis, which must be a kind of rete mucosum.

The cutis in this tribe is extremely villous on its external surface, answering to the rough surface of the cuticle, and forming in some parts small ridges, similar to those on the human fingers and toes. These villi are soft and pliable; they float in water, and each is longer or shorter, according to the size of the animal. In the spermaceti whale they were about a quarter of an inch long; in the grampus, bottle-nose, and piked whales, much shorter; in all, they are extremely vascular.

The cutis seems to be the termination of the cellular membrane of the body more closely united, having smaller interstices and becoming more compact[a]. This alteration in the texture is so sudden as to make

---

[a] [That is to say, the denser external layer or dermis, and the more open cellular and fibrous structure below, which in the Cetacea is loaded with oil, are essentially modifications of one and the same structure. It is this combination of the dermal with the adipose tissues in the blubber of the whale which serves to retain the internal heat, and at the same time resist the external pressure, which must be occasionally enormous.]

an evident distinction between what is solely connecting membrane, and skin, and is most evident in lean animals; for in the change from fat to lean the skin does not undergo an alteration equal to what takes place in the adipose membrane, although it may be observed that the skin itself is diminished in thickness.   In fat animals the distinction between skin and cellular membrane is much less, the gradation from the one to the other seeming to be slower; for the cells of both membrane and skin being loaded with fat, the whole has more the appearance of one uniform substance.   This uniformity of the adipose membrane and skin is most observable in the whale, seal, hog, and the human species, and is not only visible in the raw, but in the dressed hides; for in dressed skins the external is much more compact in texture than the inner surface, and is in common very tough.

In some animals the cutis is extremely thick, and in some parts much more so than in others : where very thick it appears to be intended as a defence against the violence of their own species or other animals.   In most quadrupeds it is muscular, contracting by cold, and relaxing by heat.   Many other stimulating substances make it contract, but cold is probably that stimulus by which it was intended to be generally affected.

The skin is extremely elastic in the greatest number of quadrupeds, and in its contracted state may be said to be rather too small for the body; by this elasticity it adapts itself to the changes which are constantly taking place in the parts, and it is from the want of it that it becomes too large in some old animals.   In all animals it is more elastic in some parts than others, especially in those where there is the greatest motion.   How far these variations take place in the whale I do not exactly know; but a loose elastic skin in this tribe would appear to be improper as an universal covering, considering the progressive motion of the animal, and the medium in which it moves; therefore it appears to be kept always on the stretch, by the adipose membrane being loaded with fat, which does not allow the skin to recede when cut.   It is, however, more elastic at the setting on of the eyelids, round the opening of the prepuce, the nipples, the setting on of the fins, and under the jaw, to allow of motion in those parts; and here there is more reticular, and less adipose membrane.   But in the piked whale there is probably one of the most striking instances of an elastic cuticular contraction; for though the whole skin of the fore part of the neck and breast of the animal, as far down as the middle of the belly, be extremely elastic; yet to render it still more so it is ribbed longitudinally, like a ribbed stocking, which gives an increased lateral elasticity.   These ribs are, when contracted, about five-eighths of an inch broad, covered with the common skin of the animal; but in the hollow part of the rib it is of a softer texture, with a thinner cuticle. This part is possessed of the greatest elasticity; why it should be so elastic is difficult to say, as it covers the thorax, which can never be increased in size; yet there must be some peculiar circumstance in the œconomy of the species requiring this structure, which we as yet know nothing of[a].

The skin is intended for various purposes. It is the universal covering given for the defence of all kinds of animals; and that it might answer this purpose well, it is the seat of one of the senses[b].

Of the Mode of catching their Food.

The mouths of animals are the first parts to be considered respecting

---

[a] [A strong and extensive cutaneous muscle is intimately connected with the skin, but is separated by a loose cellular texture from the deep-seated muscles.]

[b] [The skin of the Cetacea has been made the subject of a special and minute study by MM. Breschet and Roussel de Vauzème, who distinguish in it, as in that of other Mammalia, six chief constituents, which either penetrate or are superimposed upon one another, as follows:

1. The derm or *corium* (*le derme*), a dense fibrous cellular texture, which contains and protects all the other parts of the skin. In the whale it is constantly white and opake, and its peripheral surface presents a series of papillæ, the intervals of which are occupied by the epidermis, which forms for each a sheath.

2. The papillary bodies (*les corps papillaires*) consist of papillæ covered by the derm. They have a nacreous lustre, and are several lines in length in the whale, but are much shorter in the common dolphin and porpesse. These papillæ are composed of fibres penetrated by vessels; they originate from the subcutaneous nervous plexus, and return back again to the same; the derm serves merely as a sheath to the papillæ, the extremities of which exercise the sense of touch.

3. The sudorific apparatus (*l'appareil sudorifique*) consists of soft, elastic, spiral canals, which extend through the entire thickness of the derm, and open in the intervals of the papillæ by an orifice generally closed by a small epidermic valve.

4. The inhalent apparatus (*l'appareil d'inhalation*) is formed by extremely delicate canals, which are smooth, straight, silvery, branched, and very easily ruptured: they originate in a plexus extended in the dermis beneath the sudorific canals, anastomose together, and are provided with partitions. The lymphatic vessels have no connection with these canals, which communicate directly with the arteries and veins. They are absorbing canals.

5. The mucous apparatus (*l'appareil blennogène*). This is composed of secerning glands and excretory ducts, which open between the papillæ like the orifices of the preceding canals. It is wholly contained in the derm, and produces a mucous material, which by desiccation (or condensation) becomes the cuticle. In the whales this cuticle acquires an extreme thickness: it is much thinner in the dolphins[1].

6. The colorific apparatus (*l'appareil chromatogène*) is likewise composed of secerning glands and excretory ducts; it is situated in the first superior (peripheral) layers of the corium on the right and left sides of the outlet of the excretory ducts of the preceding apparatus, and it pours out the coloured product at the same point where the mucous matter is excreted, where it stains it.]

---

[1] [In the Cachalot the external layer of cuticle is extremely fine, resembling goldbeaters' skin.]

nourishment or food, and are so much connected with everything relative to it as not only to give good hints whether the food is vegetable
or animal, but also respecting the particular kind of either, especially
of animal food.   The mouth not only receives the food, but is the immediate instrument for catching it.   As it is a compound instrument in
many animals, having parts of various constructions belonging to it, I
shall at present consider it in this tribe no further than as connected
with their mode of catching food, and adapting and disposing it for
being swallowed.   It is probable that these animals do not require
either a division of the food, or a mastication of it in the mouth, but
swallow whatever they catch whole; for we do not find any of them
furnished with parts capable of producing either effect.   The mouth in
most of this tribe is well adapted for catching the food; the jaws spread
as they go back, making the mouth proportionally wider than in many
other animals.

There is a very great variety in the formation of the mouths of this
tribe of animals, which we have many opportunities of knowing, from
the head being often brought home when the other parts of the animal
are rejected; a circumstance which frequently leaves us ignorant of
the particular species to which it belonged.

Some catch their food by means of teeth, which are in both jaws, as
the porpoise and grampus ; in others, they are only in one jaw, as in
the spermaceti whale[a]; and in the large bottle-nose whale, described
by Dale, there are only two small teeth in the anterior part of the lower
jaw.   In the narwhale only two tusks* in the fore part of the upper
jaw[b]; while in some others there are none at all.   In those which have
teeth in both jaws, the number in each varies considerably; the small
bottle-nose had forty-six in the upper, and fifty in the lower; and in
the jaws of others there are only five or six in each.

* I call these tusks to distinguish them from common teeth.   A tusk is that kind
of tooth which has no bounds set to its growth, excepting by abrasion, as the tusk of
the elephant, boar, sea-horse, manatee, &c.

---

[a] [The large exserted teeth are confined to the lower jaw in this species, but there
are a few smaller teeth in the upper jaw of the cachalot.   They are described by Mr.
F. D. Bennett (Zoological Proceedings, December, 1836.) as sometimes occupying the
bottom of the cavities which receive the teeth of the lower jaw, but generally corresponding to the intervals between them.   They measure in length about three inches,
and are slightly curved backwards, are developed in the gum, and have only a very
slight attachment to the jaw-bone; in two instances, Mr. Bennett found eight on each
side of the upper jaw.]

[b] [The concealed rudimental tusk in the male narwhale (figured by Sir Everard
Home in the Philosophical Transactions for 1813, p. 126,) was first discovered by
Tichonius, and described by him in a dissertation entitled, *Monoceros Piscis haud Mo-
noceros*, Copenhagen, 1706.]

The teeth are not divisible into different classes, as in quadrupeds; but are all pointed teeth, and are commonly a good deal similar. Each tooth is a double cone, one point being fastened in the gum, the other projecting: they are, however, not all exactly of this shape. In some species of porpoise the fang is flattened, and thin at its extremity ; in the spermaceti whale the body of the tooth is a little curved towards the back part of the mouth; this is also the case in some others. The teeth are composed of animal substance and earth, similar to the bony part of the teeth in quadrupeds. The upper teeth are commonly worn down upon the inside, the lower on the outside ; this arises from the upper jaw being in general the largest.

The situation of the teeth, when first formed, and their progress afterwards, as far as I have been able to observe, is very different in common from those of the quadruped. In the quadruped the teeth are formed in the jaw, almost surrounded by the alveoli, or sockets, and rise in the jaw as they increase in length; the covering of the alveoli being absorbed, the alveoli afterwards rise with the teeth ; covering the whole fang; but in this tribe the teeth appear to form in the gum[a], upon the edge of the jaw, and they either sink in the jaw as they lengthen, or the alveoli rise to inclose them; this last is most probable, since the depth of the jaw is also increased, so that the teeth appear to sink deeper and deeper in the jaw. This formation is readily discovered in jaws not full grown; for the teeth increase in number as the jaw lengthens, as in other animals. The posterior part of the jaw becoming longer, the number of teeth in that part increases, the sockets becoming shallower and shallower, and at last being only a slight depression.

---

[a] [In the young porpesse the capsules and pulps of the teeth are always originally imbedded in the substance of the gum, where the first development of the tooth commences, by the formation of the crown. In this structure we see the analogy to the growth of whalebone, in which the base of the baleen-plates adhere throughout life to the gum only. A superficial or less scrupulous observer might have been led to describe the development of the teeth of the Cetacea according to the ordinary analogies ; but what are we to think of that writer who takes the opportunity to correct (!) Hunter's original and just description of this point, by informing his readers that the germs of the teeth are developed in an alveolar cavity in other mammalia? and who, in reference to the hypotheses suggested by Hunter to account for the lodgment of the teeth of the Cetacea in sockets, quotes only the first, for the purpose of contradicting it, asserting that the ' cavity for the reception of the young teeth cannot be formed by the sinking of the teeth in it,' but avoids all mention of the second hypothesis, which Hunter states to be the most probable of the two, and which is the true one? (See Knox, in the Edinburgh Philosophical Transactions, vol. xi. p. 411.) Rapp, however, seems to adopt the first view ; he says, the fangs of the teeth grow by degrees into the groove of the jaw: " Nach und nach wächst dann die Wurzel in die Rinne des Kiefers hinein." (Cetaceen, p. 127.)]

It would appear, that they do not shed their teeth, nor have they new ones formed similar to the old, as is the case with most other quadrupeds, and also with the alligator.   I have never been able to detect young teeth under the roots of the old ones; and indeed the situation in which they are first formed makes it in some degree impossible, if the young teeth follow the same rule in growing with the original ones, as they probably do in most animals.

If it is true that the whale tribe do not shed their teeth, in what way are they supplied with new ones corresponding in size with the increased size of the jaw?   It would appear that the jaw, as it increases posteriorly, decays at the symphysis, and while the growth is going on, there is a constant succession of new teeth, by which means the new-formed teeth are proportioned to the jaw.   The same mode of growth is evident in the elephant, and in some degree in many fish; but in these last the absorption of the jaw is from the whole of the outside along where the teeth are placed.   The depth of the alveoli seems to prove this, being shallow at the back part of the jaw, and becoming deeper towards the middle, where they are the deepest, the teeth there having come to the full size.   From this forwards they are again becoming shallower, the teeth being smaller, the sockets wasting, and at the symphysis there are hardly any sockets at all.   This will make the exact number of teeth in any species uncertain.

Some genera of this tribe have another mode of catching their food, and retaining it till swallowed, which is by means of the substance called whalebone.   Of this there are two kinds known; one very large, probably from the largest whale yet discovered; the other from a smaller species[a].

This whalebone, which is placed on the inside of the mouth, and attached to the upper jaw, is one of the most singular circumstances belonging to this species, as they have most other parts in common with quadrupeds.   It is a substance, I believe, peculiar to the whale, and of the same nature as horn, which I shall use as a term to express what constitutes hair, nails, claws, feathers, &c.; it is wholly composed of animal substance, and extremely elastic[*].

Whalebone consists of thin plates of some breadth, and in some of very considerable length, their breadth and length in some degree corresponding to one another; and when longest they are commonly the broadest, but not always so. (Plate L.)   These plates are very dif-

* From this it must appear, that the term bone is an improper one.

---

[a] [The largest species of whale yet discovered is distinguished by the small-sized baleen-plates, and is the *Balænoptera Boops*, as was before observed.]

ferent in size in different parts of the same mouth, more especially in the large whalebone whale, whose upper jaw does not pass parallel upon the under, but makes an arch, the semidiameter of which is about one fourth of the length of the jaw. The head in my possession is nineteen feet long, the semidiameter not quite five feet: if this proportion is preserved, those whales which have whalebone fifteen feet long must be of an immense size.

These plates are placed in several rows, encompassing the outer skirts of the upper jaw, similar to teeth in other animals. They stand parallel to each other, having one edge towards the circumference of the mouth, the other towards the centre or cavity. They are placed near together in the piked whale, not being a quarter of an inch asunder where at the greatest distance, yet differing in this respect in different parts of the same mouth; but in the great whale the distances are more considerable.

The outer row is composed of the longest plates; and these are in proportion to the different distances between the two jaws, some being fourteen or fifteen feet long, and twelve or fifteen inches broad; but towards the anterior and posterior part of the mouth, they are very short; they rise for half a foot or more, nearly of equal breadths, and afterwards shelve off from their inner side until they come near to a point at the outer: the exterior of the inner rows are the longest, corresponding to the termination of the declivity of the outer, and become shorter and shorter till they hardly rise above the gum.

The inner rows are closer than the outer, and rise almost perpendicularly from the gum, being longitudinally straight, and have less of the declivity than the outer. The plates of the outer row laterally are not quite flat, but make a serpentine line; more especially in the piked whale the outer edge is thicker than the inner. All round the line made by their outer edges, runs a small white bead, which is formed along with the whalebone, and wears down with it. The smaller plates are nearly of an equal thickness upon both edges. In all of them, the termination is in a kind of hair, as if the plate was split into innumerable small parts, the exterior being the longest and strongest.

The two sides of the mouth composed of these rows meet nearly in a point at the tip of the jaw, and spread or recede laterally from each other as they pass back; and at their posterior ends, in the piked whale, they make a sweep inwards, and come very near each other, just before the opening of the œsophagus. In the piked whale, there were above three hundred in the outer rows on each side of the mouth. Each layer terminates in an oblique surface, which obliquity inclines to the roof of the mouth, answering to the gradual diminution of their length; so that the whole surface, composed of these terminations, forms one plane rising gradually from the roof of the mouth; from this obliquity of the edge of the outer row, we may in some measure judge of the extent of the whole base, but not exactly, as it makes a hollow curve, which increases the base.

The whole surface resembles the skin of an animal covered with strong hair, under which surface the tongue must immediately lie when the mouth is shut: it is of a light brown colour in the piked whale, and is darker in the large whale.

In the piked whale, when the mouth is shut, the projecting whalebone remains entirely on the inside of the lower jaw, the two jaws meeting everywhere along their surface; but how this is effected in the large whale I do not certainly know, the horizontal plane made by the lower jaw being straight, as in the piked whale; but the upper jaw, being an arch, cannot be hid by the lower. I suppose therefore that a broad upper lip, meeting as low as the lower jaw, covers the whole of the outer edges of the exterior rows.

The whalebone is continually wearing down, and renewing in the same proportion, except when the animal is growing it is renewed faster and in proportion to the growth.

The formation of the whalebone is extremely curious, being in one respect similar to that of the hair, horns, spurs, &c.; but it has besides another mode of growth and decay equally singular.

These plates form upon a thin vascular substance, not immediately adhering to the jaw-bone, but having a more dense substance between, which is also vascular. This substance, which may be called the nidus of the whalebone, sends out (the above) thin broad processes (a. Pl. LI.), answering to each plate, on which the plate is formed, as the cock's spur, or the bull's horn on the bony core, or a tooth on its pulp; so that each plate is necessarily hollow at its growing end, the first part of the growth taking place on the inside of this hollow.

Besides this mode of growth, which is common to all such substances, it receives additional layers on the outside (B. Pl. LI.), which are formed upon the above-mentioned vascular substance extended along the surface of the jaw. This part also forms upon it a semi-horny substance between each plate, which is very white, rises with the whalebone, and becomes even with the outer edge of the jaw, and the termination of its outer part forms the bead above-mentioned. This intermediate substance (C. Pl. LI.) fills up the spaces between the plates as high as the jaw, acts as abutments to the whalebone, or is similar to the alveolar processes of the teeth, keeping them firm in their places.

As both the whalebone and intermediate substance are constantly growing, and as we must suppose a determined length necessary, a regular mode of decay must be established, not depending entirely on chance or the use it is put to.

In its growth three parts appear to be formed: one from the rising core, which is the centre; a second on the outside; and a third, being the intermediate substance. These appear to have three stages of duration; for that which forms on the core I believe makes the hair, and that on the outside makes principally the plate of whalebone; this, when got a certain length, breaks off, leaving the hair projecting, becoming at the termination very brittle; and the third, or intermediate substance, by the time it rises as high as the edge of the skin of the jaw, decays and softens away like the old cuticle of the sole of the foot when steeped in water[a].

The use of the whalebone, I should believe, is principally for the retention of the food till swallowed, and do suppose the fish they catch are small when compared with the size of the mouth.

The œsophagus, as in other animals, begins at the fauces, or posterior part of the mouth; and, although circular at this part, is soon divided into two passages by the epiglottis passing across it, as will be described hereafter. Below its attachment to the trachea, it passes down in the posterior mediastinum, at some distance from the spine, to which it is attached by a broad part of the same membrane, and its anterior surface makes the posterior part of a cavity behind the pericardium.

Passing through the diaphragm it enters the stomach, and is lined with a very thick, soft, and white cuticle, which is continued into the first cavity of the stomach.

The inner or true coat is white, of a considerable density, and not muscular, but thrown into large longitudinal folds by the contraction of the muscular fibres of the œsophagus, which are very strong. It is very glandular; for on its inner surface, especially near the fauces, orifices of a vast number of glands are visible.

The œsophagus is larger in proportion to the bulk of the animal than in the quadruped, although not so much so as it usually is in fish, which we may suppose swallow their food much in the same way. In the piked whale it was three inches and a half wide.

The stomach, as in other animals, lies on the left side of the body, and terminates in the pylorus towards the right.

---

[a] [The supplementary note appended, in the second edition of the 'Leçons d'Anatomie Comparée,' tom. iii. p. 376, to the imperfect description given by Cuvier of the formation of the whalebone, is a mere condensation of the minute, original, and accurate account in the text: to which, however, no reference is made by M. Duvernoy.]

In the piked whale the duodenum passes down on the right side, very much as in the human subject, excepting that it is more exposed, from the colon not crossing it. It lies on the right kidney, and then passes to the left side behind the ascending part of the colon and root of the mesentery, comes out on the left side, and getting on the edge of the mesentery becomes a loose intestine, forming the jejunum. In this course behind the mesentery it is exposed, as in most quadrupeds, not being covered by it as in the human. The jejunum and ileum pass along the edge of the mesentery downwards to the lower part of the abdomen. The ileum near the lower end makes a turn towards the right side, and then mounting upwards, round the edge of the mesentery, passes a little way on the right, as high as the kidney, and there enters the colon or cæcum. The cæcum lies on the lower end of the kidney, considerably higher than in the human body, which renders the ascending part of the colon short. The cæcum is about seven inches long, and more like that of the lion or seal than of any other animal I know.

The colon passes obliquely up the right side, a little towards the middle of the abdomen, and when as high as the stomach crosses to the left and acquires a broad mesocolon; at this part it lies upon the left kidney, and in its passage down gets more and more to the middle line of the body. When it has reached the lower part of the abdomen it passes behind the uterus and along with the vagina in the female, between the two testicles and behind the bladder and root of the penis in the male, bending down to open on what is called the belly of the animal, and in its whole course it is gently convoluted. In those which have no cæcum, and therefore can hardly be said to have a colon, the intestine before its termination in the rectum makes the same kind of sweep round the other intestines as the colon does where there is a cæcum.

The intestines are not large for the size of the animal, not being larger in those of eighteen or twenty-four feet long than in the horse, the colon not much more capacious than the jejunum and ileum, and very short; a circumstance common to carnivorous animals. In the piked whale the length from the stomach to the cæcum is twenty-eight yards and a half, length of cæcum seven inches, of the colon to the anus two yards and three quarters. The small intestines are just five times the length of the animal, the colon with the cæcum a little more than one half the length.

Those parts that respect the nourishment of this tribe do not all so exactly correspond as in land animals, for in these one in some degree leads to the other. Thus the teeth in the ruminating tribe point out the kind of stomach, cæcum, and colon; while in others, as the horse, hare, lion, &c., the appearances of the teeth only give us the kind of colon and cæcum; but in this tribe, whether teeth or no teeth, the stomachs do not vary much, nor does the circumstance of cæcum seem to depend on either teeth or stomach. The circumstances by which from the form of one part we judge what others are, fail us here: but this may arise from not knowing all the circumstances. The stomach in all that I have examined consists of several bags, continued from the first on the left towards the right, where the last terminates in duodenum. The number is not the same in all: for in the porpoise, grampus, and piked whale there are five; in the bottle-nose (*Hyperoodon*) seven. Their size respecting one another differs very considerably, so that the largest in one species may in another be only the second. The two first in the porpoise, bottle-nose, and piked whale, are by much the largest; the others are smaller, although irregularly so.

The first stomach has, I believe, in all very much the shape of an egg, with the small end downwards. It is lined everywhere with a continuation of the cuticle from the œsophagus. In the porpoise the œsophagus enters the superior end of the stomach. In the piked whale its entrance is a little way on the posterior part of the upper end, and is oblique.

The second stomach in the piked whale is very large, and rather longer than the first. It is of the shape of the italic *S*, passing out from the upper end of the first on its right side, by nearly as large a beginning as the body of the bag. In the porpoise it by no means bears the same proportion to the first, and opens by a narrower orifice; then passing down along the right side of the first stomach, it bends a little outwards at the lower end, and terminates in the third. Where this second stomach begins, the cuticle of the first ends[a]. The whole of the inside of this stomach is thrown into unequal rugæ, appearing like a large irregular honeycomb. In the piked whale the rugæ are longitudinal, and in many places very deep, some of them being united by cross bands; and in the porpoise the folds are very thick, massy,

---

[a] [The lining membrane of the first stomach in the porpesse sends off a number of irregular projections, where it surrounds the opening into the second stomach, whereby that opening is rendered valvular, and adapted to prevent the passage of anything but fluids or substances of very small size. The first stomach, therefore, serves not only as a reservoir, but the food undergoes a considerable change in it, probably by the action of the gastric secretion of the second cavity regurgitated into it. Thus the bones of fish have been found in the first cavity with all the flesh dissolved, and the bones themselves softened by the removal of their earthy constituent. See Preparation No. 569 c. Physiological Series, Hunterian Museum.]

and indented into one another[a]. This stomach opens into the third by a round contracted orifice, which does not seem to be valvular.

The third stomach is by much the smallest, and appears to be only a passage between the second and fourth. It has no peculiar structure on the inside, but terminates in the fourth by nearly as large an opening as its beginning. In the porpoise it is not above one, and in the bottle-nose about five, inches long.

The fourth stomach is of a considerable size; but a good deal less than either the first or second. In the piked whale it is not round, but seems flattened between the second and fifth. In the porpoise it is long, passing in a serpentine course almost like an intestine. The internal surface is regular, but villous, and opens on its right side into the fifth by a round opening smaller than the entrance from the third.

The fifth stomach is in the piked whale round, and in the porpoise oval[b]; it is small, and terminates in the pylorus, which has little of a valvular appearance. Its coats are thinner than those of the fourth, having an even inner surface, which is commonly tinged with bile.

The piked whale, and, I believe, the large whalebone whale, have a cæcum; but it is wanting in the porpoise, grampus, and bottle-nose whale[c].

The structure of the inner surface of the intestine is in some very singular, and different from that of the others.

The inner surface of the duodenum in the piked whale is thrown into longitudinal rugæ, or valves, which are at some distance from each other, and these receive lateral folds. The duodenum in the bottle-nose swells out into a large cavity, and might almost be reckoned an eighth stomach; but as the gall-ducts enter it I shall call it duodenum.

The inner coat of the jejunum, and ileum, appears in irregular folds, which may vary according as the muscular coat of the intestine acts: yet I do not believe that their form depends entirely on that circumstance, as they run longitudinally, and take a serpentine course when the gut is shortened by the contraction of the longitudinal muscular

---

[a] [It is to this stomach that the pneumogastric nerves are principally distributed; the thick and soft lining substance presents, according to the microscopical researches of Sir David Brewster, a peculiar structure, consisting of closely aggregated minute tubes placed perpendicularly between the smooth internal mucous membrane and the vascular tunic which immediately lines the muscular coat.]

[b] [This part we regard as the dilated duodenum, since the gall-ducts terminate in it, and consequently reckon but four compartments in the stomach of the porpesse.]

[c] [In all the vegetable feeding Cetacea there is a cæcum, but it is small. In the dugong it is of a simple conical form, and very muscular. In the manatee the cæcum is bifurcate.]

fibres. The intestinal canal of the porpoise has several longitudinal folds of the inner coat passing along it through the whole of its
length. In the bottle-nose the inner coat, through nearly the whole
track of the intestine, is thrown into large cells, and these again subdivided into smaller; the axis of which cells is not perpendicular to a
transverse section of the intestine, but oblique, forming pouches with
the mouths downwards, and acting almost like valves when anything
is attempted to be passed in a contrary direction: they begin faintly
in the duodenum, before it makes its quick turn, and terminate near
the anus[a]. The colon and rectum have the rugæ very flat, which
seems to depend entirely on the contraction of the gut.

The rectum in the piked whale near the anus, appears for four or
five inches much contracted, is glandular, covered by a soft cuticle,
and the anus small.

I never found any air in the intestines of this tribe; nor indeed in
any of the aquatic animals.

The mesenteric artery anastomoses by large branches.

There is a considerable degree of uniformity in the liver of this tribe
of animals. In shape it nearly resembles the human, but is not so
thick at the base, nor so sharp at the lower edge, and is probably not
so firm in its texture. The right lobe is the largest and thickest, its
falciform ligament broad, and there is a large fissure between the two
lobes, in which the round ligament passes. The liver towards the left
is very much attached to the stomach, the little epiploon being a thick
substance. There is no gall-bladder. The hepatic duct is large, and
enters the duodenum about seven inches beyond the pylorus[b].

The pancreas is a very long, flat body, having its left end attached to
the right side of the first cavity of the stomach: it passes across the
spine at the root of the mesentery, and near to the pylorus joins the
hollow curve of the duodenum, along which it is continued, and adheres to that intestine, its duct entering that of the liver near the termination in the gut.

Although this tribe cannot be said to ruminate, yet in the number of

---

[a] [See the Preparations, Nos. 709, 710, 711, 712, Physiological Series, Hunterian
Museum.]

[b] [In the dugong there is a gall-bladder of the usual dimensions, which is chiefly
peculiar for the mode in which the bile is conveyed to it; in other mammalia this
takes place by a communication between the hepatic and cystic ducts, at some distance
from the bladder, but here two large hepatic ducts open directly into the neck of the
gall-bladder, in the same way as the ureters terminate in the urinary bladder. The
cystic duct, which fulfils the office of the ductus communis, proceeds to the duodenum,
and becomes slightly dilated, before it enters that intestine. The manatee has also a
gall-bladder, but it is wanting in the northern manatee or *Rytina*.]

stomachs they come nearest to that order ; but here I suspect that the order of digestion is in some degree inverted. In both the ruminants, and this tribe, I think it must be allowed that the first stomach is a reservoir. In the ruminants the precise use of the second and third stomachs is perhaps not known; but digestion is certainly carried on in the fourth; while in this tribe, I imagine, digestion is performed in the second[a], and the use of the third and fourth is not exactly ascertained.

The cæcum and colon do not assist in pointing out the nature of the food and mode of digestion in this tribe. The porpoise, which has teeth and four cavities to the stomach, has no cæcum, similar to some land animals, as the bear, badger, racoon, ferret, polecat, &c.; neither has the bottle-nose a cæcum which has only two small teeth in the lower jaw; and the piked whale, which has no teeth, has a cæcum, almost exactly like the lion, which has teeth and a very different kind of stomach.

The food of the whole of this tribe, I believe, is fish ; probably each may have a particular kind of which it is fondest, yet does not refuse a variety. In the stomach of the large bottle-nose I found the beaks of some hundreds of cuttle-fish. In the grampus I found the tail of a porpoise; so that they eat their own genus. In the stomach of the piked whale I found the bones of different fish, but particularly those of the dog-fish[b]. From the size of the œsophagus we may conclude that they do not swallow fish so large in proportion to their size as many fish do that we have reason to believe take their food in the same way; for fish often attempt to swallow what is larger than their stomachs can at one time contain, and part remains in the œsophagus till the rest is digested.

The epiploon on the whole is a thin membrane ; on the right side it is rather a thin network[c], though on the left it is a complete membrane, and near to the stomach of the same side becomes of a considerable thickness, especially between the two first bags of the stomach. It has little or no fat, except what slightly covers the vessels in particular parts. It is attached forwards, all along to the lower part of the different bags constituting the stomach, and on the right to the root of

[a] [It is doubtless performed in great part by the secretion of the second, but as before observed, the act is far advanced in the first cavity.]

[b] [In the stomach of the porpesse I have found the bones of an eel, and of a flounder; these were in the first cavity. The great sperm whale is nourished principally by mollusca of the class of Cephalopods, and their beaks seem to form the nuclei of the intestinal concretions, called ' ambergris.']

[c] [It presents this reticulate structure in the otter.]

the mesentery, between the stomach and transverse arch of the colon, first behind to the transverse arch of the colon and root of the mesentery, then to the posterior surface of the left or first bag of the stomach, behind the anterior attachment. In some of this tribe there is the usual passage behind the vessels going to the liver, common to all quadrupeds I am acquainted with; but in others, as the small bottle-nose, there is no such passage, by which the cavity behind the stomach in the epiploon of this animal becomes a circumscribed cavity.

The spleen, in the piked whale, is involved in the epiploon, and is very small for the size of the animal. There are in some, as the porpoise, one or two small ones, about the size of a nutmeg, often smaller, placed in the epiploon behind the other[a]. These are sometimes met with likewise in the human body.

The kidneys in the whole of this tribe of animals are conglomerated, being made up of smaller parts, which are only connected by cellular membrane, blood-vessels, and ducts, or infundibula; but not partially connected by continuity of substance, as in the human body, the ox, &c.: every portion is of a conical figure, whose apex is placed towards the centre of the kidney, the base making the external surface; and each is composed of a cortical and tubular substance, the tubular terminating in the apex, which apex makes the mamilla. Each mamilla has an infundibulum, which is long, and at its beginning wide, embracing the base of the mamilla, and becoming smaller. These infundibula unite at last, and form the ureter. The whole kidney is an oblong flat body, broader and thicker at the upper end than the lower, and has the appearance of being made up of different parts placed close together, almost like the pavement of a street.

The ureter comes out at the lower end, and passes along to the bladder, which it enters very near the urethra.

The bladder is oblong, and small for the size of the animal. In the female the urethra passes along to the external sulcus or vulva, and opens just under the clitoris, much as in the human subject.

Whether being inhabitants of the water makes such a construction of kidney necessary I cannot say; yet one must suppose it to have some connection with such situation, since we find it almost uniformly take place in animals inhabiting the water, whether wholly, as this tribe, or occasionally, as the manatee, seal, and white bear: there is, however, the same structure in the black bear, which I believe never inhabits the water[b]. This, perhaps, should be considered in another light, as Na-

---

[a] [The smaller accessory spleens are sometimes four, five, or six in number.]

[b] [In the beaver and other Rodentia of amphibious habits, the kidney presents a

ture keeping up to a certain uniformity in the structure of similar animals; for the black bear in construction of parts is, in every other respect as well as this, like the white bear.

The capsulæ renales are small for the size of the animal, when compared to the human, as indeed they are in most animals. They are flat, and of an oval figure; the right lies on the lower and posterior part of the diaphragm, somewhat higher than the kidney; the left is situated lower down, by the side of the aorta, between it and the left kidney. They are composed of two substances, the external having the direction of its fibres or parts towards the centre; the internal seeming more uniform, and not having so much of the fibrous appearance.

The blood of animals of this order is, I believe, similar to that of quadrupeds, but I have an idea that the red globules are in larger proportion. I will not pretend to determine how far this may assist in keeping up the animal heat, but as these animals may be said to live in a very cold climate or atmosphere, and such as readily carries off heat from the body, they may want some help of this kind.

It is certain that the quantity of blood in this tribe and in the seal is comparatively larger than in the quadruped, and therefore probably amounts to more than that of any other known animal.

This tribe differs from fish in having the red blood carried to the extreme parts of the body, similar to the quadruped.

The cavity of the thorax is composed of nearly the same parts as in the quadruped, but there appears to be some difference, and the varieties in the different genera are greater. The general cavity is divided into two, as in the quadruped, by the heart and mediastinum.

The heart in this tribe and in the seal is probably larger in proportion to their size than in the quadruped, as also the blood-vessels, more especially the veins.

The heart is inclosed in its pericardium, which is attached by a broad surface to the diaphragm, as in the human body. It is composed of four cavities*, two auricles, and two ventricles: it is more flat than in the quadruped, and adapted to the shape of the chest. The auricles have more fasciculi, and these pass more across the cavity from side to

* As the circulation is a permanent part of the constitution respecting the class to which the animal belongs, and as the kind of heart corresponds with the circulation, these should be considered in the classing of animals. Thus we have animals whose hearts have only one cavity, others with two, three, and four cavities.

simple undivided form; and although in the manatee and rytina the kidney presents the subdivided type of formation, yet it has a smooth unbroken external surface in the dugong, and the papillæ form two lateral series opening into a single elongated pelvis.]

side than in many other animals; besides, being very muscular they are very elastic, for being stretched they contract again very considerably. There is nothing uncommon or particular in the structure of the ventricles, in the valves of the ventricles, or in that of the arteries.

The general structure of the arteries resembles that of other animals, and where parts are nearly similar the distribution is likewise similar. The aorta forms its usual curve, and sends off the carotid and subclavian arteries[a].

Animals of this tribe, as has been observed, have a greater proportion of blood than any other known, and there are many arteries apparently intended as reservoirs, where a larger quantity of arterial blood seemed to be required in a part, and vascularity could not be the only object. Thus we find that the intercostal arteries divide into a vast number of branches, which run in a serpentine course between the pleura and the ribs, and their muscles, making a thick substance somewhat similar to that formed by the spermatic artery in the bull. Those vessels everywhere lining the sides of the thorax pass in between the ribs near their articulation, and also behind the ligamentous attachment of the ribs, and anastomose with each other. The medulla spinalis is surrounded with a network of arteries in the same manner, more especially where it comes out from the brain, where a thick substance is formed by their

---

[a] [Both the aorta and pulmonary artery are considerably dilated above their origin in the narwhal, according to Albers, Mayer, and Rapp (*Cetaceen*, p. 158.). In the porpoise the aorta sends off, as usual, first the two coronary arteries, then three branches from the convexity of the arch. The first of these is the largest; it sends off the posterior thoracic and then the right carotid, and lastly divides into the right subclavian and internal mammary arteries. The second branch sends off the left carotid, subclavian, and internal mammary arteries; but the left posterior thoracic arises, as a third branch, immediately from the arch of the aorta. Notwithstanding the shortness of the neck, the common carotid, on each side, sends off a branch, as in most mammalia, before dividing into the external and internal carotids; and the subordinate branches of both these vessels form plexuses in various parts of the head, especially at the basis cranii, and around the optic nerve.

The abdominal aorta lies deep in the cleft between the right and left psoæ muscles. It gives off the cæliac, and close to it the superior mesenteric, then, at a greater distance, a small inferior mesenteric artery; also a right and left renal artery, which, in the true Cetacea, enter the upper or anterior extremity of the kidney, and subdivides to distribute branches to the different lobules, like the stalk of a bunch of grapes. The spermatic arteries are quickly resolved into plexuses. The lumbar arteries are given off as usual in pairs; and a little anterior to the pelvic bones the aorta divides into two hypogastric arteries (which send off the umbilical arteries to the sides of the bladder), and a middle caudal artery, which is the largest, and passes, as a continuation of the aortic trunk, through the arches of the inferior spines. There are no branches analogous to common iliac and crural arteries.]

ramifications and convolutions; and these vessels most probably anastomose with those of the thorax[a].

The subclavian artery in the piked whale, before it passes over the
first rib, sends down into the chest arteries which assist in forming the
plexus on the inside of the ribs[b]; I am not certain but the internal mammary arteries contribute to form the anterior part of this plexus. The
motion of the blood in such must be very slow, the use of which we do
not readily see.

The descending aorta sends off the intercostals, which are very large,
and give branches to this plexus; and when it has reached the abdomen,
it sends off, as in the quadruped, the different branches to the viscera
and the lumbar arteries, which are likewise very large for the supply
of that vast mass of muscles which moves the tail.

In our examination of particular parts, the size of which is generally
regulated by that of the whole animal, if we have only been accustomed
to see them in those which are small or middle-sized, we behold them
with astonishment in animals so far exceeding the common bulk as the
whale. Thus the heart and aorta of the spermaceti whale appeared
prodigious, being too large to be contained in a wide tub, the aorta
measuring a foot in diameter. When we consider these as applied to

---

[a] [Tyson, who was the first discoverer and describer of this structure (Anatomy of a
Porpesse, p. 32, pl. 2, fig. 7, 4to, 1680), speaks of it as a ‘ glandulous body,’ but describes
it as a curious contexture of blood-vessels variously contorted and winding, emerging
from the medulla spinalis at the holes where the nerves come out between the ribs; and
he observes, “the same substance likewise for a good thickness covered the medulla
spinalis throughout.” Hunter first determined the exact nature of this structure, and
that it was a reservoir of arterial blood. It is from this reservoir that the central
axis of the nervous system receives its appropriate stimulus, and the powerful muscles
of the tail their supply of oxygenated blood during the period of submersion and consequent interruption of the respiratory function. M. Breschet, in a treatise *ex professo*
on this structure, gives some beautiful figures of it. (See *Histoire Anatomique et Phy-
siologique d'un Organe de Nature vasculaire découvert dans les Cetacés*, par G. M.
Breschet; 4to, 1836.) He detected it in the *Delphinus Delphis* and *Delphinus Globiceps*, and in a fœtus of the *Balæna Mysticetus*; but in reasoning on the physiology of
the great arterial reservoirs which thus seem to be common to the true Cetacea, it is
necessary to bear in mind that the structure does not exist in the herbivorous Cetacea.]

[b] [It also gives off external thoracics to the pectoral muscles, a subscapular branch,
and one to the supraspinal fossa: these arteries supply the moving powers of the fin:
the trunk then divides in two branches, which almost immediately subdivide, and form
plexuses upon the humerus, which are expended in nourishing the bones and their
ligaments and the enveloping integument. This disposition is but remotely analogous
to the condition of the axillary artery in the slow lemurs and sloths, where a plexus
is formed by a sudden subdivision of the trunk into numerous small branches, which
after a brief course reunite into the common trunk, which then proceeds, as brachial
artery, to supply the muscles of the forearm and hand.]

the circulation, and figure to ourselves that probably ten or fifteen gallons of blood are thrown out at one stroke, and moved with an immense velocity through a tube of a foot diameter, the whole idea fills the mind with wonder.

The veins, I believe, have nothing particular in their structure, excepting in parts requiring a peculiarity, as in the folds of the skin on the breast in the piked whale, where their elasticity was to be increased[a].

Of the Larynx.

The larynx in most animals living on land is a compound organ, adapted both for respiration, deglutition, and sound, which last is produced in the actions of respiration; but in this tribe the larynx I suppose is only adapted to respiration, as we do not know that they have any mode of producing sound[b].

It is composed of os hyoides, thyroid, cricoid, and two arytenoid cartilages, with the epiglottis. It varies very much in structure and size, when compared in animals of different genera. These cartilages were much smaller in the bottle-nose of twenty-four feet long than in the piked whale of seventeen feet, while the os hyoides was much larger.

In the bottle-nose the os hyoides is composed of three bones, besides two whose ends are attached to it, being placed above the os hyoides, making five in all. In the porpoise, piked whale, &c. it is but one bone, slightly bent, having a broad thin process passing up, which is a little

---

[a] [Hunter has previously noticed the great capacity of the veins; they are also remarkable for their number and the immense plexuses which they form in different parts of the body, but above all for the almost total absence of valves. Tyson has given a figure of the extensive venous plexus situated on the membrane investing the psoas muscles (*ibid.*, pl. 1, fig. 2, H.), and these have recently occupied the attention of Breschet, *loc. cit.*, and V. Baer (*Acta Acad. Nat. Cur.*, vol. xvii. p. 1, 1834.) The inferior and superior venæ cavæ are not brought into communication by the vena azygos, as in other mammalia; such veins in the usual situation in the chest would have been subject to compression between the arterial plexuses and the lungs. The venæ azygos are therefore represented by two venous trunks situated in the interior of the vertebral canal, where they receive the intercostal and lumbar veins, and finally communicate with the superior cava by means of a short single large trunk, which penetrates the parietes of the posterior and right side of the chest. The non-valvular structure of the veins in the Cetacea, and the pressure of the sea-water at the depths to which they retreat when harpooned, explain the profuse and deadly hemorrhage which follows a wound that in other mammalia would be by no means fatal.]

[b] [My learned friend and colleague in the present work, Mr. T. Bell, considers the evidence to be strong, if not incontestable, in favour of the existence of a voice in the Cetacea. It is variously described as a bellow, a grunt, or a melancholy cry; of which he cites several instances in his beautiful work on British quadrupeds, pp. 460, 475.]

forked: it has no attachment to the head by means of other bones, as in many quadrupeds.

The thyroid cartilage in the piked whale is broad from side to side, but not from the upper to the lower part: it has two lateral processes, which are long, and pass down the outside of the cricoid, near to its lower end, and are joined to it much as in the human subject. These differ in shape in different animals of this tribe.

The cricoid cartilage is broad and flat, making the posterior and lateral part of the larynx, and is much deeper behind, and laterally, than before. It is extremely thick and strong, flattened on the posterior surface, and hollowed from the upper edge to the lower. It terminates by a thick edge on the posterior part above, but irregularly at the lower edge, in the cartilages of the larynx.

The two arytenoid cartilages are extremely projecting, and united to each other till near their ends; are articulated on the upper edge of the cricoid, but send down a process, which passes on the inside of the cricoid, being attached to a bag in the piked whale, which is formed below the thyroid and before the cricoid cartilages; they cross the cavity of the larynx obliquely, making the passage at the upper part a groove between them: the cavity at this place swells out laterally, but is very narrow between the anterior and posterior surfaces. The passage above between the arytenoid and thyroid cartilages is wide from side to side, and is continued down on the outside of the processes of the arytenoid cartilage, as well as between them, ending below the thyroid, which is folliculated on its inner surface on the fore part of the cricoid cartilage.

The epiglottis makes a third part of the passage, and completes the glottis by forming it into a canal, in several of this tribe; but in the piked whale it was not attached to the two arytenoid cartilages, but only in contact, or inclosing them at their base, so as to make them form a complete canal.

I could not observe anything like a thyroid gland[a].

From the glottis and epiglottis being so connected as to make but one canal, and from the thyroid and cricoid cartilages being so flattened in some between the anterior and posterior surface, the passage through these parts is very small or contracted; but the trachea swells out again into a very considerable size. Its larger branches are in proportion to the trunk, and enter the lungs at the upper end along with the blood-vessels.

---

[a] [This body certainly exists both in the porpoise and bottle-nose dolphin; it is bilobed, and placed transversely across the trachea. Below this body is the thymus, which extends into the chest and is much subdivided.]

Of the Lungs.

The lungs are two oblong bodies, one on each side of the chest, and are not divided into smaller lobes, as in the human subject. They are of considerable length, but not so deep between the fore and back part as in the quadruped, from the heart being broad, flat, and of itself filling up the fore part of the chest. They pass further down on the back part than in the quadruped, by which their size is increased, and rise higher up in the chest than the entrance of the vessels, coming to a point at the upper end. From the entrance of the vessels they are connected downwards, along their whole inner edge, by a strong attachment (in which there are in some lymphatic glands) to the posterior mediastinum. The lungs are extremely elastic in their substance, even so much so as to squeeze out any air that may be thrown into them, and to become almost at once a solid mass, having a good deal the appearance, consistence, and feel of an ox's spleen. The branches of the bronchiæ which ramify into the lungs have not the cartilages flat, but rather rounded; a construction which admits of greater motion between each[a].

The pulmonary cells are smaller than in quadrupeds, which may make less air necessary, and they communicate with each other, which those of the quadruped do not; for by blowing into one branch of the trachea, not only the part to which it immediately goes, but the whole lungs are filled.

As the ribs in this tribe do not completely make the cavity of the thorax, the diaphragm has not the same attachments as in the quadruped, but is connected forwards to the abdominal muscles, which are very strong, being a mixture of muscular and tendinous fibres.

The position of the diaphragm is less transverse than in the quadruped, passing more obliquely backwards, and coming very low on the spine, and higher up before; which makes the chest longest in the direction of the animal at the back, and gives room for the lungs to be continued along the spine.

The parts immediately concerned in inspiration are extremely strong; the diaphragm remarkably so. The reason of this must at once appear; it necessarily requiring great force to expand in a dense medium like water, especially too when the vacuity is to be filled with one which is rarer, and is to water a species of vacuum, the pressure being much

---

[a] [The cartilaginous hoops of the bronchiæ are continued to their extreme ramifications. The pleura costalis is denser and stronger in the porpoise than serous membranes usually are.]

greater on the external surface than the counter-pressure from within. But expiration on the other hand must be much more easily performed ; the natural elasticity of the parts themselves, with the pressure of the water on the external surface of the body, being greater than the resistance of the air within, will both tend to produce expiration without any immediate action of muscles[a].

The diaphragm, in these animals, appears to be the principal agent in inspiration ; and the cavity of the thorax not being entirely surrounded by bony parts, is of course less easily expanded, and the apparatus for its expansion in all directions, as in the quadruped, does not exist here.

The Blow-hole, or Passage for the Air.

As the nose in every animal that breathes air is a common passage for the air, and is also the organ of smelling ; I shall describe it in this tribe as instrumental to both these purposes.

There is a variety in some species of this animal which is, I believe, peculiar to this order; that is, the want of the sense of smelling ; none of those which I have yet examined having that sense, except the two kinds of whalebone whale : such of course have neither the olfactory nerves, nor the organ; therefore in them, the nostrils are intended merely for respiration ; but others have the organ placed in this passage as in other animals.

The membranous portion of the posterior nostrils is one canal ; but when in the bony part, in most of them, it is divided into two; the spermaceti whale, however, is an exception. In those which have it divided, it is in some continued double through the anterior soft parts, opening by two orifices, as in the piked whale ; but in others, it unites again in the membranous part, making externally only one orifice, as in the porpoise, grampus, and bottle-nose. At its beginning in the fauces, it is a roundish hole, surrounded by a strong sphincter muscle, for grasping the epiglottis ; beyond this, the canal becomes larger, and opens into the two passages in the bones of the head. This part is very glandular, being full of follicles, whose ducts ramify in the surrounding substance, which appears fatty and muscular like the root of the tongue, and these ramifications communicate with one another, and contain a viscid slime. In the spermaceti whale, which has a single canal, it is thrown a little to the left side.

---

[a] [Professor Mayer, of Bonn, has however recently described a muscular membrane as immediately investing the lungs in the dolphin.]

After these canals emerge from the bones near the external opening, they become irregular, and have several sulci passing out laterally, o irregular forms, with corresponding eminences. The structure of these eminences is muscular and fatty, but less muscular than the tongue of a quadruped.

In the porpoise there are two sulci on each side; two large and two small, with corresponding eminences of different shapes, the large ones being thrown into folds.

The spermaceti whale has the least of this structure; the external opening in it comes further forwards towards the anterior part of the head, and is consequently longer than in others of this order. Near to its opening externally, it forms a large sulcus, and on each side of this canal is a cartilage, which runs nearly its whole length. In all that I have examined, this canal, forwards from the bones, is entirely lined with a thick cuticle of a dark colour.

In those which have only one external opening, it is transverse, as in the porpoise, grampus, bottle-nose and spermaceti whale, &c.: where double, they are longitudinal, as in the piked whale, and the large whalebone whale. These openings form a passage for the air in respiration to and from the lungs: for it would be impossible for these animals to breathe air through the mouth; indeed, I believe the human species alone breathe by the mouth, and in them it is mostly from habit; for in quadrupeds the epiglottis conducts the air into the nose.

In the whole of this tribe, the situation of the opening on the upper surface of the head is well adapted for this purpose, being the first part that comes to the surface of the water in the natural progressive motion of the animal; therefore it is to be considered principally as a respiratory organ, and where it contains the organ of smell, that is only secondary.

As the animals of this order do not live in the medium which they inspire, the organs conducting the air to the lungs are in some sort particularly constructed, that the water in which they live may not interfere with the air they breathe.

The projecting glottis, which has been described, passes into the posterior nostrils, by which means it crosses the fauces, dividing them into two passages. The enlargement of the termination of the glottis, observed in some of them, would seem to be intended to prevent its retraction: but, as it seems confined to the porpoise and grampus, it may, perhaps, in them answer some other purpose.

The beginning of the posterior nostrils, which answers to the palatum molle in the quadruped, having a sphincter, the glottis is grasped by it, which renders its situation still more secure, and the passages through the head, across the fauces and along the trachea, are rendered one continued canal ; this union of glottis and epiglottis with the posterior nostril, making only a kind of joint, admits of motion, and of dilatation and contraction of the fauces, in deglutition, from the epiglottis moving more in or out of the posterior nostril.

This construction of parts answers a purpose similar to that of the epiglottis in the quadruped; it may be considered as the epiglottis and the arytenoid cartilages joining to make a tubular or cylindrical epiglottis, instead of a valvular one.

The reasons why there should be so peculiar a construction of parts do not at first appear; but we certainly see by it an absolute guard placed upon the lungs, that no water should get into them.

This tribe being without the projecting tongue of the quadruped, and wanting its extensive motion and the power of sucking things into the mouth, may probably require the construction between the air and lungs to be more perfect; but how far it is so I will not pretend to say.

The Brain and Medulla Spinalis.

The size of the brain differs much in different genera of this tribe, and likewise in the proportion it bears to the bulk of the animal. In the porpoise, I believe, it is the largest, and perhaps in that respect comes nearest to the human.

The size of the cerebellum in proportion to that of the cerebrum is smaller in the human subject than in any animal with which I am acquainted. In many quadrupeds, as the horse, cow, &c. the disproportion in size between cerebellum and cerebrum is not great, and in this tribe it is still less; yet not so small as in the bird, &c.

The whole brain in this tribe is compact, the anterior part of the cerebrum not projecting so far forwards as in either the quadruped or in the human subject; neither is the medulla oblongata so prominent, but flat, lying in a kind of hollow made by the two lobes of the cerebellum[a].

The brain is composed of cortical and medullary substances, very distinctly marked; the cortical being in colour like the tubular substance of a kidney, the medullary very white. These substances are nearly in the same proportion as in the human brain. The two lateral ventricles are large, and in those that have olfactory nerves are not continued into them as in many quadrupeds; nor do they wind so much outwards as in the human subject, but pass close round the posterior ends of the tha-

---

[a] [The most characteristic feature of the brain of the Cetacean is its great breadth, which exceeds its length. Each hemisphere is divided below by a *fissura magna* into an anterior and middle lobe, which extends over the cerebellum, so as to form a posterior lobe.]

lami nervorum opticorum[a]. The thalami themselves are large, the corpora striata small[b]; the crura of the fornix are continued along the windings of the ventricles, much as in the human subject[c]. The plexus choroides is attached to a strong membrane which covers the thalami nervorum opticorum, and passes through the whole course of the ventricle, much as in the human subject[d].

The substance of the brain is more visibly fibrous than I ever saw it in any other animal, the fibres passing from the ventricles as from a centre to the circumference, which fibrous texture is also continued through the cortical substance. The whole brain in the piked whale weighed four pounds ten ounces[e].

The nerves going out from the brain, I believe, are similar to those of the quadruped, except in the want of the olfactory nerves in the genus of the porpoise.

The medulla spinalis is much smaller in proportion to the size of the body than in the human species, but still bears some proportion to the quantity of brain; for in the porpoise, where the brain is largest, the medulla spinalis is largest; yet this did not hold good in the spermaceti whale, the size of the medulla spinalis appearing to be proportionally larger than the brain, which was small when compared to the size of the animal. It has a cortical part in the centre, and terminates about the twenty-fifth vertebra, beyond which is the cauda equina, the dura mater going no lower. The nerves which go off from the medulla spi-

[a] [They extend, as in the human subject, into an anterior, descending, and posterior horn; but the latter is very small.]

[b] [The smallness of size of these parts, and the shortness of the anterior lobes of the brain are in relation with the absence of olfactory nerves. The corpora striata are brought into communication with each other by an anterior commissure.]

[c] [The fornix sends down two slender anterior pillars to the corpora albicantia, and is continued into the anterior part of the corpus callosum; it then bends backwards along the under surface of the corpus callosum and above the thalami, and its posterior crura sink down, and diverge from each other to form the hippocampi.]

[d] [The hemispheres of the brain are united by a corpus callosum, chiefly remarkable for its position, being much inclined downwards and forwards; its size is large, bearing the usual proportion to that of the hemispheres. The bigeminal bodies are large; the anterior pair are rounded and lie close together; the posterior are oval, and are separated by a depression which receives the anterior part of the vermiform process of the cerebellum. The medulla oblongata is characterized by the absence of the trapezoid bodies, in which respect it resembles that in the human subject and orang. The remarkable number and depth of the cerebral convolutions have been noticed by Tyson in the porpoise, by Scoresby in the whale, and by Tiedemann in the dolphin.]

[e] [Scoresby found the brain of the mysticete whale (*Balæna Mysticetus*) to weigh three pounds twelve ounces. Tyson found the brain of a porpoise, which weighed ninety-six pounds avoirdupoise, to weigh sixteen ounces and a half. I found the weight of the brain of an adult male porpoise to be one pound two ounces and three quarters avoirdupois.]

nalis are more uniform in size than in the quadruped, there being no
such inequality of parts, nor any extremities to be supplied, except the
fins[a]

The medulla spinalis is more fibrous in its structure than in other
animals; and when an attempt is made to break it longitudinally it tears
with a fibrous appearance, but transversely it breaks irregularly.[b]

The dura mater lines the skull, and forms in some the three processes
answerable to the divisions of the brain, as in the human subject; but
in others this is bone.   Where it covers the medulla spinalis it differs
from all the quadrupeds I am acquainted with, inclosing the medulla
closely, and the nerves immediately passing out through it at the lower
part, as they do at the upper, so that the cauda equina, as it forms, is
on the outside of the dura mater.

The Organs of Sense.

As the organs of sense are variously formed in different animals, fitted
for the various modes of impression; and as the modes are either increased or varied, according to circumstances which make no part of the
sense itself, but which are necessary for the œconomy of the animal, we
find the senses in this tribe varied in their construction, and in some a
sense is even wholly wanting.

The organs of sense which appear to be adapted to every mode of life
are those of touch and taste; but those of smell, sight, and hearing
probably require to be varied according to circumstances.   Thus smell
may be increased by a mode of impregnation, hearing by the vibration
of different mediums, and sight by the different powers of refraction of
different mediums; therefore as animals are intended by Nature to be
differently circumstanced, so are the senses formed.

Of the Sense of Touch.

The cutis in this tribe appears in general particularly well calculated
for sensation, the whole surface being covered with villi, which are so
many vessels, and we must suppose nerves.   Whether this structure is
only necessary for acute sensation, or whether it is necessary for com-

---

[a] [The anterior roots of the spinal nerves are the largest: the posterior roots, after
piercing the dura mater, are continued for a third of an inch before the gangl on is
formed upon them, in the dorsal region; and the separate roots are progressively longer
as they come off nearer the caudal extremity of the spinal chord.   In the porpoise,
from which the above description is taken, I counted forty-one pairs of spinal nerves:
the cervical are closely approximated in consequence of the shortness of the neck.]

[b] [The canal continued from the fourth ventricle is persistent in the anterior part
of the spinal chord. as in the horse.]

mon sensation, where the cuticle is thick and consisting of many layers.
I do not know. We may observe that where it is necessary the sense
of touch should be accurate the villi are usually thick and long, which
probably is necessary, because in most parts of the body, where the
more acute sensations of touch are required, such parts are covered by
a thick cuticle. Of this the ends of our fingers, toes, and the foot of
the hoofed animals, are remarkable examples.

Whether this sense is more acute in water, I am not certain; but
should imagine it is.

Of the Sense of Taste.

The tongue, which is the organ of taste, is also endowed with the
sense of touch. It is likewise to be considered, in the greatest number
of animals, as an instrument for mechanical purposes; but probably less
so in this tribe than any other. However, even in these it must have
been formed with this view, since merely as an organ of taste it would
only have required surface, yet is a projecting body endowed with motion. In some it is better adapted for motion than in others; and I
should suppose this to be requisite, on account of the difference in the
mode of catching the food and in the act of swallowing. It is most
projecting in those with teeth, probably for the better conducting the
food, step by step, to the œsophagus; whereas it does not seem so necessary to have such management of the tongue in those which have no
teeth, and catch their food by merely opening the mouth and swimming
upon it, or by having their prey carried in by the water. In the porpoise and grampus it is firm in texture, composed of muscle and fat,
being pointed and serrated on its edges, like that of the hog[a].

In the spermaceti whale the tongue was almost like a feather-bed[b].
In the piked whale it was but gently raised, hardly having any lateral
edges, and its tip projecting but little, yet, like every other tongue,
composed of muscle and fat. The extent between the two jaw-bones
in this whale was very considerable, taking in the whole width of the
head or upper jaw, and of course including the whalebone. This extent
of surface between jaw and jaw, having but little projection of tongue,
is almost flat from side to side, is extremely elastic when contracted, and
throws the inner membrane into a vast number of very small folds, that
run parallel to one another, but which are again thrown into a close
serpentine course by the elasticity of the part in a contrary direction.
From the tongue being capable of but little motion, there is only a small

[a] [We have found the marginal serration of the tongue of the hog only in the fœtus
or very young state.]

[b] [It is, however, of much smaller size in this species than in the whalebone whales.]

mass of muscle required; and, from the thinness of the jaw-bone, the distance between the lower surface of the mouth and external surface of the skin is but small; and this skin being ribbed and very elastic is capable of considerable distention, by which the cavity of the mouth can be enlarged.

The tongue of the large whalebone whale, I should suppose, rose in the mouth considerably; the two jaws at the middle being kept at such a distance on account of the whalebone, so that the space between, when the mouth is shut, must be filled up by the tongue.

Of the Sense of Smelling.

In this tribe of animals there is something very remarkable in what relates to the sense of smelling; nor have I been able to discover the particular mode by which it is performed.

When we consider these animals as mammalia, and only constructed differently in external form for progressive motion through water, we must see that it was necessary that all the senses should correspond with this medium: we must therefore be at a loss to conceive how they smell, since we may observe that the organ for smelling water, as in fish, is very different from that formed to smell air; and as we must suppose this tribe are only to smell water, being the medium in which such odoriferous particles can be diffused, we should expect their organ to be similar to that of fish; but in that case nature would have been obliged to have attached the nose of a fish to an animal constructed like a quadruped; and it is contrary to the laws which are established in the animal creation to mix parts of different animals together.

In many of this tribe there is no organ of smell at all; and in those which have such an organ, it is not that of a fish, therefore probably not calculated to smell water. It becomes difficult therefore to account for the manner in which such animals smell the water; and why the others should not have had such an organ*, which, I believe, is peculiar to the large and small whalebone whales.

Although it is not the external air which they inspire that produces smell, I believe it is the air retained in the nostril out of the current of respiration, which by being impregnated with the odoriferous particles contained in the water during the act of blowing, is applied to the organ of smell. It might be supposed that they could smell the air on

* Is the mode of smelling in fish similar to tasting in other animals? Or is the air contained in the water impregnated with the odoriferous parts, and this air the fish smells? If so, it is somewhat similar to the breathing of fish, it not being the water which produces the effect there, but the air contained in it. This I proved by experiments, and is mentioned by Dr. Priestley.

the surface of the water by every inspiration, as animals do on land;
and probably they may: but this will not give them the power to smell
the odoriferous particles of their prey in the water at any depth; and
as their organ is not fitted to be affected by the application of water,
and as they cannot suck water into the nostril without the danger of
its passing into the lungs, it cannot be by its application to this organ
that they are enabled to smell.

Some have the power of throwing the water from the mouth through
the nostril, and with such force as to raise it thirty feet high: this must
answer some important purpose, although not immediately evident to us.

As the organ appears to be formed to smell air only, and as I conceive
the smelling of the external air could not be of use as a sense, I therefore believe that they do not smell in inspiration; yet let us consider how
they may be supposed to smell the odoriferous particles of the water.

The organ of smell is out of the direct road of the current of air in
inspiration; it is also out of the current of water when they spout;
may we not suppose then, that this sinus contains air, and as the water
passes in the act of throwing it out, that it impregnates this reservoir
of air, which immediately affects the sense of smell? This operation is
probably performed in the time of expiration, because it is said that this
water is sometimes very offensive; but all this I only give as conjecture.

If the above solution is just, then only those which have the organ
of smell can spout, a fact worthy of inquiry.

The organ of smell would appear to be less necessary in these animals than in those which live in air, since some are wholly deprived of
it; and the organ in those which have it is extremely small, when
compared with that of other animals, as well as the nerve which is to
receive the impression, as was observed above[a].

---

[a] [It is singular that Mr. Hunter should not have added a description of the organ,
the function of which is the subject of so many singular and original speculations in
the preceding section.

The olfactory nerve in the whalebone whale (*Balæna Mysticetus*) is solid, as in the
human subject, but round, about half an inch in diameter at its narrowest part, and
gradually swelling into a pyriform bulbous termination, from the fundus of which the
divisions of the nerve pass off through the foramina of the cribriform plate; the larger
of these foramina are from one to two lines in diameter, about twenty in number, and
placed chiefly around the circumference of the cribriform plate; there are two large
ones in the centre which lead to the root of the middle spongy bone. The lamella
itself is concave towards the fossa of the nerve.

The nerves are lodged for some distance in a peculiar cavity, surrounded by the
cancellous diploe of the skull, leading from the cranial cavity to the cribriform plate.
The turbinated bones are three in number, but are none of them distinct, merely projections from the side of the nasal cavity into its area. The middle one is the largest;
besides its lateral adhesion, it is attached by a narrow pedicle to the cribriform plate,

Of the Sense of Hearing.

The ear is constructed much upon the same principle as in the quadruped; but as it differs in several respects, which it is necessary to
particularize, to convey a perfect idea of it the whole should be described. As this would exceed the limits of this paper, I shall content myself with a general description, taking notice of those material
points in which it differs from that of the quadruped.

This organ consists of the same parts as in the quadruped; an external opening, with a membrana tympani, an Eustachian tube, a tympanum with its processes, and the small bones[a]. There is no external
projection forming a funnel, but merely an external opening. We
can easily assign a reason why there should be no projecting ear, as it
would interfere with progressive motion; but the reason why it is not
formed as in birds, is not so evident; whether the percussions of water
could be collected into one point as air, I cannot say. The tympanum
is constructed with irregularities, so much like those of an external ear,
that I could suppose it to have a similar effect.

The external opening begins by a small hole, scarcely perceptible,
situated on the side of the head a little behind the eye[b]. It is much
longer than in other animals, in consequence of the size of the head
being so much increased beyond the cavity that contains the brain. It
passes in a serpentine course, at first horizontally, then downwards,
and afterwards horizontally again, to the membrana tympani, where it
terminates. In its whole length it is composed of different cartilages,
which are irregular and united together by cellular membrane, so as to
admit of motion, and probably of lengthening or shortening, as the
animal is more or less fat.

The bony part of the organ is not so much inclosed in the bones of

---

from which it quickly expands into a body of about one and a half inch in diameter,
having an upper, middle, and lower protuberance separated by sinuosities; but the
bone is not a convoluted plate, but solid, or having its substance of the same cellular
structure as the surrounding diploe. The inferior turbinated process is a simple elliptic
protuberance, about one inch in length and half an inch in width.

The olfactory nerves in the *Balænoptera* are somewhat larger than in the human
subject; they are of a pulpy texture, yet readily divisible into fasciculi, and terminate
in a small bulb which rests on the cribriform plate. Treviranus states that olfactory
nerves, but of very minute size, do exist in the porpoise; and V. Baer describes them
as being one sixth of a line in diameter in the *Delphinus Delphis*.]

[a] [The internal ear or labyrinth, which Hunter afterwards describes as 'the immediate
organ,' seems to have been accidentally omitted in the above enumeration.]

[b] [In the full-grown spermaceti whale Mr. F. D. Bennett found the aperture of the
meatus auditorius to form a narrow longitudinal fissure, one inch in length; it admitted with difficulty the extremity of the index finger.]

the skull as in the quadruped, consisting commonly of a distinct bone or bones, closely attached to the skull, but in general readily to be separated from it[a]; yet in some it sends off, from the posterior part, processes which unite with the skull. It varies in its shape, and is composed of the immediate organ and the tympanum.

The immediate organ is, in point of situation to that of the tympanum, superior and internal, as in the quadruped. The tympanum is open at the anterior end, where the Eustachian tube begins.

The Eustachian tube opens on the outside of the upper part of the fauces: in some higher in the nose than others; highest I believe in the porpoise. From the cavity of the tympanum, where it is rather largest, it passes forwards and inwards, and near its termination appears very much fasciculated, as if glandular[b].

The Eustachian tube and tympanum communicate with several sinuses, which passing in various directions, surround the bone of the ear. Some of these are cellular, similar to the cells of the mastoid process in the human subject, although not bony. There is a portion of this cellular structure of a particular kind, being white, ligamentous, and each part rather rounded than having flat sides*. One of the sinuses passing out of the tympanum close to the membrana tympani, goes a little way in the same direction, and communicates with a number of cells.

The whole function of the Eustachian tube is perhaps not known; but it is evidently a duct from the cavity of the ear, or a passage for the mucus of these parts; the external opening having a particular form would incline us to believe, that something was conveyed to the tympanum.

* These communications with the Eustachian tube may be compared to a large bag on the bases of the skull of the horse and ass, which is a lateral swell of the membranous part of the tube, and when distended will contain nearly a quart[c].

---

[a] [Being united to the skull by fibrous texture only, a structure which is peculiar to the Cetacea, but not universal in that order.]

[b] [The Eustachian tube in the true Cetacea is characterized by its membranous structure throughout; its parietes are nowhere supported by cartilage, nor does it traverse any bone. In the porpesse its internal surface is provided with many semilunar valves, the free margins of which are directed towards the nasal outlet of the tube.]

[c] [In a beautiful drawing of the organ of hearing in the porpoise, recently published by the College of Surgeons, Hunter gives a view of part of the sinuses which communicate with the tympanum and Eustachian tube. See Physiological Catalogue of the Hunterian Collection, vol. iii. pl. xxxiv. i. k. In the preparation (No. 1582) the sinuses are seen to contain numerous small worms (*Strongylus minor*), Kuhn, Mém. du Muséum, tom. xviii. p. 363. The same have been observed by other physiologists, as Klein, Camper, Albers, and Rudolphi, the latter of whom regards them as a small variety of the *Strongylus inflexus*.]

The bony part of the organ is very hard and brittle, rendering it even difficult to be cut with a saw, without its chipping into pieces. That part which contains the immediate organ is by much the hardest, and has a very small portion of animal substance in it; for when steeped in an acid, what remains is very soft, almost like a jelly, and laminated. The bone is not only harder in its substance, but there is on the whole more solid bone than in the corresponding parts of quadrupeds, it being thick and massy.

The part containing the tympanum is a thin bone, coiled upon itself, attached by one end to the portion which contains the organ; and this attachment in some is by close contact only, as in the narwhale; in others, the bones run into one another, as in the bottle-nose and piked whales.

The concave side of the tympanum is turned towards the organ, its two edges being close to it; the outer is irregular, and in many only in contact, as in the porpoise; while in others the union is by bony continuity, as in the bottle-nose whale, leaving a passage on which the membrana tympani is stretched, and another opening, which is the communication with the sinuses.

The surface of the bone containing the immediate organ opposite to the mouth of the tympanum is very irregular, having a number of eminences and cavities. The cavity of the tympanum is lined with a membrane, which also covers the small bones with their muscles, and appears to have a thin cuticle. This membrane renders the bones, muscles, tendons, &c. very obscure, which are seen distinctly when that is removed. It appears to be a continuation of the periosteum, and the only uniting substance between the small bones. Besides the general lining, there is a plexus of vessels, which is thin and rather broad, and attached by one edge, the rest being loose in the cavity of the tympanum, somewhat like the plexus choroides in the ventricles of the brain. The cavity we may suppose intended to increase sound, probably by the vibration of the bone; and from its particular formation we can easily conceive, that the vibrations are conducted, or reflected, towards the immediate organ, it being in some degree a substitute for the external ear.

The external opening being smaller than in any animals of the same size, the membrana tympani is nearly in the same proportion. In the bottle-nose whale, the grampus, and porpoise, it is smooth and concave externally, but of a particular construction on the inner surface; for a tendinous process passes from it towards the malleus, converging as it proceeds from the membrane, and becoming thinner till its insertion into that bone. I could not discover whether it had any muscular fibres which could affect the action of the malleus. In the piked whale, the termination of the external opening, instead of being smooth and concave, is projecting, and returns back into the meatus for above an inch in length[a], is firm in texture, with thick coats, is hollow on its inside, and its mouth communicating with the tympanum; one side being fixed to the malleus, similar to the tendinous process which goes from the inside of the membrana tympani in the others[b].

A little way within the membrana tympani, are placed the small bones, which are three in number, as in the quadruped, malleus, incus, and stapes; but in the bottle-nose whale there is a fourth, placed on the tendon of the stapedius muscle. These bones are as it were suspended between the bone of the tympanum and that of the immediate organ.

The malleus has two attachments, besides that with the incus; one close to the bone of the tympanum, which, in the porpoise, is only by contact, but in others by a bony union[c]; the other attachment is form-

---

[a] [As might be expected, the same structure exists in the whalebone whale (*Balæna Mysticetus*, Linn.), where, according to Home, the membrana tympani, "instead of being concave, as in other animals, towards the meatus externus, is convex and projects nearly an inch into that tube," Phil. Trans. 1812, p. 84. In this respect, the whalebone whales resemble the sloths, the turtle, and crocodile, and in fact the whole series of air-breathing oviparous vertebrata, which have the ear-drum convex externally. In the dolphins and porpoises, however, as also in the narwhale, the membrana tympani is concave externally, as in other Mammalia.]

[b] [This connexion between the membrana tympani and the malleus is denied by Sir Everard Home, who wrote a paper and gave two plates in support of his opinion. After quoting Mr. Hunter's description, he says, "the fact is, that there is no connection whatever between the membrana tympani and the malleus;" and adds, that "this circumstance forms the great peculiarity in the organ of hearing in this species of whale (*Balæna Mysticetus*, Linn.)." So singular an anomaly as the absence of any communication between the membrana tympani and the ossicula auditûs, would, independently of our interest in the character of Hunter as an accurate observer, have induced us to spare no pains to test the conflicting statements with the facts themselves. It fortunately happens that the preparations figured by Home are preserved (No. 1598 a. Physiological Series, Hunterian Museum); and after a careful examination of them, we find the following to be the true structure of the parts in question. The membrane marked *c* in Home's figure (Phil. Trans. 1812, pl. II.) is continuous at *d* with *e*, the convex projection of the membrana tympani; whereas, the edge of the shadow is so strong in the figure as to cause it to appear as if *c* and *e* were separate membranes, as Home describes them to be: they are, however, parts of the same membrana tympani, the attachment of which is extended inwards beyond the circumference of the termination of the bony meatus auditorius. The triangular ligament proceeding from the handle of the malleus, and which is common to all the Cetacea, is attached not only to the plane portion of the ear-drum, but to the whole of one side of the convex portion which projects into the meatus, and is affected by every motion of that portion.]

[c] [The malleus is anchylosed to the parietes of the tympanum in the dugong.]

ed by the tendon, above described, being united to the inner surface of the membrana tympani. Its base articulates with the incus.

The incus is attached by a small process to the tympanum, and is suspended between the malleus and stapes. The process by which it articulates with the stapes is bent towards that bone.

The stapes stands on the vestibulum, by a broad oval base. In many of this tribe, the opening from side to side of the stapes is so small as hardly to give the idea of a stirrup[n].

The muscles which move these bones are two in number, and tolerably strong. One arises from that projecting part of the tympanum which goes to form the Eustachian tube, and running backwards is inserted into a small depression on the anterior part of the malleus. The use of this muscle seems to be to tighten the membrana tympani; but in those which have the malleus anchylosed with the tympanum, we can hardly conjecture its use. The other has its origin from the inner surface of the tympanum, and passing backwards is inserted into the stapes by a tendon, in which I found a bone in the large bottle-nose. This muscle gives the stapes a lateral motion. What particular use in hearing may be produced by the action of these muscles, I will not pretend to say; but we must suppose, whatever motion is given to the bones must terminate in the movement of the stapes.

The immediate organ of hearing is contained in a round bony process, and consists of the cochlea and semicircular canals, which somewhat resemble the quadruped; but, besides the two spiral turns of the cochlea, there is a third, which makes a ridge within that continued from the foramen rotundum, and follows the turns of the canal.

The cochlea is much larger, when compared with the semicircular canals, than in the human species and quadruped.

We may reckon two passages into the immediate organ of hearing, the foramen rotundum, and foramen ovale. They are at a greater distance than in the quadruped. The foramen rotundum is placed much more on the outer surface of the bone, and not in the cavity of the bony tympanum; but may be said to communicate with the surrounding cellular part of the tympanum. The foramen rotundum, which is the beginning of one of these turns (the scala cochleæ, which is the central or inner canal), appears to be only one end of a transverse groove, which is afterwards closed in the middle, forming a canal with the two ends open; so that this foramen appears to have two beginnings; but the other opening is probably only a passage for blood-vessels going to the cochlea.

From this foramen begins the inner turn of the cochlea, which is

---

[a] [In the *Delphinus Leucas*, the stapes is imperforate, as in the walrus.]

the largest, especially at its beginning; the other begins from the vestibulum. The cochlea is a spiral canal coiled within itself, and divided into two by a thin spiral bony plate, which is completed in the recent subject, and forms two perfect canals.

In the recent subject, the foramen rotundum is lined with the membrane of the tympanum, which terminates in a blind end, forming a kind of membrana cochleæ. The other opening, in the recent subject, communicates with the spiral turn, beyond the membranous termination of the foramen rotundum.

The foramen ovale has a little projection inwards all round, on which the stapes stands : within this is the vestibulum, which is common to the other spiral turn of the cochlcæ, and the semicircular canals; this canal of the cochlea (scala vestibuli) passes out first in a direction contrary to its general course, but soon makes a turn into the spiral. It is round, and not merely a division of the cochlea into two by a septum [a], but has a membrane of its own, which is attached to the thin bony plate, and lines that part of the cochlea in such a manner as to retain its structure when the bone is removed. The cochlea in some completes one turn and a half; in others, more [b]. It is not a spiral on a plane, or cylinder, but on a cone.

I have already observed, that by looking in at the foramen rotundum, we see two small ridges ; the uppermost is the swell of the canal from the vestibulum just described ; the lower ridge, which is also a canal, may be observed just to pass along the foramen belonging to this canal, close to the septum between the two; a circumstance, I believe, peculiar to this tribe. Its beginning is close to the vestibulum, but does not open from it, and passes along the first-described spiral turn to its apex : when opened, it appears to be a canal full of small perforations, probably the passages of the branches from the auditory nerve.

This bony process has several perforations in it; one of them large, for the passage of the seventh pair of nerves. The size of the portio mollis, before its entrance into the organ, is very large [c], and bears no proportion to that which enters. The passage for this nerve is very wide, and seems to have an irregular blind conical, and somewhat spiral, termination ; its being spiral arises from the closeness to the point of the cochlea.

In the terminating part there are a number of perforations into the

---

[a] [*i. e.* it is a cylindrical canal, not semicylindrical as usual in quadrupeds.]

[b] [In the porpesse, the number of gyrations are two and a half. Rudolphi describes two and a half gyrations in the narwhale. Rapp describes two complete gyrations in the *Delphinus Delphis*, and Pallas the same number in the *Delph. Leucas.*]

[c] [Tiedemann particularly notices the large size of the acoustic nerve in the dolphin.]

cochlea, and one into the semicircular canals[a], which afford a passage
to the different divisions of the auditory nerve.   There is a considerable foramen in its anterior side near the bottom, for the passage of the
portio dura, and which is continued backward to the cavity of the
tympanum near the stapes, and emerges near the posterior and upper
part of this bone.

Of the Organ of Seeing.

The eye in this tribe of animals is constructed upon nearly the same
principle as that of quadrupeds, differing, however, in some circumstances; by which it is probably better adapted to see in the medium
through which the light is to pass.   It is upon the whole small for the
size of the animal[b], which would lead to the supposition that their locomotion is not great; for I believe animals that swim are in this respect similar to those that fly; and as this tribe come to the surface of
the medium in which they live, they may be considered in the same
view with birds which soar; and we find birds that fly to great heights,
and move through a considerable space in search of food, have their eyes
larger in proportion to their size.

The eyelids have but little motion[c], and do not consist of loose cellular membrane, as in quadrupeds, but rather of the common adipose
membrane of the body; the connection, however, of their circumference
with the common integuments is loose, the cellular membrane being less
loaded with oil, which allows of a slight fold being made upon the surrounding parts in opening the eyelids.   This is not to an equal degree
in them all, being less so in the porpoise than in the piked whale.

The tunica conjunctiva, where it is reflected from the eyelid to the
eyeball, is perforated all round by small orifices of the ducts of a circle
of glandular bodies lying behind it.

The lachrymal gland is small[d]; its use being supplied by those above
mentioned; and the secretion from them all I believe to be a mucus

---

[a] [The semicircular canals are chiefly remarkable for their small proportional size;
they were overlooked by Camper and Pallas, but were described by Comparetti two
years later than Hunter, in his "*Observationes anatomicæ de Aure interna*," Patavii, 1789.]

[b] [The longest diameter of the eye of the mysticete whale and of the cachalot is two
inches and a half, that of the piked whale four inches; but the eye owes much of
its bulk to the thick sclerotic.   An affinity to the elephant and other large Pachyderms is manifested in this circumstance.]

[c] [The true Cetacea have no tarsal cartilages, and no membrana nictitans, or third
eyelid; this is present in the herbivorous species, as the dugong and manatee, and is
represented by a thick duplicature of the conjunctiva at the inner canthus in the
cachalot.]

[d] [This is merely a larger development of the palpebral glands at the inner side of
the eyeball, and should therefore be regarded as analogous to a Harderian gland.]

similar to what is found in the turtle and crocodile. There are neither
puncta nor lachrymal duct, so that the secretion, whatever it be, is
washed off into the water.

The muscles which open the eyelids are very strong: they take their
origin from the head, round the optic nerve, which in some requires
their being very long, and are so broad as almost to make one circular
muscle round the whole of the interior straight muscles of the eye itself. They may be divided into four; a superior, an inferior, and one
at each angle: as they pass outwards to the eyelids, they diverge and
become broader, and are inserted into the inside of the eyelids almost
equally all round. They may be termed the dilatores of the eyelids;
and, before they reach their insertion, give off the external straight
muscles, which are small[a], and inserted into the sclerotic coat before the
transverse axis of the eye: these may be named the elevator, depressor,
adductor, and abductor, and may be dissected away from the others as
distinct muscles. Besides these four going from the muscles of the
eyelid to the eye itself, there are two which are larger, and inclose the
optic nerve with the plexus. As these pass outwards they become
broad, may in some be divided into four, and are inserted into the sclerotic coat, almost all round the eye, rather behind its transverse axis[b].

The two oblique muscles are very long; they pass through the muscles of the eyelids, are continued on to the globe of the eye, between
the two sets of straight muscles, and at their insertions are very broad;
a circumstance which gives great variation to the motion of the eye[c].

---

[a] [The word "small" is here used relatively to the palpebral muscles; for, compared
with the size of the eyeball the recti muscles in the Cetacea exceed in bulk those of
any other mammiferous animal.]

[b] [These shorter series of straight muscles correspond with the choanoid muscle or
retractor oculi of other mammalia in which (man and the quadrumana excepted), it
co-exists with a membrana nictitans, and is subservient to its motions by retracting
the globe of the eye and displacing the adipose matter posterior to the eyeball, which
then presses forward the third eyelid. In the true Cetacea where there is no third
eyelid some other uses must be assigned for the retractor oculi; it may perhaps assist
by retracting the eyeball, in closing the ordinary eyelids, which have not the advantage of an orbicularis muscle for that purpose. The retractor oculi is represented by
four short muscles in the turtle and tortoise, where the third eyelid is present, but
has a special muscle for nictitation.]

[c] [The superior oblique arises, as in other mammalia, from the posterior part of the
orbit above the foramen opticum; it passes forwards on the external surface of the conical apertor palpebrarum, which it perforates, and a kind of pulley is formed for it by
this muscle and the cellular substance beneath it, the superior oblique becoming at this
bend partially tendinous, but with little diminution of size; it then goes to be inserted
into the sclerotica, at such a direction to the ball of the eye as to act as a rotator to it, according to the use assigned by Hunter to the oblique muscles in a previous memoir.
The inferior oblique arises from the superior maxillary bone at the inner side of the
orbital space. Neither the direction of this or of the superior oblique in the whales
enables them to act as the antagonists of the recti muscles.]

The sclerotic coat gives shape to the eye, both externally and internally, as in other animals; but the external shape and that of the internal cavity are very dissimilar, arising from the great difference in the thickness of this coat in different parts. The external figure is round, except that it is a little flattened forwards; but that of the cavity is far otherwise, being made up of sections of various circles, being a little lengthened from the inner side to the outer, a transverse section making a short ellipsis.

In the piked whale the long axis is two inches and three quarters, the short axis two inches and one-eighth[a].

The posterior part of the cavity is a tolerably regular curve, answering to the difference in the two axises; but forwards, near the cornea, the sclerotic coat turns quickly in, to meet the cornea, which makes this part of the cavity extremely flat, and renders the distance between the anterior part of the sclerotic coat and the bottom of the eye not above an inch and a quarter.

In the piked whale the sclerotic coat, at its posterior part, is very thick: near the extreme of the short axis it was half an inch, and at the long axis one-eighth of an inch thick. In the bottle-nose whale (*Hyperoodon*) the extreme of the short axis was half an inch thick, and the extremes of the long axis about a quarter of an inch, or half the other.

The sclerotic coat becomes thinner as it approaches to its union with the cornea, where it is thin and soft. It is extremely firm in its texture where thick, and from a transverse section would seem to be composed of tendinous fibres, intermixed with something like cartilage: in this section four passages for vessels remain open. This firmness of texture precludes all effect of the straight muscles on the globe of the eye, by altering its shape, and adapting its focus to different distances of objects, as has been supposed to be the case in the human eye.

The cornea makes rather a longer ellipsis than the ball of the eye; the sides of which are not equally curved, the upper being most considerably so. It is a segment of a circle somewhat smaller than that of the eyeball, is soft and very flaccid[b].

The tunica choroides resembles that of the quadruped; and its inner surface is of a silver hue, without any nigrum pigmentum[c].

---

[a] [See a view of the section of the eye of a whale in Soemering's work, entitled, "*De Oculorum sectione horizontali*, tab. ii.]

[b] [In the preparation No. 1682, Physiological Series, Hunterian Museum, Hunter has displayed the laminated structure of the cornea of the whale; this was known to Leeuenhoek, who succeeded in separating it into twenty-two layers. (See Epist. Phys. 1719, p. 42,) which are united by a fine cellular tissue.]

[c] [The choroid in the cetacea is easily separable into two vascular laminæ, of which the outermost is of a blackish colour, and is composed of larger vessels, connected by cellular membrane, which gives it a tomentose appearance; the innermost (membrana

The nigrum pigmentum only covers the ciliary processes, and lines the inside of the iris[a].

The retina appears to be nearly similar to that of the quadruped.

The arteries going to the coats of the eye form a plexus passing round the optic nerve, resembling in its appearance that of the spermatic artery in the bull and some other animals[b].

The crystalline humour resembles that of the quadruped; but whether it is very convex or flattened I cannot determine, those I have examined having been kept too long to preserve their exact shape and size[c]. The vitreous humour adhered to the retina at the entrance of the optic nerve.

The optic nerve is very long in some species, owing to the vast width of the head[d].

I shall not at present consider the eye in animals of this tribe, as it respects the power of vision, that being performed on a general princi-

---

rhuischiana) is equally vascular, of a pale colour, dense, but thinner, most delicately villous and lined by a remarkable tapetum of a bluish-white colour in the whale, with a greenish and somewhat yellowish tinge in the cachalot, and of a very light blue in the porpesse. The ciliary zone is black, broad, almost flat, composed of about seventy long processes, thick, flexuous, and extending their cylindrical apices almost as far as the anterior surface of the lens.]

[a] [When this layer of pigment is removed from the iris, (as Hunter has done in the preparation 1680, Physiological Series), the fibrous structure of the posterior part of the iris becomes very apparent; the outer series of fibres converge towards the margin of the pupil, where they are concealed by the sphincter fibres which surround that part; these latter elliptically disposed fibres are stronger than the radiated ones. The posterior fibrous coat of the iris may be separated without much difficulty from the anterior vascular layer. This consists chiefly of the branches of the two long ciliary arteries, which bifurcate opposite the long axis of the pupil, and, the opposite branches anastomosing, form a canal which surrounds the pupil. Numerous tortuous or wavy branches radiate from this canal towards the outer margin of the iris.

In the preparations No. 1680 and 1683 the structure of the iris in the whale is beautifully shown.

The choroid is puckered up into numerous minute folds, which form the ciliary zone; of these folds every third, fourth, or fifth becomes enlarged, and is extended forwards in the form of a wrinkled process about three lines in length, compressed laterally, and terminating somewhat obtusely; between these larger ciliary processes, which are about seventy in number, there are shorter processes of a similar structure.]

[b] [See prep. No. 1679, Physiological Series, Hunterian Museum.]

[c] [The crystalline lens is inclosed in a strong capsule, is remarkably globose, rather more flattened anteriorly than posteriorly, placed at a very small distance from the cornea, and accordingly diminishing the space for the aqueous, while it increases that for the vitreous humour. In the preparations of the crystalline lens in the Hunterian Museum, preps. Nos. 1658—1687, the nucleus is seen to be excentric, and situated on the posterior half of the lens, and is of a dark colour.]

[d] [When this nerve is divided transversely, and the medullary substance squeezed out, the neurilema does not present the form of tubes, but of numerous septa, which converge from the circumference to the centre of the nerve.]

ple common to every animal inhabiting the water; more especially as I am only master of the construction and formation of the coats, and not of the size, shape, and densities of the humours; yet from reasoning we must suppose them to correspond with the shape of the eye, and the medium through which the light is to pass.

Of the Parts of Generation.

The parts of generation in both sexes of this order of animals come nearer in form to those of the ruminating than of any others, and this similarity is, perhaps, more remarkable in the female than in the male, for their situation in the male must vary on account of external form, as was before observed.

The testicles retain the situation in which they were formed, as in those quadrupeds in which they never come down into the scrotum[a]. They are situated near the lower part of the abdomen, one on each side, upon the two great depressors of the tail. At this part of the abdomen the testicles come in contact with the abdominal muscles anteriorly[b].

The vasa deferentia pass directly from the epididymis behind the bladder, or between it and the rectum, into the urethra; and there are no bags similar to those called vesiculæ seminales in certain other animals[c].

The structure of the penis is nearly the same in them all, and formed much upon the principle of the quadruped. It is made up of two crura, uniting into one corpus cavernosum, and the corpus spongiosum seems first to enter the corpus cavernosum. In the porpoise, at least, the urethra is found nearly in the centre of the corpus cavernosum; but towards the glans seems to separate or emerge from it, and becoming a distinct spongy body, runs along its under surface, as in quadrupeds.

---

[a] [In this respect however the cetacea differ from the ruminants, and resemble the elephant and the hyrax amongst the pachyderms.]

[b] [At the period of sexual excitement the testes acquire a great size. In a male porpoise I found them occupying almost entirely the posterior fourth part of the abdominal cavity; they measured each nine inches in length and four inches in the shortest diameter, and weighed together four pounds avoirdupois. The corpus Highmorianum occupied the middle or axis of the gland, as in all testes which are subject to considerable enlargement at the period of the rut; and the membranous septa radiate from this body to the tunica albuginea.]

[c] [The epididymis in the porpoise is of an elongated triedral form; the broadest facet is connected by a duplicature of peritonæum to the testes; the connexion is close, except at the lower part of the gland, where the membrane is half an inch broad. The vas deferens continues to be convoluted, as in other testiconda, to within two inches of its termination in the dilated bulbous part of the urethra: the lining membrane of the terminal two inches of the vas deferens is denser, and of a less glandular structure than the preceding part.]

The corpus cavernosum in some is broader from the upper part to the lower than from side to side; but in the porpoise has the appearance of being round, becoming smaller forwards, so as to terminate almost in a point some distance from the end of the penis[a]. The glans does not spread out as in many quadrupeds, but seems to be merely a plexus of veins covering the anterior end of the penis, yet is extended a good way further on, and is in some no more than one vein deep.

The crura penis are attached to two bones, which are nearly in the same situation and in the same part of the pelvis as those to which the penis is attached in quadrupeds; but these bones are only for the insertion of the crura, and not for the support of any other part, like the pelvis in those animals which have posterior extremities, neither do they meet at the fore part, or join the vertebræ of the back[b].

The erectores penis are very strong muscles, having an origin and insertion similar to those of the human subject.

The acceleratores muscles are likewise very strong; and there is a strong and long muscle, arising from the anus, and passing forwards to the bulb of the penis, that runs along the under surface of the urethra, and is at last lost or inserted in the corpus spongiosum. This muscle draws the penis into the prepuce, and throws that part of the penis that is behind its insertion into a serpentine form. It is common to most animals that draw back the penis into what is called the sheath, and may be called the retractor penis.

In all the females which I have examined, the parts of generation are very uniformly the same, consisting of the external opening, the vagina, the uterus, fallopian tubes, fimbriæ, and ovaria.

The external opening is a longitudinal slit, or oblong opening, whose edges meet in two opposite points, and the sides are rounded off, so as

---

[a] [The corpus cavernosum is remarkable for the thickness of its fibrous sheath, which equals that of the contained erectile tissue; the fibres composing the sheath affect distinctly two directions, the external ones running longitudinally, the internal circularly.]

[b] [These bones are of an elongated form, and are regarded by Cuvier as analogous to the iliac bones; but as they give attachment to the crura penis, and as the erectores penis arise from their whole outer and posterior surfaces, they would seem to be rather the homologues of the ischia. A strong tendon is continued, in the porpoise, from the anterior and internal extremity of each bone, descends obliquely inwards, and after the course of an inch and a half expands into a muscular belly, which joins its fellow in the mesial line behind the rectum. Below this fleshy belly on each side there is an oval, flattened, slightly concave bone. The commencement of the urethra is surrounded by thick capsule of muscular fibres, which arise from the inner and anterior part of the ischia, and from the inner surface of the oval bones above mentioned. These fibres seem, therefore, to correspond with Wilson's muscle combined with the muscular part of the urethra. They envelope a glandular substance analogous to a prostate.]

to form a kind of sulcus. The skin and parts on each side of this sulcus are of a looser texture than on the common surface of the animal, not being loaded with oil, and allowing of such motion of one part on another as admits of dilatation and contraction. The vagina passes upwards and backwards towards the loins, so that its direction is diagonal respecting the cavity of the abdomen, and then divides into the two horns, one on each side of the loins ; these afterwards terminating in the fallopian tubes, to which the ovaria are attached. From each ovarium there is a small fold of the peritonæum, which passes up towards the kidney of the same side, as in most quadrupeds.

The inside of the vagina is smooth for about one half of its length, and then begins to form something similar to valves projecting towards the mouth of the vagina, each like an os tincæ ; these are about six, seven, eight, or nine in number. Where they begin to form, they hardly go quite round, but the last are complete circles. At this part too the vagina becomes smaller, and gradually decreases in width to its termination[a].

From the last projecting part, the passage is continued up to the opening of the two horns, and the inner surface of this last part is thrown into longitudinal rugæ, which are continued into the horns. Whether this last part is to be reckoned common uterus or vagina, and that the last valvular part is to be considered as os tincæ, I do not know ; but from its having the longitudinal rugæ, I am inclined to think it is uterus, this structure appearing to be intended for distinction[b].

The horns are an equal division of this part ; they make a gentle turn outwards, and are of considerable length. Their inner surface is thrown into longitudinal rugæ, without any small protuberances for the cotyledons to form upon, as in those of ruminating animals[c]; and where they terminate, the fallopian tubes begin.

---

[a] [A muscle arises, on each side, from the whole length of the ischial bone, and passing inwards is inserted into the external surface of the vagina, and into the crura of the clitoris. This body is situated like a projecting ridge, without any preputial fold, between the thin labiæ. On each side of the clitoris, within the mouth of the vagina, are the orifices of sinuses, analogous to the canals of Malpighi in Ruminantia.]

[b] [From the os tincæ, which Hunter calls the last projecting part of the vagina, to the beginning of the division of the uterus, in the porpoise, is about two inches. The uterus is lined with a very smooth mucous membrane ; a thin layer of cellular substance separates this from the muscular tunic, in which the circular fibres may be clearly discerned. The external tunic is derived from the peritoneum which forms the broad ligaments.]

[c] [The fœtus has neither placenta nor colytedons, but, as in the hog and camel, the general vascularity of the chorion is subservient to its nutrition and respiration. The allantois is coextensive in its development with the chorion, and both extend into the horns of the uterus.]

In the bottle-nose whale (*Hyperoodon*), where the fallopian tubes opened into the horns of the uterus, they were surrounded by pendulous bodies hanging loose in the horns.

The fallopian tubes, at their termination in the uterus, are remarkably small for some inches, and then begin to dilate rather suddenly; and the nearer to the mouth the more this dilatation increases, like the mouth of a French horn, the termination of which is five or six inches in diameter[a]. They are very full of longitudinal rugæ through their whole length.

The ovaria are oblong bodies about five inches in length, one end attached to the mouth of the fallopian tube, and the other near to the horn of the uterus[b]. They are irregular on their external surface, resembling a capsula renalis or pancreas. They have no capsula, but what is formed by the long fallopian tube.

How the male and female copulate, I do not know; but it is alleged that their position in the water is erect at that time, which I can readily suppose may be true; for otherwise, if the connection is long, it would interfere with the act of respiration, as in any other position the upper surface of the heads of both could not be at the surface of the water at the same time. However, as in the parts of generation they most resemble those of the ruminating kind, it is possible they may likewise resemble them in the duration of the act of copulation; for, I believe, all the ruminants are quick in this act.

Of their uterine gestation I as yet know nothing; but it is very probable that they have only a single young one at a time, there being only two nipples[c]. This seemed to be the case with the bottle-nose

---

[a] [The margin of this opening, in the porpoise, is entire, without fimbriated processes.]

[b] [In the porpesse the ovaria are attached to the ovarian ligament, and are situated half way between the expanded orifice of the fallopian tube and the extremity of the uterine horn.]

[c] [The dolphin has generally one, but sometimes two at a birth, according to Aristotle. According to Pallas, the Beluga (*Delphinus Leucas*) brings forth two, but the exception to the general rule may have been observed in this case; since Fabricius describes the same species as being uniparous (Fauna Grœnlandica, p. 51.). The Greenland whale brings forth a single young one in April. The spermaceti whale produces one young one every year, according to Mr. Beale (Obs. on the Sperm. Whale, 8vo, p. 36.). Mr. F. D. Bennett found in a gravid cachalot a single fœtus fourteen feet in length, and six in girth; its position in the uterus was that of a bent bow. (Zool. Proceed., Dec. 1836.) When brought forth the young cachalot is usually twenty feet in length. And we may observe that the cetacea in general are remarkable for the large size of the fœtus at birth. Camper describes the new-born porpoise as being half the size of the parent. (Obs. Anatomiques sur les Cetaces, p. 147.) The rudimental condition of the pelvis renders the birth easy.]

whale caught near Berkeley, which had been seen for some days with one young one following it, and they were both caught together.

The glands for the secretion of milk are two, one on each side of the middle line of the belly at its lower part. The posterior ends, from which go out the nipples, are on each side of the opening of the vagina, in small sulci. They are flat bodies lying between the external layer of fat and abdominal muscles, and are of considerable length, but only one-fourth of that in breadth. They are thin, that they may not vary the external shape of the animal, and have a principal duct, running in the middle through the whole length of the gland, and collecting the smaller lateral ducts, which are made up of those still smaller. Some of these lateral branches enter the common trunk in the direction of the milk's passage, others in the contrary direction, especially those nearest to the termination of the trunk in the nipple. The trunk is large, and appears to serve as a reservoir for the milk[a], and terminates externally in a projection, which is the nipple. The lateral portions of the sulcus which incloses the nipple are composed of parts looser in texture than the common adipose membrane, which is probably to admit of the elongation or projection of the nipple. On the outside of this there is another small fissure, which, I imagine, is likewise intended to give greater facility to the movements of all these parts.

The milk is probably very rich; for in that caught near Berkeley with its young one, the milk, which was tasted by Mr. Jenner and Mr. Ludlow, surgeon, at Sodbury, was rich, like cow's milk to which cream had been added.

The mode in which these animals must suck would appear to be very inconvenient for respiration, as either the mother or young one will be prevented from breathing at the time, their nostrils being in opposite directions; therefore the nose of one must be under water, and the time of sucking can only be between each respiration. The act of sucking must likewise be different from that of land animals; as in them it is performed by the lungs drawing the air from the mouth backwards into themselves, which the fluid follows, by being forced into the mouth from the pressure of the external air on its surface; but in this tribe, the lungs having no connection with the mouth, sucking must be performed by some action of the mouth itself, and by its having the power of expansion[b].

---

[a] [From this reservoir the milk is injected into the mouth of the young by the action of powerful cutaneous muscles, arranged so as to compress the reservoir and dilated ducts of the mammary glands.]

[b] [Aided, as in the *Marsupiata* and *Monotremata*, by muscular actions on the part of the parent tending to expel the milk.]

NOTES ON THE ANATOMY OF THE JERBOA,

(*Dipus Sagitta*, GM.)

(Extracted from the Appendix to Russel's History of Aleppo, where they are thus introduced.)

" HAVING met with nothing more on the internal structure of the jerboa than what is given by Gmelin from M. Buffon (*Hist. Nat.* tom. xiii.), I applied to my worthy friend Mr. John Hunter, who very obligingly favoured me with the following circumstances from his *Adversaria* by way of supplement. He was not certain whether the animal he dissected was from Asia or Africa."

.... The meatus auditorius was large like that of a bird. The tympanum was also large[a]. There are two venæ cavæ superiores. The cæcum was four inches in length; it makes a close turn upon itself, and gradually diminishing in size, terminates in an obtuse point. The colon, which is large at its beginning, passes first upwards upon the right side, and before crossing the abdomen on the left, makes a little fold upon itself; it then crosses the spine, and making another fold shorter than the former, it passes the left side and commences rectum.

The lower part of the abdomen lies upon the anterior part of the pubes, and the bend of the penis is seen within the cavity of the abdomen, making a little projection, as it were, between the origin of the two musculi recti. The penis in a flaccid state lies reverted upon itself, but when in erection has a bone on each side of the part projecting, in the same manner as in a guinea-pig. The prepuce is furnished with a number of glands which secrete a thick mucus. The testicles are situated on each side of the symphysis, and can occasionally lie in the rings of the abdominal muscles, which are very large, but can never descend much further, there being no scrotum for their reception. The vesiculæ seminales are two long bags, which make a turn upon themselves. The anus is bent downwards towards the parts of generation[b].

---

[a] [See the preparation No. 1599 Physiological Series, Hunterian Museum, which is most probably the part here described, and if so, proves the description to be of the *Dipus Sagitta*.]

[b] [These short and simple notes are interesting as an example of the matter composing the lost " *Adversaria*," or manuscript notes of Hunter. The comparison which he makes with reference to the structure of the ear-passage shows that he was alive to those interesting points of structure which are indicative of the natural affinities of different groups of animals. The jerboa not only resembles the bird in the large size of the meatus auditorius, but also (together with the whole order of Rodentia) in the un-anchylosed state of the tympanum with the other elements of the temporal bone. In the affinity to the oviparous vertebrata manifested in the two superior cavæ the genus *Dipus* agrees with the following rodent genera: *Alactaga, Helamys, Echimys, Hystrix, Sciurus, Pteromys, Orycteropus, Bathyergus, Lepus*, and *Cœlogenys*. I have also shown that the same structure characterizes the marsupial animals. See *Proceedings of the Zoological Society*, April 1832.]

ANATOMICAL DESCRIPTION OF THE AMPHIBIOUS BIPES OF ELLIS, (*Siren Lacertina*, Linn.)

By Mr. John Hunter, F.R.S.[a]

THE tongue is broad and has very little motion. It has a bone similar to that in birds, turtles, &c. On the posterior and lateral parts of the mouth are three openings on each side; these are similar to the slits of the gills in fish, but the partitions do not resemble gills on their outer

---

[a] [This paper was read before the Royal Society June 5, 1766, and is interesting from the circumstance of its being the first which Hunter communicated to that learned body, as well as from its being the earliest contribution to the anatomy of one of the most singular tribes of animals at present in existence, viz. the *Batrachia perennibranchiata*, or true *Amphibia*. The sirens dissected by Hunter were brought from South Carolina in 1758, and purchased along with other subjects of natural history by Mr. Hunter; the specimens described by Ellis were transmitted to him by Dr. Alexander Gardner, of Charles Town, South Carolina. The natives call the siren "mud-iguana." It is found in swampy and muddy places by the sides of pools, under the trunks of old trees that hang over the water. The external description of the siren by Mr. Ellis is given in the explanation of the plate lii. p. 23.

Besides the siren, Mr. Hunter also obtained two other species of perennibranchiate reptiles, dissections of which are preserved in his museum, and recorded in his manuscripts under the names of "*Kattewagoe*," (the *Menopoma Alleghanniensis* of Dr. Harlan) and the "Amphibious quadruped," since particularly described by Cuvier under the name of "Amphiuma." Types of three other genera of perennibranchiata have subsequently been described, and the whole tribe is divided into those which retain the external branchiæ throughout life, and those which lose these vascular processes, but retain the gill apertures.

The sirens and menobranchus of the United States, the axolotl of Mexico, and the proteus of Hungary have external fimbriated branchiæ, while the amphiuma and menopoma have only the branchial arches and apertures, but not external gills. These genera are all perfectly distinct from each other both in their external and anatomical characters, and it is only with respect to one of them, viz. the axolotl, that any doubt still remains as to whether the external gills are permanent or not.

At the period of the discovery of the siren it was natural to suppose from the analogy of the newt and salamander that it was a larva, representing an immature stage of its existence, on which subject Linnæus thus cautiously expresses himself in a letter to Mr. Ellis.

" Upsal, December 27, 1765. I received Dr. Garden's very rare two-footed animal with gills and lungs. The animal is probably the larva of some kind of Lacerta, which I very much desire that he will particularly inquire into.

" If it does not undergo a change, it belongs to the order of Nantes, which have both lungs and gills; and if so, it must be a new and very distinct genus, and should most probably have the name of Siren.

" I cannot possibly describe to you how much this two-footed animal has exercised my thoughts; if it is a larva he will no doubt find some of them with four feet. It is not an easy matter to reconcile it to the larva of the lizard tribe, its fingers being

edges, for they have not the comb-like structure. Above* and close to the extremity of each of these openings externally, so many processes arise, the anterior the smallest, the posterior the largest; their anterior and inferior edges and extremity are serrated, or formed into fimbriæ; these processes fold down and cover the slits externally, and would seem to answer the purposes of the comb-like part of the gill in fish.

At the root of the tongue, nearly as far back as these openings reach, the trachea begins much in the same manner as in birds. It passes backwards above the heart, and there divides into two branches, one going to each lobe of the lungs. The lungs are two long bags, one on each side, which begin just behind the heart, and pass back through the whole length of the abdomen, nearly as far as the anus. They are largest in the middle, and honey-combed on the internal surface through their whole length. The heart consists of one auricle and one ventricle. What answers to the inferior vena cava passes forwards above,

---

* To avoid the confusion in our ideas which might arise from the use of the words anterior, posterior, upper, lower, &c., in the whole of this description the animal is considered in its natural horizontal position, so that the head is forwards, the back upwards, &c.

---

furnished with claws; all the larvas of lizards that I know are without them ("*digitis muticis.*") Then also the branchiæ or gills are not to be met with in the aquatic salamanders, which are probably the larvas of lizards. Further, the croaking noise or sound it makes does not agree with the larvas of these animals, nor does the situation of the anus. So that there is no creature that ever I saw that I long so much to be convinced of the truth as to what this will certainly turn out to be."

Doctor Pockells of Brunswick, who visited the Museum of the Royal College of Surgeons, in 1820, perceiving some specimens of Amphiuma, concluded from their having four legs and no external gills that they were the adult or perfect Siren, and Rusconi adopted this opinion without further investigation; but Cuvier has shown that the Amphiuma differs from the Siren in its osteological structure, having in one species ten, and in another twenty-two additional vertebræ, while the construction of the cranium and other parts of the skeleton are also totally different: moreover the completely ossified state of the skeleton of the Siren, without the slightest vestige of posterior extremities, proves it to be neither the larva of an Amphiuma or of any other known Amphibian.

See Rusconi, *Descr. Anat. delle larve Salamandre*, 4to, 1817 ; *Del Proteo Anguino*, 4to, 1819 ; and *Amours des Salamandres*, fol. 1826, p. 12. Cuvier, *Recherches sur les Reptiles douteux*, in Humboldt's *Obs. Zool.*, 4to, 1811—1827; *Ossemens Fossiles*, tom. v. pt. 2.; *Mém. du Mus.*, tom. xiv. See also "A Notice of a *Siren Lacertina*," kept alive at Canon Mills, Edinburgh, for more than six years, in Jamieson's Journal, 1832, p. 298. From the observations made on this animal it appears that the branchiæ are the respiratory organs most essential to its existence, and its death is supposed to have been occasioned by the fimbriæ of the gills becoming completely dried and shrivelled up, in consequence of its accidentally falling out of the box of water in which it was habitually kept. It ate worms, sticklebacks, and small minnows greedily; and showed great alertness and sagacity in concealing itself most accurately beneath a floating patch of frog-bit.]

but in a sulcus of the liver, and opens into a bag similar to the pericardium ; this bag surrounds the heart and aorta, as the pericardium does in other animals ; from this there is an opening into a vein which lies above, and upon the left of the auricle, which vein seems to receive the blood from the lungs, gills, and head, is analogous to the superior vena cava, and opens into the auricle, which is upon the left of the ventricle.   The aorta goes out, passing for a little way in a loose spiral turn, then becomes straight, where it seems to be muscular ; at this part the branches go off, between which there is a rising within the area of the aorta like a bird's tongue, with its tip turned towards the heart*.   The liver is principally one lobe, pretty close to the heart at the fore part, and passes back on the right of the stomach and intestines ; at its anterior extremity on the left side there is a very short lobe, ending abruptly.   The gall-bladder lies in a fissure on the left side of the liver near its middle ; there is no hepatic duct ; the hepato-cystic ducts, which seem to be three in number, enter the gall-bladder at its anterior end or fundus, and the cystic duct passes out from the posterior end of the gall-bladder, and terminates in the gut, about half an inch from the pylorus.   The œsophagus, which is pretty large, passes back, and is continued into the stomach in the same line.   The stomach at

* This account of the venæ cavæ opening into the cavity of the pericardium may appear incredible ; and it might be supposed that, in the natural state of the parts, there is a canal of communication going from one cava to the other, which being broken or nipped through, in the act of catching or killing the animal, would give the appearance above described.   I can only say that the appearances were what have been described in three different subjects which I have dissected ; and in all of them the pericardium was full of coagulated blood.   But besides the smallness of the subjects, it may be observed that they had been long preserved in spirits, which made them more unfit for anatomical inquiries.   They had been in my possession above seven years[a].

[a] [There is no preparation in the Hunterian Collection demonstrative of the structure described in the text, and it was in the dissections of the siren, instituted with the view to reconcile or account for Hunter's description of the heart, that I was led to the discovery of the two distinct auricles in that animal. (*Trans. Zool. Soc.* vol. i. p. 213, April, 1834.)   The inferior vena cava terminates at the lower part of a large membranous sinus, which also receives the blood from the two superior cavæ by two separate orifices.   The common trunk of the pulmonary veins seems also to end in this sinus, but it merely traverses without communicating with it, and finally opens into a distinct transverse auricular chamber, which is not separated externally from the apparently single and capacious auricle of the venæ cavæ, which is characterized by numerous elongated fimbriated processes.   The glistening fibrous coat of the pericardium closely adheres to the surrounding muscles as in fish, so that the absence of any detached bag surrounding the heart, the magnitude of the auricle, and the peculiar passage of the pulmonary veins through the great sinus of the venæ cavæ may have contributed to mislead Mr. Hunter as to the real structure of the part.]

the posterior end bends a little to the right, where it terminates in the pylorus.   The intestines pass back, making many turns ; at the poste-rior end they become pretty straight, forming what may be called the colon, or rectum, where they are a little larger, and run to the anus in a straight direction.   At the beginning of this larger part of the intes-tinal tube there is no valvular structure.   The spleen is a very small but long body ; its anterior end is attached to the upper surface of the stomach, and it is continued back along the left side of the mesentery, to which it adheres.   The pancreas is a small body lying above the duodenum, and is attached also to the mesentery.   The kidneys are situated in the upper and posterior part of the abdomen, having the rectum passing below and between them, as in the snake, &c.   Below the rectum lies a long bag, like a bladder ; it adheres all along to the inside of the abdominal muscles, and its mouth opens into the rectum ; but whether it is the bladder of urine or not I cannot tell.   On each side of the rectum, close to the lungs, there is a body, the posterior end of which rests upon the anterior end of the kidney : whether they are testicles or ovaria I cannot pretend to determine, but should imagine that they are either the one or the other[a].

---

[a] [The ovaria in the siren are irregularly shaped elongated somewhat compressed bodies, becoming smaller at the two extremities.   In a siren of two feet long they were each four inches in length, and half an inch broad, both situated at the lower and back part of the abdomen ; the left about an inch nearer the head, having a smooth surface outwardly, and moulded on the inner surface to the convolutions of the intestine.   The stroma ovarii was crowded with very numerous and minute ovisacs of a whitish colour, and was studded here and there with larger drops of a dark-coloured oil.   The oviducts extend from the cloaca, in the form of broad, flattened, membranous canals, to near the anterior ends of the ovaria, where they alter their form and become rounded tubes, each becoming folded upon itself in broad close-set plaits, and terminating, without change of dimensions, in a longitudinal slit, which occupies part of the anterior surface of the last plait.   The oviducts are attached by a broad fold of peritoneum to the dor-sal region of the abdomen.]

OF THE ELECTRIC PROPERTY OF THE TORPEDO.

In a Letter from John Walsh, Esq., F.R.S., to Benjamin Franklin, Esq., LL.D., F.R.S.; Ac. R. Par. Soc. Ext., &c. [a]

Chesterfield Street, July 1, 1773.

DEAR SIR,

I AM concerned that other engagements have prevented me from giving to the Royal Society, before their recess, a complete account of my experiments on the electricity of the torpedo; a subject not only curious in itself, but opening a large field for interesting inquiry, both to the electrician in his walk of physics, and to all who consider, particularly or generally, the animal œconomy.

To supply the deficiency in the best manner I am now able, I will request the favour of you to lay before the Society my letter from La Rochelle, of the 12th July, 1772, and such part of the letter I afterwards wrote from Paris as relates to this subject. Loose and imperfect as these informations are, for they were never intended for the public eye, they are still the most authentic, and so far the most satisfactory I can at present offer, since the notes I made of the experiments themselves remain nearly, I am sorry to say it, in that crude and bulky state in which you had the trouble to read them.

Letter from Mr. Walsh to Dr. Franklin, dated La Rochelle, July 12, 1772.

" It is with particular satisfaction I make to you my first communication, that the effect of the torpedo appears to be absolutely electrical; by forming its circuit through the same conductors with electricity, for instance, metals and water; and by being intercepted by the same non-conductors, for instance, glass and sealing-wax. I will not at present trouble you with the detail of our experiments, especially as we are daily advancing in them, but only observe that we have discovered the back and breast of the animal to be in different states of electricity; I mean in particular the upper and lower surfaces of those two assemblages of pliant cylinders of which you have seen engravings in Lorenzini*. By the knowledge of this circum-

---

* Observazioni intorno alle Torpedini di Stef. Lorenzini, 1678.
Redi appears to be the first who remarked these singular parts of the torpedo in 1666. Franc. Redi, Exper. Nat.

---

a [This letter is prefixed to Mr. Hunter's description of the Electric Organs, in the Philosophical Transactions, vol. lxiii.]

stance we have been able to direct his shocks, though they were very small, through a circuit of four persons, all feeling them ; likewise through a considerable length of wire held by two insulated persons, one touching his lower surface and the other his upper. When the wire was exchanged for glass or sealing wax no effect could be obtained, but as soon as it was resumed the two persons became liable to the shock. These experiments have been varied many ways and repeated times without number, and they all determined the choice of conductors to be the same in the torpedo as in the Leyden phial. The sensations likewise occasioned by one and the other in the human frame are precisely similar. Not only the shock, but the numbing sensation which the animal sometimes dispenses, expressed in French by the words *engourdissement* and *fourmillement*, may be exactly imitated with the phial, by means of Lane's electrometer, the regulating rod of which, to produce the latter effect, must be brought almost into contact with the prime conductor which joins the phial. We have not yet perceived any spark to accompany the shock, nor the pith balls to be ever affected[a]. Indeed, all our trials have been done on very feeble subjects, whose shock was seldom sensible beyond the touching finger. I remember but one, of at least two hundred that I myself must have received, to have extended above the elbow. Perhaps the Isle of Ré, which we are about to visit, may furnish us with torpedos fresher taken and of more vigour, by which a further insight into these matters may be had. Our experiments have been chiefly in the air, where the animal was more open to our examination than in water. It is a sin-

---

[a] [Gardini and Galvani, and more recently Matteuci, concur in stating that they have seen a feeble spark from the discharge of a torpedo, but other philosophers have not been so successful. The observations of Dr. John Davy on this point (Philos. Trans., 1834) particularly deserve attention. He experimented on very active fish, and varied his trials, with every endeavour to obtain the required result, but never procured a spark. By means of Harris's electrometer, however, he saw proof of the evolution of heat during the torpedo's discharge. Abundant evidence of the chemical effects of animal electricity has been obtained by the same philosopher. He applied golden wires, one to the dorsal, the other to the ventral surface of the torpedo, and passed the discharge through solutions of nitrate of silver, common salt, and superacetate of lead, and found that all were decomposed, but the latter substance only when the fish seemed to put forth all its energy, after being much irritated (Philos. Trans., 1832). In resuming the inquiry instituted by Sir Humphry Davy, relative to the magnetical effects of the torpedo's discharge, Dr. John Davy ascertains in the most satisfactory manner that these effects were produced by animal electricity. He placed eight needles within a spiral of fine copper wire, containing about one hundred and eighty convolutions, and having passed through this a single discharge from a torpedo six inches long, the contained needles were all converted into magnets, and the ends of the needles which were nearest the ventral surface of the fish had received the southern polarity. See Phil. Trans., 1829.]

gularity that the torpedo, when insulated, should be able to give to us, insulated likewise, forty or fifty successive shocks from nearly the same part, and these with little, if any, diminution in their force; indeed, they were all very minute. Each effort in the animal to give the shock is conveniently accompanied with a depression of his eyes, by which even his attempts to give it to non-conductors can be observed. The animal, with respect to the rest of his body, is in a great degree motionless, but not wholly so. You will please to acquaint Dr. Bancroft of our having thus verified his suspicion concerning the torpedo *, and make any other communication of this matter you may judge proper. Here I shall be glad to excite, as far as I am able, both electricians and naturalists to push their inquiries concerning this extraordinary animal, whilst the summer affords them the opportunity."

Extracts of a Letter from Mr. Walsh to Dr. Franklin, dated Paris, August 27, 1772.

" ...... I spent a complete week in my experiments at the Isle of Ré, and had there every convenience for prosecuting them to their extent, except that I was restrained by the jealousy of the government from making them where the animal was caught. At my return to La Rochelle, I communicated to the members of the Academy of that place and to many of the principal inhabitants all that I had observed concerning the torpedo, in the intention of stirring up a spirit of inquiry both as to its electricity and general œconomy.

" ...... The vigour of the fresh-taken torpedos at the Isle of Ré was not able to force the torpedinal fluid across the minutest tract of air; not from one link of a small chain, suspended freely to another; not through an almost invisible separation, made by the edge of a penknife, in a slip of tinfoil pasted on sealing-wax. The spark, therefore (of course the attendant snapping noise), was denied to all our attempts to discover it, not only in daylight, but in complete darkness. I observed to you in my last the singularity of the torpedo being able, when insulated, to give to an insulated person a great number of successive shocks: in this situation I have taken no less than fifty from him in the space of a minute and a half. All our experiments confirmed that his electricity was condensed in the instant of its explosion by a sudden energy of the animal, and as there was no gradual accumulation nor retention of it, as in the case of charged glass, it is not at all surprising that no signs of attraction nor repulsion were perceived in the pith

* Bancroft's Natural History of Guiana, p. 191.

balls. In short, the effect of the torpedo appears to arise from a compressed elastic fluid, restoring itself to its equilibrium in the same way and by the same mediums as the elastic fluid compressed in charged glass. The skin of the animal, bad conductor as it is, seems to be a better conductor of his electricity than the thinnest plate of elastic air. Notwithstanding the weak spring of the torpedinal electricity, I was able, in the public exhibitions of my experiments at La Rochelle, to convey it through a circuit, formed from one surface of the animal to the other, by two long brass wires and four persons, which number at times was increased even to eight. The several persons were made to communicate with each other, and the two outermost with the wires, by means of water contained in basins, properly disposed between them for the purpose, each person dipping his hands in the nearest basins, connectively with his neighbour on either side . . . .

" The effect produced by the torpedo when in air appeared, on many repeated experiments, to be about four times as strong as when in water."

A clear and succinct narrative of what passed at one of the public exhibitions alluded to in the last letter appeared in the French Gazette of the 30th October, 1772. As it came from a very respectable quarter, not less so from the private character of the gentleman than from the public offices he held, I must desire leave of the Society to avail myself of such a testimony to the facts I have advanced by giving a translation of that narrative.

Extract of a Letter from the Sieur Seignette, Mayor of La Rochelle, and Second Perpetual Secretary of the Academy of that City, to the publisher of the French Gazette.

" In the Gazette of the 14th August, you mentioned the discovery made by Mr. Walsh, member of the parliament of England, and of the Royal Society of London. The experiment of which I am going to give you an account, was made in the presence of the Academy of this city. A live torpedo was placed on a table. Round another table stood five persons insulated. Two brass wires, each thirteen feet long, were suspended to the ceiling by silken strings. One of these wires rested by one end on the wet napkin on which the fish lay ; the other end was immersed in a basin full of water placed on the second table, on which stood four other basins likewise full of water. The first person put a finger of one hand in the basin in which the wire was immersed, and a finger of the other hand in the second basin. The second person put a finger of one hand in this last basin, and a finger of the other hand in the third; and so on successively, till the five persons communicated with one another by the water in the basins. In the last basin one end of the second wire was immersed; and with the other end Mr. Walsh touched the back of the torpedo, when the five persons felt a commotion which differed in nothing from that of the Leyden experiment, except in the degree of force. Mr. Walsh, who was not in the circle of conduction, received no shock. This experiment was repeated several times, even with eight persons, and always with the same success. The action of the torpedo is communicated by the same mediums as that of the electric fluid. The bodies which intercept the action of the one, intercept likewise the action of the other. The effects produced by the torpedo resemble in every respect a weak electricity."

This exhibition of the electric powers of the torpedo before the Academy of La Rochelle, was at a meeting held for the purpose in my apartments, on the 22nd July, 1772, and stands registered in the journals of the Academy.

The effect of the animal was, in these experiments, transmitted through as great an extent and variety of conductors as almost at any time we had been able to obtain it, and the experiments included nearly all the points in which its analogy with the effect of the Leyden phial had been observed. These points were stated to the gentlemen present, as were the circumstances in which the two effects appeared to vary. It was likewise represented to them, that our experiments had been almost wholly with the animal in the air; that its action in water was a capital desideratum; that indeed all as yet done was little more than opening the door to inquiry; that much remained to be examined by the electrician as well as by the anatomist; that as artificial electricity had thrown light on the natural operation of the torpedo, this might in return, if well considered, throw light on artificial electricity, particularly in those respects in which they now seemed to differ; that for me, I was about to take leave of the animal, as nature had denied it to the British seas; and that the prosecution of these researches rested in a particular manner with them, whose shores abounded with it.

The torpedo on this occasion dispensed only the distinct, instantaneous stroke so well known by the name of the electric shock. That protracted but lighter sensation, that torpor or numbness which he at times induces, and from which he takes his name, was not then experienced from the animal; but it was imitated with artificial electricity, and shown to be producible by a quick consecution of minute shocks. This in the torpedo may perhaps be effected by the successive dis-

charge of his numerous cylinders, in the nature of a running fire of
musketry: the strong single shock may be his general volley. In the
continued effect, as well as in the instantaneous, his eyes, usually prominent, are withdrawn into their sockets.

The same experiments, performed with the same torpedos, were on
the two succeeding days repeated before numerous companies of the
principal inhabitants of La Rochelle. Besides the pleasure of gratifying the curiosity of such as entertained any on the subject, and the desire I had to excite a prosecution of the inquiry, I certainly wished to
give all possible notoriety to facts, which might otherwise be deemed
improbable, perhaps by some of the first rank in science. Great authorities had given a sanction to other solutions of the phænomena of
the torpedo; and even the electrician might not readily listen to assertions, which seemed in some respects to combat the general principles of electricity. I had reason to make such conclusions from different conversations I had held on the subject with eminent persons
both at London and Paris. It is but justice to say, that of all in that
class you gave me the greatest encouragement to look for success in
this research, and even assisted me in forming hypotheses, how the
torpedo, supposed to be endued with electric properties, might use them
in so conducting an element as water.

After generally recommending to others an examination of the electric powers of these animals when acting in water, I determined, before I took my final leave of them, to make some further experiments
myself with that particular view; since, notwithstanding the familiarity
in which we may be said to have lived with them for near a month,
we had never detected them in the immediate exercise of their electric
faculties against other fish, confined with them in the same water,
either in the circumstance of attacking their prey, or defending themselves from annoyance; and yet that they possessed such a power, and
exercised it in a state of liberty, could not be doubted.

A large torpedo, very liberal of his shocks, being held with both
hands by his electric organs above and below, was briskly plunged into
water to the depth of a foot, and instantly raised an equal height into
air; and was thus continually plunged and raised, as quick as possible,
for the space of a minute. In the instant his lower surface touched
the water in his descent, he always gave a violent shock, and another
still more violent in the instant of quitting the water in his ascent;
both which shocks, but particularly the last, were accompanied with a
writhing in his body, as if meant to force an escape: besides these two
shocks from the surface of the water, which may yet be considered as

delivered in the air, he constantly gave at least two when wholly in
the air, and constantly one, and sometimes two, when wholly in the
water. The shocks in water appeared, as far as sensation could decide, not to have near a fourth of the force of those at the surface of
the water, nor much more than a fourth of those entirely in the air.

The shocks received in a certain time were not on this occasion
counted by a watch, as they had been on a former, when fifty were delivered in a minute and a half by the animal in an insulated and un-
agitated state : but from the quickness with which the immersions were
made, it may be presumed there were full twenty of these in a minute;
from whence the number of shocks in that time must have amounted
to above a hundred. This experiment, therefore, while it discovered
the comparative force between a shock in water and one in air, and between a shock delivered with greater exertion on the part of the animal
and one with less, seemed to determine, that the charge of his organs
with electricity was effected in an instant, as well as the discharge.

The torpedo was then put into a flat basket, open at top, but se-
cured by a net with wide meshes, and in this confinement was let
down into the water about a foot below the surface : being there
touched through the meshes with only a single finger on one of his
electric organs, while the other hand was held at a distance in the
water, he gave shocks which were distinctly felt in both hands.

The circuit for the passage of the effect being contracted to the finger
and thumb of one hand, applied above and below to a single organ,
produced a shock, to our sensation, of twice the force of that in the
larger circuit by the arms.

The torpedo, still confined in the basket, being raised to within three
inches of the surface of the water, was there touched with a short iron
bolt, which was held half above and half in the water by one hand,
while the other hand was dipped as before at a distance in the water;
and strong shocks, felt in both hands, were thus obtained through the
iron.

A wet hempen cord being fastened to the iron bolt, was held in the
hand above water, while the bolt touched the torpedo; and shocks were
obtained through both those substances.

A less powerful torpedo, suspended in a small net, being frequently
dipped into water and raised again, gave from the surface of the water
slight shocks through the net to the person holding it.

These experiments in water manifested that bodies immersed in that
element might be affected by immediate contact with the torpedo;
that the shorter the circuit in which the electricity moved, the greater

would be the effect; and that the shock was communicable from the animal in water to persons in air through some substances.

How far harpoons and nets, consisting of wood and hemp, could in like circumstances, as it has been frequently asserted, convey the effect, was not so particularly tried as to enable us to confirm it. I mention the omission in the hope that some one may be induced to determine the point by express trial.

We convinced ourselves on former occasions that the accurate Kæmpfer*, who so well describes the effect of the torpedo, and happily compares it with lightning, was deceived in the circumstance that it could be avoided by holding in the breath, which we found no more to prevent the shock of the torpedo when he was disposed to give it, than it would prevent the shock of the Leyden phial.

Several persons, forming as many distinct circuits, can be affected by one stroke of the animal, as well as when joined in a single circuit. For instance, four persons, touching separately his upper and lower surfaces, were all affected; two persons likewise, after the electricity had passed through a wire into a basin of water, transmitted it from thence, in two distinct channels, as their sensation convinced them, into another basin of water, from whence it was conducted, probably in a united state, by a single wire. How much further the effect might be thus divided and subdivided into different channels was not determined; but it was found to be proportionably weakened by multiplying these circuits, as it had been by extending the single circuit.

Something may be expected to be said of the parts of the animal immediately concerned in producing the electrical effect. The engraving which accompanies this letter, while it shows the general figure of the torpedo, gives an internal view of his electric organs. The Society will, besides, have a full anatomical description of these parts from the ingenious Mr. John Hunter, in a paper he has expressly written on the subject at my request. It would therefore be superfluous for me to say anything either in regard to their situation or structure.

I have to observe, however, that in these double organs resides the electricity of the torpedo, the rest of his body appearing to be no otherwise concerned in his electrical effect than as conducting it: that they are subject to the will of the animal; but whether, like other double parts so controlable, they are exercised at times singly as well as in concert, is difficult to be ascertained by experiment: that their upper and under surfaces are capable, from a state of equilibrium with re-

* Kæmpf. Amœn. Exot. 1712, p. 511.

spect to electricity, of being instantly thrown, by a mere energy, into an opposition of a *plus* and *minus* state, like that of the charged phial : that, when they are thus charged, the upper surfaces of the two are in the same state of electricity; as are the under surfaces of the two, though in a contrary to that of the upper ; for no shock can be obtained by an insulated person touching both organs above, or both below : and that the production of the effect depends solely on an intercourse being made between the opposite surfaces of the organs, whether taken singly or jointly.

All the parts bordering on the organs act more or less as conductors, either through their substance or by their superficies.   While an insulated person, placing two fingers on the same surface of one or both organs, cannot be affected, if he removes one of his fingers to any such contiguous part he will be liable to a shock ; but this shock will not be near, perhaps not half so violent as one taken immediately between the opposite surfaces of the organ, which shows the conduction to be very imperfect.

The parts which conduct the best are the two great lateral fins bounding the organs outwardly, and the space lying between the two organs inwardly.   All below the double transverse cartilages scarcely conduct at all, unless when the fish is just taken out of water and is still wet, the mucus with which he is lubricated showing itself as it dries to be of an insulating nature.

The organs themselves when uncharged appeared to be, not interiorly we might suppose, but rather exteriorly, conductors of a shock. An insulated person touching two torpedos, lying near one another on a damp table, with fingers placed, one on the organ of one fish, and another on the organ of the other, was sensible of shocks, sometimes delivered by one fish, and sometimes by the other, as might be discovered by the respective winking of their eyes.   That the organs uncharged served some way or other as conductors, was confirmed with artificial electricity, in passing shocks by them, and in taking sparks from them when electrified.

The electric effect was never perceived by us to be attended with any motion or alteration in the organs themselves, but was frequently accompanied with a little transient agitation along the cartilages which surround both organs : this is not discernible in the plump and turgid state of the animal while he is fresh and vigorous; but as his force decays, from the relaxation of his muscles, his cartilages appear through the skin, and then the slight action along them is discovered.

May we not from all these premises conclude, that the effect of the torpedo proceeds from a modification of the electric fluid ?   The torpedo

resembles the charged phial in that characteristic point of a reciproca-
tion between its two surfaces.   Their effects are transmitted by the
same mediums; than which there is not perhaps a surer criterion to
determine the identity of subtile matter : they besides occasion the same
impression on our nerves.   Like effects have like causes.   But it may
be objected, that the effects of the torpedo, and of the charged phial,
are not similar in all their circumstances ; that the charged phial occasions attractive or repulsive dispositions in neighbouring bodies ; and
that its discharge is obtained through a portion of air, and is accompanied with light and sound; nothing of which occurs with respect to
the torpedo.

The inaction of the electricity of the animal in these particulars,
whilst its elastic force is so great as to transmit the effect through an
extensive circuit and in its course to communicate a shock, may be a
new phænomenon, but is no ways repugnant to the laws of electricity,
for here too the operations of the animal may be imitated by art.

The same quantity of electric matter, according as it is used in a dense
or rare state, will produce the different consequences.   For example,
a small phial, whose coated surface measures only six square inches,
will, on being highly charged, contain a dense electricity capable of
forcing a passage through an inch of air, and afford the phænomena of
light, sound, attraction, and repulsion.   But if the quantity condensed
in this phial be made rare by communicating it to three large connected
jars, whose coated surfaces shall form together an area four hundred
times larger than that of the phial (I instance these jars because they
are such as I use); it will, thus dilated, yield all the negative phænomena, if I may so call them, of the torpedo ; it will not now pass the
hundredth part of that inch of air, which in its condensed state it
sprung through with ease ; it will now refuse the minute intersection
in the strip of tinfoil ; the spark and its attendant sound, even the attraction or repulsion of light bodies, will now be wanting ; nor will a
point brought however near, if not in contact, be able to draw off the
charge : and yet, with this diminished elasticity, the electric matter
will, to effect its equilibrium, instantly run through a considerable circuit of different conductors, perfectly continuous, and make us sensible
of an impulse in its passage.

Let me here remark, that the sagacity of Mr. Cavendish in devising
and his address in executing electrical experiments, led him the first to
experience with artificial electricity, that a shock could be received
from a charge which was unable to force a passage through the least
space of air.

But after the discovery that a large area of rare electricity would imitate the effect of the torpedo, it may be inquired, where is this large area to be found in the animal? We here approach to that veil of nature which man cannot remove. This, however, we know, that from infinite division of parts infinite surface may arise, and even our gross optics tell us that those singular organs, so often mentioned, consist like our electric batteries of many vessels, call them cylinders or hexagonal prisms, whose superficies taken together furnish a considerable area.

ANATOMICAL OBSERVATIONS ON THE TORPEDO[a].

By John Hunter, F.R.S.

I WAS desired some time since, by Mr. Walsh, whose experiments at La Rochelle had determined the effect of the torpedo to be electrical, to dissect and examine the peculiar organs by which that animal produces so extraordinary an effect. This I have done in several subjects furnished to me by that gentleman.

I am now desired by him to lay before the Society the observations I have made ; and for the better understanding of them, to present, on his part, a male and female torpedo in spirits; in the latter of which the electric organs are exposed in different views and sections; likewise a copper-plate, which he took care to have engraved, exhibiting those organs.

Of the general structure and anatomy of the torpedo I say nothing, since the animal does not differ very materially, excepting in its electric organs (as they have been properly named by Mr. Walsh), from the rest of the rays, of which family it is well known to be. I will only premise that the torpedo, of which I treat, is about eighteen inches long, twelve broad, and in its central or thickest part two inches thick ; which is nearly the size of the female specimen now presented to the Society, as well as of that from which the plate was taken : but where there is any difference in the organ arising from difference in size, notice will be taken of it in this account.

The electric organs of the torpedo[b] are placed on each side of the cranium and gills, reaching from thence to the semicircular cartilages of each great fin, and extending longitudinally from the anterior extremity of the animal to the transverse cartilage which divides the thorax from the abdomen ; and within these limits they occupy the whole space between the skin of the upper and of the under surfaces : they are thickest at the edges near the centre of the fish, and become gradually thinner towards the extremities. Each electric organ, at its inner longitudinal edge, is unequally hollowed, being exactly fitted to the irregular projections of the cranium and gills. The outer longitudinal edge is a convex elliptic curve. The anterior extremity of each organ makes the section of a small circle ; and the posterior extremity

---

[a] [This paper was read before the Royal Society July 1, 1773, and published in the 63rd volume of the Philosophical Transactions.]

[b] [Pl. liii., fig. 1, 2, *a a*.]

makes nearly a right angle with the inner edge. Each organ is attached to the surrounding parts by a close cellular membrane, and also by short and strong tendinous fibres which pass directly across from its outer edge to the semicircular cartilages.

They are covered above and below by the common skin of the animal[a], under which there is a thin fascia spread over the whole organ. This is composed of fibres, which run longitudinally, or in the direction of the body of the animal : these fibres appear to be perforated in innumerable places, which gives the fascia the appearance of being fasciculated; its edges all around are closely connected to the skin, and at last appear to be lost, or to degenerate into the common cellular membrane of the skin.

Immediately under this is another membrane exactly of the same kind, the fibres of which in some measure decussate those of the former, passing from the middle line of the body outwards and backwards. The inner edge of this is lost with the first described; the anterior, outer, and posterior edges are partly attached to the semicircular cartilages, and partly lost in the common cellular membrane.

This inner fascia appears to be continued into the electric organ by so many processes, and thereby makes the membranous sides or sheaths of the columns, which are presently to be described ; and between these processes the fascia covers the end of each column, making the outermost or first partition.

Each organ of the fish under consideration[b] is about five inches in length, and at the anterior end three in breadth, though it is but little more than half as broad as at the posterior extremity.

Each consists wholly of perpendicular columns, reaching from the upper to the under surface of the body, and varying in their lengths according to the thickness of the parts of the body where they are placed; the longest column being about an inch and a half, the shortest about one-fourth of an inch in length, and their diameters about two tenths of an inch.

The figures of the columns are very irregular, varying according to situation and other circumstances. The greatest number of them are either irregular hexagons or irregular pentagons; but from the irregularity of some of them it happens that a pretty regular quadrangular column is sometimes formed. Those of the exterior row are either quadrangular or hexagonal, having one side external, two lateral,

---

[a] [Pl. liii., *b b*.]

[b] [This specimen was eighteen inches long, twelve inches broad, and in its central or thickest part two inches thick.]

and either one or two internal. In the second row they are mostly pentagons.

Their coats are very thin, and seem transparent, closely connected with each other, having a kind of loose network of tendinous fibres, passing transversely and obliquely between the columns, and uniting them more firmly together. These are mostly observable where the large trunks of the nerves pass. The columns are also attached by strong inelastic fibres, passing directly from the one to the other.

The number of columns in different torpedos of the size of that now offered to the Society appeared to be about 470 in each organ, but the number varies according to the size of the fish*. These columns increase, not only in size, but in number, during the growth of the animal; new ones forming perhaps every year on the exterior edges, as there they are much the smallest. This process may be similar to the formation of new teeth in the human jaw as it increases.

Each column is divided by horizontal partitions (Pl. liv. fig. 3, H. H.), placed over each other, at very small distances, and forming numerous interstices, which appear to contain a fluid. These partitions consist of a very thin membrane, considerably transparent. Their edges appear to be attached to one another, and the whole is attached by a fine cellular membrane to the inside of the columns. They are not totally detached from one another: I have found them adhering at different places by blood-vessels passing from one to another.

The number of partitions contained in a column of one inch in length, of a torpedo which had been preserved in proof spirit, appeared on a careful examination to be one hundred and fifty; and this number in a given length of column appears to be common to all sizes in the same state of humidity, for by drying they may be greatly altered; whence it appears probable that the increase in the length of a column, during the growth of the animal, does not enlarge the distance between each partition in proportion to that growth; but that new partitions are formed, and added to the extremity of the column from the fascia.

The partitions are very vascular[a]; the arteries are branches from the vessels of the gills which convey the blood that has received the influence

---

* In a very large Torpedo, (see the preparation No. 2176, Physiological Series,) the number of columns in one electric organ were 1182.

---

[a] [See prep. No. 2176, which is the section of a Torpedo, of very large size, taken in Torbay in August, 1774. It weighed fifty-three pounds, was four feet in length, two feet and a half in breadth, and four inches and a half in thickness. Mr. Hunter having received this fish in a recent state was enabled to inject it, and thus demonstrate the vascularity of the electrical organs.]

of respiration. They pass along with the nerves to the electric organ, and enter with them; then they ramify in every direction into innumerable small branches upon the sides of the columns, sending in from the circumference all around upon each partition small arteries, which ramify and anastomose upon it, and passing also from one partition to another, anastomose with the vessels of the adjacent partitions.

The veins of the electric organ pass out close to the nerves and run between the gills to the auricle of the heart.

The nerves inserted into each electric organ arise by three very large trunks from the lateral and posterior part of the brain. The first of these in its passage outwards turns round a cartilage of the cranium and sends a few branches to the first gill, and to the anterior part of the head, and then passes into the organ towards its anterior extremity[a]. The second trunk enters the gills between the first and second openings, and after furnishing it with small branches passes into the organ near its middle. The third trunk, after leaving the skull, divides itself into two branches, which pass to the electric organ through the gills; one between the second and third openings, the other between the third and fourth, giving small branches to the gill itself. These nerves having entered the organs ramify in every direction between the columns, and send in small branches upon each partition, where they are lost.

The magnitude and the number of the nerves bestowed on these organs, in proportion to their size, must on reflection appear as extraordinary as the phenomena they afford. Nerves are given to parts either for sensation or action. Now if we except the more important senses of seeing, hearing, smelling, and tasting, which do not belong to the electric organs, there is no part even of the most perfect animal which, in proportion to its size, is so liberally supplied with nerves; nor do the nerves seem necessary for any sensation which can be supposed to belong to the electric organs. And with respect to action, there is no

---

[a] [This nerve (A, fig. 2, pl. liv.) is a part of the third division of the fifth pair, and does not greatly exceed the size of the corresponding nerve in other species of the ray tribe; it distributes branches to the mucous tubes (F fig. 1), which are fewer in number in the torpedo than in the ordinary rays, before it penetrates the electric organ. The other great fasciculi of nerves (B C D, fig. 2, pl. liv.) correspond with the pneumogastric, or eighth pair of nerves; a large branch is continued from the most posterior to the stomach, where it is spread over the great arch. Dr. John Davy conjectures that the superfluous electricity when not required for the defence of the animal may be directed to this organ to promote digestion. In the instance of a Torpedo which he preserved alive for many days, and which was frequently excited to give shocks, digestion appeared to have been completely arrested; when it died, a small fish was found in its stomach, much in the same state in which it was swallowed; no portion of it had been dissolved.]

part of any animal with which I am acquainted, however strong and constant its natural actions may be, which has so great a proportion of nerves.

If it be then probable that those nerves are not necessary for the purposes of sensation or action, may we not conclude that they are subservient to the formation, collection, or management of the electric fluid? especially as it appears evident, from Mr. Walsh's experiments, that the will of the animal does absolutely control the electric powers of its body, which must depend on the energy of the nerves.

How far this may be connected with the power of the nerves in general, or how far it may lead to an explanation of their operations, time and future discoveries alone can fully determine.

AN ACCOUNT OF THE GYMNOTUS ELECTRICUS[a].

By JOHN HUNTER, F.R.S.

To Mr. Walsh, the first discoverer of animal electricity, the learned will be indebted for whatever the following pages may contain, either curious or useful. The specimen of the animal which they describe was procured by that gentleman, and at his request this dissection was performed and this account of it is communicated.

This fish on the first view appears very much like an eel, from which resemblance it has most probably got its name; but it has none of the specific properties of that fish. This animal may be considered, both anatomically and physiologically, as divided into two parts, viz. the common animal part, and a part which is superadded, viz. the *peculiar organ*. I shall at present consider it only with respect to the last, as the first explains nothing relating to the other, nor any thing relating to the animal œconomy of fish in general. The first, or common animal part, is so contrived as to exceed what was necessary for itself, in order to give situation, nourishment, and most probably the peculiar property to the second. The last part, or peculiar organ, has an immediate connexion with the first, the body affording it a situation, the heart nourishment, and the brain nerves, and probably its peculiar powers. For the first of these purposes the body is extended out in length, being much longer than would be sufficient for what may be called its progressive motion. For the real body, or that part where the viscera and parts of generation lie, is situated, with respect to the head, as in other fish, and is extremely short, so that, according to the ordinary proportions, this should be a very short fish. Its great length, therefore, seems chiefly intended to afford a surface for the support of the peculiar organ; however, the tail part is likewise adapted to the progressive motion of the whole and to preserve the specific gravity; for the spine, medulla spinalis, muscles, fin, and air-bladder[b] are continued through its whole length. Besides which parts there is a mem-

---

a [This paper was read before the Royal Society May 11, 1775, and published in the 65th volume of the Philosophical Transactions.]

b [The *Gymnotus electricus* has two air-bladders, one of which, of an oval form and bilobed, is situated at the anterior part of the abdomen, beneath the œsophagus; the other is the elongated sac described by Hunter, and extended through the posterior part of the body. In another species, the *Gymnotus æquilabiatus* of Humboldt, the posterior elongated air-bladder is wanting.]

brane passing from the spine to that fin which runs along the belly or lower edge of the animal. This membrane is broad at the end next to the head, terminating in a point at the tail; it is a support for the abdominal fin, gives a greater surface of support for the organ, and makes a partition between the organs of the two opposite sides.

The Organs.

The organs which produce the peculiar effect of this fish constitute nearly one half of that part of the flesh in which they are placed, and perhaps make more than one-third of the whole animal. There are two pair of these organs, a larger and a smaller, one being placed on each side. The large pair occupy the whole lower or anterior, and also the lateral part of the body, making the thickness of the fore or lower parts of the animal; and run almost through its whole length, viz. from the abdomen to near the end of the tail*. It is broadest on the sides of the fish at the anterior end, where it incloses more of the lateral parts of the body, becomes narrower towards the end of the tail, occupying less and less of the sides of the animal, till at last it ends almost in a point. These two organs are separated from one another at the upper part by the muscles of the back, which keep their posterior or upper edges at a considerable distance from one another†; below that, and towards the middle, they are separated by the air-bag‡, and at their lower parts they are separated by the middle partition §. They begin forwards by a pretty regular edge, almost at right angles with the longitudinal axis of the body, situated on the lower and lateral parts of the abdomen. Their upper edge is a pretty straight line, with small indentations made by the nerves and blood vessels which pass round it to the skin. At the anterior end they go as far towards the back as the middle line of the animal, but in their approach towards the tail they gradually leave that line, coming nearer to the lower surface of the animal. The general shape of the organ, on an external or side view, is broad at the end next to the head of the animal, becoming gradually narrower towards the tail, and ending there almost in a point. The other surfaces of the organ are fitted to the shape of the parts with which they come in contact, therefore on the upper and inner surface it is hollowed to receive the muscles of the back. There is also a longitudinal depression on its lower edge, where a substance lies which di-

* Pl. LVI. fig. 1. K K K.   † Pl. LVII. fig. 5. c c c c.   ‡ Pl. LVII. fig. 5. D.
§ Pl. LVII. fig. 5. K.

vides it from the small organ, and which gives a kind of fixed point for the lateral muscles of the fin*. Its most internal surface is a plane adapted to the partition which divides the two organs from one another†. The edge next to the muscles of the back is very thin, but the organ becomes thicker and thicker towards its middle, where it approaches the centre of the animal. It becomes thinner again towards the lower surface or belly, but that edge is not so thin as the other. Its union with the parts to which it is attached is in general by a loose but pretty strong cellular membrane, except at the partition, to which it is joined so close as to be almost inseparable.

The small organ lies along the lower edge of the animal, nearly to the same extent as the other ‡. Its situation is marked externally by the muscles which move the fin under which it lies. Its anterior end begins nearly in the same line with the large organ, and just where the fin begins. It terminates almost insensibly near the end of the tail, where the large organ also terminates. It is of a triangular figure, adapting itself to the part in which it lies §. Its anterior end is the narrowest part; towards the tail it becomes broader; in the middle of the organ it is thickest, and from thence becomes gradually thinner to the tail, where it is very thin. The two small organs are separated from one another by the middle muscles, and by the bones upon which the bones of the fins are articulated ‖. The large and the small organ on each side are separated from one another by a fatty membrane, the inner edge of which is attached to the middle partition, and its outer edge is lost on the skin of the animal ¶. To expose the large organ to view nothing more is necessary than to remove the skin, which adheres to it by a loose cellular membrane; but to expose the small organ it is necessary to remove the long row of small muscles which move the fin.

Of the Structure of these Organs.

The structure is extremely simple and regular, consisting of two parts, viz. flat partitions of septa, and cross divisions between them. The outer edges of these septa appear externally in parallel lines nearly in the direction of the longitudinal axis of the body**. These septa are thin membranes, placed nearly parallel to one another. Their lengths are nearly in the direction of the long axis, and their breadth is nearly

---

* Pl. LVII. fig. 4. p p.　　† Pl. LVII. fig. 4. o o.　　‡ Pl. LVI. l l l.
§ Pl. LVII. fig. 5. i i.　　‖ Pl. LVII. fig. 4. e.　　¶ Pl. LVII. fig. 4. r.
** Pl. LVI. k k k.

the semi-diameter of the body of the animal. They are of different lengths, some being as long as the whole organ. I shall describe them as beginning principally at the anterior end of the organ, although a few begin along the upper edge, and the whole, passing towards the tail, gradually terminate on the lower surface of the organ; the lower-most at their origin terminating soonest. Their breadths differ in different parts of the organ. They are in general broadest near the anterior end, answering to the thickest part of the organ, and become gradually narrower towards the tail; however, they are very narrow at their beginnings or anterior ends. Those nearest to the muscles of the back are the broadest, owing to their curved or oblique situation upon these muscles, and grow gradually narrower towards the lower part, which is in a great measure owing to their becoming more transverse, and also to the organ becoming thinner at that place*. They have an outer and an inner edge; the outer is attached to the skin of the animal, to the lateral muscles of the fin, and to the membrane which divides the great organ from the small, and the whole of their inner edges are fixed to the middle partition formerly described, also to the air-bladder, and three or four terminate on that surface which inclose the muscles of the back. These septa are at the greatest distance from one another at their exterior edges near the skin, to which they are united; and as they pass from the skin towards their inner attachments they approach one another. Sometimes we find two uniting into one. On that side next to the muscles of the back they are hollow from edge to edge, answering to the shape of those muscles, but become less and less so towards the middle of the organ, and from that towards the lower part of the organ they become curved in the other direction. At the anterior part of the large organ, where it is nearly of an equal breadth, they run pretty parallel to one another, and also pretty straight, but where the organ becomes narrower it may be observed in some places that two join or unite into one, especially where a nerve passes across. The termination of this organ at the tail is so very small that I could not determine whether it consisted of one septum or more. The distances between these septa will differ in fishes of different sizes. In a fish of two feet four inches in length I found them $\frac{1}{7}$ of an inch distant from one another, and the breadth of the whole organ, at the broadest part, about an inch and a quarter, in which place were thirty-four septa. The small organ has the same kind of septa, in length passing from end to end of the organ, and in breadth passing quite across; they run somewhat serpentine, not exactly in straight

* Pl. LVII. fig. 4. 11., where the different breadths are seen in one view.

lines *.   Their outer edges terminate on the outer surface of the organ, which is in contact with the inner surface of the external muscle of the fin, and their inner edges are in contact with the centre muscles. They differ very much in breadth from one another, the broadest being equal to one side of the triangle, and the narrowest scarcely broader than the point or edge.   They are pretty nearly at equal distances from one another, but much nearer than those of the large organ, being only about $\frac{1}{30}$ part of an inch asunder; but they are at a greater distance from one another towards the tail, in proportion to the increase of breadth of the organ.   The organ is about half an inch in breadth, and has fourteen septa.   These septa, in both organs, are very tender in consistence, being easily torn.   They appear to answer the same purpose with the columns in the torpedo, making walls or butments for the subdivisions, and are to be considered as making so many distinct organs.   These septa are intersected transversely by very thin plates or membranes, whose breadth is the distance between any two septa, and therefore of different breadths in different parts, broadest at that edge which is next to the skin, narrowest at that next to the centre of the body, or to the middle partition which divides the two organs from one another.   Their lengths are equal to the breadths of the septa, between which they are situated.   There is a regular series of them continued from one end of any two septa to the other.   They appear to be so close as even to touch.   In an inch in length there are about two hundred and forty, which multiplies the surface in the whole to a vast extent.

Of the Nerves.

The nerves in this animal may be divided into two kinds, the first appropriated to the general purposes of life, the second for the management of this peculiar function, and very probably for its existence. They arise in general from the brain and medulla spinalis, as in other fish, but those from the medulla are much larger than in fish of equal size, and larger than is necessary for the common operations of life. The nerve which arises from the brain and passes down the whole length of the animal (which I believe exists in all fish) is larger in this than in others of the same size, and passes nearer to the spine †. In the common eel it runs in the muscles of the back, about midway between the skin and spine.   In the cod it passes immediately under the skin.   From its being larger in this fish than in others of the same size one might suspect that it was intended for supplying the organ in

* Pl. LVI. κ ι.   † Pl. LVII. fig. 4. τ.

some degree; but this seems not to be the case, as I was not able to trace any nerves going from it to join those from the medulla spinalis, which run to the organ. This nerve is as singular an appearance as any in this class of animals; for surely it must appear extraordinary that a nerve should arise from the brain to be lost in common parts while there is a medulla spinalis giving nerves to the same parts. It must still remain one of the inexplicable circumstances of the nervous system [a]. The organ is supplied with nerves from the medulla spinalis,

[a] [This remarkable nerve, the nervus lateralis, is, in the *Gymnotus*, a branch of the nervus vagus. It does not exist in the myxine, but in the higher cartilaginous fishes it is largely developed. In the rays it extends from the occiput to the end of the tail, even where this, as in the *Raia fasciata*, is six times the length of the body; and in the trunk the two nerves exceed the size of the spinal chord.

In osseous fishes it is relatively smaller, and in some species, as the cod, is formed by a combination of a branch of the fifth with a filament of the eighth or nervus vagus.

Besides the class of fishes (with the exception of the myxine), the lateral nerve is also present in those reptiles which preserve throughout life the external branchiæ or the branchial apertures, and which reside habitually in water, and move, like fish, by the actions of a caudal fin. In the *Menobranchus* the nervus lateralis forms a large branch of the nervus vagus, and passes superficially beneath the skin as far back as the middle of the tail, where it joins the filaments of the spinal nerves. In the proteus the nervus vagus sends off on each side two nervi laterales, one deep-seated, the other superficial. In the menopome the lateral nerve is likewise present, but is much more delicate than in the Perennibranchiata with external gills. In the larva of the *Rana paradoxa* the lateral nerve may be observed beneath the skin in the longitudinal fissure which separates the two large muscular fasciculi of the tail on each side. After the full formation of the anterior extremities this nerve becomes gradually more attenuated, and finally disappears with the absorption of the tail. It does not exist in the anourous batrachia. We may thus perceive a relationship of co-existence to subsist between these enigmatical nerves and branchial respiration. This imperfect kind of respiration is assisted by the vascularity and active powers of excreting mucus in the whole or a part of the external tegument. In the osseous fishes a linear series of mucous follicles is extended along each side of the body, and the lateral nerves, which run parallel with these lines give numerous branches to the mucous sacs and the neighbouring skin; and in the *Perennibranchiata* the lateral nerves are exclusively distributed to the skin: hence they might be termed the cutaneous respiratory nerves. They do not supply the muscles along which they pass; these derive their nervous energy from the ordinary spinal nerves. When irritated or galvanized the lateral nerves excite no contractions in the muscles; they are therefore not analogous to the spinal accessory nerves in the mammalia. In the *Gymnotus* Mr. Hunter was not able to trace any nerves going from the lateral nerve to join those from the medulla spinalis which supply the electric organ, but it anastomoses with the spinal nerves which supply the caudal fin. And in the cod, where this anastomosis takes place at each of the numerous fins, Mr. Swan conjectures that its function may be to produce sympathy and harmonious cooperation, and to regulate and produce, independently of the will, the action of the muscles of these parts. (See his accurate and beautiful Illustrations of the Comparative Anatomy of the Nervous System, p. 26, pl. vii.) And this theory equally agrees with the laws of co-existence of the lateral nerves as established by an extensive induction of particular dissections.]

from which they come out in pairs between all the vertebræ of the spine*. In their passage from the spine they give nerves to the muscles of the back, &c. They bend forwards and outwards upon the spine, between it and the muscles, and send out small nerves to the external surface, which join the skin near to the lateral lines. These ramify upon the skin, but are principally bent forwards between it and the organ, into which they send small branches as they pass along. They seem to be lost in these two parts. The trunks get upon the air-bladder, or rather dip between it and the muscles of the back, and continuing their course forwards upon that bag, they dip in between it and the organ, where they divide into smaller branches; then they get upon the middle partition, on which they continue to divide into still smaller branches; after which they pass on and get upon the small bones and muscles, which are the bases for the under fin, and at last they are lost on that fin. After having got between the organ and the above-mentioned parts they are constantly sending small nerves into the organs, first into the great organ and then into the small one; also into the muscles of the fin, and at last into the fin itself. These branches, which are sent into the organ as the trunk passes along, are so small that I could not trace their ramifications in the organs. In this fish, as well as in the torpedo, the nerves which supply the organ are much larger than those bestowed on any other part for the purposes of sensation and action; but it appears to me that the organ of the torpedo is supplied with much the largest proportion. If all the nerves which go to it were united together they would make a vastly greater chord than all those which go to the organ of this eel. Perhaps when experiments have been made upon this fish, equally accurate with those made upon the torpedo, the reason for this difference may be assigned.

Blood Vessels.

How far this organ is vascular I cannot positively determine, but from the quantities of small arteries going to it I am inclined to believe that it is not deficient in vessels. The arteries arise from the large artery which passes down the spine; they go off in small branches like the intercostals in the human subject, pass round the air-bladder, and get upon the partition together with the nerves, and distribute their branches in the same manner. The veins take the same course backwards, and enter the large vein which runs parallel with the artery[a].

* Pl. LVII. fig. 4. s.

---

[a] [A vivid and interesting account of the mode of capture of the gymnotus, and the

power of its electric shocks, is given by Humboldt in his *Observations de Zoologie et d'Anatomie Comparée*, vol. i. p. 49.   An abstract of these observations will be found in the Cyclopædia of Anatomy and Physiology, art. 'Animal Electricity,' from which, towards completing the view of this interesting subject, we quote the following description of the electrical organs in the *Silurus* or *Malapterurus electricus*, a fish inhabiting the rivers Nile and Niger.

" *The electrical organs in the Silurus.*

" The only organ that can be regarded as connected with the electrical function in this fish is a thick layer of dense cellular tissue, which completely surrounds the body immediately beneath the integuments.   So compact is it that at first sight it might be mistaken for a deposit of fatty matter.   But under the microscope it appears to be composed of tendinous fibres, closely interwoven, the meshes of which are filled with a gelatinous substance.

" This organ is divided by a strong aponeurotic membrane into two circular layers, one outer lying immediately beneath the corion, the other internal, placed above the muscles.

" Both organs are isolated from the surrounding parts by a dense fascia, excepting where the nerves and blood-vessels enter.   The cells or meshes in the outer organ, formed by its reticulated fibres, are rhombic in shape, and very minute, so as to require a lens to see them well.   The component tissue of the inner organ is somewhat flaky, and also cellular.

" The nerves of the outer organ are branches of the fifth pair, which runs beneath the lateral line, and above the aponeurotic covering of the organ.   This aponeurosis is pierced with many holes for the transmission of the nerves, which are lost within the cellular tissue of the organ.   The intercostals supply the inner organ: their electrical branches are numerous, and remarkably fine.   The organs of the other known electrical fishes have not yet come under the notice of any anatomist.   In taking a general view of these interesting organs, we are struck with the existence of a certain degree of analogy amongst them, and yet we fail to discover such resemblances as might be expected, and such as exist between the structures of other organs performing the same functions in different animals.   Here we have tendinous membranes variously arranged, yet all so as to form a series of separate cells, filled with a gelatinous matter.   But how great is the difference between the large columnar cell in the torpedo, full of delicate partitions, and the minute rhombic cells of the silurus !

" All, however, are equally supplied with nerves of very great size, larger than any others in the same animals, and indeed we may venture to say, larger than any nerve in any other animal of like bulk.   The organs vary in different fishes; first, in situation, relatively to other organs.   They bound the sides of the head in the torpedo, run along the tail of the gymnotus, and surround the body of the silurus : secondly, in having different sources of nervous energy : and thirdly, in the form of the cells.   No other fishes have aponeuroses so extensive, or such an accumulation of gelatine and albumen in any cellular organ.   Broussonet remarked that all the electrical fishes at present known to us, although all belonging to different classes, have yet certain characters in common.   All, for instance, have the skin smooth, without scales, thick, and pierced with small holes, most numerous about the head, and which pour out a peculiar fluid.   Their fins are formed of soft and flexible rays, united by means of dense membranes.   Neither the gymnotus nor torpedo has any dorsal fin ; the silurus has only a small one without rays, situated near the tail.   All have small eyes."]

OBSERVATIONS ON BEES[a].

By John Hunter, F.R.S.

Of the Common Bee.

THE common bee, from a number of peculiarities in its œconomy, has called forth the attention of the curious, and from the profit arising from its labours, it has become the object of the interested; therefore no wonder it has excited universal attention, even from the savage to the most civilized people; but it has hardly been considered by the anatomist, at least the two modes of investigation have not gone so much hand in hand as they ought to have done.

The history of the bee has rather been considered as a fit subject for the curious at large, whence more has been conceived than observed. Swammerdam, indeed, has rather erred on the other side, having with great industry been very minute on the particular structure of the bee. I shall here observe that it is commonly not only unnecessary to be minute in our description of parts in natural history, but in general improper. It is unnecessary when it does not apply to anything but the thing itself, more especially if it be of no consequence; but whenever it applies, then it should so far be treated accurately. Minutiæ beyond what is essential, tire the mind, and render that which should entertain along with instruction heavy and disagreeable; the more so too if the parts are small, where the sense can only take them in singly, and the mind can hardly comprehend the whole or apply all the parts combined to any consequent action. This has been too much the case with Swammerdam: he often attempted too much accuracy in his description of minute things[b]. But the natural history of insects has not been sufficiently understood at large, so as to throw light on this subject where there was an analogy, and where without such analogy, it must appear

---

[a] [This paper was read before the Royal Society, February 23, 1792, and published in the 82nd volume of the Philosophical Transactions.]

[b] [If the objects of the comparative anatomist were limited to the elucidation of the function of the organs he dissected, there might then, perhaps, be some reason in the animadversions in the text; but his researches have a still higher aim, viz. to trace the general plan which pervades the construction of animals amidst the various modifications to which each organ is subject in reference to particular functions; and the study of organic homologies requires that attention be paid to the minutest particulars, independently of consideratiions as to the uses in the œconomy to which they may be subservient.]

in the bee alone unintelligible, from the obscurity attending some parts of their œconomy; for there is hardly any species of animals but what has some part of its œconomy obscure, and probably this is as much so in this insect as in any other class of animals we are at one season of the year almost daily seeing; yet these parts of the œconomy may be evident in some other species of the same tribe or genus, and thus be cleared up, from analogy, so that the species assist each other in their demonstration. This is evident in the whole tribe of flying insects, for what is lost or cannot be made out in the one may be demonstrated in another; and we find there are some things in the œconomy of the bee that cannot be seen or demonstrated in it alone, but which are evident in some other insects; and while they possess the same parts, and other circumstances are similar, we must conclude the uses of those parts are similar in both; for whenever a circumstance in one animal cannot be found out in that animal, but can in another, then the natural conclusion is that the uses are similar in both.

Though the bee may classed in some degree among the domestic animals, yet from there being such a cluster of them, and because they are an offensive and irritable animal, their actions are rendered very obscure, and can only be observed by little starts; often we can only see the effects, which renders the knowledge of their œconomy still imperfect: they would in many cases seem to evade our wishes; they often remove out of our sight part of their œconomy when they can. Thus they often remove their eggs and young. Many quadrupeds do this, as cats, &c., and I have reason to believe that birds can remove their eggs, at least I have reason to suspect the sparrow of this.

As the bee is an insect, it has most things peculiar to that class of animals: such as are common are not to be taken notice of in the history of this insect, but only its peculiarities which distinguish it from all others, and constitute it to be a bee; and as bees form a large tribe of insects, it is the more singular peculiarities that constitute a distinct species of this tribe. As most parts of the œconomy of insects have not been in every respect understood, and although now known in some insects yet cannot be observed in the bee, but which accord with many circumstances attending this insect, therefore such must be brought into the present history of the bee to render it more complete. I shall not be minute in the anatomy of this animal, as that would be too tedious and uninteresting. When we talk of the œconomy of the colony, such as the secreting wax, making combs, collecting farina, honey, feeding the maggots, covering in the chrysalis and the honey, stinging, &c., it is the labouring bees that are meant.

In pursuing any subject most things come to light as it were by accident, that is, many things arise out of investigation that were not at first conceived, and even misfortunes in experiments have brought things to our knowledge that were not and probably could not have been previously conceived: on the other hand, I have often devised experiments by the fire-side or in my carriage, and have also conceived the result; but when I tried the experiment the result was different, or I found that the experiment could not be attended with all the circumstances that were suggested.

As bees, from their numbers, hide very much their operations, it is necessary to have such contrivances as will explore their œconomy. Hives with glass lights in them often show some of their operations, and when wholly of glass still more; but as they form such a cluster, and begin their comb in the centre, little can be seen till their work becomes enlarged, and by that time they have produced a much larger quantity of bees, so as still to obscure their progress. Very thin glass hives are the best calculated for exposing their operations; the distance from side to side about three inches; of a height and length sufficient for a swarm of bees to complete one summer's work in. As one perpendicular comb, the whole length and height of the hive, in the centre, dividing it into two, is the best position for exposing their operations; it is necessary to give them a lead or direction to form it so; therefore it is proper to make a ridge along the top from end to end, in the centre, between the two sides, for they like to begin their comb from an eminence; if we wished to have them transverse or oblique, it would only be necessary to make transverse or oblique ridges in the hive. I had one made of two broad pieces of plate-glass, with glass ends, which answered for simple exposure very well; but I often saw operations going on when I wished to have caught some of the bees, or to take out a piece of comb, &c.; therefore I had hives made of the same shape and size, but with different panes of glass, each pane opening with hinges, so that if I saw anything going on that I wished to examine more minutely or immediately, I opened the pane at this part and executed what I wished as much as was in my power; this I was obliged to do with great caution, as often the comb was fastened to the glass at this part. When I saw some operations going on, the dates or periods of which I wished to ascertain, such as the time of laying eggs, of hatching, &c., I made a little dot with white paint opposite to the cell where the egg was laid and put down the date.

From these animals forming colonies, and from a vast variety of effects being produced, and with a degree of attention and nicety that seem even to vie with man, man, not being in the least jealous, has wished to bestow on them more than they possess, viz. a reasoning faculty;

while every action is only instinctive, and what they cannot avoid or alter except from necessity, not from fancy. They have been supposed to be legislators, even mathematicians; indeed, upon a superficial view there is some show of reason for such suppositions; but people have gone much further, and have filled up from their imagination every blank, but in so unnatural a way that one reads it as if it were the description of a monster. Probably the best way of treating the history of this insect is only to describe what is, and the reader will immediately see where authors have been inventing; however, there are some assertions that should be particularly taken notice of, such as forming queen bees at pleasure.

Countries that have but little variety in their seasons may have insects whose œconomy is well adapted to this uniformity, and which would not be suited to a climate whose seasons are very different; for insects of countries, whose seasons are strongly marked, as in this, have a period in their life which it is little in our power to investigate, and can scarcely be discovered but by accident, for experiments often give little assistance; therefore we are obliged to fill up this blank by reasoning, and from analogy, where we have any. This period is principally the winter, in those insects which live through that season. Animals of season are somewhat like most vegetables, while the common bee is only an animal of seasons in the common actions of life, or what may be called its voluntary actions, and therefore it is somewhat like the human species, suited to every country, which may be the reason why it is so universally an animal, for I believe bees are one of the most universal animals known[a]; yet this may arise from cultivation, in consequence of which they have been brought into climates where of themselves they would not have come[b].

Insects are so small and so few of them are capable of being domesticated, that the duration of their life is not easily ascertained; therefore we are to rely more on circumstantial than on positive or demonstrative proof, and perhaps the life of the common bee may be least in our power to know, for their numbers in the same society make it almost impossible to be ascertained. From their forming a colony or society, which keeps stationary, the continuance of this society is known,

---

[a] [The humble bee was found by Captain Parry in Melville Island, Arctic circle.]

[b] [The true honey bee (*Apis mellifica*) was originally limited in its geographical range to the old world, whence it has been transported to America and other colonies, where it is now acclimated. The distinguished entomologist Latreille, on whose authority we state this fact, finds that the hive bee of the south and east of Europe and that of Egypt differ specifically from the *Apis mellifica* of the west of Europe.]

but to what age the individual lives is not known; we are certain, however, that it is only the labourers and queens that continue the society, for the males die the same year they are formed. From their fixing on the branches of trees, under projecting exposed surfaces, when they swarm, we should be inclined to suppose that they were animals of a warm climate; yet their providing liberally for the change of climate, or rather for a change of season, would, on the contrary, make us believe they were adapted for changeable climates, or rather these two circumstances should make us suppose they were fitted for both, and their universality proves it. And I do conceive that in a pretty uniform warm climate their œconomy may be somewhat different from what it is in the changeable, as they would not be under the same necessity to lay up so much store, and probably might employ their cells in breeding, for a much longer period; however, a good climate agrees with them best, as also a good season in an indifferent climate, such as Britain. We find the common bee in Europe, Asia, Africa, and America. That they may be, or should be, in the three first is easily supposed, but how they came to America is not so readily conceived; for although a kind of manageable animal, yet they do not like such long confinement in their hives as would carry them to the West Indies, excepting in an ice-house; for when I have endeavoured to confine them in their hives they have been so restless as to destroy themselves.

The female and the working bee, I believe in every species, have stings, which renders them an animal of offence, indeed, but rather of defence; for although they make an attack, I believe it is by way of defence, excepting when they attack one another, which is seldom or never with their stings. As this belongs more to the labourers, it shall be considered when I treat of them in particular. Of the whole bee tribe, the common bee is the easiest irritated; for as they have property, they are jealous of it, and seem to defend it; but when not near it they are quiet, and must be hurt before they will sting; with all this disposition for defence, which is only to secure their property or themselves, when more closely attacked, yet they have no covetousness, nor a disposition to obstruct others. Thus two bees or more will be sucking at the same flower, without the first possessor claiming it as his right; a hundred may be about the same drop of honey, if it is beyond the boundaries of their own right; but what they have collected they defend. It is easily known when they mean to sting; they fly about the object of their anger very quickly, and by the quickness of their motion evade being struck or attacked; which is discovered by the sound of their wings, as if going to give a stroke as they fly, a very different noise from that of the wings when coming home of a fine evening loaded with farina or honey; it is then a soft contented noise. When a single bee is attacked by several others, it seems the most passive animal possible, making no resistance, and even hardly seeming to wish to get away; and in this manner they allow themselves to be killed. They are perhaps the only insect that feeds in the winter, and therefore the only one that lays up external store; and as all animals, whether insects or not, that keep quiet in the winter, without either eating at all, or eating very little in proportion to what they do in the summer, grow fat and muscular in the summer (which I term internal store), we see why the common bee need not be fatter at one time than another; and accordingly we find them nearly of the same fatness the year round.

There are accidents befalling hives of bees that are not easily accounted for. I had a hive, which in the month of November was become quite empty of bees, and upon examination had no honey in it, which was strong in the summer, and had violent attacks made upon it in October by wasps belonging to a nest in the garden, but appeared quiet when that nest was removed. Upon examining this hive, I found only five dead bees, and not a drop of honey in any one cell: there was a good deal of bee bread in different cells scattered up and down the comb, which was become white with mould on its surface. On the other hand, I have had swarms die in the winter in the hives, while there was great plenty of honey in the combs; what seemed remarkable, they all died with their proboscides elongated, and in those which I opened, I found the stomachs full of honey, and their intestines full also of excrement, especially the last part.

Of the Heat of Bees.

Bees are perhaps the only insect that produces heat within itself[a], and

---

[a] [It has long been known that other social insects besides the bee maintain, when congregated in their habitations, a higher temperature than that of the external atmosphere. In an excellent and highly important series of experiments on this subject recently communicated by Mr. Newport to the Royal Society, it is shown that insects in general have the power of generating animal heat; that that power in the solitary insects is greatest in the diurnal species of flying insects, especially such as reside most constantly in the open air. The law that the mature or more perfect animal is " more capable of generating heat than when it it is younger " (see p. 135), is well exemplified by Mr. Newport in the class of insects.

In the Lepidoptera, the average elevation of the temperature of the body above that of its surrounding medium is in the larvæ from $0°·9$ to $1°·5$, while in the imago it is from $5°$ to $10°$. Among the Hymenoptera it is from $2°$ to $4°$ in the larva, and in the imago from $4°$ to $15°$, or even $20°$. In all these cases the amount of animal heat developed is in the ratio of the consumption of oxygen and the quantity of carbonic acid formed in the change of the arterial into serous blood: or in other words,

were therefore intended to have a tolerably well-regulated warmth, without which, of course, they are very uncomfortable and soon die; and which makes not only a part of their internal œconomy respecting the individual, but a part of their external or common œconomy, and is therefore necessary to be known.   The heat of bees is ascertainable by the thermometer, and I shall give the result of experiments made at two different seasons of the year.

July 18th, at ten in the evening, wind northerly, thermometer at 54° in the open air, I introduced it into the top of a hive full of bees, and in less than five minutes it rose to 82°.   I let it stand all night; at five in the morning it was down at 79°; at nine the same morning it had risen to 83°, and at one o'clock to 84°; and at nine in the evening it was down to 78°.

December 30th, air at 35°, bees at 73°.

Although bees support a heat nearly equal to that of a quadruped, yet their external covering is not different from that of insects which do not; there is no difference between their coat and a common fly's or wasp's, nor are they fatter, all which makes them bad retainers of heat; therefore they are chilly, and in a cold too severe for them to be comfortable in, they make up for their want of size singly and get into clusters.   A single bee has so little power of keeping itself warm, that it presently becomes numbed, and almost motionless : a common night in summer will produce this effect.   A cold capable of producing such effects kills them soon, by which means vast numbers die; therefore a common bee is obliged to feed and live in society to keep itself warm in cold weather.

We know that the consumption of heat may be greater than the power of forming it; when that is the case we become sensible of it, and then take on such actions as are either instinctive, such as arise naturally out of the impression, or as reason, custom, or habit direct.   Many animals upon the impression of cold, coil themselves up in their own fur, bringing all their extremities into the centre or hollow of the belly; birds bring their feet under the belly, and thrust their bill between their wing and body; many, if not all, go to the warmest places, either from instinctive principle or habit; but the bees have no other mode but forming clusters, and the larger the better.   As they are easily affected by cold, their instinctive principle respecting cold is very strong, as likewise with regard to wet.   I have seen a swarm hanging out at the door of a hive ready to take flight, and then return; a chill has come on of which I was not sensible, and in a few

in proportion to the energy with which the functions of respiration and locomotion go on in the insect.]

minutes the whole has gone back into the hive; and by the cold increasing, I have at length perceived the cause of their return. If rain is coming on, we observe them returning home in great quantities, and hardly any abroad. The eggs of bees require this heat as much as themselves, nor will the maggot live in a cold of 60° or 70°, nor even their chrysalis. This warmth keeps the wax so soft as to allow them to model it with ease. In glass hives, or those that have windows of glass in them, we often find a dew on the inside of the glass, especially when the glass is colder than the air within; whether this is perspiration from the bees, both from their external surface and lungs, or evaporation from the honey, I cannot say.

Bees are very cleanly animals respecting themselves, although not so respecting the remains of their young. They, I believe, seldom or never evacuate their excrement in the hive. I have known them confined many days without discharging the contents of the rectum, and the moment they got abroad they evacuated in the air when flying; and they appear to be very nice in their bodies, for I have often detected them cleaning one another, more especially if by accident they are besmeared with honey.

This animal may be considered alone, or so far as concerns its own œconomy as an individual, which is common to the most solitary animals; but it can also be considered as a member of society, in which it is taking an active part, and in which it becomes an object of great curiosity.

To consider this society individually, it may be said to consist of a female breeder, female non-breeders, and males; but to consider it as a community, it may be said to consist only of female breeders and non-breeders, the males answering no other purpose than simply as a male, and are only temporary; and it is probable the female breeder is to be considered in no other light than as a layer of eggs, and that she only influences the non-breeders by her presence, being only a bond of union, for without her they seem to have no tie; it is her presence that makes them an aggregate animal. May we not suppose that the offspring of the queen have an attachment to the mother, somewhat similar to the attachment of young birds to the female that brings them up? for although the times of their attachment are not equal, yet it is the dependence which each has on its mother that constitutes the bond; for bees have none without her: however, the similarity is not exact, for young animals who have lost their nurse will herd together, and jointly make the best shifts they can, because in future they are to become single animals; but bees have an eternal instinctive dependence on the mother, probably from there not being distinct sexes. When the queen is lost, this attachment is broke ; they give up industry, probably die, or we may suppose, join some other hive. This is not the case with those of this tribe whose queen singly forms a colony ; for although the queen is destroyed, yet they go on with that work which is their lot, as the wasp, hornet, and humble bee. Most probably the whole œconomy of the bee, which we so much admire, belongs to the non-breeders, and depends on their instinctive powers being set to work by the presence of the breeders, that being their only enjoyment; therefore when we talk of the wonderful œconomy of bees, it is chiefly the labourers at large we are to admire, although the queen gets the principal credit for the extent of *their* instinctive properties.

This œconomy, in its appearances and operations, is somewhat similar to human society, but very different in its first causes and mode of conduct. The human species sets up its own standard; the bee has one set up by nature, and therefore fulfils all the necessary purposes. This standard of influence, which is the breeder, is called the queen, and I shall keep to the name, although I do not allow her voluntary influence or power.

The non-breeders are what compose the hive, or what may be called the community at large ; and the males are mere males : each of these parts of the community I shall hereafter consider separately.

To take up the common bee in any one period of the year, or in other words, in any one month, and carry it round to the same, and observe what happens in that time, is probably including the whole œconomy of bees ; for although they may live more than one year, which I believe is not known, from its not being easily ascertained, yet each year can only be a repetition of the last, as I conceive they are complete in the first; therefore the history of one year may be said to make a whole, and of course it is not material at what time in the circle we begin the history.

Perhaps the best time to begin the history of such insects as only come to full growth the season they are bred, and live through the winter, and breed the summer following, is when they emerge from the torpid state, and begin to breed ; but it might be thought that the common bee is an exception to this rule, because they begin early in the spring to breed, generally before they can be observed ; and as they breed to form a colony, which is to go off from the old stock, in order to set out anew, it might seem most natural to begin with this colony, and trace it through its various actions of life for one year, when it as it were regenerates itself, and comes round to the same point again that the old stock was in when it threw off this colony.

Bees, like every other animal that is taken care of in the time of breeding or incubation, and nursed to the age of taking care of itself, cannot be said to have a period in which we can begin its natural history; but in some other insects there is such a period, for they can be traced from an egg, becoming totally independent of the parent from the moment of being laid, as the silk-worm, &c. There are three periods at which the history of the bee may commence: first, in the spring, when the queen begins to lay her eggs; in the summer, at the commencement of a new colony; or in the autumn, when they are going into winter-quarters. I shall begin the particular history of the bee with the new colony, when nothing is formed; for it then begins everything that can possibly happen afterwards.

When a hive sends off a colony it is commonly in the month of June; but that will vary according to the season, for in a mild spring bees sometimes swarm in the middle of May, and very often at the latter end of it. Before they come off they commonly hang about the mouth of the hole or door of the hive for some days, as if they had not sufficient room within for such hot weather, which I believe is very much the case; for if cold or wet weather come on, they stow themselves very well, and wait for fine weather. But swarming appears to be rather an operation arising from necessity, for they would seem not naturally to swarm, because if they have an empty space to fill, they do not swarm; therefore by increasing the size of the hive, the swarming is prevented. This period is much longer in some than in others. For some evenings before they come off, is often heard a singular noise, a kind of ring, or sound of a small trumpet; by comparing it with the notes of the piano-forte, it seemed to be the same sound with the lower A of the treble.

The swarm commonly consists of three classes; a female, or females*, males, and those commonly called mules, which are supposed to be of no sex, and are the labourers; the whole about two quarts in bulk, making about six or seven thousand. It is a question that cannot easily be determined, whether this old stock sends off entirely young of the same season, and whether the whole of their young ones, or only part. As the males are entirely bred in the same season, part go off; but part must stay, and most probably it is so with the others. They commonly come off in the heat of the day, often immediately after a shower; who takes the lead I do not know, but should suppose it was the queen. When one goes off they all immediately follow, and fly about seemingly in great confusion, although there is one principle actuating the whole. They soon appear to be directed to some fixed place, such as the

* I have reason to believe that never more than one female comes off with a swarm.

branch of a tree or bush, the cavities of old trees, holes of houses leading into some hollow place; and whenever the stand is made, they all
immediately repair to it, till they are all collected. But it would seem
in some cases that they had not fixed upon any resting place before
they came off, or if they had, that they were either disturbed, if it was
near, or that it was at a great distance; for after hovering some time,
as if undetermined, they fly away, mount up into the air, and go off
with great velocity. When they have fixed upon their future habita-
tion, they immediately begin to make their combs, for they have the
materials within themselves. I have reason to believe that they fill
their crops with honey when they come away; probably from the stock
in the hive. I killed several of those that came away, and found their
crops full, while those that remained in the hive had their crops not
near so full: some of them came away with farina on their legs, which
I conceive to be rather accidental. I may just observe here, that a
hive commonly sends off two, sometimes three swarms in a summer;
but that the second is commonly less than the first, and the third less
than the second; and this last has seldom time to provide for the winter: they shall often threaten to swarm, but do not; whether the
threatening is owing to too many bees, and their not swarming is owing
to there being no queen, I do not know. It sometimes happens that
the swarm shall go back again; but in such instances I have reason to
think that they have lost their queen, for the hives to which their swarm
have come back do not swarm the next warm day, but shall hang out
for a fortnight or more, and then swarm; and when they do, the swarm
is commonly much larger than before, which makes me suspect that
they waited for the queen that was to have gone off with the next swarm.

So far we have set the colony in motion. The materials of their
dwelling, or comb, which is the wax, is the next consideration, with the
mode of forming, preparing, or disposing of it. In giving a totally new
account of the wax, I shall first show it can hardly be what it has been
supposed to be. First I shall observe that the materials, as they are
found composing the comb, are not to be found in the same state (as a
composition) in any vegetable, where they have been supposed to be
got. The substance brought in on their legs, which is the farina of the
flowers of plants, is, in common, I believe, imagined to be the materials
of which the wax is made, for it is called by most the wax: but it is
the farina, for it is always of the same colour as the farina of the flower
where they are gathering; and indeed we see them gathering it, and
we also see them covered almost all over with it, like a dust; nevertheless, it has been supposed to be the wax, or that the wax was extracted from it. Reaumur is of this opinion. I made several experi-

ments to see if there was such a quantity of oil in it as would account for the quantity of wax to be formed, and to learn if it was composed of oil. I held it near the candle; it burnt, but did not smell like wax, and had the same smell when burning, as farina when it was burnt. I observed that this substance was of different colours on different bees, but always of the same colour on both legs of the same bee[a]; whereas new-made comb was all of one colour. I observed that it was gathered with more avidity for old hives, where the comb is complete, than for those hives where it is only begun, which we could hardly conceive if it was the materials of wax : also we may observe that at the very beginning of a hive, the bees seldom bring in any substance on their legs for two or three days, and after that the farina gatherers begin to increase; for now some cells are formed to hold it as a store, and some eggs are laid, which when hatched will require this substance as food, and which will be ready when the weather is wet. I have also observed, that when the weather has either been so cold, or so wet, in June, as to hinder a young swarm from going abroad, they have yet in that time formed as much new comb as they did in the same time when the weather was such as allowed them to go abroad. I have seen them bring it in about the latter end of March, and have observed in glass hives the bees with the farina on their legs, and have seen them disposing of it, as will be described hereafter.

The wax is formed by the bees themselves; it may be called an external secretion of oil, and I have found that it is formed between each scale of the under side of the belly[b]. When I first observed this sub-

---

[a] [Aristotle, who describes many interesting particulars of the œconomy of the bee, and knew something of the structure of the interior of the hive, was the first to observe that a bee in each single excursion from the hive always visits the same species of flower, and consequently comes home laden with pollen of the same colour. This has been confirmed by all subsequent observers, and, as we see, did not escape Mr. Hunter. The necessity for this instinct arises out of the operation which the pollen first undergoes; the bee rakes out the pollen with incredible quickness by means of its first pair of legs, then passes it to the middle pair, which transfer it to the hind legs, by which it is wrought up into little pellets. Now if the pollen were taken indiscriminately from different flowers, the difference in the size and shape of the pollen-grains would probably prevent them cohering together sufficiently to allow of the pellet being formed. Hence it is that in watching the return of bees to the hive some may be seen laden with yellow-coloured pellets, others with orange, pink, white, or greenish-coloured ones. The grains of pollen are not changed by the operation of kneading when detached from the pellet; under a microscope they are seen to possess their original figure.]

[b] [Huber first confirmed this statement by actual observation, but the merit of the discovery is entirely Hunter's. The only approach to it is in the observation by Morley, who says that he has taken bees with six pieces of wax within the plaits of the abdomen, three on each side (*Female Monarchy*, 1771,) but without knowing the source of these pieces of wax.]

stance, in my examination of the working bee, I was at a loss to say what it was: I asked myself if it was new scales forming, and whether they cast the old, as the lobster, &c. does? But it was to be found only between the scales, on the lower side of the belly. On examining the bees through glass hives while they were climbing up the glass I could see that most of them had this substance, for it looked as if the lower or posterior edge of the scale was double, or that there were double scales; but I perceived it was loose, not attached. Finding that the substance brought in on their legs was farina, intended, as appeared from every circumstance, to be the food of the maggot, and not to make wax, and not having yet perceived anything that could give me the least idea of wax, I conceived these scales might be it, at least I thought it necessary to investigate them. I therefore took several on the point of a needle, and held them to a candle, where they melted, and immediately formed themselves into a round globe; upon which I no longer doubted but this was the wax, which opinion was confirmed to me by not finding those scales but in the building season. In the bottom of the hive we see a good many of the scales lying loose, some pretty perfect, others in pieces. I have endeavoured to catch them, either taking this matter out of themselves, from between the scales of the abdomen, or from one another, but never could satisfy myself in this respect: however I once caught a bee examining between the scales of the belly of another, but I could not find that it took anything from between. We very often see some of the bees wagging their belly, as if tickled, running round and to and fro for only a little way, followed by one or two other bees, as if examining them. I conceived they were probably shaking out the scales of wax, and that the others were ready upon the watch to catch them, but I could not absolutely determine what they did. It is with these scales that they form the cells called the comb, but perhaps not entirely, for I believe they mix farina with it; however, this only occasionally, when probably the secretion is not in great plenty. I have some reason to think that where no other substance is introduced the thickness of the scale is the same with that of the sides of the comb; if so, then a comb may be no more than a number of these united; but a great deal of the comb seems to be too thick for this, and, indeed, would appear to be a mixture similar to the covering of the chrysalis. The wax naturally is white, but when melted from the comb at large it is yellow. I apprehended this might arise from its being stained with honey, the excrement of the maggots, and with the bee-bread. I steeped some white comb in honey, boiled some with farina as also with old comb, but I could not say that it was made yellower. Wax, by bleaching, is brought back to its natural colour, which is also a proof that its colour is derived from some mixture. I have reason to believe that they take the old comb, when either broken down, or by any accident rendered useless, and employ it again; but this can only be with combs that have had no bees hatched in them, for the wax cannot be separated from the silk afterwards. Reaumur supposed that they new worked up the old materials, because he found the covering of the chrysalis of a yellower colour than the other parts of the new comb; but this is always so, whether they have old yellow comb to work up or not, as will be shown.

The bees who gather the farina also form the wax, for I found it between their scales.

The cells, or rather the congeries of cells, which compose the comb, may be said to form perpendicular plates or partitions, which extend from top to bottom of the cavity in which they build them, and from side to side. They always begin at the top or roof of the vault in which they build, and work downwards; but if the upper part of this vault, to which their combs are fixed, is removed, and a dome is put over, they begin at the upper edge of the old comb and work up into the new cavity at the top. They generally may be guided as to the direction of their new plates of comb, by forming ridges at top, to which they begin to attach their comb. In a long hive, if these ridges are longitudinal, their plates of comb will be longitudinal; if placed transverse, so will be the plates; and if oblique, the plates of comb will be oblique. Each plate consists of a double set of cells, whose bottoms form the partition between each set. The plates themselves are not very regularly arranged, not forming a regular plane where they might have done so; but are often adapted to the situation or shape of the cavity in which they are built. The bees do not endeavour to shape their cavity to their work, as the wasps do, nor are the cells of equal depths, also fitting them to their situation; but as the breeding cells must all be of a given depth, they reserve a sufficient number for breeding in, and they put the honey into the others, as also into the shallow ones. The attachment of the comb round the cavity is not continued, but interrupted so as to form passages; there are also passages in the middle of the plates, especially if there be a cross stick to support the comb; these allow of bees to go across from plate to plate. The substance which they use for attaching their combs to surrounding parts is not the same as the common wax; it is softer and tougher, a good deal like the substance with which they cover in their chrysalis or the humble bee surrounds her eggs. It is probably a mixture of wax with farina. The cells are placed nearly horizontally, but not exactly so; the mouth raised a little. which probably may be to retain the honey the better; however, this rule is not strictly observed, for often they are horizontal, and towards the lower edge of a plane of comb they are often declining. The first combs that a hive forms are the smallest, and much neater than the last or lowermost. Their sides or partitions between cell and cell are much thinner, and the hexagon is much more perfect. The wax is purer, being probably little else but wax, and it is more brittle. The lower combs are considerably larger, and contain much more wax, or perhaps, more properly, more materials; and the cells are at such distances as to allow them to be of a round figure: the wax is softer, and there is something mixed with it. I have observed that the cells are not all of equal size, some being a degree larger than the others; and that the small are the first formed, and of course at the upper part where the bees begin, and the larger are nearer the lower part of the comb, or last made: however, in hives of particular construction, where the bees may begin to work at one end, and can work both down and towards the other end, we often find the larger cells both on the lower part of the combs and also at the opposite end.

These are formed for the males to be bred in; and in the hornets' and wasps' combs there are larger cells for the queens to be bred in: these are also formed in the lower tier, and the last formed.

The first comb made in a hive is all of one colour, viz. almost white; but it is not so white towards the end of the season, having then more of a yellow cast.

Of the Royal Cell.

There is a cell which is called the royal cell, often three or four of them, sometimes more; I have seen eleven, and even thirteen in the same hive; commonly they are placed on the edge of one or more of the combs, but often on the side of a comb; however, not in the centre along with the other cells, like a large one placed among the others, but often against the mouths of the cells, and projecting out beyond the common surface of the comb; but most of them are formed from the edge of the comb, which terminates in one of these cells. The royal cell is much wider than the others, but seldom so deep: its mouth is round, and appears to be the largest half of an oval in depth, and is declining downwards, instead of being horizontal or lateral. The materials of which it is composed are softer than common wax, rather like the last mentioned, or those of which the lower edge of the plate of comb is made, or with which the bees cover the chrysalis: they have very little wax in their composition, not one-third; the rest I conceive to be farina.

This is supposed to be the cell in which the queen is bred, but I have reason to believe that this is only imagination : for, first, it is too large, and, moreover, seldom so deep as the large cells in which the males are bred; whereas, if proportioned to the length of the queen, it ought to be deeper, for length of body is her greatest difference. In the second place, its mouth is placed downwards; and in the third place, it is never lined with the silken covering of the chrysalis, similar to the cells of the males and labourers; nor do we find excrement at the bottom of it. The number of these cells is very different in different hives. I think I have seen hives without any, and I have seen them with eleven or twelve, sometimes more. I have examined them at all times through the summer, but never found any alteration in them.

The comb seems at first to be formed for propagation, and the reception of honey to be only a secondary use ; for if the bees lose their queen they make no combs; and the wasp, hornet, &c. make combs, although they collect no honey; and the humble bee collects honey, and deposits it in cells she never made.

I shall not consider the bee as an excellent mathematician, capable of making exact forms, and having reasoned upon the best shape of the cell for capacity, so that the greatest number might be put into the smallest space (for the hornet and the wasp are much more correct, although not seemingly under the same necessity, as they collect nothing to occupy their cells); because, although the bee is pretty perfect in these respects, yet it is very incorrect in others, in the formation of the comb : nor shall I consider these animals as forming comb of certain shape and size, from mere mechanical necessity, as from working round themselves ; for such a mould would not form cells of different sizes, much less could wasps be guided by the same principle, as their cells are of very different sizes, and the first by much too small for the queen wasp to have worked round herself : but I shall consider the whole as an instinctive principle, in which the animal has no power of variation or choice, but such as arises from what may be called external necessity. The cell has in common six sides, but this is most correct in those first formed ; and their bottom is commonly composed of those sides or planes, two of the sides making one; and they generally fall in between the bottoms of three cells of the opposite side ; but this is not regular, it is only to be found where there is no external interruption.

I have already observed, that the last-formed cells in the season are not so well made ; that their partitions are thicker, and more of a yellow colour: this arises, I imagine, from the wax being less pure, having more alloy in it ; and therefore, not being so strong, more of it is required.   The bees would appear to reserve many of their cells for honey, and those are mostly at the upper part.   In old hives, of several years' standing, I have found the upper part of the comb free from the consequences of having bred, such as the silk lining, and the excrement of the maggots at the bottom ; while the lower part, for probably more than one half of the plane of cells, showed strong marks of having contained many broods of young bees.   In such the lining of silk is thick at the sides, composed of many laminæ; and in many, the bottom is half filled up with excrement; and I observed at such parts, the comb was thickest at its mouth, which inclines me to think, that when a cell becomes shallow, by the bottom being in some degree filled up, the bees then add to its mouth.   Such also they seem to reserve principally for the bee-bread; so that to lay up a greater store of honey is an object to them.

Of the Laying of Eggs.

As soon as a few combs are formed, the female bee begins laying of eggs.   As far as I have been able to observe, the queen is the only bee that propagates, although it is asserted that the labourers do.   Her first eggs in the season are those which produce labourers ; then the males, and probably the queen; this is the progress in the wasp, hornet, humble bee, &c.   However, it is asserted by Riem, that when a hive is deprived of a queen, labourers lay eggs; also, that at this time, some honey and farina are brought in as store for a wet day.   The eggs are laid at the bottom of the cell, and we find them there before the cells are half completed, so that propagation begins early and goes on along with the formation of the other cells.   The egg is attached at one end to the bottom of the cell, sometimes standing perpendicularly, often obliquely; it has a glutinous or slimy covering, which makes it stick to anything it touches.   It would appear that there was a period or periods for laying eggs; for I have observed in a new swarm that the great business of laying eggs did not last above a fortnight; although the hive was not half filled with comb, it began to slacken.   Probably that end of the egg which is first protruded is that which sticks to the bottom of the cell ; and probably the tail of the maggot is formed at that end : when they move the egg, how they make it stick again, I do not know.   I have just observed, that they often move the egg out of a cell to some other, we may suppose; why they do this I cannot say; whether it is because we have been exposing this part, is not easily determined. In those new-formed combs, as also in many not half finished, we find the substance called bee-bread, and some of it is covered over with wax, which will be considered further. By the time they have worked above half way down the hive with the comb, they are beginning to form the larger cells, and by this time the first broods are hatched, which were small or labourers; and now they begin to breed males, and probably a queen, for a new swarm; because the males are now bred to impregnate the young queen for the present summer, as also for the next year. This progress in breeding is the same with that of the wasp, hornet, and humble bee*. Although *this account* is commonly allowed, yet writers on this subject have supposed another mode of producing a queen, when the hive is in possession of maggots, and deprived of their queen.

What may be called the complete process of the egg, namely, from the time of laying to the birth of the bee, (that is, the time of hatching,) the life of the maggot, and the life of the chrysalis, is, I believe, shorter than in most insects. It is not easy to fix the time when the eggs hatch; I have been led to imagine it was in five days. When they hatch, we find the young maggot lying coiled up in the bottom of the cell, in some degree surrounded with a transparent fluid. In many of cells, where the eggs have just hatched, we find the skin standing in its place, either not yet removed, or not pressed down by the maggot. There is now an additional employment for the labourers, namely, the feeding and nursing the young maggots. We may suppose the queen has nothing to do with this, as there are at all times labourers enough in the hive for such purposes, especially too as she never does bring the materials, as every other of the tribe is obliged to do at first; therefore she seems to be a queen by hereditary, or rather by natural right, while the humble bee, wasp, hornet, &c. seem rather to work themselves into royalty, or mistresses of the community. The bees are readily detected feeding the young maggot; and indeed a young maggot might easily be brought up by any person who would be attentive to feed it. They open their two lateral pincers to receive the food, and swallow it. As they grow, they cast their coats or cuticles; but how often they throw their coats, while in the maggot state, I do not

---

* Reaumur on Bees says that the drone eggs, when laid in small cells, produce drones; and Wilhelmi says that it is the labourers only that lay drone eggs. Mr. Riem says that queens are never reared in any but royal cells, although males sometimes in common cells; and workers in old queen cells, but never in those recently made.

know[a]. I observed that they often removed their eggs; I also find they very often shift the maggot into another cell, even when very large. The maggots grow larger and larger till they nearly fill the cell; and by this time they require no more food, and are ready to be inclosed for the chrysalis state: how this period is discovered I do not know, for in every other insect, as far as I am acquainted, it is an operation of the maggot or caterpillar itself; but in the common bee it is an operation of the perfect animal; probably it arises from the maggot refusing food. The time between their being hatched and their being inclosed is, I believe, four days; at least, from repeated observations, it comes nearly to that time. When ready for the chrysalis state, the bees cover over the mouth of the cell with a substance of a light brown colour, much in the same manner that they cover the honey, excepting that in the present instance the covering is convex externally, and appears not to be entirely wax, but a mixture of wax and farina. The maggot is now perfectly inclosed, and it begins to line the cell and covering of the mouth above-mentioned with a silk it spins out similar to the silkworm, and which makes a kind of pod for the chrysalis. Bonnet observed that in one instance the cell was too short for the chrysalis, and it broke its covering, and formed its pod higher or more convex than common: this I can conceive possible; we often see it in the wasp. Having completed this lining, they cast off, or rather shove off, from the head backwards, the last maggot coat, which is deposited at the bottom of the cell, and then they become chrysalises.

Of the Food of the Maggot, or what is commonly called Bee-Bread.

One would naturally suppose that the food of the maggot bee should be honey, both because it is the food of the old ones, and it is what they appear principally to collect for themselves; however, the circumstance of honey being food for the old ones is no argument, because very few young animals live on the same food with the old, and therefore it is probable the maggot bee does not live upon honey; and if we reason from analogy, we shall be led to suppose the bee-bread to be the food of the maggot. It is the food of the maggot of the humble bee,

---

[a] [It has not yet been ascertained that the larva of the bee sheds its skin, as the lepidopterous caterpillars do, except when on the point of becoming a pupa, at which period a thin pellicle is also thrown out by each of the stigmata from the tracheal tubes.]

who feeds upon honey, and even lays up a store of honey for a wet day, yet does not feed the young with it. It is the food of the maggot of a black bee, and also of several others of the solitary kind who also feed upon honey; and wasps, &c. who do not bring in such materials, do not feed themselves upon honey. We cannot suppose that the bee-bread is for the food of the old bees, when we see them collecting it in the months of June, July, &c., at which time they have honey in great plenty; this substance is as common to a hive as any part belonging to the œconomy of bees. Before they have formed five or six square inches of comb in a young hive, we shall find eggs, honey, and bee-bread; and at whatever time of the year we kill a hive, we shall find this substance; and if a hive is short of honey and dies in the winter, we find no honey, but all the bee-bread, which was laid up in store for the maggots in the spring. They take great care of it, for it is often covered over with wax as the honey, and I believe more especially in the winter; probably with a view to preserve it till wanted. In April I have found some of the cells full, others only half full. If we slit down a cell filled with this substance, we shall commonly find it composed of layers of different colours; some a deep orange, others a pale brown. In glass hives we often find that the glass makes one side of the cell, and frequently in such we shall see at once the different strata above mentioned. This is the substance which they bring in on their legs, and consists of the farina of plants. It is not the farina of every plant that the bee collects, at least they are found gathering it from some with great industry, while we never find them on others: St. John's wort is a favourite plant, but that comes late. The flower of the gourd, cucumber, &c., they seem to be fond of. What they do collect must be the very loose stuff, just ready to be blown off to impregnate the female part of the flower; and to show that this is the case, we find bees impregnate flowers that have not the male part. It is in common of a yellow colour, but that of very different shades, often of an orange; and when we see bees collecting it on bushes that have a great many flowers, so as to furnish a complete load, it is then of the colour of the farina of that bush. It is curious to see them deposit this substance in the cell. On viewing the hives, we often see bees with this substance on their legs, moving along on the combs, as if looking out for the cell to deposit it in. They will often walk over a cell that has some deposited in it, but shall leave that, and try another, and so on till they fix; which made me conceive that each bee had its own cell. When they come to the intended cell, they put their two hind legs into it, with the two fore legs and the trunk out on the mouth of the neighbouring cell, and then the tail or belly is thrust down into the intended cell; they then bring the leg under the belly, and turning the point of the tail to the outside of the leg, where the farina is, they shove it off by the point of the tail. When it is thus shoved off both legs, the bee leaves it, and the two pieces of farina may be seen lying at the bottom of the cell; another bee comes almost immediately, and creeping into the cell, continues about five minutes, kneading and working it down into the bottom, or spreads it over what was deposited there before, leaving it a smooth surface.

It is of a consistency like paste, burns slightly, and gives a kind of unusual smell, probably from having been mixed with animal juice in the act of kneading it down, for when brought in it is rather a powder than a paste. That it is the food of the maggot is proved by examining the animal's stomach; for when we kill a maggot full grown, we find its stomach full of a similar substance, only softer, as if mixed with a fluid, but we never find honey in the stomach; therefore we are to suppose it is collected as food for the maggot, as much as honey is for the old bee. Mr. Schirach imagines that the semen of the male is the food of the maggot; but the food of the male and the queen maggot has been supposed to be different from that of the labourers. Reaumur says the food of the queen maggot is different in taste from that of the common ones. How he knew this, who was unacquainted with the food of the others, I cannot conceive.

Of the Excrement of the Maggot.

They have very little excrement, but what they do discharge is deposited at the bottom of the cell; and what at first will appear rather extraordinary, it is never cleared away by the bees, but allowed to dry along with the maggot coats; and both fresh eggs and honey are deposited in these cells so circumstanced, every future year; so that in time the cells become nearly half full.

Of the Chrysalis State.

In this state they are forming themselves for a new life; they are either entirely new built, or wonderfully changed, for there is not the smallest vestige of the old form remaining; yet it must be the same materials, for now nothing is taken in. How far this change is only the old parts new modelled, or gradually altering their form, is not easily determined. To bring about the change, many parts must be removed, out of which the new ones are probably formed[a]. As bees are not different in this state from the common flying insects in general, I shall not pursue the subject of their changes further; although it makes a very material part in the natural history of insects.

When the chrysalis is formed into the complete bee, it then destroys the covering of its cell, and comes forth. The time it continues in this state is easier ascertained than either in that of the egg or the maggot: for the bees cannot move the chrysalis as they do the two others. In one instance it was thirteen days and twelve hours exactly; so that an egg in hatching being five days, the age of the maggot being four days, and the chrysalis continuing thirteen and a half, the whole makes twenty-two days and a half: but how far this is accurate I will not pretend to say. I found that the chrysalis of a male was fourteen days, but this was probably accidental. When they first come out they are of a greyish colour, but soon turn brown.

When the swarm of which I have hitherto been giving the history has come off early and is a large one, more especially if it was put into too small a hive, it often breeds too many for the hive to keep through

---

[a] [It is in the determination of these interesting questions that the minute researches of Swammerdam manifest their importance. His figures demonstrate that the larva of the bee consists of thirteen annular segments, of which one corresponds to the head, three to the thorax, and nine to the abdomen of the perfect insects.

The cephalic segment supports the rudimental eyes, which resemble the ocelli of other insects in structure, but are colourless and semi-transparent. The antennæ are represented by two small organs placed at the anterior angles of the head; the oral organs are also indicated; there is a small transverse upper lip or labrum, beneath which are two little horny parts, afterwards destined to become the mandibles; then "two little parts which seem as if they were articulated;" these are subsequently developed into the *maxillæ*; and between these is a mesial "small, and somewhat prominent part, which resembles a trunk or tongue, and this increasing by degrees, at length indeed constitutes," says Swammerdam, "the trunk of the bee."

We thus have evidence that the parts which so conspicuously distinguish the imago from the larva, are not "entirely new built," but are "wonderfully changed" by gradually altering their form and relative dimensions.

With respect to the rest of the larva, we find that the body is furnished on each side with ten minute circular spiracles, a pair being placed on each segment, with the exception of that which immediately follows the head, and the terminal one which bears the arms. Previous to shedding the skin, the first three segments of the body begin to swell, and make room for the aggregated muscles which are to put in motion the locomotive organs, attached, in the perfect insect, exclusively to these segments.

The larva being apodal, both the legs and wings may be regarded as being "entirely new built," and the pupa of the bee then presents an elegant disposition and well-ordered representation of all the limbs and parts of the future bee. The antennæ and the tongue are seen lying along the breast, and the wings and legs bent from the sides of the thorax along the belly. Some of the segments of the larva are "removed," and out of these the organs of generation appear to be formed.]

the winter; and in such case a new swarm is thrown off, which, how-ever, is commonly not a large one, and generally has too little time to complete its comb, and store it with honey sufficient to preserve them through the winter. This is similar to the second or third swarm of the old hives.

Of the Seasons when the different operations of Bees take place.

I have already observed that the new colony immediately sets about the increase of their numbers, and everything relating to it. They had their apartments to build, both for the purpose of breeding, and as a storehouse for provisions for the winter. When the season for laying eggs is over, then is the season for collecting honey; therefore when the last chrysalis for the season comes forth its cell is immediately filled with honey, and as soon as a cell is full it is covered over with pure wax, and is to be considered as store for the winter. This covering answers two very essential purposes: one is to keep it from spilling, or daubing the bees; the other to prevent its evaporation, by which means it is kept fluid in such a warmth. They are also employed in laying up a store of bee-bread for the young maggots in the spring, for they begin to bring forth much earlier than probably any other insect, because they retain a summer heat and store up food for the young.

In the month of August we may suppose the queen or queens are impregnated by the males; and as the males do not provide for them-selves, they become burdensome to the workers, and are therefore teazed to death much sooner than they otherwise would die; and when the bees set about this business of providing their winter store, every ope-ration is over, except the collecting of honey and bee-bread. At this time it would seem as if the males were conscious of their danger, for they do not rest on the mouth of the hive in either going out or coming in, but hurry either in or out; however, they are commonly attacked by one, two, or three at a time: they seem to make no resistance, only getting away as fast as possible. The labourers do not sting them, only pinch them, and pull them about as if to wear them out; but I suspect it may be called as much a natural as a violent death.

The whole of the males are now destroyed, and indeed it would have been useless to have saved any to impregnate the queen in the spring. That there may be many more than may be wanted I can easily believe, for this we see throughout nature; but she always times her operations well, although there may be supernumeraries.

When the young are wholly come forth, and either the cells entirely filled, or no more honey to be collected, then is the time or season for remaining in their hives for the winter.

Although I have now completed a hive, and no operations are going on in the winter months, yet the history of this hive is imperfect till it sends forth a new swarm.

As the common bee is very susceptible of cold, we find as soon as the cold weather sets in they become very quiet or still, and remain so throughout the winter, living on the produce of the summer and autumn; and indeed a cold day in the summer is sufficient to keep them at home more so than a shower in a warm day; and if the hive is thin and much exposed, they will hardly move in it, but get as close together as the comb will let them, into a cluster. In this manner they appear to live through the winter; however, in a fine day they become very lively and active, going abroad, and appearing to enjoy it, at which time they get rid of their excrement; for I fancy they seldom throw out their excrement when in the hive. To prove this, I confined some bees in a small hive, and fed them with honey for some days, and the moment I let them out they flew, and threw out their excrement in large quantities; and therefore in the winter, I presume, they retain the contents of their bowels for a considerable time. Indeed, when we consider their confinement in the winter, and that they have no place to deposit their excrement, we can hardly account for the whole of this operation in them. Their excrement is of a yellow colour, and according to their confinement it is found higher and higher up in the intestine, almost as high as the crop.

Their life at this season of the year is more uniform, and may be termed simple existence, till the warm weather arrives again. As they now subsist on their summer's industry, they would seem to feed in proportion to the coldness of the season; for from experiment I found the hive grow lighter in a cold week than it did in a warmer, which led to further experiments. I first made an experiment upon a bee-hive, to ascertain the quantity of honey lost through the winter. The hive was put into the scale November 3, 1776.

			oz.	drams.
November 10th,	it had lost	———	2	7
17th,	———		4	$2\frac{1}{2}$
24th,	———		3	$7\frac{1}{2}$
December 1st,	———		8	2
8th,	———		2	1
15th,	———		5	2
22nd,	———		4	3
29th,	———		5	4
1777. January 1st,	———		2	5
12th,	———		5	2
19th,	———		3	4

		oz.	drams.
January 26th,	it had lost	3	1½
February 2nd,	————	5	0
9th,	————	7	0
	The whole	72	1½

Although an indolent state is very much the condition of bees through the winter, yet progress is making in the queen towards a summer's increase. The eggs in the oviducts are beginning to swell, and I believe in the month of March she is ready to lay them, for the young bees are to swarm in June; which constitutes the queen bee to be the earliest breeder of any insect we know. In consequence of this, the labourers become sooner employed than any other of this tribe of insects This both queen and labourers are enabled to accomplish, from living in society through the winter; and it becomes necessary in them, as they have their colony to form early in the summer, which is to provide for itself for the winter following. All this requires the process to be carried forward earlier than by any other insect, for these are only to have young which are to take care of themselves through the summer, not being under the necessity of providing for the winter.

In the month of April I found in the cells young bees, in all stages, from the egg to the chrysalis state, some of which were changed in colour, therefore were nearly arrived at the fly state, and probably some might have flown.

As this season is too early for collecting the provision of the maggot abroad, the store of farina comes now into use; but as soon as flowers begin to blow, the bees gather the fresh, although they have farina in store, giving the fresh the preference.

Of the Queen.

The queen bee, as she is termed, has excited more curiosity than all the others, although much more belongs to the labourers. From the number of these, and from their exposing themselves, they have their history much better made out; but as there is only one queen, and she scarcely ever seen, it being only the effects of her labour we can come at, an opportunity has been given to the ingenuity of conjecture, and more has been said than can well be proved. She is allowed to be bred in the common way, only that there is a peculiar cell for her in her first stage; and Reaumur says, " her food is different when in the maggot state;" but as there is probably but one queen, that the whole might not depend on one life, it is asserted that the labourers have a power of forming a common maggot into a queen. If authors had given us this as an opinion only, we might have passed it over as improbable; but they have endeavoured to prove it by experiments, which require to be examined. And for that purpose I shall give what they say on that head, with my remarks upon it.

Abstracts from Mr. Schirach.

The following experiments were made to ascertain the origin of the queen bee:—" In twelve wooden boxes were placed twelve pieces of comb, four inches square, each containing both eggs and maggots, so suspended that the bees could come round every part of the comb: in each box was shut up a handful of working bees. Knowing that when bees are forming a queen they should be confined*, the boxes were kept shut for two days. When examined at the end of that period (six boxes only were opened), in all of them royal cells were begun, one, two, or three in each; all of these containing a maggot four days old. In four days, the other six boxes were opened, and royal cells found in each, containing maggots five days old, surrounded by a large provision of jelly; and one of these maggots examined in the microscope, in every respect resembled a working bee.

" This experiment was repeated, and the maggots selected to be made queens were three days old; and in seventeen days there were found in the twelve boxes fifteen lively, handsome queens†. These experiments were made in May, and the bees were allowed to work great part of the summer; the bees were examined one by one, but no drone could be discovered, and yet the queens were impregnated, and laid their eggs‡.

" The above experiment was repeated with pieces of comb containing eggs only, in six boxes, but no preparations were made towards producing a queen§.

* How he came to know this I cannot conceive, for nothing *a priori* could give such information.

† Now this account is not only improbable, but it does not tally with itself. First, it is not probable that a handful of bees should or would set about making two, three, or four queens, when we do not find that number in a large hive; and secondly, it seems inconsistent that only fifteen should be formed out of twelve parcels, when some of the former parcels had four young queens.

‡ Here is a wonder of another kind: queens laying eggs, which (we must suppose Mr. Schirach meant we should believe) they hatched, without the influence of the male.

§ Why eggs, which we must conceive hatched, and produced maggots, did not form queens, one cannot imagine.

" The experiment of producing a queen bee from a maggot was repeated every month of the year, even in November*.

" A maggot three days old was procured from a friend, inclosed in an ordinary cell, and shut up with a piece of comb, containing eggs and maggots. That three days old was formed into a queen, and all the other maggots and eggs were destroyed†.

" In above a hundred experiments a queen has been formed from maggots three days old‡."

Wilhelmi observes that a queen cell, which is made while the bees are shut up, is formed by breaking down three common cells into one, when the maggot is placed in the centre, after which the sides are repaired.

A young queen lately hatched was put into a hive, which had been previously ascertained to contain no drones, and whose queen was removed; and yet the young queen laid eggs§. In repeating Mr. Schirach's experiment, he shut up four pieces of comb, with one maggot in each; after two days the maggots were all dead, and the bees had desisted from labour‖.

A piece of comb from which all the eggs and maggots had been removed, was shut up with some honey and a certain number of workers: in a short time they became very busy, and upon the evening of the second day three hundred eggs were found in the cells¶. He repeated this experiment with the same result, and the bees were left to themselves; they placed queen maggots in the queen cells, newly constructed, and others in male cells; the rest were left undisturbed. He again took two pieces of comb which contained neither eggs nor maggots, and shut them up with a certain number of workers, and carried the box into a stove; next evening, one of the pieces of comb contained several eggs, and the beginning of a royal cell that was empty.

* In which month, as bees never swarm, there could be no occasion for mothers, or supernumerary queens, and still each experiment produced a handsome queen. This is as singular an observation as any. In this country, and in all similar ones, bees hardly breed after July, and by the beginning of September there is hardly a chrysalis to be seen; yet these bred till November, and even laid eggs.

† Why did the bees destroy them in this experiment, and not in others?

‡ The working bees from the above experiments are considered as all females, although the ovaria are too small for examination.

It would appear that a maggot three days old was of the best age for this experiment, yet one should have conceived that a maggot two days old would soon be fit.

§ There is no mystery in this; but did they hatch?

‖ This is the most probable event in the whole experiments.

¶ This would show that labourers can be changed into queens at will, and that neither they nor their eggs require to be impregnated; if this was the case, there would be no occasion for all the push in making a queen or a male.

Besides the short observations contained in the notes, I beg leave to observe that I have my doubts respecting the whole of these experiments, from several circumstances which occurred in mine. The three following facts appear much against their probability; first, a summer's evening in this country is commonly too cold for so small a parcel of bees to be lively, so as to set about new operations; they get so benumbed that they hardly recover in the day, and I should suspect that where these experiments were made (and indeed some are said to have been tried in this country), it is also too cold: secondly, if the weather should happen to be so warm as to prevent this effect, then they are so restless that they commonly destroy themselves, or wear themselves out; at least, after a few days' confinement we find them mostly dead: and thirdly, the account given of the formation of a royal cell, without mentioning the above inconvenience, which is natural to the experiment, makes me suspect the whole to be fabricated. To obviate the first objection, which I found from experiment to prevent any success that otherwise might arise, I put my parcel of bees, with their comb, in which were eggs, as also maggots, and in some of the trials there were chrysalises*, into a warmer place, such as a glass frame over tan, the surface of which was covered with mould to prevent the rising of unwholesome air; but from knowing that the maggot was fed with beebread, or farina, I took care to introduce a cell or two with this substance, as also the flowers of plants that produce a great deal of it, likewise some honey for the old ones. In this state my bees were preserved from the cold, as also provided with necessaries; but after being confined several days, upon opening the door of the hive, what were alive came to the door, walked and flew about, but gradually left it, and on examining the combs, &c., I found the maggots dead, and nothing like any operation going on.

The queen, the mother of all, in whatever way produced, is a true female, and different from both the labourers and the male. She is not so large in the trunk (abdomen) as the male, and appears to be rather larger in every part than the labourers. The scales on the under surface of the belly of the labourers, are not uniformly of the same colour over the whole scale; that part being lighter which is overlapped by the terminating scale above, and the uncovered part being darker; this

---

* I chose to have some chrysalises, for I supposed that if my bees died or flew away, the chrysalises when they came out, which would happen in a few days, not knowing where to go, might stay and take care of the maggots that might be hatched from the eggs; but to my surprise, I found that neither the eggs hatched, nor did the chrysalises come forth; all died; from which I began to suspect that the presence of the bees was necessary for both.

light part does not terminate in a straight line, but in two curves, making a peak, all which gives the belly a lighter colour in the labouring bees; more especially when it is pulled out or elongated.

The tongue of the female is considerably shorter than that of the labouring bee, more like that of the male; however, the tongues of the labourers are not in all of an equal length, but none have it so short as the queen.

The size of the belly of the female of such animals varies a little, according to the condition they are in; but the belly of the male and the labourer has but little occasion to change its size, as they are at all times nearly in the same condition with regard to fat, having always plenty of provision; but the true female varies very considerably; she is of a different size and shape in the summer to what she is in the winter; and in the winter she has what may be called her natural size and shape; she is upon the whole rather thicker than the labourer, and this thickness is also in the belly, which probably arises from the circumstance of the oviduct being in the winter pretty large, and the reservoir for semen full. The termination of the belly is rather more peaked than in the labourers, the last scale being rather narrower from side to side, and coming more to a point at the anus. The scales at this season are more overlapped, which can only be known by drawing them out. In the spring and summer she is more easily distinguished; the belly is not only thicker, but considerably longer than formerly, which arises from the increase of the eggs. We distinguish a queen from the working bee simply by size, and in some degree by colour; but this last is not so easily ascertained, because the difference in the colour is not so remarkable in the back, and the only view we can commonly get of her is on this part; but when a hive is killed, the best way is to collect all the bees, and spread them on white paper, or put them into water in a broad, flat-bottomed, shallow white dish, in which they swim; and by looking at them singly, she may be discovered. As the queen breeds the first year she is produced, and the oviducts never entirely subside, an old queen is probably thicker than a new-bred one, unless indeed the oviducts and the eggs form in the chrysalis state, as in the silk-worm, which I should suppose they did. The queen is perhaps at the smallest size just as she has done breeding, for as she is to lay eggs by the month of March, she must begin early to fill again; but I believe her oviducts are never emptied, having at all times eggs in them, although but small. She has fat in her belly, similar to the other bees.

It is most probable that the queen which goes off with the swarm is a young one, for the males go off with the swarm to impregnate her, as she must be impregnated the same year, because she breeds the same year.

The queen has a sting similar to the working bee.

Of the Number of Queens in a Hive.

I believe a hive or swarm has but one queen, at least I have never found more than one in a swarm, or in an old hive in the winter; and probably this is what constitutes a hive; for when there are two queens, it is likely that a division may begin to take place. Supernumerary queens are mentioned by Riem, who asserts he has seen them killed by the labourers, as well as the males.

November 18th, 1788, I killed a hive that had not swarmed the summer before, and which was to appearance ready to swarm every day; but when I supposed the season for swarming was over, and it had not swarmed, I began to suspect that the reason why it did not was owing to there being no young queen or queens; and I found only one. This is a kind of presumptive proof that I was right in my conjecture; unless it be supposed, that when they were determined not to swarm, they destroyed every queen except one. In a hive that died, I found no males, and only one queen. This circumstance, that so few queens are bred, must arise from the natural security the queen is in from the mode of their society; for although there is but one queen in a wasp's, hornet's, and humble bee's nest or hive, yet these breed a great number of queens; the wasp and hornet some hundreds; but not living in society during the winter, they are subject to great destruction, so that probably not one in a hundred lives to breed in the summer. I have said that the queen leaves off laying in the month of July; and now she is to be impregnated by the males before they die. Mr. Riem asserts, he has seen the copulation between the male and the female, but does not say at what season. I should doubt this; but Mr. Schirach supposes the queen impregnated without copulation. I know not whether he means by this that she is not impregnated at all, and supposes, like Mr. Debraw, that the eggs are impregnated after they are laid, by a set of small drones, who pass over the cells, and thrust their tails down into the cell, so as to besmear the egg*. Mr. Bonnet does not consider it necessary that the drones should be small for this purpose, for he saw a large drone passing over the cells of a piece of comb,

---

* Mr. Debraw, knowing the drones died in the latter end of summer or the autumn, was obliged to suppose a small set of males, that lived through the winter, for that purpose.

stopping at every one which contained an egg, but at no other, and giving a knock with his tail on the mouth of the cell three times; this he supposed was the mode of impregnating the eggs. The number three has always been a famous number; but it will not do where there are no males, which is the case of a hive in the spring, the time when the queen is most employed in laying eggs; which made him suppose the use of the males was to feed the maggots with their semen. It is probable that the copulation is like that of most other insects. The copulation of the humble bee I have seen, it is similar to the common fly. The sting is extended at the time, and turned up on the back, between the two animals: they are some time in this act. In the hornet it is the same. The circumstances relative to the impregnating the queen not being known, great room has been given for conjecture, which, if authors had presented as conjectures only, it would have shown their candour; but they have given, what in them were probably conceits, as facts.

Of the Male Bee.

The male bee is considerably larger than the labourers: he is even larger than the queen, although not so long when she is in her full state with eggs: he is considerably thicker than either, but not longer in the same proportion: he does not terminate at the anus in so sharp a point; and the opening between the two last scales of the back and belly is larger, and more under the belly than in the female. His proboscis is much shorter than that of the labouring bee, which makes me suspect he does not collect his own honey, but takes that which is brought home by the others; especially as we never find the males abroad on flowers, &c. only flying about the hives in hot weather, as if taking an airing; and when we find that the male of the humble bee, which collects its own food, has as long a proboscis or tongue as the female, I think it is from all these facts reasonable to suppose the male of the common bee feeds at home. He has no sting.

The males, I believe, are later in being bred than the labouring bee. As they are only produced to go off with a hive, they are not so early brought forth; for in the month of April I killed a hive, in which I found maggots and chrysalises, but did not find any males among the latter: the maggots are too young for such investigation; but about the 20th of May we observed males: they are all very much of the same size. In the month of August, probably about the latter end, we may suppose they impregnate the queen for the next year, and about

the latter end of the same month, and beginning of September, they are
dying, but seem to be hastened to their end by the labourers. In 1791,
as early as the 19th of June, I saw the labourers killing the males of a
hive, or rather of a swarm, that had not yet swarmed, but was hanging
out; this, however, was out of the common course. They appear to
be sensible of their fate, for they hurry in and out of the hive as quick
as possible, seemingly with a view to avoid the labourers; and we find
them attacked by the labourers, who pinch them with their forceps,
and when they are so hurt, and fatigued with attempts to make their
escape, as not to be able to fly, they are thrown over on the ground
and left to die. That this is the fate of every male bee is easily ascertained, by examining every bee in the hive when killed for the honey,
which is after this season; no male being then found in it. Bonnet
supposes them starved to death, as he never saw wounds on them. In
the course of a winter I have killed several hives, some as late as April,
and in such a way as to preserve every bee, and after examining every
one entirely, I never perceived one male of any kind; although it has
been asserted there are two sizes of males, and that the small are preserved through the winter to impregnate the queen.

Of the Labouring Bee.

This class, for we cannot call it either sex or species, is the largest
in number of the whole community; there are thousands of them to
one queen, and probably some hundreds to each male, as we shall see
by and by. It is to be supposed they are the only bees which construct
the whole hive, and that the queen has no other business but to lay the
eggs: they are the only bees that bring in materials; the only ones we
observe busy abroad; and, indeed, the idea of any other is ridiculous,
when we consider the disproportion in numbers as well as the employment of the others, while the working bee has nothing to take off its
attention to the business of the family. They are smaller than either
the queen or the males: not all of equal size, although the difference is
not very great.

The queen and the working bees are so much alike that the latter
would seem to be females on a different scale: however, this difference
is not so observable in the beginning of winter as in the spring, when
the queen is full of eggs. They are all females in construction, having
the female parts, which are extremely small, and would be easily overlooked by a person not very well acquainted with the parts in the queen:
this has been observed by Mr. Riem; indeed, one might suppose that

they were only young queens, and that they became queens after a certain age; but this is not the case. They all have stings, which is another thing that makes them similar to the queen. From their being furnished with an instrument of defence and offence, they are endowed with such powers of mind as to use it, their minds being extremely irritable; so much so that they make an attack when not meddled with, simply upon suspicion, and when they do attack they always sting; and yet, from the circumstance of their not being able to disengage the sting, one should suppose they would be more cautious in striking with it. When they attack one another, they seldom use it, only their pincers: yet I saw two bees engaged, and one stung the other in the mouth, or thereabouts, and the sting was drawn from the body to which it belonged, and the one who was stung ran very quickly about with it; but I could not catch that bee to observe how the sting was situated.

As they are the collectors of honey, much more than what is for their own use, either immediately or in future, their tongue is proportionably fitted for that purpose: it is considerably longer than that of either the queen or the male, which fits them to take up the honey from the hollow parts of flowers, of considerable depth. The mechanism is very curious, as will be explained further on.

The number of labourers in a hive varies very considerably.

In one hive that I killed there were	3338
In another	4472
In one that died there were	2432
That I might guess at the number of bees from a given bulk, I counted what number an alehouse pint held, when wet, and found it contained	2160
Therefore, as some swarms will fill two quarts, such must consist of near	9000

Of the Parts concerned in the Nourishment of the Bee.

Animals which only swallow food for themselves, or whose alimentary organs are fitted wholly for their own nourishment, have them adapted to that use only; but in many, these organs are common for more purposes, as in the pigeon, and likewise in the bee. In this last, some of the parts are used as a temporary reservoir, holding both that which is for the immediate nourishment of the animal, and also that which is to be preserved for a future day, in the cells formerly described; this last portion is therefore thrown up again, or regurgitated. As it is the labourers alone in the common bee that are so employed, we might conceive this reservoir would belong only to them; but both the queen and males, both in the common and humble bee, have it, as also, I believe, every one of the bee tribe.

As the bee is a remarkable instance of regurgitation, it is necessary the structure of the parts concerned in this operation, and which are also connected with digestion, should be well considered. Ruminating animals may be reckoned regurgitating animals, but in them it is for the purpose of digestion entirely in themselves. But many birds may be called regurgitating animals, and in them it is for the purpose of feeding their young. Crows fill their fauces, making a kind of craw, out of which they throw back the food when they feed their young; but the most remarkable is the dove tribe, who first fill their craw, and then throw it up into the beak of their young*. The bee has this power to a remarkable degree, not however for the purpose of feeding the young, but it is the mode of depositing their store in the cells when brought home.

In none of the above-mentioned regurgitating animals are the reservoirs containing the food the immediate organ of digestion; nor does the reservoir for the honey in the bee appear to be its stomach.

The tongue[a] of the bee is the first of the alimentary organs to be considered: it is of a peculiar structure, and is probably the largest tongue of any animal we know, for its size. It may be said to consist of three parts respecting its length, having three articulations. One, its articulation with the head, which is in some measure similar to our larynx (*mentum*). Then comes the body of the tongue, which is composed of two parts; one, a kind of base (*labium*), on which the other, or true tongue (*lingua*), is articulated. The first part (*labium*) is principally a horny substance, in which there is a groove, and it is articulated with the first or larynx (*mentum*); on the end of this is fixed the true tongue, with its different parts. These two parts of the tongue are as it were inclosed laterally by two horny scales (*maxillæ*), one on each side, which are concave on that side next to the tongue; one edge

---

* See Observations on certain parts of the Animal Œconomy, p. 191 [p. 122 of the present edition].

---

[a] [The part which Hunter so calls includes the maxillæ and their rudimental palpi, the labium and its palpi, as well as the tongue properly so called, which seems, indeed, to be strictly an inordinate development of the labium, or lower lip of the ordinary trophi. I have inserted in the text the terms by which the different parts described by Hunter are known to entomologists.]

is thicker than the other, and they do not extend so far as the other parts. Each of these scales is composed of two parts, or scales, respecting its length, one articulated with the other : the first of those scales (*cardo*) is articulated with the common base, at the articulation of the first part of the tongue, and incloses laterally the second part of the tongue, coming as far forwards as the third articulation : on the end of this is articulated the second scale (*lobus*), which continues the hollow groove that incloses the tongue laterally ; this terminates in a point. These scales have some hairs on their edge.

On the termination of the second part is placed the true tongue, having two lateral portions or processes on each side, one within the other : the external (*palpus labialis*) is the largest, and is somewhat similar to the before-mentioned scales. This is composed of four parts, or rather of one large part, on which three smaller are articulated, having motion on themselves. The first, on which the others stand, is articulated at the edges of the tongue, on the basis or termination of the last-described part of the tongue ; this has hairs on its edge.

A little further forwards on the edges of the tongue are two small thin processes (*paraglossæ*), so small as hardly to be seen with the naked eye. The middle part of all, of which these lateral parts are only appendages, is the true tongue (*lingua*). It is something longer than any of the before-mentioned lateral portions, and is not horny as the other parts are, but what may be called fleshy, being soft and pliable. It is composed of short sections, which probably are so many short muscles, as in fish, for they are capable of moving it in all directions. The tongue itself is extremely villous, having some very long villi at the point, which act, I conceive, somewhat like capillary tubes [a].

This whole apparatus can be folded up, into a very small compass, under the head and neck. The larynx falls back into the neck, which brings the extreme end of the first portion of the tongue within the upper lip, or behind the two teeth ; then the whole of the second part, which consists of five parts, is bent down upon and under this first part, and the two last scales are also bent down over the whole, so that the true tongue is inclosed laterally by the two second horny scales, and over the whole lie the two first.

The œsophagus, in all this tribe of insects, begins just at the root of

---

[a] [Mr. Kirby observes, "The upper part of this tongue is cartilaginous, and remarkable for a number of transverse rings : below the middle it consists of a membrane, longitudinally folded in inaction, but capable of being distended to a considerable size. This membranous bag receives the honey, which the tongue, as it were laps from the flowers, and conveys it to the pharynx."]

the tongue, as in other animals [a], covered anteriorly by a horny scale, which terminates the head, and which may be called the upper lip or the roof of the mouth.   It passes down through the neck and thorax, and when got into the abdomen it immediately dilates into a fine transparent bag, which is the immediate receiver of whatever is swallowed.   From this the food (whatever it be) is either carried further on into the stomach to be digested, or is regurgitated for other purposes.   To ascertain this in some degree in living bees, I caught them going out early in the morning, and found this bag quite empty: some time after I caught others returning home and found the bag quite full of honey, and some of it had got into the stomach.   Now I suppose that which was in the crav⁻ was for the purpose of regurgitation, and as probably they had fasted during the night, part had gone on further for digestion.   Whatever time the contents of this reservoir may be retained, we never find them altered, so as to give the idea of digestion having taken place : it is pure honey.   From this bag the contents can be moved either way ; either downwards to the stomach, for the immediate use of the animal itself, or back again, to be thrown out as store for future aliment.

The stomach arises from the lower end and a little on the right side of this bag.   It does not gradually contract into a stomach, nor is the outlet a passage directly out, but in the centre of a projection which enters some way into the reservoir, being rather an inverted pylorus, thickest at its most projecting part, with a very small opening in the centre, of a peculiar construction.   This inward projecting part is easily seen through the coats of the reservoir, especially if full of honey.

The stomach begins immediately on the outside of the reservoir, and the same part which projects into the reservoir is continued some way into the stomach, but appears to have no particular construction at this end, and therefore it is only fitted to prevent regurgitation into the reservoir, as such would spoil the honey.   This construction of parts is well adapted for the purpose, for the end projecting into the reservoir prevents any honey from getting into the stomach, because it acts there

---

[a] [This observation appears to have been overlooked by entomologists, who continued to believe that the opening of the pharynx was situated below the proboscis in bees, until the researches of Savigny on the oral organs of these insects and of the Lepidoptera were made public.   Cuvier, in his *Analyse des Travaux de la Classe des Sciences Mathématiques et Physiques de l'Institut, pendant l'Année* 1814, observes, "On avait cru voir que l'ouverture du pharynx était située en dessous de cette trompe ou de cette lévre, tandis que dans les masticateurs ordinaires elle l'est en dessous ; mais c'était une erreur ; le pharynx est toujours sur la base de la trompe, et il y est meme garnis de parties intéressantes à reconnaitre, et dont M. Savigny donne une déscription détaillée." p. 25.]

as a valve; therefore whatever is taken in must be by an action of this valvular part. The stomach has a good deal the appearance of a gut, especially as it seems to come out from a bag. It passes almost directly downwards in the middle of the abdomen. Its inner surface is very much increased, by having either circular valves, somewhat like the valvulæ conniventes in the human jejunum, or spiral folds, as in the intestine of the shark, &c.; these may be seen through the external coats. In this part the food undergoes the change. Where the stomach terminates is not exactly to be ascertained, but it soon begins to throw itself into convolutions and becomes smaller.

The intestine makes two or three twists upon itself, in which part it is enveloped in the ducts, constituting the liver and probably the pancreas, and at last passes on straight to the termination of the abdomen. Here it is capable of becoming very large, to serve upon occasion as a reservoir, containing a large quantity of excrement; it then contracts a little, and opens under the posterior edge of the last scale of the back, above the sting in the female and labourers, and the penis in the male [a].

Of the Senses of Bees.

Bees certainly have the five senses. Sight none can doubt. Feeling they also have; and there is every reason for supposing they have likewise taste, smell, and hearing. Taste we cannot doubt; but of smell we may not have such proofs; yet, from observation, I think they give strong signs of smell. When bees are hungry, as a young swarm in wet weather, and are in a glass hive so that they can be examined, if we put some honey into the bottom it will immediately breed a commotion; they all seem to be upon the scent; even if they are weak and hardly able to crawl, they will throw out their proboscides as far as possible to get to it, although the light is very faint. This last appears to arise more from smell than seeing. If some bees are let loose in a bee-hive, and do not know from which house they came, they will take their stand upon the outside of some hive or hives, especially when the evening is coming on; whether this arises from the smell of the hives or sound I can hardly judge.

Of the Voice of Bees.

Bees may be said to have a voice. They are certainly capable of form-

---

[a] [See Preps. 476, 477, 601, 602, 603, 604, 605. Physiological Series, Hunterian Museum.]

ing several sounds. They give a sound when flying, which they can vary according to circumstances. One accustomed to bees can immediately tell when a bee makes an attack by the sound. These are probably made by the wings. They may be seen standing at the door of their hive, with the belly rather raised, and, moving their wings, making a noise. But they produce a noise independent of their wings; for if a bee is smeared all over with honey, so as to make the wings stick together, it will be found to make a noise which is shrill and peevish. To ascertain this further, I held a bee by the legs with a pair of pincers, and observed it then made the peevish noise, although the wings were perfectly still: I then cut the wings off, and found it made the same noise. I examined it in water, but it then did not produce the noise till it was very much teased, and then it made the same kind of noise, and I could observe the water, or rather the surface of contact of the water, with the air at the mouth of an air-hole at the root of the wing, vibrating. I have observed that they, or some of them, make a noise the evenings before they swarm, which is a kind of ring, or sound of a small trumpet: by comparing it with the notes of the piano-forte, it seemed to be the same with the lower A of the treble.

Of the Female Parts.

I may here observe that insects differ from most of the classes of animals above them in having their eggs formed in the ducts along which they pass, not in a cluster on the back, as in some fish (for instance, all of the ray kind, or what are called the amphibia), in the bird, and as is supposed in the quadruped[a]; from thence the eggs are taken up, and by the ducts are carried along to their places of destination.

Of the Oviducts.

The female of the common bee, similar to all the females of the bee tribe, has six oviducts on each side, beginning by very small and almost imperceptible threads, as high as the chest; they then form one cord coiled up, or pass very serpentine, and become larger and larger as they approach the anus, owing to the gradual increased size of the eggs in

[a] [This supposition, that the ova of the mammalia are formed in the ovaria, i. e. in a cluster attached to the dorsal aspect of the abdomen, and not in the ducts along which they pass, is now proved incontestably by the researches of V. Baer and other physiologists.]

them, which are now more distinct, and give the duct a sort of interrupted appearance toward the lower end.   The six ducts, when full of
eggs, make a kind of quadrangle, then all unite into one duct, which
enters the duct common to it and the oviducts of the other side.   The
ducts common to the six oviducts on each side are extremely tender, so
much so that it is difficult to save them.   The duct common to those
on both sides may be called the vagina, and it is continued to the
anus or termination of the belly.

Of the Male Parts.

The male parts of generation in the common bee are much larger than
in the humble bee.   This we suppose necessary, considering the vast
number of eggs the common bee lays more than the humble bee does.

The external parts of generation of the male bee are rather more under the belly than in the others of this tribe, not so much at the termination of the belly, and they are rather more exposed, the two last scales,
especially the under one, not projecting so much ; the two holders are
not so projecting beyond their base, nor are they so hooked or sharp
as in the humble bee ; hardly deserving the name of holders.   From
the external parts passes up into the abdomen a pretty large sheath,
whose termination incloses the glans penis. It is a bulbous part, having
a dark-coloured horny part upon it, which has two processes near its
opening externally, one on each side, of a yellow colour ; it has another
process, which is white, and seems to be a gland.   It can be made to
pass along this sheath or prepuce, and appear externally : I have been
able, with a pair of forceps, to invert the sheath, beginning externally
at the mouth, and pulling out a little at a time, by shifting my hold, till
the glans has appeared externally.

The internal parts are the testicles, with their appendages. The testicles are two small oblong bodies, lying near the back, having a vast
number of air-vessels passing into them, and ramifying upon them.
They are of a pale yellowish colour.   From their lower ends pass down
ducts, which may be called vasa deferentia, and which enter two bags :
these two bags, into which the vasa deferentia enter, are probably reservoirs for the semen.   From the union of these two bags passes out
a duct, which runs towards the termination of the abdomen, and ends
in the penis. These three parts, namely, testicles with their ducts, the
two bags, and the duct arising from them, which I have termed urethra,
are all folded on each other, so as to appear as one body.

In the introduction to this account of bees I observed, that several things in their œconomy might escape us if we considered them alone, but might be made out in other insects : an instance of this occurs in the impregnation of the female bee. The death of the males in the month of August, so that not one is left, and yet the queen to breed in the month of March, must puzzle any one not acquainted with the mode of impregnation of the females of most insects. Insects, respecting the males, are of two kinds : one, where the male lives through the winter, as well as the female ; and the other, where every male of that species dies before the winter comes on ; among which may be considered, as a third, those where both male and female die the same year. Of the first, I shall only give the common fly as an instance ; of the second, I shall just mention all of the bee tribe ; and the third may be illustrated in the silk-worm moth. The mode of impregnation in the first is its being continued uninterruptedly through the whole period of laying eggs ; .while in the second, the copulation is in store ; and in the third the female lays up, by the copulation, a store of semen, although the male is alive. Of this I shall now give an explanation in the silk-moth, which may be applied to the bee, and many other insects.

In dissecting the female parts in the silk-moth, I discovered a bag lying on what may be called the vagina, or common oviduct, whose mouth or opening was external, but it had a canal of communication between it and the common oviduct. In dissecting these parts before copulation I found this bag empty, and when I dissected them after, I found it full. Suspecting this to contain the semen of the male, I immediately conceived the following experiment. I opened the female as soon as the male had united to her, and found the penis in the opening of this bag, and by opening the duct where the penis lay I observed the semen lying on the end of the penis. In another, I observed the bag to fill in the time of copulation ; and in a pair that died in the act, I found the penis in this passage.

When we consider the impregnation of the egg in the silk-worm, we may observe the following circumstances :

First, many of the ova are completely formed, and covered with a hard shell, before copulation ; secondly, the animals are a vast while in the act of copulation ; and, thirdly, the bags at the anus are filled during the time of copulation. From the first observation it appears that the egg can receive the male influence through the hard or horny part of the shell. To know how far the whole, or only a part of the eggs, were impregnated by each copulation, I made the following experiments*. I took a female just emerged out of her cell, and put a male to her, and

* All these experiments on the silk-moth were begun in the summer 1767, and repeated by Mr. Bell in the year 1770.

allowed them to be connected their full time. They were in copulation ten hours. I then put her into a box by herself, and when she
laid her eggs, I numbered the different parcels as she laid them, viz.
1, 2, 3, 4, 5; these eggs I preserved, and in the summer following I
perceived that the No. 5 was as prolific as the No. 1; so that this one
copulation was capable of impregnating the whole brood; and therefore
the male influence must go either along the oviduct its whole length, and
impregnate the incomplete eggs as well as the complete, which appears
to me not likely, or those not yet formed were impregnated from the
reservoir in the act of laying: for I conceived that these bags, by containing semen, had a power of impregnating the egg as it passed along
to the anus, just as it traversed the mouth of the duct of communication.

Finding that eggs completely formed could be impregnated by the
semen, and also finding that the before-mentioned bag was a reservoir for
the semen till wanted, I wished next to discover if they could be impregnated from the semen of this bag; but as this must be done without the act of copulation, I conceived it proper, first, to see whether the
ova of insects might be impregnated without the natural act of copulation, by applying the male semen over the ova, just as they were laid.
The following experiments were made on the silk-moth.

Experiment I. I took a female moth, as soon as she escaped from
her pod, and kept her carefully by herself upon a clean card, till she
began to lay; then I took males that were ready for copulation, opened
them, exposing their seminal ducts, and after cutting into these, collected their semen with a hair pencil: with this semen I covered the
ova, as soon as they passed out of the vagina. The card with these
eggs, having a written account of the experiment upon it, I kept in a
box by itself. In the ensuing season eight of the ova hatched at the
same time with others naturally impregnated. Thus then I ascertained
that the eggs could be impregnated by art, after they were laid[a].

The ova laid by females that had not been impregnated did not stick
where they were laid; so that the semen would appear not only to impregnate the ova, but also to be the means of attaching them.

To know whether that bag in the female silk-moth which increased
at the time of copulation, was filled with the semen of the male, I made
the following experiment.

Experiment II. I took a female moth, as soon as she had escaped
from the pod, and kept her on a card till she began to lay. I then took
females that were fully impregnated before they began to lay, and dis-

---

[a] [This circumstance was proved, as regards the ova of fishes, by Gleditsch. See
Mémoires de l'Acad. de Berlin, 1764.]

sected out that bag which I supposed to be the receptacle for the male
semen; and wetting a camel-hair pencil with this matter, covered the
ova as soon as they passed out of the vagina. These ova were laid
carefully on the clean card, and kept till the ensuing season, when they
all hatched at the same time with those naturally impregnated.

This proves that this bag is the receptacle for the semen, and gradually decreases as the eggs are laid.

Of the Sting of the Bee.

I have observed that it is only the queen and the labourers that have
stings; and this provision of a sting is perhaps as curious a circumstance
as any attending the bee, and probably is one of the characters of the
bee tribe.

The apparatus itself is of a very curious construction, fitted for in-
flicting a wound, and at the same time conveying a poison into that
wound. The apparatus consists of two piercers, conducted in a groove,
or director, which appears to be itself the sting. This groove is somewhat thick at its base, but terminates in a point; it is articulated to the
last scale of the upper side of the abdomen by thirteen thin scales, six
on each side, and one behind the rectum. These scales inclose, as it
were, the rectum or anus all round; they can hardly be said to be articulated to each other, only attached by thin membranes, which allow
of a variety of motions; three of them, however, are attached more
closely to a round and curved process, which comes from the basis of
the groove in which the sting lies, as also to the curved arms of the
sting, which spread out externally. The two stings may be said to begin
by those two curved processes at their union with the scales, and converging towards the groove at its base, which they enter, then pass
along it to its point. They are serrated on their outer edges, near to
the point. These two stings can be thrust out beyond the groove
although not far, and they can be drawn within it; and, I believe, can
be moved singly. All these parts are moved by muscles, which we may
suppose are very strong in them, much stronger than in other animals;
and these muscles give motion in almost all directions, but more particularly outwards. It is wonderful how deep they will pierce solid
bodies with the sting. I have examined the length they have pierced
the palm of the hand, which is covered with a thick cuticle: it has often
been about the $\frac{1}{17}$ of an inch. To perform this by mere force two things
are necessary, power of muscles and strength of the sting, neither of
which they seem to possess in sufficient degree. I own I do not un-

derstand this operation. I am apt to conceive there is something in it distinct from simple force applied to one end of a body; for if this was simply the case, the sting of the bee could not be made to pierce by any power applied to its base, as the least pressure bends it in any direction; it is possible the serrated edges may assist by cutting their way in, like a saw.

The apparatus for the poison consists of two small ducts, which are the glands that secrete the poison: these two lie in the abdomen, among the air-cells, &c.: they both unite into one, which soon enters into, or forms, an oblong bag, like a bladder of urine; at the opposite end of which passes out a duct, which runs towards the angle where the two stings meet; and entering between the two stings, is continued between them in a groove, which forms a canal by the union of the two stings to this point. There is another duct on the right of that described above, which is not so circumscribed, and contains a thicker matter, which, as far as I have been able to judge, enters along with the other: but it is the first that contains the poison, which is a thin, clear fluid. To ascertain which was the poison, I dipped points of needles into both, and pricked the back of the hand; and those punctures that had the fluid from the first-described bags in them grew sore and inflamed, while the others did not. From the stings having serrated edges, it is seldom the bees can disengage them; and they immediately upon stinging endeavour to make their escape, but are generally prevented, as it were caught in their own trap; and the force they use commonly drags out the whole of the apparatus for stinging, and also part of the bowels; so that the bee most frequently falls a sacrifice immediately upon having effected its purpose. Upon a superficial view one conceives that the first intention of the bee having a sting is evident; one sees it has property to defend, and that therefore it is fitted for defence: but why it should naturally fall a sacrifice in its own defence, does not so readily appear: besides, all bees have stings, although all bees have not property to defend, and therefore are not under the same necessity of being so provided. Probably its having a sting to use was sufficient for nature to defend the bee without using it liberally; and the loss of a bee or two, when they did sting, was of no consequence; for it is seldom that more die.

I have now carried the operations of a hive, or the œconomy of the bee, completely round the year; in which time they revolve to the first point we set out at, and the continuance is only a repetition of the same revolutions as I have now described: but those revolutions occasion a series of effects in the comb, which effects in time produce variations in the life of the hive. Besides, there are observations that have little to do with the œconomy of a year, but include the whole of the life of this insect, or at least its hive.

Of the Life of the Bee.

I have observed that the life of the male is only one summer, or rather a month or two ; and this we know from there being none in the winter, otherwise their age could not be ascertained, as it is impossible to learn the age of either the queen or labourers. Some suppose that it is the young bees which swarm ; and most probably it is so : but I think it is probable also, that a certain number of young ones may be retained to keep up the stock, as we must suppose that many of the old ones are, from accidents of various kinds, lost to the hive ; and we could conceive, that a hive three or four years old might not have an original bee in it, although a bee might live twice that time. But there must be a period for a bee to live ; and if I were to judge from analogy, I should say that a bee's natural life is limited to a certain number of seasons ; viz. one bee does not live one year, another two, another three, &c. I even conceive that no individual insect of any species lives one month longer than the others of the same species. I believe this is the case with all insects ; but the age of either a labourer or a queen may never be discovered. One might suppose that the life of a bee, and the time a hive can possibly last, would be nearly equal : although this is not absolutely necessary, because they can produce a succession, which they probably do ; for I am very ready to imagine, that after the first brood in the season, all the last winter bees die, and the hive is occupied with this first brood ; and that they breed the first swarm, or that the old breed the whole of this season's breeding, and then die, and those that continue through the winter are the young, and if so, then they follow the same course with their progenitors.

The comb of a hive may be said to be the furniture and storehouse of the bees, which by use wear out ; and from the description I have given, it will appear that the comb in time will be rendered unfit for use. I observed that they did not clean out the excrement of the maggot, and that the maggot, before it moved into the chrysalis state, lined the cell with a silk, similar to many other insects. It lines the whole cell, top, sides, and bottom ; the two last are permanent ; and at the bottom it covers with this lining its own excrement*. Why the bee maggot is formed to do this is probably because honey afterwards is to be put into the cell ; so that the honey is laid into this last silken bag.

---

* This neither the wasp nor the hornet do, although they do not clean out the excrement of their maggots.

How often they may breed in the same cell I do not know, but I have known them three times in the same season; each time the excrement has been accumulating, and the cell has been lined three times with silk. From this account we must see that a cell in time will be so far filled up as to render it unfit for breeding. On separating the lining of silk, which is easiest done at the bottom, on account of the dried excrement between each lining, I have counted above twenty different linings in one cell, and found the cell about one quarter, or one third filled up; when such a cell, or a piece of comb with such cells, is steeped in water, so as to soften the excrement between the linings, they are separated from each other at the bottom by the swelling of the excrement, so that they can be easily counted. A piece of comb so circumstanced, when boiled for the wax, will keep its form, and the small quantity of wax is squeezed out of different parts as if squeezed out of a sponge, and runs together into the crevices; while a piece of comb, that never has been bred in, even of the same hive, melts almost wholly down. It is this wax that has the fine yellow, while the other of the same hives, although brown, yet shall be white when melted; so that I was led to imagine the wax took its tinge from the farina, excrement, &c., but upon boiling pure wax with such materials it was not tinged with this transparent yellow, only became dirty. In some of those cells that had probably been bred in twenty times or more, when soaked so as to make the excrement swell, I have seen the bottom of the last lining rise even with the mouth, or top of the cell, so that the cavity of the cell was now full: in others, I have seen it rise higher than the mouth, so that the last-formed layers were almost inverted, and turned inside out. A piece of such comb, consisting of two rows of cells, is to be considered as a mould, and the lining of silk and the excrement as the cast; when this is boiled, so as either to extract all the wax or mould, or to destroy its original regular formation which constituted the comb, and nothing is left but the cells of silk, &c., they all easily separate from each other, being only so many casts, with the mould destroyed; and the bottoms, which were indented into each other, are very perfect.

From the above account we must see that the combs of a hive can only last a certain number of years; however, to make them last longer, the bees often add a little to the mouth of the cell, which is seldom done with wax alone, but with a mixture; and they sometimes cover the silk lining of the last chrysalis; but all this makes such cells clumsy, in comparison to the original ones.

ANATOMICAL REMARKS ON A NEW MARINE ANIMAL[a].

ANIMALS which come from foreign countries, and cannot be brought to England alive, must be kept in spirits to preserve them from putrefaction, which makes them less fitted for anatomical examination; for the spirits which preserve them produce a change in many of their properties, and alter the natural colours and texture of their parts, so that often the structure alone of the animal can be ascertained; and where this is not naturally distinct it becomes frequently entirely obscured, and the texture of the finer parts is wholly destroyed, requiring a very extensive knowledge of such parts in animals at large, to assist us in bringing them to light: this happens to be the case with the animal whose dissection is the subject of this postscript.

The animal (Pl. LVIII.) may be said to consist of a fleshy covering, a stomach and intestinal canal, and the two cones with their tentacula and moveable shell, which last may be considered as appendages.

The body of the animal is flattened, and terminates in two edges, which are intersected by rugæ, the fasciculi of transverse muscular fibres which run across the back being continued over them. Upon each of these edges is placed a row of fine hairs, which project to some distance from the skin.

The fleshy covering consists principally of muscular fibres: those upon the back are placed transversely, to contract the body laterally; those on the belly longitudinally, to shorten the animal when stretched out, and to draw it into the shell.

The stomach and intestine make one straight canal: the anterior end of this forms the mouth, which opens into the grooves made by the spiral turns of the tentacula round the stem of each of the cones; and the intestine at the posterior end opens externally, forming the anus. From the contracted state of the animal the intestine is thrown into a number of folds.

On examining the cones and the tentacula I at first believed that the spiral form arose from their being in a contracted state; and that when the tentacula were erected the cone untwisted, forming a longer cone

---

[a] [This animal was sent to Mr. Hunter from Barbadoes by Sir Everard (then Mr.) Home, who described it in the Philosophical Transactions for 1784 as a species of *Actinia*, and the anatomical remarks in the text form the postscript to that Paper. The same species had been, however, previously described and figured by Pallas in the *Miscellanea Zoologica*, p. 139, tab. x. fig. 2—10, (1766), and had been more correctly referred by that distinguished naturalist to the genus *Serpula*, under the name of *Serpula gigantea*. It still retains this denomination, and is placed among the tubicular *Anellides* in the latest edition of the *Règne Animal* of Cuvier.]

with the tentacula arising from its sides, like the plume from the stem of a feather; and that this stem was drawn in or shortened by means of a muscle passing along the centre, which threw the tentacula into a spiral line, similar to the penises of many birds; but how far this is really the case I have not been able to ascertain.

The internal structure of this animal, like most of those which have tentacula, is very simple; it differs, however, materially from many, in having an anus, most animals of this tribe, as the polypi, having only one opening, by which the food is received, and the excrementitious part of it also afterwards thrown out[a]. This we might have supposed, from analogy, to take place in the animal which is here described, more particularly since it is inclosed in a hard shell, at the bottom of which there appears to be no outlet; but as there is an anus this cannot be the case.

It is very singular that in the leech[b], polypi, &c., where no apparent inconvenience can arise from having an anus, there is not one; while in this animal, where it would seem to be attended with many, we find one; but there being no anus in the polypi, &c. may depend upon some circumstance in the animal œconomy which we are at present not fully acquainted with.

The univalves, whose bodies are under similar circumstances respecting the shell with this animal, have the intestine reflected back, and the anus by that means brought near to the external opening of the shell, the more readily to discharge the excrement; and although this structure in these animals appears to be solely intended to answer that purpose, yet when we find the same structure in the black snail, which has no shell, this reasoning will not wholly apply, and we must refer it to some other intention in the animal œconomy[c].

In this animal we must therefore rest satisfied that the disadvantageous situation of the anus, with respect to the excrement's being discharged from the shell, answers some purpose in the œconomy of the animal which more than counterbalances the inconveniences produced by it.

It would appear, from considering all the circumstances, that the excrement thrown out at the anus must pass from the tail along the inside of the tube, between it and the body of the animal, till it comes to the

---

[a] [This is not the case with those Polypi which have the tentacula beset with vibratile cilia, as the *Flustræ*, *Escharæ*, *Vesculariæ*, &c., as in these there is a reflected intestinal canal, terminating by a distinct anus, opening near the mouth.]

[b] [In the leech the alimentary canal terminates by a minute anus, situated above the caudal sucker.]

[c] [The reflected disposition of the intestinal canal is, in a greater or less degree, common to all molluscous animals. and the anus is thus brought into communication with the respiratory cavity.]

external opening of the shell, as there is no other evident mode of discharging it.

How the tube or shell is formed in stone or coral is not easily ascertained. It may be asked whether this animal has the power of boring backwards, as the *Teredo navalis* probably does, or whether the stone or coral is formed at the same time with the animal, and grows and increases with it; and if we consider all the circumstances, this last would appear to be most probable, and agree best with the different phænomena; for the coral is lined with a shell, which could not be the case if the animal was continually increasing this hole, both in length and breadth, in proportion to its growth; but if the coral and the animal increase together, it is then similar to the growth of all shells, whether bivalve or univalve.

The animal does not appear to have the power of increasing its canal, being only composed of soft parts. This, however, is no argument against its doing it, for every shellfish has the power of removing a part of its shell, so as to adapt the new and the old together, which is not done by any mechanical power, but by absorption[a].

The tribe of animals which have tentacula consists of an almost infinite variety, and many of the species have been described. Of that kind, however, which has the double cones, I believe hitherto no account has been given. It is most probably to be found in the seas surrounding the different islands in the West Indies, for I received an animal some years ago from Mr. Oliver, surgeon, at Tenby in Pembrokeshire, which he had procured from a gentleman at St. Vincent's, which, upon examination, proves to be the same animal with that above described, only that the moveable shell is wanting.

Since I began this Postscript I find there is a description of a double-coned Terebella, published by the Rev. Mr. Cordiner, at Banff in Scotland, which was found upon that coast, in which the cones have their tentacula passing out from the end, and when erected they spread from the cone as from a centre. This proves that the animals with double-coned tentacula also have different species.

---

[a] [This is best illustrated in the thinning of the septa between the different whorls of the *cones* and *olives*. If the margins of these septa be examined with a pocket lens, after a section of the shell has been made, it will be found that two out of the three layers of which they were originally composed have been removed. The absorption of shell is also illustrated in the removal or the smoothing down of the spines of the *Murices*; in the flattening of the inner lip of the mouth of the *Purpuræ*; in the widening of the fœcal aperture of the *Fissurellæ*, &c. &c. These instances were doubtless well known to Hunter; but the doctrine of the absorption of shell has been lately adduced as a new discovery, in a recent volume of the Philosophical Transactions. See Mr. J. E. Gray 'On the Power possessed by Mollusca of dissolving Shells.' Phil. Trans. 1833. p. 796.]

OBSERVATIONS ON THE FOSSIL BONES PRESENTED TO
THE ROYAL SOCIETY BY HIS MOST SERENE HIGHNESS
THE MARGRAVE OF ANSPACH, &c.

By THE LATE JOHN HUNTER, Esq., F.R.S.

[Communicated by Everard Home, Esq., F.R.S.[a]]

THE bones which are the subject of the present paper are to be considered more in the light of incrusted bodies than extraneous fossils, since

---

[a] [From the Philosophical Transactions, vol. lxxxiv.; read May 8th, 1794.

The following description, by the Margrave of Anspach, of the caves from which
the fossils described in the text were taken, precedes the original memoir.

" A ridge of primæval mountains runs almost through Germany, in a direction nearly
from west to east; the Hartz, the mountains of Thuringia, the Fichtelberg in Fran-
conia, are different parts of it, which in their further extent constitute the Riesenberg,
and join the Carpathian mountains.   The highest parts of this ridge are granite, and
are flanked by alluvial and stratified mountains, consisting chiefly of limestone, marl,
and sandstone; such at least is the tract of hills in which the caves to be spoken of
are situated; and over these hills the main road leads from Bayreuth to Erlang, or
Nurenberg.   Half-way to this town lies Streitburg, where there is a post, and but
three or four English miles distant from thence are the caves mentioned, near Gailenreuth and Klausstein, two small villages, insignificant in themselves, but become famous
for the discoveries made in their neighbourhood.

" The tract of hills is there broken off by many small and narrow valleys, confined
mostly by steep and high rocks, here and there overhanging, and threatening, as it
were, to fall and crush all beneath; and everywhere thereabouts are to be met with
objects which suggest the idea of their being evident vestiges of some general and
mighty catastrophe which happened in the primæval times of the globe.

" The strata of these hills consist chiefly of limestone of various colour and texture,
or of marl and sandstones.   The tract of limestone hills abounds with petrifactions of
various kinds.

" The main entrance to the caves at Gailenreuth opens near the summit of a limestone hill towards the east.   An arch, near seven feet high, leads into a kind of antechamber, eighty feet in length, and three hundred feet in circumference, which constitutes the vestibule of four other caves.   This antechamber is lofty and airy, but has
no light except what enters by its open arch; its bottom is level, and covered with
black mould, although the common soil of the environs is loam and marl.

" By several circumstances, it appears that it has been made use of in turbulent
times as a place of refuge.

" From this vestibule, or first cave, a dark and narrow alley opens in the corner at
the south end, and leads into the second cave, which is about sixty feet long, eighteen
high, and forty broad.   Its sides and roof are covered, in a wild and rough manner,
with stalactites, columns of which are hanging from the roof, others rising from the
bottom, meeting the first in many whimsical shapes.

" The air of this cave, as well as of all the rest, is always cool, and has, even in the

their external surface has only acquired a covering of crystallized earth, and little or no change has taken place in their internal structure.

---

height of summer, been found below temperate. Caution is therefore necessary to its visitors; for it is remarkable that people, having spent any time in this or the other caverns, always on their coming out again appear pale, which in part may be owing to the coolness of the air, and in part likewise to the particular exhalations within the caves. A very narrow, winding, and troublesome passage opens further into a

" Third cave or chamber, of a roundish form, and about thirty feet diameter, covered all over with stalactites. Very near its entrance there is a perpendicular descent of about twenty feet, into a dark and frightful abyss; a ladder must be brought to descend into it, and caution is necessary in using it, on account of the rough and slippery stalactites. When you are down, you enter into a gloomy cave, of about fifteen feet diameter and thirty feet high, making properly but a segment of the third cave.

" In the passage to this third cave, some teeth and fragments of bones are found; but coming down to the pit of the cave, you are every way surrounded by a vast heap of animal remains. The bottom of this cave is paved with a stalactical crust of near a foot in thickness; large and small fragments of all sorts of bones are scattered everywhere on the surface of the ground, or are easily drawn out of the mouldering rubbish. The very walls seem filled with various and innumerable teeth and broken bones. The stalactical covering of the uneven sides of the cave does not reach quite down to its bottom, whereby it plainly appears that this vast collection of animal rubbish some time ago filled a higher space in the cave, before the bulk of it sunk by mouldering.

" This place is in appearance very like a large quarry of sandstones; and indeed the largest and finest blocks of osteolithical concretes might be hewn out in any number, if there was but room enough to come to them, and to carry them out. This bony rock has been dug into in different places, and everywhere undoubted proofs have been met with, that its bed, or this osteolithical stratum, extends every way far beneath and through the limestone rock into which and through which these caverns have been made; so that the queries suggesting themselves about the astonishing numbers of animals buried here confound all speculation.

" Along the sides of this third cavern there are some narrower openings, leading into different smaller chambers, of which it cannot be said how deep they go. In some of them bones of smaller animals have been found, such as jaw-bones, vertebræ, and tibiæ, in large heaps. The bottom of this cave slopes toward a passage seven feet high, and about as wide, being the entrance to a

" Fourth cave, twenty feet high and fifteen wide, lined all round with a stalactical crust, and gradually sloping to another steep descent, where the ladder is wanted a second time, and must be used with caution as before, in order to get into a cave forty feet high and about half as wide. In those deep and spacious hollows, worked out through the most solid mass of rock, you again perceive with astonishment immense numbers of bony fragments of all kinds and sizes, sticking everywhere in the sides of the cave, or lying on the bottom. This cave also is surrounded by several smaller ones; in one of them rises a stalactite of uncommon bigness, being four feet high and eight feet diameter, in the form of a truncated cone. In another of those side grottos, a very neat stalactical pillar presents itself, five feet in height, and eight inches in diameter.

" The bottom of all these grottos is covered with true animal mould, out of which may be dug fragments of bones.

" Besides the smaller hollows, spoken of before, round this fourth cave, a very narrow opening has been discovered in one of its corners. It is of very difficult access,

The earths with which bones are most commonly incrusted are the calcareous, argillaceous, and siliceous, but principally the calcareous; and this happens in two ways: one, the bones being immersed in water in which this earth is suspended; the other, water passing through masses of this earth, which it dissolves, and afterwards deposits upon bones which lie underneath.

Bones which are incrusted seem never to undergo this change in the earth, or under the water, where the soft parts were destroyed; while bones that are fossilized become so in the medium in which they were deposited* at the animal's death.   The incrusted bones have been previously exposed to the open air: this is evidently the case with the bones at present under consideration, those of the rock of Gibraltar, and those found in Dalmatia; and, from the account given by the Abbé Spallanzani, those of the island of Cerigo are under the same circumstances.   They have the characters of exposed bones, and many of them are cracked in a number of places, particularly the cylindrical bones, similar to the effects of long exposure to the sun.   This circumstance appears to distinguish them from fossilized bones, and gives us some information respecting their history.

If their numbers had corresponded with what we meet with of recent bones, we might have been led to some opinion of their mode of accumulation; but the quantity exceeds anything we can form an idea of. In an inquiry into their history three questions naturally arise: Did the animals come there and die? or, Were their bodies brought there, and lay exposed? or, Were the bones collected from different places?   The

---

* Bones that have been buried with the flesh on acquire a stain which they never lose, and those which have been long immersed in water receive a considerable tinge.

---

as it can be entered only in a crawling posture.   This dismal and dangerous passage leads into a fifth cave, of near thirty feet high, forty-three long, and of unequal breadth. To the depth of six feet this cave has been dug, and nothing has been found but fragments of bones and animal mould.   The sides are finely decorated with stalactites of different forms and colours; but even this stalactical crust is filled with fragments of bones sticking in it, up to the very roof.

" From this remarkable cave another very low and narrow avenue leads into the last discovered, or the

" Sixth cave, not very large, and merely covered with a stalactical crust, in which, however, here and there bones are seen sticking. And here ends this connected series of most remarkable osteolithical caverns, as far as they have been hitherto explored; many more may for what we know exist, hidden, in the same tract of hills.

" Mr. Esper has written a history in German of these caves; and given descriptions and plates of a great number of the fossil bones which have been found there. To this work we must refer for a more particular account of them."]

first of these conjectures appears to me the most natural; but yet I am by no means convinced of its being the true one.

Bones of this description are found in very different situations, which makes their present state more difficultly accounted for. Those in Germany are found in caves; the coast of Dalmatia is said to be almost wholly formed of them; and we know that this is the case with a large portion of the rock of Gibraltar.

If none were found in caves, but in solid masses covered with marl or limestone, it would then give the idea of their having been brought together by some strange cause, as a convulsion in the earth, which threw these materials over them; but this we can hardly form an idea of. Or if they had all been found in caves, we should have imagined these caves were places of retreat for such animals, and had been so for some thousands of years; and if the bones were those of carnivorous animals and herbivorous, we might have supposed that the carnivorous had brought in many animals of a smaller size which they caught for food. And this, upon the first view, appears to have been the case with those which are the subject of this paper; yet when we consider that the bones are principally of carnivorous animals, we are confined to the supposition of their being only places of retreat. If they had been brought together by any convulsion of the earth, they would have been mixed with the surrounding materials of the mountains, which does not appear to be the case; for although some are found sticking in the sides of the caves incrusted in calcareous matter, this seems to have arisen from their situation in the cave. Such accumulation would have made them coeval with the mountains themselves, which from the recent state of the bones I should very much doubt.

The difference in the state of the bones shows that there was probably a succession of them for a vast series of years; for if we consider the distance of time between the most perfect having been deposited, which we must suppose were the last, and the present time, we must consider it to be many thousand years. And if we calculate how long these must still remain to be as far decayed as some others are, it will require many thousand years, a sufficient time for a vast accumulation. From this mode of reasoning, therefore, it would appear that they were not brought here at once in a recent state.

The animal earth, as it is called, at the bottom of these caves, is supposed to be produced by the rotting of the flesh, which is supposing the animals brought there with the flesh on; but I do conceive that, if the caves had been stuffed with whole animals, the flesh could not have produced one tenth part of the earth; and, to account for such a quan-

tity as appears to be the produce of animals, I should suppose it the remains of the dung of animals who inhabited the caves, and the contents
of the bowels of those they lived upon.   This is easily conceived from
knowing that there is something similar to it, in a smaller degree, in
many caves in this kingdom, which are places of retreat for bats in the
winter, and even in the summer, as they only go abroad in the evenings.
These caves have their bottoms covered with animal earth, for some feet
in depth, in all degrees of decomposition, the lowermost the most pure,
and the uppermost but little changed, with all the intermediate degrees;
in which caves are formed a vast number of stalactites, which might incrust the bones of those that die there[a].

The bones in the caves in Germany are so much the object of the
curious that the specimens are dispersed throughout Europe, which
prevents a sufficient number coming into the hands of any one person
to make him acquainted with the animals to which they belong.

From the history and figures given by Esper it appears that there are
the bones of several animals; but what is curious, they all appear to
have been carnivorous, which we should not have expected.   There are
teeth, in number, kind, and mode of setting, exactly similar to the white
bear, others more like those of the lion; but the representations of parts,
however well executed, are hardly to be trusted to for the nicer characters, and much less so when the parts are mutilated[b].

The bones sent by his Highness the Margrave of Anspach agree with
those described and delineated by Esper as belonging to the white bear;
how far they are of the same species among themselves I cannot say.
The heads differ in shape from each other; they are, upon the whole,
much longer for their breadth than in any carnivorous animal I know of:
they also differ from the present white bear, which, as far as I have seen,

---

[a] [Hunter probably little suspected that there were caves in this kingdom, like those
of Germany, abounding with the remains of extinct mammalia.   These caves, especially
that of Kirkdale in Yorkshire, and the fossils discovered in them, are admirably described in the ‘Reliquiæ Diluvianæ’ of Dr. Buckland; and it is gratifying to find that
the conclusion which Hunter adopted, out of the different hypotheses which he suggests
to account for the presence of the bears’ bones in the Bayreuth caverns, viz. that these
had served as an habitual retreat to the living animals, and had thus become the depository of the remains of successive generations, agrees with the theory proposed by
Dr. Buckland with reference to the bones of the hyænas, accumulated at Kirkdale, the
chief argument in support of which is derived from the abundance of earthy or bony
dung with which the fossils are associated.]

[b] [Remains of an indubitably large feline animal have been found associated with
the bears’ bones in the Bayreuth and Gaybureuth caverns.   The mutilated cranium
figured by Leibnitz in his Protogæa, Pl. XI., is considered by Soemmering to have belonged to a lion.]

has a common proportional breadth. It is supposed, indeed, that the heads of the present white bear differ from one another; but the truth of this assertion I have not seen heads enough of that animal to determine.

The heads not only vary in shape but also in size; for some of them, when compared with the recent white bear, would seem to have belonged to an animal twice its size: while some of the bones correspond in size with those of the white bear, and others are even smaller*.

There are two ossa humeri, rather of a less size than those of the recent white bear; a first vertebra, rather smaller; the teeth also vary considerably in size, yet they are all those of the same tribe; so that the variety among themselves is not less than between them and the recent.

In the formation of the head, age makes a considerable difference: the skull of a young dog is much more rounded than an old one; the ridge leading back to the occiput, terminating in the two lateral ones, hardly exists in a young dog; and among the present bones there is the back part of such a head, yet it is larger than the head of the largest mastiff; how far the young white bear may vary from the old, similar to the young dog, I do not know, but it is very probable[a]. Drawings of the different heads and ossa humeri, done in a very masterly manner by Mr. Batty, surgeon, in Great Marlborough-street, who was so obliging as to take that trouble, are annexed to this account. See Tab. LIX. and LX.

Bones of animals under circumstances so similar, although in different parts of the globe, one would have naturally supposed to consist chiefly of those of one class or order in every place, one principle acting in all places[b]. In Gibraltar they are mostly of the ruminating tribe, of

---

* It is to be understood that the bones of the white bear that I have, belonged to one that had been a show, and had not grown to the full or natural size; and I make allowance for this in my assertion that the heads of those incrusted appear to belong to an animal twice the size of our white bear.

---

[a] [There are now skulls of the young and old white bear in the Collection of the College of Surgeons in London which confirm Hunter's conjecture respecting the difference of form which is due to age in this genus. It will be seen that Hunter adduces this circumstance merely as one which must be taken into consideration in comparing recent and fossil crania of the same genus; and that he by no means asserts, as Cuvier states he does, that the differences which he had detected between the fossil and recent skulls, and between the different fossil skulls of the cave bears, are of the same nature and degree.—*Ossemens Fossiles*, 6me Ed., tom. vii. p. 236.]

[b] [This sagacious conjecture has received remarkable confirmation from recent discoveries; the fossil bones that have been found in Australia appertain for the most part to animals of the marsupial order, and those collected in South America contain

the hare kind, and the bones of birds; yet there are some of a small dog or fox, and likewise shells. Those in Dalmatia appear to be mostly of the ruminating tribe; yet I saw a part of the os hyoides of a horse; but those from Germany are mostly carnivorous. From these facts we should be inclined to suppose that their accumulation did not arise from any instinctive mode of living, as the same mode could not suit both carnivorous and herbivorous animals[a].

In considering animals respecting their situation upon the globe, there are many which are peculiar to particular climates, and others that are less confined, as herrings, mackerel, and salmon; others again which probably move over the whole extent of the sea, as the shark, porpus, and whale tribe; while many shellfish must be confined to one spot[b]. If the sea had not shifted its situation more than once, and was to leave the land in a very short time, then we could determine what the climate had formerly been by the extraneous fossils of the stationary animals, for those only would be found mixed with those of passage; but if the sea moves from one place to another slowly, then the remains of animals of different climates may be mixed, by those of one climate moving over those of another, dying, and being fossilized; but this I am afraid cannot be made out. By the fossils we may, however, have some idea how the bones of the land animals fossilized may be disposed with respect to those of the sea.

If the sea should have occupied any space that never had been dry land prior to the sea's being there, the extraneous fossils can only be those of sea animals; but each part will have its particular kind of those that are stationary mixed with a few of the amphibia, and of sea birds, in those parts that were the skirts of the sea. I shall suppose that when the sea left this place it moved over land where both vegetables and land animals had existed, the bones of which will be fossilized, as also those of the sea animals; and if the sea continued long here, which

a remarkable proportion of Edentata, some of them of gigantic proportions, but all protected by a bony armour analogous to that of the armadillos, which are peculiar to South America.]

[a] [Mr. Lyell thus describes some of the circumstances under which the bones of animals are accumulated at Gibraltar: "At the north extremity of the rock are perpendicular fissures, on the ledges of which a number of hawks nestle and rear their young in the breeding season. They throw down from their nests the bones of small birds, mice, and other animals, on which they feed, and these are gradually united into a breccia of angular fragments of the decomposing limestone with a cement of red earth." (Principles of Geology, vol. iii. p. 158.)]

[b] [For a full development of the relation which the geographical distribution of animals bears to the science of Oryctology, or Fossil Remains, the reader is referred to the second and third volumes of Lyell's Principles of Geology.]

there is reason to believe, then those mixed extraneous fossils will be covered with those of sea animals. Now if the sea should again move, and abandon this situation, then we should find the land and sea fossils above mentioned disposed in this order; and as we begin to discover extraneous fossils in a contrary direction to their formation, we shall first find a stratum of those of animals peculiar to the sea, which were the last formed, and under it one of vegetables and land animals, which were there before they were covered by the sea, and among them those of the sea, and under this the common earth. Those peculiar to the sea will be in depth in proportion to the time of the sea's residence and other circumstances, as currents, tides, &c.

From a succession of such shiftings of the situation of the sea we may have a stratum of marine extraneous fossils, one of earth, mixed probably with vegetables and bones of land animals, a stratum of terrestrial extraneous fossils, then one of marine productions; but from the sea carrying its inhabitants along with it, wherever there are those of land animals there will also be a mixture of marine ones ; and from the sea commonly remaining thousands of years in nearly the same situation, we have marine fossils unmixed with any others[a].

All operations respecting the growth or decomposition of animal and vegetable substances go on more readily on the surface of the earth than in it; the air is most probably the great agent in decomposition and combination, and also a certain degree of heat. Thus the deeper we go into the earth we find the fewer changes going on ; and there is probably a certain depth where no change of any kind can possibly take place. The operation of vegetation will not go on at a certain depth, but at this very depth a decomposition can take place, for the seed dies, and in time decays ; but at a still greater depth the seed retains its life for ages, and when brought near enough to the surface for vegetation it grows. Something similar to this takes place with respect to extraneous fossils; for although a piece of wood or bone is dead when so situated as to be fossilized, yet they are sound and free from decomposition, and the depth, joined with the matter in which they are often found, as stone, clay, &c. preserves them from putrefaction, and their dissolution requires thousands of years to complete it; probably they may be under the same circumstances as in a vacuum ; the heat in such

---

[a] [The importance of the study of fossil remains in the elucidation of the nature of the changes to which the earth's surface has been subject, here dwelt upon by Hunter, was placed in a strong light by the subsequent researches of Cuvier and Brogniart on the structure of the Paris Basin, and the fossils which have rendered it so famous. By the aid of these fossils Cuvier was enabled to refer the succession of strata to several distinct alternations of marine and freshwater formations.]

situations is uniform, probably in common about 52° or 53°, and in the colder regions they are still longer preserved.

I believe it is generally understood that in extraneous fossils the animal part is destroyed, but I find that this is not the case in any I have met with.

Shells, and bones of fish, most probably have the least in quantity, having been longest in that state; otherwise they should have the most; for the harder and more compact the earth, the better is the animal part preserved, which is an argument in proof of their having been the longest in a fossil state. From experiment and observation the animal part is not allowed to putrefy; it appears only to be dissolved into a kind of mucus, and can be discovered by dissolving the earth in an acid: when a shell is treated in this way the animal substance is not fibrous or laminated, as in the recent shell, but without tenacity, and can be washed off like wet dust; in some, however, it has a slight appearance of flakes.

In the shark's tooth, or glosso-petra, the enamel is composed of animal substance and calcareous earth, and is nearly in the same quantity as in the recent; but the central part of the tooth has its animal substance in the state of mucus interspersed in the calcareous matter.

In the fossil bones of sea animals, as the vertebræ of the whale, the animal part is in large quantity, and in two states, the one having some tenacity, but the other like wet dust; but in some of the harder bones it is more firm. In the fossil bones of land animals, and those which inhabit the waters, as the sea-horse, otter, crocodile, and turtle, the animal part is in considerable quantity. In the stags' horns dug up in Great Britain and Ireland, when the earth is dissolved, the animal part is in considerable quantity, and very firm. The same observations apply to the fossil bones of the elephant found in England, Siberia, and other parts of the globe; also those of the ox kind; but more particularly to their teeth, especially those from the lakes in America, in which the animal part has suffered very little; the inhabitants find little difference in the ivory of such tusks from the recent, but its having a yellow stain; the cold may probably assist in their preservation.

The state of preservation will vary according to the substance in which they have been preserved; in peat and clay I think the most; however, there appears in general a species of dissolution, for the animal substance, although tolerably firm, in a heat a little above 100° becomes a thickish mucus, like dissolved gum, while a portion from the external surface is reduced to the state of wet dust.

In incrusted bones the quantity of animal substance is very different in different bones. In those from Gibraltar there is very little; it in part retains its tenacity, and is transparent, but the superficial part dissolves into mucus.

Those from Dalmatia give similar results when examined in this way.

Those from Germany, especially the harder bones and teeth, seem to contain all the animal substance natural to them; they differ, however, among themselves in this respect.

The bones of land animals have their calcareous earth united with the phosphoric acid instead of the aerial[a], and I believe retain it when fossilized, nearly in proportion to the quantity of animal matter they -contain.

The mode by which I judge of this is by the quantity of effervescence; when fossil bones are put into the muriatic acid it is not nearly so great as when a shell is put into it, but it is more in some, although not in all, than when a recent bone is treated in this way, and this I think diminishes in proportion to the quantity of animal substance they retain; as a proof of this, those fossil bones which contain a small portion of animal matter produce in an acid the greatest effervescence when the surface is acted on, and very little when the centre is affected by it; however, this may be accounted for by the parts which have lost their phosphoric acid, and acquired the aerial, being easiest of solution in the marine acid, and therefore dissolved first, and the aerial acid let loose.

In some bones of the whale the effervescence is very great; in the Dalmatia and Gibraltar bones it is less; and in those the subject of the present paper it is very little, since they contain by much the largest proportion of animal substance[b].

---

[a] [Carbonic.]

[b] [In this Paper we may perceive that Hunter appreciated the value of the study of Fossil Remains, and their application to the elucidation of many important subjects. First, with reference to the extension of our ideas respecting the zoology of this planet, we find him comparing the fossils which are the subject of the text, with their recent analogues, and he shows that they differ both from them and among themselves: his observations and comparisons are, it is true, too general and summary, and it was left to his successors in this field of inquiry to pursue the comparison with the requisite minuteness and precision, and to give names to the distinct but extinct species. Hunter next briefly alludes to the different situations and climates in the globe, to which animals are more or less confined; and this subject, or the geographical distribution of animals, considered in relation to fossil remains, elucidates, amongst other interesting questions, the changes of temperature to which different parts of the earth have been subject at different epochs. Hunter points out more distinctly, and with more detail, the evidence which extraneous fossils afford respecting the alternations of land and sea, of which the earth's surface has been the theatre; and by his frequent allusion to the "many thousand years" which must have elapsed during these periods, seems to have fully appreciated the necessity of an ample allowance of past time in order to account philosophically for the changes in question. Lastly, he treats of the nature and causes of the different states in which the remains of extinct animals are found; and

many of the fossil bones which were the subject of his chemical experiments are still preserved in his museum (see Nos. 118—130, Physiological Series).

When we turn from the perusal of this highly philosophical memoir to the notice of it in the *Ossemens Fossils* of Cuvier, we must suppose that it could have been but very imperfectly known to the great founder of oryctological science.   In the chapter on the ' Ours Fossiles,' Cuvier says : " Le célèbre chirurgeon anglais, J. Hunter, dans un Mémoire sur les os fossiles, *qui n'a que leur analyse chimique pour objet*, et qui est inséré dans les Transactions Philosophiques, donne deux belles figures de crânes d'ours fossiles les meillures qui aient paru jusque là, mais sans déscription détaillée, et en disant pour toute comparaison que les différentes têtes *d'ours de cavernes* diffèrent autant entre elles qu'elles diffèrent de *l'ours polaire*, et que toutes ces différences ne surpassent point 'celles que l'âge peut produire dans les animaux carnassiers; assertion vague et même erronée."—*Loc. cit.*, p. 236.

A careful and candid perusal of Hunter's Memoir would doubtless have exonerated the author from this charge in the mind of Cuvier, as it must do in that of every unprejudiced reader.   But it would still afford a very inadequate notion of the extent to which Hunter had pursued his study of fossil remains.   The interest that he took in them is shown by the frequent exhortations towards their collection in his letters to Jenner, and his collection at his decease included about 1050 specimens, of which there are 259 belonging to the vertebrate classes (including 70 specimens of fossil fishes, and 40 of reptiles), 116 cephalopods, 166 univalves, 143 bivalves, 35 crustacea, 163 echinodermata, 109 zoophytes, and 50 fossil vegetable productions.]

DESCRIPTIONS OF SOME ANIMALS FROM NEW SOUTH WALES.

By John Hunter, F.R.S.

[The following descriptions are interesting, not less from being the first that appeared of some of the most singular of the quadrupeds which characterize the Fauna of Australia, than from the celebrity of their author, of whose contributions to descriptive zoology they are almost the only examples. They form part of the zoological appendix to a "Journal of a voyage to New South Wales, 4to, 1790," published by John White, Esq., Surgeon-General to the settlement, who thus acknowledges the assistance which he derived from the gentlemen by whose cooperation he was " enabled to surmount those difficulties that necessarily attended the description of so great a variety of animals, presented for the first time to the observation of the naturalist, and consequently in the class of nondescripts. Among those gentlemen he has the honour particularly to reckon the names of Dr. Shaw, Dr. Smith, the possessor of the celebrated Linnæan Collection ; and John Hunter, Esq., who to a sublime and inventive genius, happily unites a disinterested and generous zeal for the promotion of natural science."

Dr. Shaw, who superintended the publication of White's Zoological Appendix, thus introduces the observations contributed by Hunter :—

" The nondescript animals of New South Wales occupied a great deal of Mr. White's attention, and he preserved several specimens of them in spirits, which arrived in England in a very perfect state. There was no person to whom these could be given with so much propriety as Mr. Hunter, he perhaps, being most capable of examining accurately their structure, and making out their place in the scale of animals ; and it is to him that we are indebted for the following observations upon them, in which the anatomical structure is purposely avoided, as being little calculated for the generality of readers of a work of this kind."]

IT is much to be wished that those gentlemen who are desirous of obliging their friends, and promoting the study of natural history, by sending home specimens, would endeavour to procure all the information they can relating to such specimens as they may collect, more especially animals.

The subjects themselves may be valuable, and may partly explain their connection with those related to them, so as in some measure to establish their place in nature[a], but they cannot do it entirely; they only give us the form and construction, but leave us in other respects to conjecture, many of them requiring further observation relative to their œconomy.

A neglect in procuring this information has left us almost to this day very ignorant of that part of the natural history of animals which is the most interesting.   The Opossum is a remarkable instance of this. There is something in the mode of propagation in this animal, that deviates from all others; and although known in some degree to be extraordinary, yet it has never been attempted, where opportunity offered, to complete the investigation.   I have often endeavoured to breed them in England; I have bought a great many, and my friends have assisted me by bringing them or sending them alive, yet never could get them to breed; and although possessed of a great many facts respecting them, I do not believe my information is sufficient to complete the system of propagation in this class[b].

---

[a] [It is interesting to meet with these indications of the spirit in which Hunter prosecuted his zoological researches.   To ascertain the affinities of the animals whose structure he explored, or, in other words, to establish a natural system of classification, was not less the aim of Hunter than the determination of the functions of the different organs in the animal frame; and the truth of the remark of the necessity of combining observation of the living habits of animals, with anatomical and zoological research, in order to establish entirely their place in nature, as well as to fully understand their œconomy, is now universally admitted.]

[b] [Since the time of Mr. Hunter, the kangaroo by breeding in this country has afforded the opportunity of elucidating many of the peculiarities of the generative œconomy of the Marsupial quadrupeds.   These peculiarities are not confined to the female. In the male, the testicles are situated in an external fold of the integument, corresponding in situation to the internal fold which constitutes the marsupial pouch in the female, and the scrotum thus formed is consequently anterior to the penis.   The cremaster muscles wind round the supplementary bones attached to the pubis, which act as fulcra to the muscles, and enable them to compress the gland with a force which seems to be demanded in consequence of the tortuosity of the double vagina along which the semen has to be propelled.   The coitus is of long duration in the kangaroo, and the scrotum disappears during the forcible retraction of the testes against the marsupial bones.

The female kangaroo is pregnant for the space of thirty-eight days, when uterine birth takes place, and the embryo, now about an inch in length, is transferred, I suspect, by the mouth of the parent, from the vulva to the nipple, where it hangs, protected and concealed by the pouch for about six months.

Only two opportunities have as yet occurred for the examination of the uterine fœtus.

In collecting animals, even the name given by the natives if possible should be known, for a name to a naturalist should mean nothing but

---

These show that it is nourished chiefly by means of omphalo-mesenteric vessels, which ramify over a large vitelline sac. When the extremities are formed, and the uterine fœtus has attained about two-thirds its size as such, an allantois is developed ; the umbilical arteries co-extended with this sac do not, however, as in the placental mammalia, pass to the chorion ; but this membrane continues unorganized, as in the ovoviviparous and oviparous classes, and consequently there is no adhesion of the fœtal membranes to the uterine parietes, and therefore no obstruction to the escape of the embryo (at the premature period destined for its birth) from the uterus into the va-gina.

The uterus is double in all the marsupiata, and each cavity is of small size, and of a simple elongated form. In the *Didelphis dorsigera*, each os tincæ opens into a long vagina, which makes a sweep outwards, and then converging towards its fellow, opens into the upper end of a cloacal passage, common to the two vaginæ and the urethra. In the Virginian opossum, each vagina, before describing the outward curvature, sends down a cul-de-sac, which is closely united to the one on the opposite side, but the cavities are distinct. In the kangaroo, the two cul-de-sacs are blended together, so that the vaginæ communicate together both at their commencement, and also at their termination in the meatus communis. The size of the vaginal cul-de-sacs seems to be in the ratio of the capacity of the external pouch.

The embryo is adapted to its intra-marsupial existence by a precocious development of the respiratory and circulating organs, by a peculiar tubular form of the mouth, and a grooved tongue calculated to retain a firm hold on the elongated nipple ; it has also a peculiar construction of the larynx, somewhat analogous to that of the whale, by which respiration may be safely continued in the fœtus while the mother injects the milk down its pharynx. It would seem that the new-born marsupial is incompetent from its feeble and incomplete structure to the office of forcing a stream of milk through the long and tortuous lacteal ducts, since the mammary gland is embraced by a muscle, corresponding to the cremaster in the male, and winding in a similar manner round the marsupial bones ; these therefore aid the expulsion of the milk in the female, as they do that of the se-men in the male ; they also in the female add to the power of the mammary muscles in sustaining a portion of the weight of the fœtus which is attached to the nipple.

Many have been the conjectures respecting the final intention of the premature birth of the marsupial animal, and of the various singular modifications of structure necessitated by, and adapted to that circumstance. Since it obtains in quadrupeds of almost every variety of form, and with various modes of locomotion and diversity of diet, it must result from some more general law than individual proportions or habits of the parent. It is associated with a marked inferiority of cerebral organiza-tion ; but the final purpose will be most probably discovered to relate to some pecu-liarity in the physical geography of that portion of the globe in which the quadrupeds almost exclusively exhibit the marsupial organization. Long-continued droughts and a scarcity of freshwater streams are amongst the most striking features of the cli-mate and territory of Australia ; and when we reflect that the principal exceptions to the marsupial organization, viz., the Ornithorhynchus and the Hydromys, or water-rat of the colonists, habitually inhabit the freshwater ponds, the peculiarities of the re-production above described may have reference to the great distances which the mammalia of New South Wales are generally compelled to traverse in order to quench their thirst.]

that to which which it is annexed, having no allusion to anything else, for when it has it divides the idea. This observation applies particularly to the animals which have come from New Holland; they are, upon the whole, like no other that we yet know of, but as they have parts in some respects similar to others, names will naturally be given to them expressive of those similarities, which has already taken place ; for instance, one is called the kangaroo rat, but which should not be called either kangaroo or rat ; I have therefore adopted such names as can only be appropriated to each particular animal, conveying no other idea [a].

Animals admit of being divided into great classes, but will not so di-

---

[a] [The evils of implying false affinities and of suppressing differences of primary importance, which would have resulted from referring the newly discovered quadrupeds of Australia to the known Linnæan genera, as was afterwards done by Dr. Shaw, were sagaciously avoided by Hunter. And had the same expanded views been taken by his colleague, zoology would not at the present time have been burdened with such useless synonyms as *Didelphys petaurus*, *Didelphys penicillata*, *Didelphys viverrina*, *Didelphys obesula*, &c., and the zoologists of the continent might have been spared the task of rectifying the errors of that arrangement, which arising from an ignorance of the anatomical distinctions of the animals in question, and from a disregard of the modifications presented by their teeth and locomotive extremities, consisted in grouping with the American opossums the species above quoted,—species which now form respectively the types of the genera *Petaurus*, *Phascogale*, *Dasyurus* and *Perameles*. Hunter, on the contrary, adopted the more natural and philosophical method of accurately pointing out the differences and resemblances of each species, retaining for them, like Adanson with reference to the nondescripts of Senegal, the native names, instead of applying to them Linnæan generic appellatives, which could only serve to propagate erroneous ideas of the objects to which they were attached. These reflections are so obviously suggested by the text, that the following is offered as an apology for their insertion : the writer of a volume entitled a " Discourse on the Study of Natural History", which by some unfortunate casualty has appeared in the same series of publications as that which contains Herschel's admirable Discourse on Natural Philosophy, introduces the name of John Hunter in his account of the naturalists who have contributed to the rise and progress of zoology for the sole purpose of instituting a disparaging comparison between that great and original thinker and the author of the General Zoology. " Dr. Shaw", Mr. Swainson observes, " was unquestionably the writer of nearly all the zoological descriptions in White's Voyage to New South Wales, whereas he (John Hunter) merely wrote the account of five of the quadrupeds and these are neither named nor scientifically characterized."

Now the fact is that Hunter's descriptions of the parts best adapted for zoological characters are so exact and so minute that a zoologist has no difficulty in assigning the species to the most recent zoological subdivisions, as any one may convince himself who compares the account of the *Tapao Tafa* with the characters assigned by Temminck to his genus *Phascogale*. But Hunter added also observations on the differences and peculiarities of the internal structure of the marsupial quadrupeds, yet Dr. Shaw was so blind to the true methods of advancing the science of zoology, and so little able to appreciate the labours of his colleague to this end, that science was deprived of the benefit of Hunter's anatomical description of five marsupial genera, because they were, in Dr. Shaw's estimation, little calculated for the readers of a zoological appendix !]

stinctly admit of subdivision without interfering with each other. Thus the class called quadrupeds is so well marked that even the whole is justly placed in the same class, birds the same, amphibia (as they are called) the same, and so of fishes, &c.; but when we are subdividing these great classes into their different tribes, genera and species, then we find a mixture of properties, some species of one tribe partaking of similar properties with a species of another tribe.

Of the Kangaroo[a].

This animal (probably from its size) was the principal one taken notice of in this island; the only parts at first brought home were some skins and skulls, and I was favoured with one of the skulls from Sir Joseph Banks. As the teeth of such animals as are already known in some degree point out their digestive organs, I was in hopes that I might have been able to form an opinion of the particular tribe of the animals already known to which the kangaroo should belong; but the teeth did not accord with those of any one class of animals I was acquainted with, therefore I was obliged to wait with patience till I could get the whole; and in many of its other organs the deviation from other animals is not less than in its teeth. In its mode of propagation it very probably comes nearer to the opossum than any other animal, although it is not at all similar to it in other respects. Its hair is of a greyish brown colour, similar to that of the wild rabbit of Great Britain, is thick and long when the animal is old; but it is late in growing, and when only begun to grow it is like a strong down; however, in some parts it begins earlier than others, as about the mouth, &c. In all of the young kangaroos yet brought home (although some as large as a full-grown rat) they have all the marks of a fœtus : no hair; ears lapped close over the head; no marks on the feet of having been used in progressive motion : the large nail on the great toe sharp at the point, and the sides of the mouth united something like the eyelids of a puppy just whelped, having only a passage at the anterior part. This union of the two lips on the sides is of a particular structure; it wears off as it grows up, and by the time it is the size of a small rabbit, disappears.

Of the Teeth of the Kangaroo.

The teeth of this animal are so singular that it is impossible from them to say what tribe it is of. There is a faint mixture in them, corresponding to those of different tribes of animals. Take the mouth at large,

---

[a] [The species here for the first time described is the *Macropus major* of modern systems : several other species of the same genus have since been discovered.]

respecting the situation of the teeth, it would class in some degree
with the *Scalpris dentata* [n], in a fainter degree with the horse and ruminants; and with regard to the line of direction of all the teeth, they are
very like those of the *Scalpris dentata*. The fore teeth in the upper jaw
agree with the hog, and those in the lower, in number, with the *Scalpris
dentata*, but with regard to position, and probably use, with the hog.
The grinders would seem to be a mixture of hog and ruminant, the enamel on their external and grinding surfaces rather formed into several
cutting edges than points.   There are six incisors in the upper jaw and
only two in the lower, but these two are so placed as to oppose those of
the upper; five grinders in each side of each jaw, the most anterior of
which is small [b].

The proportions of some of the parts of this animal bear no analogy
to what is common in most others.   The disproportions in the length
between the fore legs and the hind are very considerable, also in their
strength, yet perhaps not more than in the jerboa.   This disproportion
between the fore legs and the hind is principally in the more adult; for
in the very young, about the size of a half-grown rat, they are pretty
well proportioned; which shows that at the early period of life they
do not use progressive motion [c].   The proportions of the different parts

---

[a] [This tribe includes the rat, &c. (it corresponds to the order *Glires* of Linnæus
and the *Rodentia* of Cuvier).]

[b] [Hunter appears to have taken this description from a skull in which the first deciduous molar was still retained. The total number of molares which are developed in
the jaws of a kangaroo are seven on each side of each jaw; the greatest number in use
at any given time is four on each side of each jaw; a posterior or fifth molar may be
visible above the socket in the dry skull, but it does not cut the gum for use till the
anterior one is pushed out.

The succession of the molares is from behind forwards in both jaws. The first deciduous molar, upper jaw, resembles the first permanent false molar in the potoroo; it is
elongated, compressed, and traversed by a longitudinal sharp middle ridge, at the internal base of which are three small tubercles. It is for cutting rather than bruising. The
corresponding tooth, lower jaw, is similar in form, but smaller, and has one tubercle in
the posterior part of the inner side of the base. In some species of kangaroo, as the *Macropus elegans*, the false molar is permanent, but its earlier loss in *Macr. major* does not
warrant a generic distinction. The second deciduous molar has the form of the ordinary
grinders, but is smaller; it is shed before the first.   The third is similar, but somewhat
larger; and so also of the fourth: this grinder is much worn in old skulls, and in the
lower jaw is lost, leaving then only $\frac{4 \cdot 4}{3 \cdot 3}$ molares in aged individuals. The fifth,
sixth, and seventh follow each other from behind forwards, and are of equal size.

Before the fourth grinder is in place the permanent incisores are gained; these
closely resemble their predecessors, but are somewhat larger. In the *Macropus major*
the exterior incisor upper jaw presents two inflected folds of enamel; these are wanting in the corresponding teeth of the smaller species, which retain the spurious molares.]

[c] [At a still earlier period the fore legs, following the usual law of development, exceed the hind legs in length.]

of which the hind legs are composed are very different. The thigh of the kangaroo is extremely short, and the leg is very long. The hind foot is uncommonly long, on which, to appearance, are placed three toes, the middle toe by much the largest and the strongest, and looks something like the long toe of an ostrich. The outer toe is next in size ; and what appears to be the inner toe, is two inclosed in one skin or covering. The great toe nail much resembles that of an ostrich, as also the nail of the outer toe; and the inner, which appears to be but one toe, has two small nails, which are bent and sharp[a]. From the heel along the under side of the foot and toe, the skin is adapted for walking upon.

The fore legs, in the full-grown kangaroo, are small in proportion to the hind, or the size of the animal ; the feet, or hands, are also small. The skin on the palm is different from that on the back of the hand and fingers. There are five toes or fingers on this foot, the middle rather the largest ; the others become very gradually shorter, and are all nearly of the same shape. The nails are sharp, fit for holding. The tail is long in the old, but not so long, in proportion to the size of the animal, in the young. It would seem to keep pace with the growth of the hind legs, which are the instruments of progressive motion in this animal, and which would also show that the tail is a kind of second instrument in this action[b]. The under lip is divided in the middle, each side rounded off at the division. It has two clavicles, but they are short, so that the shoulders are not thrown out.

The Potoroo or Kangaroo Rat[c].

The head is flat sideways, but not so much so as in the true *Scalpris dentata*. The ears are neither long nor short, but much like those of a mouse in proportion to the size of the animal.

---

[a] [Each of these toes has its proper metatarsal and phalangeal bones.]

[b] [It must be remembered that at this time Hunter had never seen the living kangaroo, but the numerous opportunities of witnessing the locomotion of this remarkable animal afforded to subsequent observers have all testified to the sagacity of his prevision of the use of the tail.]

[c] [This animal differs from the kangaroo in having two small canines, in addition to the six incisors in the upper jaw. The first compressed or false molar on each side of each jaw, which is shed in the great kangaroo, is here retained. The first incisors of the upper jaw are also relatively longer and more curved. The potoroo, therefore, forms the type of a distinct genus, which was named by Illiger ' Hypsiprymnus,' from the Greek word Ὑψιπρυμνος, signifying the hinder parts raised. Of this genus three or four species have been indicated. The skin and cranium of the individual described

The fore legs are short in comparison to the hind. There are four toes on the fore feet[a], the two middle are long, and nearly of equal lengths, with long narrow nails, slightly bent ; the two side toes are short, and nearly equal in size, but the outer rather the largest. From the nails on the two middle toes one would suppose that the animal burrowed. Their hind legs are long, and it is in their power to stand either on the whole foot, or on the toes only. On the hind legs are three toes, the middle one large, and the two side ones short[b]; the tail is long. The hair on the body is rather thin ; it is of two kinds, a fur, and a long hair, which last becomes exterior from its length. The fur is the finest, and is composed of serpentine hairs ; the long hair is stronger, and is also serpentine, for more than two-thirds of its length near to the skin, and terminates in a pretty strong pointed end, like the quill of a hedgehog ; it is of a brownish grey colour, something like the brown or grey rabbit, with a tinge of a greenish yellow.

It has a pouch on the lower part of the belly ; the mouth opens forwards, and the cavity extends backwards to the pubis, where it terminates ; on the abdominal surface of this pouch are four nipples or two pair, each pair placed very near the other[c].

The Hepoona Roo[d].

This animal is of the size of a small rabbit ; it has a broad flat body ; the head a good deal resembles that of the squirrel ; the eyes are full,

---

by Hunter, and figured in the Appendix to White's Voyage, are preserved in the Museum of the College of Surgeons. The skull agrees in size and form, as also the proportions of the stuffed skin, with the skeleton of the Hypsiprymnus murinus, given in Pander and D'Alton's ' Skelete der Beutelthiere,' tab. iii.

We give the following admeasurements from the original specimen :

	ft.	in.	ln.
From the end of the nose to the vent	1	3	0
Length of the tail	0	8	7½
Length of the skull	0	3	3
Length of the foot	0	3	3

The *Hypsiprymnus murinus* of Illiger is the *Hypsiprymnus White* of Quoy and Gaimard, the *Macropus minor* of Shaw.]

[a] [In the specimen here described, as in the rest of the genus, there are five toes on the fore foot, but the fifth is so small as scarcely to perform any part of the office of a toe.]

[b] [There are four toes on this foot, as in the great kangaroo, but the two inner ones are so conjoined by a common sheath of integument as to act as but one.]

[c] [The genera Macropus and Hypsiprymnus are principally distinguished from the other marsupialia anatomically by having a large stomach, complicated with sacculi, produced as in the colon, by being puckered upon longitudinal bands.]

[d] [This animal is the type of the genus *Petaurus*, which is characterized by the following dental formula : incisors $\frac{6}{2}$, molares spuriæ $\frac{2.2}{3.3}$, molares tuberculati $\frac{4.4}{4.4} = 34$.

prominent, and large; the ears broad and thin; its legs short, and its tail very long. Between the fore and hind legs, on each side, is placed a doubling of the skin of the side, which, when the legs are extended laterally, is as it were pulled out, forming a broad lateral wing or fin, and when the legs are made use of in walking, this skin, by its elasticity, is drawn close to the side of the animal, and forms a kind of ridge, on which the hair has a peculiar appearance. In this respect it is very similar to the flying squirrel of America.

It has five toes on each fore foot, with sharp nails. The hind-foot has also five toes, but differs considerably from the fore-foot; one of the toes may be called a thumb, having a broad nail, something like that of the monkey or opossum. What answers to the fore and middle toes are united in one common covering, and appear like one toe with two nails; this is somewhat similar to the kangaroo. The two other toes are in the common form; these four nails are sharp, like those on the fore foot. This formation of the foot is well calculated for holding anything while it is moving its body or its fore foot to other parts; a property belonging (probably) to all animals which move from the hind parts, such as the monkey, mocock, mongoose, opossum, parrot, leech, &c. Its hair is very thick and long, making a very fine fur, especially on the back. It is of a dark brown grey on the upper part, a light white grey on the lower side of what may be termed the wing, and white on the under surface, from the neck to the parts adjacent to the anus.

Wha Tapoua Roo[a].

This animal, is about the size of a racoon, is of a dark grey colour on the back, becoming rather lighter on the sides, which terminates in a rich brown on the belly. The hair is of two kinds, a long hair and a kind of fur, and even the long hair at the roots is of the fur kind. The head is short, the eyes rather prominent; the ears broad, not peaked. The teeth resemble those of all the animals from that country I have hitherto seen. The incisors are not continued into the

It is the largest known species, and is the *Petaurus Taguanoides* of Desmarest, and the *Didelphys Petaurus* of Shaw.

The original specimen, described and figured in White's Appendix, is preserved in the Museum of the Royal College of Surgeons.]

[a] [This species is now called the vulpine opossum, or vulpine phalanger (*Phalangista Vulpina*), and is the type of a genus of which the species are not confined to Australia, but some were known, as inhabitants of the Indian isles, to the older naturalists. The dental characters are described in the text.]

grinders by intermediate teeth, although there are two teeth in the intermediate space in the upper jaw, and one in the lower. The incisors are similar to those of the kangaroo, and six in number in the upper jaw, opposed by two in the lower, which have an oblique surface extending some distance from their edge, so as to increase the surface of contact. There are two cuspidati on each side in the upper jaw, and only one in the lower; five grinders on each side of each jaw, the first rather pointed, the others appear nearly of the same size, and quadrangular in their shape, with a hollow running across their base from the outside to the inner, which is of some depth; and another which crosses it, but not so deep, dividing the grinding surface into four points. On the fore foot there are five toes, the inner the shortest, resembling, in a slight degree, a thumb. The hind foot resembles a hand, or that of the monkey and opossum, the great toe having no nail, and opposing the whole sole of the foot, which is bare. The nails on the other toes, both of the fore and hind foot, resemble in a small degree those of the cat, being broad and covered; and the last bone of the toe has a projection on the under side, at the articulation. Each nail has, in some degree, a small sheath, covering its base when drawn up[a]. The tail is long, covered with long hair, except the under surface of that half towards the termination, of the breadth of half an inch, becoming broader near the tip or termination : this surface is covered with a strong cuticle, and is adapted for laying hold.

The Tapoa Tafa, or Tapha[b].

This animal is the size of a rat, and has very much the appearance of the martin cat, but hardly so long in the body in proportion to its size. The head is flat forwards, and broad from side to side, especially between the eyes and ears; the nose is peaked, and projecting beyond the teeth, which makes the upper jaw appear to be considerably longer than the lower; the eyes are pretty large; the ears are broad, especially

---

[a] [In the hinder foot the two toes next the thumb are inclosed in a common sheath of integument as far as the ungual phalanx : this is the commencement of that peculiar degradation of the second and middle toe which is carried to so great an extreme in the kangaroos and potoroos. The term *Phalangista* was given to the genus in question in consequence of this binding together of the phalanges of two of the toes in the hind-feet.]

[b] [This animal is the *Phascogale penicillata* of Temminck, (*Monographies de Mammalogie*, p. 58.), *Dasyurus Tafa* of Geoffroy, *Didelphis penicillata* of Shaw.]

at their base, not becoming regularly narrower to a point[a], nor with a very smooth edge, and having a small process on the concave or inner surface, near to the base. It has long whiskers from the sides of the cheeks, which begin forwards, near the nose, by small and short hairs, and become longer and stronger as they approach the eyes[b]. It has very much the hair of a rat, to which it is similar in colour; but near to the setting on of the tail it is of a lighter brown, forming a broad ring round it. The fore feet are shorter than the hind, but much in the same proportion as those of the rat; the hind feet are more flexible. There are five toes on the fore feet, the middle the largest, falling off on each side nearly equally; but the fore or inner toe is rather shortest; they are thin from side to side; the nails are pretty broad, laterally, and thin at their base; not very long, but sharp: the animal walks on its whole palm, on which there is no hair. The hind feet are pretty long, and have five toes; that which answers to our great toe is very short, and has no nail; the next is the longest in the whole, falling gradually off to the outer toe; the shape of the hind toes is the same as in the fore feet, as are likewise the nails; it walks nearly on the whole foot. The tail is long, and covered with long hair, but not all of the same colour. The teeth of this creature are different from any other animal yet known. The mouth is full of teeth; the lower jaw narrow, in comparison to the upper, more especially backwards, which allows of much broader grinders in this jaw than in the lower, and which occasions the grinders in the upper jaw to project considerably over those in the lower. In the middle the *cuspidati* oppose one another; the upper piercers or holders go behind those of the lower; the second class of incisors in the lower jaw overtop those of the upper, while the two first in the lower go within, or behind those of the upper. In the upper jaw, before the holders ‘(canines)’, there are four teeth ‘(incisors)’ on each side, three of which are pointed, the point standing on the inner surface; and the two in front are longer, stand more obliquely forwards, and appear to be appropriated for a particular use[c].

The holders ‘(canines)’ are a little way behind the last fore teeth, to allow those of the lower jaw to come between; they are pretty long.

The cuspidati (spurious molares) on each side become longer and larger towards the grinders (true molares); they are points or cones placed on a broad base.

---

[a] [Temminck describes the ears of *Phascogale penicillata* as being “arrondies par le haut.”—*Loc. cit.*, p. 59.]

[b] [“Les moustaches des lèvres sont placés plus près des yeux que de nez.”—*Ibid.*]

[c] [This superiority of size of the two middle incisors of the two jaws is one of the characters which distinguish *Phascogale* from *Dasyurus.*]

There are four grinders on each side, the middle two the largest, the last the least; their base is a triangle, of the scalenus kind, or having one angle obtuse and two acute. Their base is composed of two surfaces, an inner and an outer, divided by processes or points : it is the inner that the grinders of the lower jaw oppose, when the mouth is regularly shut.

The lower jaw has three fore teeth, or incisors, on each side, the first considerably the largest, projecting obliquely forwards; the other two of the same kind, but smaller; the last the smallest.

The holder (canine) in this jaw is not so large as in the upper jaw, and close to the incisors.

There are three cuspidati ' (false molares) [a], the middle one the largest, the last the least; these are cones standing on their base, but not on the middle, rather on the anterior side.

There are four grinders, the two middle the largest, and rather quadrangular, each of which has a high point or cone on the outer edge, with a smaller, and three more diminutive on the inner edge.

It is impossible to say critically what the various forms of these teeth are adapted for, from the general principles of teeth. In the front we have what may divide and tear off; behind those there are holders or destroyers; behind the latter, such as will assist in mashing, as the grinders of the lion, and other carnivorous animals; and last of all, grinders, to divide parts into smaller portions, as in the graminivorous tribe : the articulation of the jaw, in some degree, admits of all those motions.

---

[a] [This is the second and most decisive distinguishing generic character between *Phascogale* and *Dasyurus*, the latter having only two false molars on each side of each jaw, instead of three. Had Fischer, Lesson, and other zoologists compared the description of the teeth in the text with that given by Temminck in his *Monographies de Mammalogie*, as characterizing his genus *Phascogale*, they could not have hesitated to refer the Tapoa tafa of Hunter to that genus, and the catalogues of mammalia need not have contained the imaginary species *Dasyurus Tafa*, which M. Temminck observes "n'a point été vue depuis par aucun naturaliste," and which species Lesson suspects to be founded on the immature state of the spotted Dasyure (*Dasyurus viverrinus*). But neither observation nor analogy favour the idea of spots being acquired by age; on the contrary, the examples of the lion and the puma, which are spotted only when young, show that they are more likely to be lost.

In the Hunterian collection the posterior half of the body of the individual described by Hunter is preserved, to show the marsupium and teats; these are eight in number, and arranged in a circle. The tail perfectly corresponds with the specimens of *Phascogale penicillata*, and with M. Temminck's description, being "couverte de poils assez courts à la base, tres-long, raides, et en pinceau vers la pointe" (*loc. cit.*, p. 59,); and the long hairs are black].

A Dingo, or Dog of New South Wales.

This animal is a variety of the dog, and, like the shepherd's dog in most countries, approaches near to the original of the species, which is the wolf; but is not so large, and does not stand so high on its legs. The ears are short and erect, the tail rather bushy; the hair, which is of a reddish dun colour, is long and thick, but straight. It is capable of barking, although not so readily as the European dog, is very ill-natured and vicious, and snarls, howls, and moans like dogs in common. Whether this is the only dog in New South Wales, and whether they have it in a wild state, is not mentioned, but I should be inclined to believe they had no other, in which case it will constitute the wolf of that country; and that which is domesticated is only the wild dog tamed, without having yet produced a variety, as in some parts of America.

THE END.

INDEX TO THE FOURTH VOLUME.

A.

ABSORPTION, experiments on lacteal, 301—307. Observations on, 299, 300. Veins have the power of, 310, note; 311, note. Supposed by Majendie to be the effect of mechanical imbibition, 312, 313. Arguments in disproof of Majendie's theory, 314, note. Is a vital selective or attractive action, 314, note. Of shell, 469.
Acrita, diffused condition of the nervous and other systems in, 198, note.
Actinia, the *Serpula gigantea* described as a species of, 467.
Adversaria anatomica of Hunter, specimen of the destroyed, 393.
Air-bags, experiments on, in fishes, 182.
Air-cells, in birds, 176. Description of, 178—180. Their final intention, 184, 185, note. In insects, 185.
Air in the stomach and other cavities, 97. Peculiar case of a woman afflicted with, 98, 99.
Alligator, sheds and renews its teeth, 354.
Allotriandrous (αλλοτριος, another; ανηρ, male) hermaphroditism explained, 35.
Ambergris, the intestinal concretions so called have the beaks of cuttle-fish for their nuclei, 362, note.
Amphibia, and birds, great similarity between, xxxvi. In the absence of vesiculæ seminales, 28; and in the presence of abdominal air-cells, 183, 184.
Amphibious bipes, anatomical description of, 394.
Animal-earth, immense accumulation of at the bottom of bone caves, 473.
Animal flower; new marine, 467. (See *Serpula gigantea*.)
Animals, the lower, allow of a considerable variation in their temperature of heat and cold, 133. Experiments on, *ib*. The higher have greater power of retaining heat than the lower, 137. In a torpid state digestion, sensation, &c. do not go on, 144. Their food may be divided into two kinds, 126. Variety in the mode of the nourishment of, 122. Life of, its state or stages, *ib*. Subject to great changes by culture, 277.
Animals with tentacula, an almost infinite variety of, 469.
Anspach, Margrave of, his description of the bone-caves of Gailenreuth, 470.
Aristotle, the author of the theory of the vital principle, iv, x. His classes Zootoka and Ootoka, xxviii.
Argala, or adjutant crane, its air-cells, 179, note.
Arteries; not uniform in their distribution, and why, 187, 188. Contractility and structure of, 253, 254, note.

B.

Banks, Sir Joseph, P.R.S., Mr. Hunter's letter to, on the structure of the crystalline lens, 287, 288.
Barberry, irritability of filaments of, 210, note.
Bats; in general have no air-cells, except in the lungs, 183. But in the genus *Nycteris* large air-cells extend under the skin, 183, note.
Beaumont, *Dr.*; his experiments on the gastric juice in a man with a fistulous opening into stomach, 96.
Bees; observations on, 422. Their anatomy and physiology better understood by the analogies of other insects, 423. Best hives for observing their operations, 424. Their actions arise out of an instinctive necessity, 425, 437. They are not legislators nor mathematicians, 425, 437. Geographical distribution of, 425, and note; 426. Have property to defend, and therefore a sting, 426. Feed in winter, and

retain a high temperature, 427. Power of generating heat in other insects, 427, note; 428. Are very susceptible of change of temperature, 429. Are cleanly, 429, 445. The society consists of a female breeder, female nonbreeders, and males, 429, 431. Their swarming, 431, 432. Formation of wax, 433. Mode of collecting farina, 433, note; 441. Formation and structure of comb, 435. Royal cell, 436. Oviposition, 438, 446. Larvæ, 439, 465, 442. Pupæ, 440, 442, Bee-bread, 440. Metamorphosis, 443, and note. Seasons of impregnation, oviposition, mellification, and mariticide, 444. Quantity of honey consumed in winter, 445. Queen bee, 446. Abortive experiment, to form, 449. Description of, 449, 450. Number of queens in a hive, 451. Copulation of, 452. Male bee, ib. Labourer, 453. Have the female parts, but extremely small, ib. Their number in a hive, 454. Tongue, 455. Œsophagus, 456. Honey-bag, 457. Stomach, 457. Intestine, 458. Senses, ib. Voice, ib. Female organs, 459. Male organs, 460. Sting, 463. Period of life, 465.

Belchier on madder, 315, note.
Bell, Thos., F.R.S.; his description of the cutaneous air-cells of Nycteris quoted, 183, note.
Bell, Wm., viii. His experiments on the silk-moth, 461.
Birds; similarity of, to reptiles, xxxvi. Characters of the class of, xxxiv. Account of certain receptacles of air in, which communicate with the lungs and Eustachian tube, 176. Before the year 1774, the air-cells of the lungs, and other. cavities of the body, not clearly explained, 176. Experiments upon the breathing of, 181.
Bivalves; adductor muscle of, 233. Antagonized by elastic ligament, 252. Quantity of contraction of adductor muscle greater than is required, 263.
Blagden, Dr. C.; his experiments in a heated room, 131, 132, note.
Blood; its coagulation depends on the fibrine, xii. Red globules of, are latest formed, xiii. Its transparency and want of colour in the lobster and snail, its milk-white colour in the slug, its red colour in the earth-worm, 218. Is more loaded with red particles in the higher than the inferior classes, 219. Living principle supposed to be inherent in the, 167.
Boerhaave on muscular action, 258.
Bone; experiments and observations on the growth of, 315; by means of madder, 315, 316. By inserting shots, 317.
Bones; description of, in birds, 178.
Borelli, observations on air-cells of birds quoted, 176, note. Experiment on muscular contraction, 257.
Brain, its fibrous structure, xvi, 373. Classes of animals according to modifications of, xvi—xviii.
Brewster, Sir David, F.R.S., his observations on the structure of the lens quoted, 289, note.
Brodie, Sir B. C., F.R.S., his experiments on the brain's influence upon the heart's action and the production of heat, 136, note.
Buffon, his observations on a wolf and dog quoted, 322.
Bulb of urethra, subservient to distention of glans, 33. Double bulb coexists with double glans in opossum, 33, note.

C.

Cachalot, difference of size in two sexes, 335, note.
Calendula pluvialis, 201.
Camper; his observations on the air-cells of birds, 176. Erroneously supposes air to enter cranial cells by the meatus auditorius, 180, note. Denies that birds have an Eustachian tube, 181, note. Not acquainted with the external opening of the organ of hearing in fishes, 298; nor with the semicircular canals in the Cetacea, 384.
Carlisle, Sir A., F.R.S.; his observations on tæniæ quoted, xxviii. His Croonian Lecture, 256.
Carp, experiments on, 132, 147.
Castrated animals, of either sex, approach each other in appearances, and have a resemblance to the unnatural hermaphrodite. 47.
Cetacea (cete, a whale) are true Testiconda, 6, note. Species dissected by Hunter, 332. Constitute an order of animals, 334; which includes the largest, 334, 335; with less variety of form than in the terrestrial orders, 337. Herbivorous species of, 335, note;

have lungs, warm blood, and other essential characteristics of quadrupeds, 336. Characteristic form of, 337. Why the tail is horizontal, 338 and note, 339. Pectoral fins analogous to anterior extremities in quadrupeds, 338. Differences *inter se* in number of ribs, structure of larynx, and cœcum, 339. Flesh of, has greater specific gravity than beef, *ib.* Bones of, 340—344. Construction of tail of, 344. Fat of, 344, 345. Cellular membrane of, 349. Skin of, 349, 351, note. Cutis is compact cellular membrane, 349. Final intention of its combination with the blubber, 349, note. Elasticity of skin in piked whale, 350; their mode of catching food, 351; teeth of, 352; peculiar mode of development of, 353, 354; mode of shedding and succession resembles those in the elephant, 354. Substitute for teeth in the whales, *ib.* Œsophagus, 357. Stomachs, 357—360. Intestines, 360—362; never contain air, 361. Liver, *ib.* Pancreas, *ib.* Food of, 362. Epiploon, *ib.* Spleens, 363. Kidneys, *ib.* Bladder, *ib.* Capsulæ renales, 364. Blood, *ib.* Heart, *ib.* Arteries, 365, 366, and note. Arterial intercostal plexuses, 365; do not exist in herbivorous species, 366, note. Veins, 367, note. Larynx, 367. Os hyoides, 367. Lungs, 369. Diaphragm, 369. Blow-hole, 370. Brain and spinal chord, 372, 373 and note. Organ of touch, 374. Of taste, 375. Of smell, 376. Of hearing, 378—384. Peculiar sinuses communicating with Eustachian tube, 379. Worms infesting those sinuses, 379, note. Membrana tympani convex outwardly, 381, and note. Discovery of semicircular canals in, 384, and note. Organ of seeing, 384, 388. Absence of lachrymal gland in, 384, note. Muscles of eye and eyelids, 385 and note. Generative organs of, 388—392. Testes always abdominal, 388 and note; their great enlargement, 388, note. Analogies of pelvic bones, 389 and note. Muscles of clitoris and Malpighian canals, 390, note. Fœtal membranes, 390, note. Gestation and number of young, 391 and note. Lactation, 392.

Chimpanzee; peritoneal canal of tunica vaginalis obliterated in, 12, note.

Chylification; process of, described, 108, note.

Circulation of the blood in insects, xxii.

Classes of animals according to the brain, xvi. Generative function, xxviii. Heart. xxix. Respiratory organs, xxxii. General structure, xxxiii.

Clift, Wm., F.R.S.; his copies of the Hunterian manuscripts include the Croonian Lectures, p. 195 to 267. Experiments on Absorption in Birds, 309. Schemes of the Classification of the Animal Kingdom, xvi. xxviii—xxxvii. Observations on the Anatomy of a Turtle, vi.

Clitoria, 200.

Clitoris; its specific use, 36.

Cock; experiments on a, 153.

Cold; how produced, 131. Effects on animals; rather rouses than depresses, 132.

Convolvulus, 200, 201.

Cooper, Sir Astley, F.R.S.; his experiments on the relative digestibility of different substances, 111, note.

Coughing; how performed, 91.

Cowper; quoted, 33, note.

Cremaster; its use, 5. Its nerves, 6, and note. Does not exist in true testiconda, 6, note. Is supplied by nerves of voluntary motion, *ib.* Some persons retain a voluntary control over it, *ib.* note. Is connected to the testis previous to its descent, 8, and note.

Crocodile; approaches the bird in the structure of brain, xix. Its single penis, xxxv. Its organ of hearing, 295.

Croonian Lectures on Muscular Motion, No. I. 195; No. II. 224; No. III. 242; No. IV. 251; No. V. 255; No. VI. 267. Some facts relative to Hunter's preparation for, 286.

Crows; regurgitate food for their young from the fauces, 455.

Cryptandrous (κρυπτος, hidden; ανηρ, man,) *hermaphroditism*; explained, 35, note.

Crystals of different oils; advantage of determining exact form of, 348.

Cuckoo; hair in stomach whence derived, 93, note.

Cuscuta, 200, note.

Cuticle; considered as a dead covering, and capable of receiving greater degrees of heat and cold than the living parts underneath, 138.

Cuttle-fish; structure of lens in, 286. Hunter's preparations of eye of, 286, note. Organ of hearing of, 294.

Cuvier; his opinion of Hunter, v. On the circulation in insects, xxiii. His observations on existing Cetacea, 333, note. On Hunter's paper on fossil bones, 480, note.

Cyclostomum thermale, a snail living in thermal springs of 100° Fahr., 134, note.

D.

Dalmatia; fossils of, chiefly ruminant, 472, 476.
Davy, Dr. John, F.R.S.; his observations on the double auricle of anourous Batrachia, xxx. His experiments on the heat of the bonito, 147, note. His experiments on the torpedo, 399, note.
Decidua; formation of, compared to the effusion of lymph in inflammation by Hunter and V. Baer, 58, note. Cylindrical villi in, described by Weber, 58, note.
Diadelphia, 201.
Diaphragm; its rudimentary existence in birds, xxxiv. 177.
Digestion; observations on, 81 to 121. Of the stomach after death, 116. Its appearances are most frequent in those who die by sudden violence, 119. Different power of in cardiac and pyloric portions of stomach, 107, note. Coagulation of substances not essential to their, 109, note.
Dingo, 493.
Dionœa muscipula, 200.
Dog; experiments on heat of, 145. Observations on the species of, 319. Propagates with the wolf, 320, 323. Same species as the wolf, 328. Variety of, with supernumerary toe, 329, note.
Dormice; experiments on, 132, 133, 141, 142.
Drowned persons; observations on, 165. Their situation similar to that of a person in a trance, 166, note. Method of treating, 170, 171, 173, 174.
Dugong, pp. 360, 361, note.
Duhamel's theory of growth of bone contrasted with Hunter's, p. 318, note.
Duodenum, digestion is carried on in, 103, note.

E.

Earth-worm; experiments on heat of, 147, 154. Red blood of, 218.
Eel; experiments on an, 148.
Eggs; experiments on, 146, 149, 150.
Elephant; its cranial air-cells, 180, note. Fossil bones of, found in England, Siberia, &c. 478.
Embryo state, or first organization of higher animals analogous in construction to full-grown state of lowest animals, xxvi. 243, 268.
Entozoa; stated by Rudolphi to revive after having been completely frozen, 152, note.
Erection of penis; caused by compression of the vena dorsalis, 32. Experiment to prove, 32. Cowper's account of muscles causing the compression in opossum, 32.
Eustachian tube; air received by the, in birds, 180.
Eye; the pigmentum of, in different animals, 277. Muscles of the, 274, 385. Power of adjustment of, 289, note.
Experiments; reflection upon, 424.

F.

Feathers; contain a considerable quantity of air, 182.
Female; when the powers of propagation cease loses many of her peculiar properties, and approaches towards the hermaphrodite, 49.
Feræ; (the name of a Linnæan order of Mammalia, corresponding with the Carnivora of Cuvier,) periodical passage of testes in insectivorous, 6, note. Vesiculæ seminales limited to insectivorous, 27, note.
Fifth pair; description of some branches of, 193, 194, note.
Fishes; account of the organ of hearing in, 292. Organ of hearing discovered by Hunter before the year 1760, 293. And described and figured by Casserius in the year 1600, 292, note. Reasons for publishing an account of it, 294. Experiments on the hearing of, 296. On the temperature of, 132, 147. The appearance of the stomachs of, after death, 120.
Flesh-fly; Hunter's experiment to prove the use of the crop, and the digestive power of the intestine, 105, note.
Fœtus; contents of the pelvis much higher than in the adult, 3.
Fox, further removed than jackall or wolf from dog, 319.

Fossil-bones; description of, from the caverns at Gailenreuth, 470. Have undergone little change of internal structure, 471. Earths which commonly incrust, 472. Three hypotheses of, proposed, *ib.* Proofs of their accumulation during many thousand years, 473. Referred to species of bear different from the present, 474; and to a lion, *ib.* Geographical distribution of animals in relation to, 476. Changes of land and sea indicated by, 476, 477. Proportion of animal matter and earth in, 478.

Frauenhofer corrects the dispersive property of the lens in his achromatic object glasses, 289, note.

Free-martins; account of, 34. Origin of, 38. Do not breed, 39. A similar circumstance met with in sheep; but they are not free-martins, 40. Description of, 41—43.

Frogs, experiment on, 148.

Frost-bitten, manner of treating the, 171.

Functions, Hunter's classification of, 336.

G.

Gailenreuth, bone caves of, 470—472.

Gastric-juice; its use, 96. Its action on the villous coat after death, 119. Dr. Stevens' opinion of the, 115. Observations and experiments in proof of its acidity, 106, note. Contains hydrochloric acid, 121, note.

Generation; classification of animals according to, xxviii. Organs of, in whales, 388. In bees, 459. In the silk-moth, 461.

Geoffroi's (Mons.) opinion on the organ of hearing in fishes, 297.

Geoffroy St. Hilaire, his theory of the cause (*l'ordonnée*) of monstrosities contrasted with Hunter's, 45, note.

Gestation; period of, the same in all the varieties of same species, 319. Of wolf is sixty-three days, 324. Of jackall is fifty-nine days, 326.

Gibraltar; fossils of, mostly carnivora, 472, 473. Mr. Lyell's account of, 476.

Gillaroo Trout; observations on, 126.

Giraffe; use of tendon exemplified in the sterno-thyroidei of, 229.

Gizzard; description of the, 127, 128. Its motion, 91, and note.

Glosso-petræ, what, 478.

Glires (*glis*, a dormouse), the name of a Linnæan order of Mammalia, corresponding with the *Scalpris dentata* of Hunter, and the *Rodentia* of Cuvier, periodical passage of testes in, 6, note.

Gray, Mr. J. E., reproduces Hunter's observation on the absorption of shell as a new discovery, 469, note.

Grew, on the colour of muscles, quoted, 220, note.

Guinea-pig; experiments on vesiculæ seminales, 27.

Gymnotus; greater part of appropriated to electric apparatus, 414. Air-bladders of, *ib.* The posterior wanting in *Gymn. æquilabiatus*, *ib.*, note. Description of electric organs, 415—418. Nerves of, 418, 419. Lateral nerve in fish, 419, note. Blood-vessels of, 420.

H.

Hale, his Veg. Statics quoted, 203.

Hall, Dr. M., F.R.S.; his observation on the difference between the sleep of hybernating and that of non-hybernating animals, p. 144, note. On the state of circulation and sensation during torpidity, 144, note. On the reflex function, 201, note.

Haller, on the Hernia congenita, 2, note. His description of olfactory nerve quoted, 191. His queries on muscular action, 257.

Hambergerus on muscular action, 258.

Harvey; a vital principle is the cause of organization, iv, x. Exists in the egg, x. And in the blood, xi. Ascertains the movements of the gizzards of birds by auscultation, 91, note. Discovers the abdominal air-cells of birds, 176, note. Compares them with the abdominal lungs of serpents and the air-bladder of fish, 184, note.

Hearing; organ of in the sepia, 294. In fishes is a link in the chain of varieties which it presents in different animals, 293. Is placed in the cranial cavity in bony fishes, 294; but in the cranial parietes in sharks and rays, 294. In the turtle and crocodile, 295. In whales, 378.

Heart; in insects, xxii. In reptiles, xxiv, xxx. Classes of animals according to the

structure of, xxix—xxxi. Its muscular fibre is striated, 261, note. Soonest acquires
   due firmness, 271. Of the siren, 396, note.
Heat; experiments and observations on animals, with respect to their power of producing it, 131. Variation of, in the same experiment, 136. Young animals and
   newly formed parts have less power of generating, 134, 135, and note. Power of
   generating modified by nervous influence, 136. Less evolved during sleep, 144.
   Power of generating in some fishes, 147, note. In bees, 151; and other insects, 427,
   note. Power of maintaining in the living egg, 149. In vegetables, 156—164.
Heautandrous (ἑαυτος, himself; ανηρ, man,) hermaphroditism explained, 35, note.
Hedgehog; periodical enlargement and displacement of testes, 7, and note. Its vesiculæ seminales, 27. Experiments on, 143. Its heat diminishes when it is at rest,
   150.
Hedysarum gyrans, 200.
Hens, experiments on, 146.
Hepoona-roo, description of, 488.
Hermaphrodite; classes of, 35, note. Natural and unnatural, *ib.* Dimidiate and quar-
   tered, *ib.* note. Description of, 36. Appear externally to be females, 37. Particular description of in black cattle, 41. In insects, 35, note. In a lobster, *ib.* In
   a dog, 36, note.
Hernia congenita; caused by the falling down of the intestine into the scrotum, after
   the testis, 14. And true hydrocele cannot exist together in the same side of the
   scrotum, 15.
Hornbill, its air-cells extend into all the bones, 180, note.
Human body, a knowledge of its construction essential to medicine, 1.
——— *subject*; experiments on a, 138—141.
——— *hand*, quoted as a remarkable instance of mechanical construction, 202.
Humboldt, on the gymnotus, 414, and 420, note.
Humulus, 200.
Hunter, Dr. William; his observations on the descent of the testis, 2. On absorption,
   299, 300.
Hypsiprymnus, 487.

                              I.

Ichthyosaurus; relation of its hinder paddles to lungs, 338, note.
Incubation; description of the crop of a pigeon during, 124.
Inflammation; does not excite the part to a degree of heat beyond the standard heat of
   the animal, 143, note.
Insects; nervous system of, xvii. Circulation in, xxii. Temperature of, 427. All
   their joints are ginglymoid, 236, note.
Internal organs; modified in shape and position by external form, 336.
Intestine of a hog, containing air, see plate xxxvii.

                              J.

Jackal; observations on, 319. History of a bitch impregnated by a spaniel dog, 325.
   A hybrid female is fertile with a dog, 326.
Jaw (lower) in birds, is supplied with air, 180.
Jenner, Dr.; his experiments quoted, p. 142.
Jerboa; its anatomy, 393. Affinities to bird, 393, and note.

                              K.

Kangaroo; described, 485. Its teeth, 485, 486, and note. Mammary fœtus of, 485.
   Disproportion of hind legs less in young, 486.
Keill; his observations on optics, 275.
Knox, Dr.; criticizes Hunter's account of the development of the teeth in the Cetacea,
   353, note.

                              L.

Leeches; experiments on, 147, 148.
Leeuwenhoek; his observations on the fibrous structure of the lens, 289. And on the
   laminated structure of the whale's cornea, 386.

Lens, crystalline; its laminated and fibrous texture, 286, 289, note. Its supposed muscularity, 288, 290, note. Is not perfectly achromatic, 289; nor is such a lens required in the eye, 290. Its layers do not progressively increase in density as they approach the centre in the horse, 290, note.

Life; power of preserving less in young animals and new-formed parts, 134, 158. Principle of, defined, 167.

Linnæus; characters of the classes of animals, xxix. Quoted, 201.

Lister, and *Musgrave, Dr. Wm.*; their experiments on the absorption of coloured matters by the lacteals, 303, note. Did not consider whether the veins had or had not any share in absorption, 304, note.

Locomotion; not given to all animals, 203. Chief purposes for which designed, 203. External resistance essential to, 246.

Lonicera, 200.

Lungs; description of, in birds, 177.

Lyell; his Principles of Geology quoted, 476.

M.

Macropus, 485, note.

Majendie, M.; his experiments on vomiting, 91, note. Experiments on digestive power in small intestines, 103, note. On the fifth pair of nerves, 190, note. His opinions on absorption, 312–313, note.

Mammalia; Linnæus's class of, adduced by Hunter with reference to their mode of nourishing the young, 123.

Marchantia; irritability of filaments in, 210.

Marks, distinguishing; belonging equally to both sexes, 45.

Marshall, On Recruits, quoted, 6, note.

Marsupiata; their mammary muscle, 392, note. Their double superior cavæ, 393, note. Their mode of propagation described, 482, note.

Mayo, H., F.R.S.; his Physiology quoted, 205, note; 259, note.

Medusa; exhibits an early stage in the development of muscular fibre, 268.

Mesembryanthemum, 201.

Mice (common); experiments on, 145.

Miles, Henry; his eye retained its power of adjustment after extraction of lens, 290, note.

Mimosa pudica, 200. Experiments on, 205. Structure of irritable intumescence of leafstalk, 204, note.

Mirabilis, 201.

Monotremata (μονος, unicus; τρημα, foramen,); an order of ovoviviparous mammalia, so called, because in them the fæces, urine, and generative products are expelled by one and the same foramen, 6.

Monro, Prof. A.; argues against lymphatic absorption, from supposed absence of lymphatics in oviparous animals, 308.

Monstrous appearances; definition of, 44. Classification of, *ib.*, note. Not a matter of mere chance, 45. Their cause lies in the original germ, *ib.*

Mule; its occasional fertility conjectured to depend on a monstrous condition of its generative organs, 319.

Mullet; description of its gizzard, which is lined with cuticle, 129, and note.

Muscles; microscopic structure of voluntary and involuntary fibre, 260, note. Condition of contracted and relaxed fibre, 261, note. Muscles involuntarily contracted will not relax by the will, 262. Contraction or stiffening of after death, 264, 267. Relaxation of, 265, 266. Elasticity of, 265. Relation of density of to strength, 267. Fallacy of experiments on muscles in the dead body, 268. Density of particular muscles according to use, 269, 270. Increased by constant exercise, 271. Use of oblique, 274. Their different specific gravity in different animals, 182. Contractility of muscular fibre known to Lycus of Macedon and Herophilus, 195, note. Self-motion most conspicuous in animals, but exists in vegetables, 196. Three kinds of self-motion, 197, 199. Muscles act by vibration, 207. Vibrations longer as muscle is weaker, 208. Contraction of, stronger than their mechanical resistance in dead body, 267. Four kinds of stimulus to the contraction of, 210. Causes of contraction of, 264. Actions of involuntary muscles never tire, 211. Nor involuntary actions of voluntary, 212. Sensation of fatigue is therefore in the mind or nerves, though referred to the muscles, 212. Performing voluntary actions have large nerves, 212. Voluntary power lost with the division of the nerve, but not the susceptibility of impressions, 213. Power of involuntary muscles illustrated by the colon of the horse, 213. Their sphinctorial power of contraction or tonicity, 214. Violent voluntary actions will produce the involuntary, 215. Fat in muscles characteristic of age, 216. Muscles of respiration must be involuntary for breathing, voluntary for uttering vocal sounds, 217. Colour of muscles, *ib.* Its relation to the colour and quantity of blood distributed to them, 219; and to their action, *ib.* Paralytic muscles become pale, and somewhat gelatinous and transparent, 220. Swelling of muscles, 221. Temporary and permanent increase from action, *ib.* Effects of habit on muscles, 222. Permanent increase of size greater in involuntary than voluntary, 223. Mechanical effects of muscles, 224. Their external figure, 225. Their different constructions, 226; and their effects, 239. Their situation, 227. Their attachment to tendons, 232. Their origin and insertion, 233. Their adaptation to joints, 235–238. Mechanical effects of, 242. Divided into three kinds, 246. Gradational development of muscles in animals, 244. Impossible to ascertain absolute force of, 248. Combination of elasticity with muscularity in blood-vessels, 253. Contraction of a muscle results from uniform approximation of its particles, 255. Increases in thickness, density, and specific gravity during contraction, 256. Experiments with the heart of dog and sheep, to ascertain whether a muscle loses bulk during contraction, 259.

N.

Narwhal; tusks of, 352, and note.
Natural history, 292.
Negro; muscular part of gastrocnemius of, shorter than in European, 263.
Nerves; description of the, which supply the organ of smelling, 187. Constancy in their different origins and distributions indicate particular uses, 187. Organs with different sensitive endowments have nerves from different parts of the brain, 189, 190. Nerves give the sensations they are destined to convey in whatever part of their course the impression is made, 191. Some animals devoid of, 198.
New South Wales; description of some animals of, 481.

O.

Oblique muscles; the use of the, 274. In the Cetacea, 385, note.
Ogle, Thomas; his case of a young woman who poisoned herself in the first month of pregnancy, 55.
Oil; its different situation in the bodies of different fishes described, 182.
Opossum; Mr. Hunter's experiments to determine mode of generation in, 482.
Orang-utan; tunica vaginalis communicates with abdomen, 12, note.
Organ of hearing; in fishes is placed on the side of the cavity of the skull, 294. Increases in dimension with the animal, 295. Described in the cod, salmon, ling, ray, and jack, 295. Nerves of the, 296, and note. Experiments on, 296.
Ornithorhynchus (ορνις, avis; ρυγχος, a beak,); its penis relates solely to the passage of the semen, 30, note. Ovum of, 58, note.
Ostrich; its abdominal air-cells figured in Perault's Memoirs, 176, note. Mentioned by Hunter, 182. Has no air in the humerus, 179.
Ovarium; experiments on extirpating it, 50.
Ovum, human, 59, note.
Owl; air admitted to interior of cranial bone by Eustachian tube, 180. Compared with hawk with reference to stimulus to action, 202.

P.

Pea-hen; change of plumage in, from female to male, 49.
Peccari; its vesiculæ seminales, 26, note. Its stomach, 103.
Pelican; its air-cells described, 185.

Pelvis; side view of, in which the vasa deferentia did not communicate with the vesiculæ, and the vesiculæ did not communicate with the urethra, 23.
Penis; small in castrated animals, 30. Description of, 30. Not so large in erection in
a cold as a warm day, 30. In a horse just killed the cells appear muscular,
and contracted upon being stimulated, *ib.* note. Erection, how produced, experiment
on, 32, note. Its specific use, 36. Impossible for one animal to have a penis and
clitoris, *ib.* Case of a gentleman who had the nerves of the glans destroyed, 191,
note. Case of a serjeant of marines who lost the greater part of the body of the, 191,
note.
Perennibranchiata; structure of heart in, 395, note. Nervus lateralis in, 419, note.
Petaurus, 488, note.
Phalæna, 201.
Phalangista, 489, note.
Phascogale, 490, note.
Pheasant; an account of an extraordinary, 44. Change in feather from a hen to a cock,
48. Does not generally take place till an advanced period of the animal's life, 48.
Supposed to be merely the effect of age, and obtain to a certain degree in every class
of animals, *ib.* May be produced by injury or disease of ovarium at any period of
life, 48, note.
Philosophical Transactions; Hunter's papers are printed in those for the years 1766,
1772, 1773, 1774, 1775, 1776, 1778, 1779, 1780, 1782, 1785, 1787, 1792, 1793, 1794.
Pigeon; change in structure of crop when breeding, 124.
Pigmentum of the eye; always corresponds with the hair and skin, 278, 279. Description of various, 277 to 285.
Placenta; structure of the, 60. Dissection of a, 61. Description of a, 63 to 65; note
on, p. 67. Of a monkey, described, 72. Modifications of in the feræ, rodentia, ru-
minants, mare, and sow, 70, note.
Polypus; gemmiparous offspring, compared with the young of mammalia while nou-
rished by the parent's secretion, 122. Moves from stimuli without sensation, 200.
Its actions contrasted with those of the mimosa, 200, note. Does not sleep, 206. Is
little more than a muscular bag, 244. Has no anus, 468. The ciliobrachiate have,
468, note.
Porcupine; its cranial air-cells, 180, note.
Porpoise; digestion carried on in first cavity of stomach, 104, note.
Potoroo; description of, 487.
Pregnancy; appearances after death in first month of, described, 55. No ovum de-
tected, 57.
Principle of life; not wholly confined to animals, or animal substance, 149. Possessed
by eggs, *ib.* Definition of, 167.
Prostate gland; wanting (or rather is bifid) in the bull, buck, and all ruminating ani-
mals, 31, note.
Prout; Observations on Digestion quoted, 108, 109, note. Difference of contents of
rectum in dogs fed on animal and vegetable food, 114, note.
Puppy; experiments on a, 143.

Q.

Quadrumana (four-handed: the name of an order of mammalia, including apes, monkeys, and lemurs,); position of testes in, 10.

R.

Rabbit; experiment on a, 146.
Raptorial birds; female larger than the male in most, 46, note.
Reaumur; his Experiments on Digestion quoted, 81, 84, 86.
Recurrent arteries; mechanical cause of, 13. Recurrent nerves explained on similar
principles, 13, note.
Regurgitating animals, 455.
Relaxation in vegetables, 206.
Reptiles; the creeping invertebrata, so called by Hunter, 104.

Retina; observations on the, 284. Is so transparent as to allow light to pass through, 284.

Rodentia; genera of, with two superior venæ cavæ, 393, note.

Rumination; experiments on, 94, note.

Ruptures; the intestines sometimes in contact with the testis, 2.

Russell, Dr.; Hunter's anatomy of the jerboa quoted from his History of Aleppo, 393.

S.

Sauvages, on muscular action, 258.

Scarpa; communicates to Hunter his intention to publish on the olfactory nerves in 1782, 189.

Secretion; in the crop of breeding pigeons, 124.

Seed; explanation of, 34.

Seeds; of vegetables, same experiments on, as on eggs of animals, 164.

Semen; described, 20. Can be absorbed in the body of the testicle, and in the epididymus, 25.

Senses; defined, 198. Consciousness in animals of atmospheric changes not referable to any of the senses, 199.

Sepia; the class so called has the organ of hearing, 296; its difference from that of fishes, 294, note.

Serpula gigantea; anatomical remarks on, 467, note.

Sexes; difference of size of the different, 46, and note.

Shark; its muscle denser than that of cod or salmon, 182.

Shaw, Dr.; considers Mr. Hunter as the person most capable of determining the natural affinities of the nondescripts from New South Wales, 481. Refers the marsupiata of New South Wales to the Linnæan genus, Didelphys, 484, note.

Shell-fish; have the power of removing part of the shell by absorption, 469.

Shirach; his Observations on Bees, quoted, 447.

Silk-Moth; experiments on impregnation of, 461—463.

Silurus electricus; electric organs of, 421, note.

Siren lacertina; anatomical description of, 394. Where found, *ib.* Linnæus' opinion of, 394, note. Has both lungs and gills, 395. Respires principally by the branchiæ, 395, note. Structure of its heart, 396, note. Of its female organs, 397, note.

Skull; manner of dissecting the nerves out of the, 189.

Sleep of plants, 201.

Sloth; speculation on the tenderness of its flesh, 272.

Slugs, black; experiments on, 147.

Smallpox; communicated by mother to fœtus, 74. Death of the part is produced by variolous inflammation, which is the best characteristic of the disease, 76. Is confined to external surfaces, the mouth and throat, 77.

Snail; its kidney discovered by Hunter, xxiv. Experiments on, 147.

Snakes; in general have but one lung, 183, note.

Soft palate; use of its muscles in violent exertions of the body, 249.

Song of birds; use of air-cells in, 185, 186, note.

Spallanzani; his Observations on Digestion quoted, 81, 86, 94. Assigns heat as an immediate aid to digestion in the snake, 87.

Sparrow; periodical variation in size of testes, 29. Sometimes removes its eggs, 423.

Species; incapacity of propagation in two proves them distinct, 319. Capacity in the hybrids of propagating *inter se* an intermediate variety establishes the identity of two supposed distinct; but this proof is yet to be obtained in reference to dog and wolf, 324, note.

Spermaceti; description of, 346, 348. Teeth of whale, 352, and note.

Spermatic artery; its origin, 3. Its course, 4.

Spiders; have not air-cells diffused through the body, as in flying insects, 185.

Squatina, or monk-fish; external orifices of the ears, 296, note.

Stimulus and irritation; difference between, 197.

Stomach; is not much excited when exposed and handled, 91. Need not act in vomiting, *ib.* Different forms of, 103.

Subordinate groups; difficulty of determining, from intermixture of characters, 484.

Susceptibility of impressions, while retained, may lead to recovery of vital actions, 169.

Sympathy, in vegetables, 207.

Swammerdam; his experiment on a frog's heart, proving that a muscle diminishes in bulk when it contracts, 257. His minute observations on the structure of the bee, 422.

Swan, Joseph, Esq., his Illustrations of the Comparative Anatomy of Nervous System quoted, 419, note.

T.

Tænia hydatigenia, 286.

Tapao-tafa, description of, 490.

Tench, experiments on, 149, 154.

Tendons and fasciæ, their uses explained, 228. Bone substituted for tendon in legs of birds and bodies of fish, 231. Attachment of muscles to, 232.

Teredo navalis, supposed to bore backwards, 469.

Testiconda, what animals are truly so called, 7.

Testis; its situation in the fœtus, with its descent into the scrotum, 1. Formed in the abdomen, *ib.* In the fœtus, explains several things in ruptures and hydrocele, 2. its shape and figure, 3. Reckoned among the abdominal viscera, *ib.* Situated immediately below the kidneys, *ib.* Is attached to the psoas-muscle, *ib.* The trunk of the aorta more distant from the right testis than the left, *ib.* Its arteries, *ib.* Its veins are analogous to its arteries, 4. Its nerves, *ib.* Its epididymis, 5. Its vas deferens, *ib.* Testicles—the cremaster-muscle different in the fœtus and in the adult, *ib.* Testis, connected with the parietes of the abdomen, 6. Testes of the hedge-hog and sheep described, 7. Its peritonæal coat, 8. Its descent, 9. Frequently happens between the second and tenth year; the failure in their descent originates in themselves, 16. Not therefore necessarily incapable of performing their function, 18, note. Method of treatment, 16, 18. Variations of, in the sparrow, buck, land-mouse, &c., 29. Penis, urethra, and all the parts connected with them, subservient to them, *ib.* An animal deprived of his when young retains more of the original youthful form, and resembles the female, 47.

Thermometer; explanation of a, 136.

Thompson, Prof. John, demonstrates experimentally the muscularity of small arteries, 254, note.

Tiger-lily, irritability of style, 210, note.

Torpedo; its large nerves in relation to voluntary power of giving shocks, 212, 409. Mr. Walsh's account of, 398. Hunter's anatomical observations on, 409. Large size of nerves supplying electric organs, 412.

Torpidity of animals; in warm climates, instances of, 88, note. No chemical change in the circulating blood during, 135, note. And sleep, difference between, 144. Different effects produced by, natural and superinduced, 151.

Tragopogon, 201.

Trout, Gillaroo (alias *Gizzard*), description of the, 126, 129.

Tubuli uriniferi, injected by Hunter, xxiv.

Tusk, definition of, 352.

Tyson; his opinion of the independent function of the vesiculæ seminales, and reasons for, from comparative anatomy, 26, note. Assigns a solvent menstruum as the cause of digestion, 84, note. His discovery of the arterial plexuses in Cetacea, 366, note.

U.

Univalves, characterized by having the intestine reflected, 468.

V.

Vallisneri, his observation on the gizzard of birds quoted, 83.

Vegetables, their power of producing heat, 156. Comparison with animals in respect to age of parts, 158. Experiments on seeds of, alluded to, 164.

Vesiculæ seminales; described, 20. Considered as reservoirs of the semen, *ib.* This opinion erroneous, *ib.* Compared with the semen of a living man, different from the mucus found in these vesiculæ, 21. Discharge from them not seminal, *ib.* In the human subject do not contain the semen, *ib.* In some animals no duct leading from them to the prostate glands, 26. No peculiar sensation of any kind felt in them, 25.

In the horse, boar, rat, beaver, guinea-pig, and hedge-hog, 26—27. Third vesicula in the horse, 26, note. Nothing analogous to them in birds, 27. This is equally applicable to amphibious animals, and to that order of fish called rays, 28. Not for the purpose of containing semen, 28; but are subservient to generation, 29, 148. Their function considered, by J. V. Horn and Tyson, to be to add an independent secretion to the semen, 26, note.

Viper, experiment on a, 147.

Vomiting, how performed, 92.

W.

Walsh, John, F.R.S., on the electric property of the torpedo, 398.

Whalebone, description of, 354—357.

Whales; on the structure and œconomy of, 331—392. (See *Cetacea*.) Difficulty of investigating their structure, 331. Hunter engages a surgeon to go out to Greenland to dissect, 332. Ribbed and elastic skin in piked, 350. The largest species, 354, note. Description of whalebone of, 354. Piked and Mysticete have a cæcum, 360; as also the herbivorous Cetacea, 360, note. Their olfactory nerves, 377, note.

Wha-Tapoua-Roo, 489.

White, John, Esq., zoological appendix of his voyage quoted, 481.

Wolf; observations on the, 319. Is impregnated by a greyhound; brought forth four puppies, 323. A hybrid female is fertile with a dog, 324.

Wollaston, Dr., F.R.S., on the vibratory nature of muscular action, 208, note.

Woodcock, its air-cells compared with those of the ostrich, 182.

Y.

Yarrell, Wm., S.Z.S., on the change of plumage of hen pheasants quoted, 48, note. On the varieties of the trout, 130, note.

Yolk, a subsance originally formed with the primordial germ; but reserved for the nourishment of the ovipara after exclusion from the egg, 122.

Young, Dr. Thomas, S.R.S., his theory of the muscularity of the lens, 290, note.

Z.

Zoological Society, Proceedings of, quoted, 352, note; 393, note.

FINIS.

PRINTED BY RICHARD AND JOHN E. TAYLOR,
RED LION COURT, FLEET STREET.

Printed in the United States
By Bookmasters